Smoking Prevention and Cessation

Giuseppe La Torre

Smoking Prevention and Cessation

Springer

Giuseppe La Torre
Department of Public Health and Infectious Diseases
"Sapienza" University of Rome
Rome, Italy

ISBN 978-1-4614-7045-8 ISBN 978-1-4614-7046-5 (eBook)
DOI 10.1007/978-1-4614-7046-5
Springer New York Heidelberg Dordrecht London

Library of Congress Control Number: 2013937315

Printed on acid-free paper

Springer is part of Springer Science+Business Media (www.springer.com)

Contents

Contributors

Stefania Boccia Institute of Hygiene, Catholic University of the Sacred Heart, Rome, Italy

Claudio Bontempi Department of Public Health and Infectious Diseases, “Sapienza” University of Rome, Rome, Italy

Luca Calzoni Department of Public Health and Infectious Diseases, “Sapienza” University of Rome, Latina, LT, Italy

Silvio Capizzi Institute of Hygiene, Catholic University of the Sacred Heart, Rome, Italy

Guido Citoni Department of Molecular Medicine, “Sapienza” University of Rome, Rome, Italy

Antonio Giulio De Belvis Institute of Hygiene - Department of Public Health, Faculty of Medicine, Università Cattolica del Sacro Cuore, Rome, Italy

Guglielmo Giraldi Section of Hygiene, Department of Public Health and Infectious Diseases, “Sapienza” University of Rome, Rome, Italy

Maria Caterina Grassi Department of Public Health and Infectious Diseases, “Sapienza” University of Rome, Rome, Italy

Maria Rosaria Gualano Department of Public Health Sciences, University of Turin, Turin, Italy

Flavia Kheiraoui Institute of Hygiene, Catholic University of the Sacred Heart, Rome, Italy

Giuseppe La Torre Department of Public Health and Infectious Diseases, “Sapienza” University of Rome, Rome, Italy

Alice Mannocci Department of Public Health and Infectious Diseases, “Sapienza” University of Rome, Rome, Italy

Marta Marino Institute of Hygiene - Department of Public Health, Faculty of Medicine, Università Cattolica del Sacro Cuore, Rome, Italy

Silvia Miccoli Department of Public Health and Infectious Diseases, "Sapienza" University of Rome, Rome, Italy

Nicola Nicolotti Local Health Unit - Massa and Carrara, P.zza Sacco e Vanzetti, 5, Carrara (MS) 54033, Italy

Ferruccio Pelone Institute of Hygiene - Department of Public Health, Faculty of Medicine, Università Cattolica del Sacro Cuore, Rome, Italy

Rosella Saulle Department of Public Health and Infectious Diseases, "Sapienza" University of Rome, Rome, Italy

Leda Semyonov Section of Hygiene, Department of Public Health and Infectious Diseases, "Sapienza" University of Rome, Rome, Italy

Maria Lucia Specchia Istituto di Igiene, Università Cattolica del Sacro Cuore, Rome, Italy

Domitilla Di Thiene Department of Public Health and Infectious Diseases, "Sapienza" University of Rome, Rome, Italy

Brigid Unim Department of Public Health and Infectious Diseases, "Sapienza" University of Rome, Rome, Italy

Chiara de Waure Institute of Hygiene, Catholic University of the Sacred Heart, Rome, Italy

Chapter 1
From Nicotine Dependence to Genetic Determinants of Smoking

Giuseppe La Torre, Rosella Saulle, Nicola Nicolotti, Chiara de Waure, Maria Rosaria Gualano, and Stefania Boccia

Objective The goal of this chapter is to introduce the reader to the world of tobacco smoking, the role of nicotine in inducing a nicotine addiction, as well as to be confident with some tools in measuring nicotine dependence and motivation to quit.

Moreover, it will serve to give an update overview about genetic risk factors for smoking behavior going in depth with molecular and biological aspects and to describe the role of genetic determinants in initiation and cessation of cigarette smoking.

Learning Outcome

At the end of this chapter the reader will be able to:

- Increase knowledge on nicotine dependence and nicotine withdrawal.
- Measure nicotine dependence.
- Measure the motivation to quit.
- Know what is the impact of genetic factor on smoking behavior both for initiation and cessation.

G. La Torre (✉) • R. Saulle
Department of Public Health and Infectious Diseases, "Sapienza" University of Rome, Piazzale Aldo Moro 5, Rome 00185, Italy
e-mail: giuseppe.latorre@uniroma1.it; rosella.saulle@uniroma1.it

N. Nicolotti
Local Health Unit - Massa and Carrara, P.zza Sacco e Vanzetti, 5, Carrara (MS) 54033, Italy
e-mail: nicola.nicolotti@gmail.com

C. de Waure • S. Boccia
Institute of Hygiene, Catholic University of the Sacred Heart, L.go F. Vito 1, Rome 00168, Italy
e-mail: chiara.dewaure@rm.unicatt.it; sboccia@rm.unicatt.it

M.R. Gualano
Department of Public Health Sciences, University of Turin, via Santena 5 bis, 10126 Turin, Italy
e-mail: mariarosaria.gualano@unito.it

G. La Torre, *Smoking Prevention and Cessation*, DOI 10.1007/978-1-4614-7046-5_1,

1.1 Introduction: Denial and Delay

The role of tobacco smoking as cause of many diseases is now well established from the scientific point of view. It is well recognized that tobacco consumption is the leading cause of preventable deaths in the majority of high-income nations and increasingly in low- and middle-income nations (Jha and Chaloupka 1999), and that it causes disability and productivity losses because of premature deaths (US Department of Health and Human Services 2004). Nevertheless, it is a common experience to see smokers in different settings. Smokers smoke even if for most of them it is dangerous for their health. Why?

This book wants to give answers to this question and to give the best available evidence concerning smoking prevention and cessation strategies.

First of all, we have to recognize that tobacco smoking is a disease for many smokers (International Classification of Disease 10th revision: F17Nicotine dependence) (See Box 1.1).

Moreover, in introducing this chapter we have to recognize that for many years smoking, and above all, smoking cigarettes, has not been considered as a health problem.

In the UK, as reported by Pollock (1999), a delay between the evidence of smoking as a cause of disease and the implementation of public health norms has occurred. Even if the evidence was strong, in some cases the political will was split between ban and denial of the problem.

"Fourteen years after Hill and Doll were 'satisfied that the case against smoking as such is proven,' ten years after the publication of the first report on their study of

Box 1.1 Nicotine dependence codes according to the ICD 10th revision (in parentheses ICD-9)

F17.201 Nicotine dependence, unspecified, in remission (ICD-9 Code: 305.1)
F17.203 Nicotine dependence unspecified, with withdrawal (ICD-9 Code: 292.0)
F17.208 Nicotine dependence, unspecified, with other nicotine-induced disorders (ICD-9 Code: 292.89)
F17.209 Nicotine dependence, unspecified, with unspecified nicotine-induced disorders (ICD-9 Code: 292.9)
F17.21 Nicotine dependence, cigarettes
F17.210 Nicotine dependence, cigarettes, uncomplicated (ICD-9 Code: 305.1)
F17.211 Nicotine dependence, cigarettes, in remission (ICD-9 Code: 305.1)
F17.213 Nicotine dependence, cigarettes, with withdrawal (ICD-9 Code: 292.0)

(continued)

Box 1.1 (continued)

F17.218 Nicotine dependence, cigarettes, with other nicotine-induced disorders (ICD-9 Code: 292.89)
F17.219 Nicotine dependence, cigarettes, with unspecified nicotine-induced disorders (ICD-9 Code: 292.9)
F17.22 Nicotine dependence, chewing tobacco
F17.220 Nicotine dependence, chewing tobacco, uncomplicated (ICD-9 Code: 305.1)
F17.221 Nicotine dependence, chewing tobacco, in remission (ICD-9 Code: 305.1)
F17.223 Nicotine dependence, chewing tobacco, with withdrawal (ICD-9 Code: 292.0)
F17.228 Nicotine dependence, chewing tobacco, with other nicotine-induced disorders (ICD-9 Code: 292.89)
F17.229 Nicotine dependence, chewing tobacco, with unspecified nicotine-induced disorders (ICD-9 Code: 292.9)
F17.29 Nicotine dependence, other tobacco product
F17.290 Nicotine dependence, other tobacco product, uncomplicated (ICD-9 Code: 305.1)
F17.291 Nicotine dependence, other tobacco product, in remission (ICD-9 Code: 305.1)
F17.293 Nicotine dependence, other tobacco product, with withdrawal (ICD-9 Code: 292.0)
F17.298 Nicotine dependence, other tobacco product, with other nicotine-induced disorders (ICD-9 Code: 292.89)
F17.299 Nicotine dependence, other tobacco product, with unspecified nicotine-induced disorders (ICD-9 Code: 292.9)

British doctors, seven years after the Medical Research Council told the Government that ‘the evidence now available is stronger than that which, in comparable matters, is commonly taken as the basis for definite action’ and two years after the Royal College of Physicians in exasperation produced a popular summary of the evidence with specific policy recommendations, the Government was still equivocal about taking effective action against this egregious cause of disease and premature death” (Fig. 1.1) (Pollock 1999).

However, the scientific awareness on the effect of tobacco smoking has been increased for several years. In his Nobel Lecture in 1975 (see Box 1.2), Renato Dulbecco, talking about the molecular biology of oncogenic DNA Viruses, made a strong attack to the role of tobacco in the field of cancer, calling for increased restrictions on tobacco use due to its carcinogenic potential.

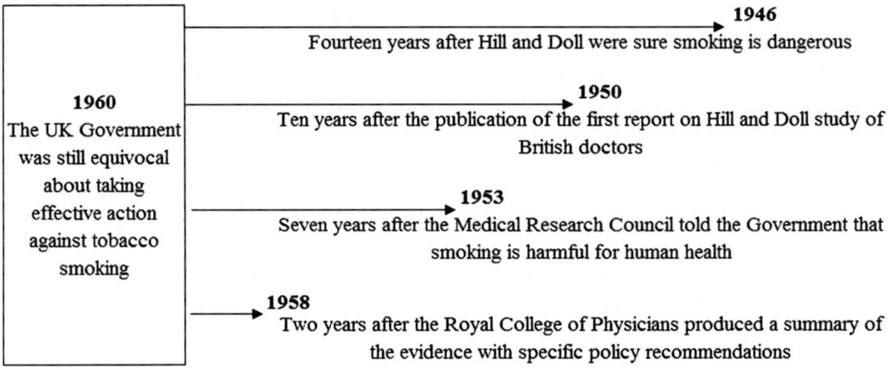

Fig. 1.1 Tobacco smoking: denial and delay in the UK [from Pollock (1999)]

Box 1.2 The role of tobacco in cancer prevention (from Dulbecco, R. (1975). From the molecular biology of oncogenic DNA viruses to cancer. Nobel Lecture, December 12, 1975) Prospects for cancer prevention

….. somatic mutations are one of the fundamental ingredients of cancer although they appear to require the occurrence of several other events not yet understood. The role of mutations in turn suggests that the incidence of cancer in man could be reduced by identifying as many promutagens as possible, and by eliminating them from the environment. One important feature of this approach to cancer prevention is that it can be started now, since these substances can be identified with simple bacterial tests suitable for mass screening. The feasibility of prevention is shown by the fact that the promutagens already identified in a preliminary screening, such as tobacco or some hair dyes, are inessential for human life.

However, it is practically difficult to achieve a substantial reduction of the use of these substances, as shown by the example of tobacco. According to

(continued)

Box 1.2 (continued)

epidemiological evidence, tobacco smoke is the agent of lung cancer in man, which in Britain is responsible for one in eight of all male deaths. Yet only mild sanctions have been imposed on tobacco products, such as a vague health warning on cigarette packets, which sounds rather like an official endorsement. Any limitation on the use of tobacco is left to the individual, although it is clear that the individual cannot easily exercise voluntary restraint in the face of very effective advertisements, especially as he does not usually appreciate the danger of a cumulative action over a long period of time.

The lax attitude of governments towards tobacco probably also derives from the difficulty of appreciating epidemiological evidence, especially since this evidence is contradicted from time to time by single-minded individuals who use incomplete or even erroneous analyses of the data and whose views are magnified out of all proportion by the media. However, the recent recognition that tobacco smoke contains promutagens contributes direct experimental evidence on the dangers of tobacco smoke, on which there cannot be any equivocation. I, therefore, call on governments to act towards severely discouraging tobacco consumption and to act now because it will be at least 30 years before their action has its full effect.

1.2 Tobacco and Nicotine

Several components of cigarettes are toxic, but they are not addictive. The addiction is caused by nicotine (one of the cigarette component). Nicotine, in fact, is the primary addictive agent in all tobacco products (cigarettes, chewing tobacco, cigars, pipe tobacco) and it acts in particular on nicotinic acetylcholine receptor (nAChR) in the central nervous system (CNS), the part of the human nervous system that integrates the information received from the body and coordinates the great part of our activities (Laviolette and van der Kooy 2004; Henningfield and Slade 1998). This binding is at the base of the neurobiology of tobacco dependence and it is the major obstacle for smokers who try to quit (Slama 2008).

1.2.1 What Is Tobacco?

Tobacco is an agricultural product and an end product of the fresh tobacco leaf in the genus Nicotiana (*64 established species*) of the Solanaceae family plants (dried leaves are used to realize tobacco products).

In Table 1.1 some details on tobacco products are illustrated.

Table 1.1 Smoking tobacco products (modified from IARC monograph production, composition, use, and regulations)

Combustible tobacco products		Nicotine content
Manufactured cigarettes	Any roll of tobacco wrapped generally in paper, with or without filter. Approximately 6–8 mm in diameter and 70–120 mm in length Cigarettes account for the 96 % of the total manufactured tobacco products sale (Mackay et al. 2006)	10 mg (typical cigarette)
Roll-your own cigarettes	Hand-filled cigarettes. They are produced combined loose tobacco and cigarette paper, sometimes with the help of a hand-held rolling machine. *They aren't more natural and safer than manufactured cigarettes*!	
Cigars	Any roll of tobacco wrapped in leaf tobacco or in any other substance containing tobacco There are several types of cigars: little cigar, small cigars ("cigarillos"), regular cigars (up to 17 mm in diameter and 110–150 mm in length) and premium cigars The users typically do not inhale the cigar smoke (Burns 1998)	From 6 to over 300 mg
Pipes and water piper	Pipes are made of a variety of substances (wood, briar, slate, or clay). Tobacco is placed in the bowl of the pipe and the smoke is inhaled through the stem. Many smokers believe that water in the hookah filters out harmful toxins (WHO 2010). But this *is false*! (Loffredo 2006)	It vary from the quantity of tobacco used (generally 3–4 g of tobacco, 20 g in a water pipe) and the time of smoking.
Bidis (*pronounced "bee-dees"*)	Hand-rolled Indian cigarette. Sun-dried temburni leaf rolled into a conical shape together with flaked tobacco and secured with a thread. Bidi smoke contains higher concentrations of nicotine than manufactured cigarettes. They are widely used in India	15.7–27 mg/g of product
Kreteks	Small cigars containing tobacco (60–80 %), cloves, and cocoa	1–3.3 mg
Smokeless tobacco products		**Nicotine content**
Chewing tobacco	It is used orally. A pinch of tobacco is placed between the cheek and the gum. The user chews and sucks it. Other names for chewing tobacco are plug, loose-leaf, chimo, toobak, gutkha, and twist (Mackay et al. 2006)	3.4–39.7 mg/g of product
Moist and dry snuff	A small amount of snuff (ground or powdered tobacco) is placed between the cheek and gum in the mouth. Snuff can be moist or dry	3.4–11.5 mg/g of product (*higher in dry snuff*)

Tobacco for cigarettes is generally derived from two varieties of plants:

1. Virginia, with a yellowish "bright" leaf (about 3 % of nicotine)
2. Burley, with higher quantity of nicotine

A tobacco of good quality seems to be produced in Cuba.

During different periods of time, people have used tobacco in several forms. In the past, tobacco was chewed or smoked in pipes. Now, it is mainly manufactured in cigarettes (Brandt 2007). Starting from the documents of the World Health Organization (Samet and Yoon 2010), tobacco products could be categorized in two principal categories: as combustible (smoked tobacco) or noncombustible (chewing and snuff tobacco).

In addition to nicotine, tobacco smoke contains thousands of potentially noxious chemical substances. They are the consequences of the burning of tobacco products (tobacco smoking).

Compounds include particulates (or tar) of sticky solids, gases such as carbon monoxide, and volatiles.

About 3,044 constituents have been isolated from tobacco and 3,996 from the mainstream smoke of cigarettes, a total of 1,172 constituents are present both in tobacco and tobacco smoke (Roberts 1988). This mixture changes as the smoke "ages": chemical substances in the smoke react with air and change under the effect of UV light (IARC 2004). In particular tar is the brown substance that stains smokers' teeth, fingers, and lungs. Up to 70 % of the tar in cigarettes remains inside the smokers lungs.

In 2001, Hoffmann and Hoffmann identified 69 carcinogens in tobacco smoke (and tar). These carcinogens include ten species of polynuclear aromatic hydrocarbons (PAHs), six heterocyclic hydrocarbons, four volatile hydrocarbons, three nitrohydrocarbons, four aromatic amines, eight *N*-heterocyclic amines, ten *N*-nitrosamines, two aldehydes, ten miscellaneous organic compounds, nine inorganic compounds, and three phenolic compounds (Hoffmann and Hoffmann 2001). The really final chemical composition of tobacco smoke is influenced by the specific manner in which an individual smokes, the type of tobacco, the design of the smoking device or product and, last but not least, by the presence of a filter (IARC 2002).

Carcinogens have been classified by the International Agency for Research on Cancer (IARC) into four different groups:

- Group 1: Carcinogenic to humans (107 agents)
- Group 2A: Probably carcinogenic to humans (63)
- Group 2B: Possibly carcinogenic to humans (271)
- Group 3: Not classifiable as to its carcinogenicity to humans (509)
- Group 4: Probably not carcinogenic to humans (1)

Since 1987, 11 compounds of tobacco smoke have been classified as IARC Group 1 human carcinogens (2-naphthylamine, 4-aminobiphenyl, benzene, vinyl chloride, ethylene oxide, arsenic, beryllium, nickel compounds, chromium, cadmium, and polonium-210) (Hoffmann and Hoffmann 2001). Starting from this year, the attention of researchers has been focused on some components of established carcinogenicity: benzo-[a]pyrene (a PAHs surrogate), tobacco-specific *N*-nitrosamines (TSNA), and aromatic amines. These components represent a serious problem from the public health perspective. In fact, the exposure to these substances is linked with several

Table 1.2 Carcinogens in cigarette smoke [modified from: IARC Monographs on the evaluation of carcinogenic risks to humans. Tobacco Smoke and Involuntary Smoking. Vol. 83 (2004)]

Agent	IARC group	Agent	IARC group
Polynuclear aromatic hydrocarbons		Glu-P-1	2B
Benz[a]anthracene	2A	Glu-P-2	2B
Benzo[b]fluoranthene	2B	PhIP	2B
Benzo[j]fluoranthene	2B	*Aldehydes*	
Benzo[k]fluoranthene	2B	Formaldehyde	2A
Benzo[a]pyrene	2A	Acetaldehyde	2B
Dibenz[a,h]anthracene	2A	*Phenolic compounds*	
Dibenzo[a,i]pyrene	2B	Catechol	2B
Dibenzo[a,e]pyrene	2B	Caffeic acid	2B
Indeno[1,2,3-cd]pyrene	2B	*Volatile hydrocarbons*	
5-Methylchrysene	2B	1,3-Butadiene	2A
Heterocyclic hydrocarbons		Isoprene	2B
Furan	2B	Benzene	1
Dibenz(a,h)acridine	2B	*Nitrohydrocarbons*	
Dibenz(a,j)acridine	2B	Nitromethane	2B
Dibenzo(c,g)carbazole	2B	2-Nitropropane	2B
Benzo(b)furan	2B	Nitrobenzene	2B
N-Nitrosamines		*Miscellaneous organic compounds*	
N-Nitrosodimethylamine	2A	Acetamide	2B
N-Nitrosoethylmethylamine	2B	Acrylamide	2A
N-Nitrosodiethylamine	2A	Acrylonitrile	2B
N-Nitrosopyrrolidine	2B	Vinyl chloride	1
N-Nitrosopiperidine	2B	1,1-Dimethylhydrazine	2B
N-Nitrosodiethanolamine	2B	Ethylene oxide	1
N′-Nitrosonornicotine	2B	Propylene oxide	2B
4-(Methylnitrosamino)-1-(3-pyridyl)-1-butanone	2B	Hydrazine	2B
Aromatic amines		Urethane	2B
2-Toluidine	2A	*Metals and metal compounds*	
2,6-Dimethylaniline	2B	Arsenic	1
2-Naphthylamine	1	Beryllium	1
4-Aminobiphenyl	1	Nickel	1
N-Heterocyclic amines		Chromium (hexavalent)	1
A-α-C	2B	Cadmium	1
MeA-α-C	2B	Cobalt	2B
IQ	2A	Lead (inorganic) 2A	2A
Trp-P-1	2B	Radio-isotope Polonium-210	1
Trp-P-2	2B		

human cancers, particularly with lung, urinary tract, head and neck, esophagus, stomach, and liver cancers.

Table 1.2 shows carcinogens of unfiltered mainstream cigarette smoke [modified from: IARC Monographs on the Evaluation of Carcinogenic Risks to Humans. Tobacco Smoke and Involuntary Smoking. Volume 83 (2004)].

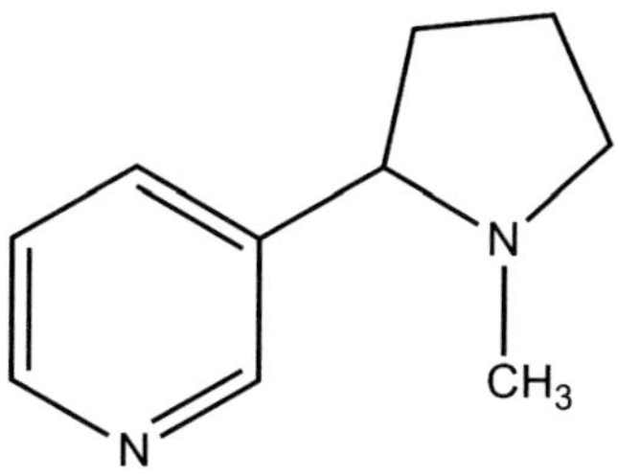

Fig. 1.2 Nicotine formula

1.2.2 What Is Nicotine?

Nicotine (Fig. 1.2) is the major cause of tobacco dependence. Understanding the neural substrates of nicotine dependence is for researchers the first step to develop antismoking medications (D'Souza and Markou 2011).

It is the principal tobacco alkaloid and its biosynthesis and accumulation take place, respectively, in the roots and in the leaves (1.5 % by weight in commercial cigarette tobacco).

In the human body, there are two major types of cholinergic receptors (i.e., receptors for acetylcholine): the muscarinic and the nicotinic. Nicotinic acetylcholine receptors (nAChRs) are selective ligand-gated ion channels (LGICs).

As reported by D'Souza and Markou (2011), "*Nicotine influences mood, cognition, and body function by binding to and activating nicotinic acetylcholine receptors (nAChRs) located on neurons in the brain. When activated by either nicotine or the endogenous neurotransmitter acetylcholine, the nAChR opens a channel that allows ions to pass through the neuron's membrane from the exterior to the interior of the cell and trigger changes that activate the cell*" (D'Souza and Markou 2011).

The ability of nicotine to activate a particular nAChR depends on the subunits that make up the receptor. nAChR subunits exist in 12 isoforms (variant forms), labeled α2–α10 and β2–β4. Every nAChR consists of five subunit molecules arranged in a ring around a central channel that opens to admit ions when the receptor is activated (Figs. 1.3 and 1.4). In this way, nicotine enhances dopamine levels in the CNS (brain's mesolimbic reward system).

Three phases characterize Nicotine dependence:

- *Acquisition and maintenance of nicotine-taking behavior*. Nicotine effects on human: mild pleasurable rush, mild euphoria, increased arousal, decreased fatigue, and relaxation (Henningfield et al. 1985). These play an important role in the initiation and maintenance of tobacco smoking (Markou 2008).
- *Withdrawal symptoms upon cessation of nicotine intake*: Chronic use of nicotine induces neuroadaptations in the brain (nicotine dependence). Thus, nicotine-dependent smokers must continue nicotine intake to avoid distressing somatic and affective withdrawal symptoms (depressed mood, anxiety, irritability, difficulty concentrating, craving, bradycardia, insomnia, gastrointestinal discomfort, and weight gain) (Hughes et al. 1991)

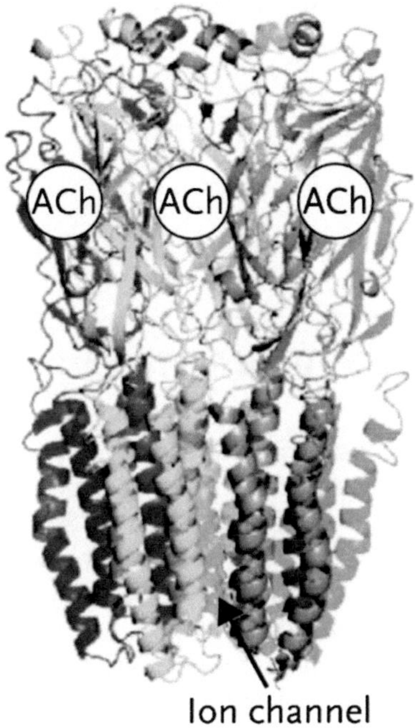

Fig. 1.3 nACh receptor seen from one side [from D'Souza and Markou (2011)]

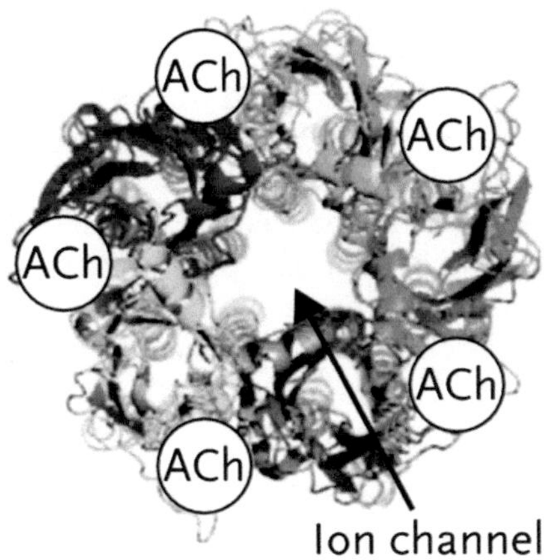

Fig. 1.4 nACh receptor seen from above [from D'Souza and Markou (2011)]

- *Vulnerability to relapse*: Abstinent smokers remain prone to relapse for weeks, months, or even years after cessation of tobacco smoking. Stress and cigarette smoking itself can also precipitate resumption of habitual smoking.

1.3 Addiction and Nicotine Addiction

Substance abuse involves the use of a substance despite social, interpersonal, or other problems caused by the use of the substance, while dependence is a more severe disorder entailing signs of physical or psychological tolerance. Dependence refers to compulsive drug use that is derived by strong and often irresistible urge that persist despite a desire to quit or even repeated attempts to quit. From behavioral point of view, addiction or dependence to a drug can be defined as repeated self-administration of a drug or substance despite of adverse medical and social consequences and attempts to abstain from it. At the cost of social and occupational commitments, an addict's daily activities center on obtaining and consuming the drug. Addictive behavior like human behavior in general is the outcome of genetic and biochemical characteristics, past learning experiences, motivational states, psychosocial antecedents, and cultural context in which it unfolds. Initial decision to use a drug is generally influenced by genetic, psychosocial, and environmental factors that initiate smoking in an individual. Therefore, substance dependence or addiction is a primary brain disease, determined genetically, expressed biochemically, and has psychosocial consequences. These consequences can and do occur in all aspects of the addict's life, influencing the social, vocational, legal, family, spiritual, psychological, and physical spheres. The disease is characterized by its chronic, progressive, relapsing, and lethal nature. There are four cardinal features generally seen in drug addiction:

- Loss of control over the use of drug
- Continuous use despite of adverse consequences
- Compulsive use
- Craving when the drug is withheld

American Psychiatric Association's internationally used Diagnostic and Statistical Manual for Mental Disorders (1994), 4th Edition (DSM-IV) outlines the criteria for substance dependence and includes nicotine dependence and nicotine withdrawal as disorders. The Diagnostic and Statistical Manual of Mental Disorders, 4th Edition (DSM-IV) 1994 classifies nicotine addiction as Nicotine Use Disorder. The criteria for diagnosis include any three of the following within a 1-year time span:

- Tolerance to nicotine with decreased effect and increasing dose to obtain same effect
- Smoking more than the usual
- Persistent desire to smoke despite efforts to decrease intake
- Extensive time spent smoking or purchasing tobacco
- Postponing work, social, and recreational events in order to smoke
- Continuing to smoke despite health hazards

Nicotine abuse is not included because clinically significant psychosocial problems from tobacco use are rare (Hughes et al. 1991). Nicotine intoxication is also not included as it is very rare (Table 1.3).

Table 1.3 The characteristic withdrawal

A.	Daily use of nicotine for at least several weeks
B.	Abrupt cessation or reduction of nicotine use, followed within 24 h by four or more of:
	1. Dysphoric or depressed mood
	2. Insomnia
	3. Irritability, frustration, or anger
	4. Anxiety
	5. Difficulty concentrating
	6. Restlessness
	7. Decreased heart rate
	8. Increased appetite or weight gain
C.	The above symptoms cause clinically sufficient distress or impairment in social, occupational, or other important areas of functioning
D.	The symptoms are not due to a general medical condition and are not better accounted for by another mental disorder

As identified by the Diagnostic and Statistical Manual (DSM-IV)

Table 1.3 illustrates how the generic DSM IV criteria for substance dependence apply to nicotine dependence. The applicability and reliability of DSM diagnosis of nicotine dependence appear high.

International Classification of Diseases (1992), 10th Revision (ICD-10) by World Health Organization (WHO) defines drug dependence as "a state psychic and sometimes also physical, resulting from the interaction between a living organism and a drug, characterized by behavioral and other responses that always include a compulsion to take the drug on a continuous or periodic basis in order to experience its psychic effects, and sometimes to avoid discomfort of its absence…" Tolerance may or may not be present. According to all these parameters, nicotine is an addictive substance and nicotine addiction has been classified as a disease by the WHO's International Classification of Diseases (ICD) 10th Revision.

Based on the WHO criteria for drug dependence, the US Surgeon General has concluded that tobacco-delivered nicotine is addictive and the Food and Drug Administration (FDA) has declared nicotine as an addictive drug on 12th July, 1996 (Table 1.4).

The American Psychiatric Association (APA) and the World Health Organization (WHO) have refined their definitions of drug dependence; they have issued criteria for specific behavioral and psychological identifiers that can be used as diagnostic criteria. The various sets of criteria change slightly as succeeding versions of the diagnostic categories are issued, reflecting growth in scientific understanding of addiction and in societal comprehension of its impact. One comprehensive definition addiction model: tobacco use as drug dependence of addiction comes from a report issued to the Royal Society of Health and Welfare Canada. In this report, addiction or dependence on a drug is described as a strongly established pattern of behavior characterized by:

(a) The repeated self-administration of a drug in amounts which reliably produce reinforcing psychoactive effects.
(b) Great difficulty in achieving voluntary long-term cessation of use, even when the user is strongly motivated to stop.

Table 1.4 Tobacco use as drug dependence

Addiction model: Tobacco use as drug dependence	
Markedly diminished effect with continued use of the same amount of the substance	Absence of nausea, dizziness, etc
Withdrawal as manifested by either	
The characteristic withdrawal syndrome for the substance. The substance is taken to relieve or avoid withdrawal symptoms	Known nicotine withdrawal symptoms are experienced by a dependent smoker
The substance if often taken in large amounts or over a longer period than intended	Most smokers do not intend to smoke 5 year later, but in fact, over 70 % continue to use
There is persistent desire or unsuccessful effort to cut down substance use	77 % of the smokers have tried to stop, 55% of these have not been able to stop despite repeated attempts and only 5–10 % of self-quitters are successful
A great deal of time is spent in activities necessary to obtain the substance, use the substance, or recover from its effects. Important social, occupational, or recreational activities are given up or reduced because of substance use	Leaving worksite to smoke. Not taking a job due to on-job smoking restrictions
The substance use is continued despite knowledge of having a persistent or recurrent physical or psychological problem that is likely to have been caused or exacerbated by the substance	Many smokers have heart disease, chronic obstructive pulmonary disease, or ulcers and continue to smoke

Diagnostic and Statistical Manual (4th Edition) American Psychiatric Association, 1994

Therefore, tobacco use is not just a random or capricious activity of human beings that simply occurs at will or pleasure of those who use it. It is a repetitive, stereotypic, and compulsive behavior characteristic of drug dependence.

This apparently irrational behavior is strongly driven by the pharmacological actions of nicotine on the brain and that cigarette and smokeless tobacco products are extraordinarily effective at maximizing the addictive effects of nicotine.

Tobacco dependence or addiction is presently a problem of many millions world wide who indulge in tobacco smoking, chewing, snuffing, or taking it inside their body in various other forms. Vulnerability to tobacco dependence is almost universal, based on the effects of nicotine on the brain and the body. Tobacco dependence has been a complex and challenging phenomenon to describe aetiologically, psychologically, and behaviorally. Tobacco-intake behavior and its remarkable difficulty to change is addiction to nicotine with wider ramifications. Addictive properties of tobacco are similar to those of other dependence producing drugs (Hughes et al. 1991) such as heroin and cocaine. Although the psychoactive effect of nicotine is less dramatic than that of heroin or cocaine, the strength of addiction is as powerful or more powerful.

Nicotine generates dependence by producing centrally mediated reinforcing effects, by regulating elements such as body weight and mood in ways that are perceived as useful or desirable by tobacco user and by leading to a physical dependence such that abstinence may result in adverse symptoms. In a cigarette smoker, following initiation of smoking a gradual increase in cigarette intake over time can be observed until he/she achieves the level that remains stable, day after day, during the smoker's life. The first cigarette of the day is smoked soon after waking (Fagerstrom 1978).

If nicotine was not absorbed quickly from the lungs, people would not take it in the form of smoke; if it was not taken up into the brain, it would not exert its psychopharmacological effects; if it was not rapidly metabolized and excreted, it would probably not be taken in such often-repeated doses.

1.4 Nicotine Withdrawal

It is obvious that smokers, just to avoid withdrawal symptoms, prefer continuing to smoke!

However, nicotine withdrawal syndrome is complex. While multiple withdrawal symptoms exist, over 65 % of smokers cite changes in recognition as a serious withdrawal symptom (Ward et al. 2001). The most frequently reported abstinence effects are anger, anxiety, depression, difficulty concentrating, irritability, and restlessness. These mood and cognitive disturbances each showed a transient increase after smoking cessation.

As studied by Ward and colleague (Ward et al. 2001), these mood and cognitive disturbances showed a transient increase after smoking cessation (Fig. 1.5).

During the withdrawal period (Days 1, 2, and 3), 50 % of the quitters reported feeling depression, 60 % anger, 66 % difficulty concentrating, 80 % anxiety, 86 % restlessness and 88 % irritability. Cognitive changes observed in abstinent smokers include deficits in working memory, verbal memory, digit recall, and associative learning.

Considering physical abstinence effects, cough and headache met the criteria for offset effects and dizziness and nausea met the criteria for transient effects. Other possible physical symptoms could be constipation, cramps, diarrhea, dry mouth, mouth ulcers, palpitations, skin rash, sore throat, stomach complaints, sweating, tremors, and fatigue (Ward et al. 2001).

The degree of all these symptoms depends on some factors, such as the age of the person, how long it has been smoking during the past and the daily average frequency of smoking.

Chain smokers are affected much more than occasional or social smokers. They smoke as first task in the morning or during coffee breaks, for them it's impossible to live without smoking. People tend to suffer from loss of concentration, restlessness, panting and perspiration, tension, insomnia, dizziness, irregular sleeping patterns, lowering levels of physical activity, constant fatigue and drowsiness, increased appetite as well as frequent headaches.

The withdrawal symptoms are generally at peak during the first 24 h of abstinence. Then, symptoms are very high during the first week of quitting and during the next 2–4 weeks, hunger levels are high and the craving for cigarettes becomes very intense. This is a challenging period for smokers.

Many people can quit smoking by themselves, other with the help of their friends. Generally, chain smokers can quit smoking within 30 days of determination. Severe addiction cases require the help of specialized therapeutic centers (Pitts 2012).

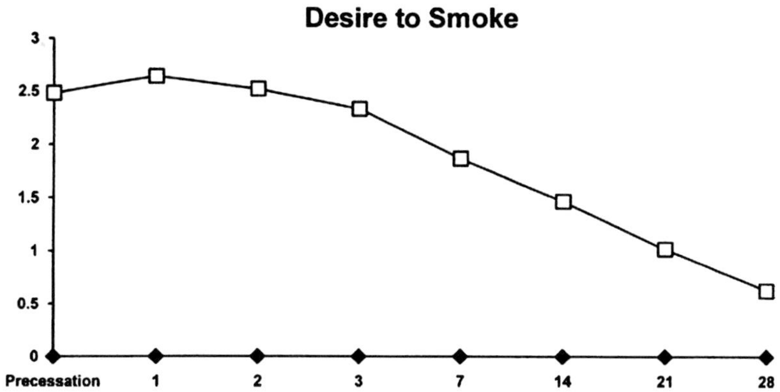

Fig. 1.5 Mean abstinence effect severity rating for desire to smoke in abstainers (*open square*) and nonsmokers (*closed square*) at precessation and days 1, 2, 3, 7, 14, 21, and 28 after cessation [from: Ward et al. (2001)]

nAChR upregulation contributes to withdrawal symptoms. Nicotine, in fact, directly enhances dopamine levels in the mesolimbic system by interacting with nAChRs on the dopaminergic neurons and causing them to release more of the neurotransmitter (to increases dopamine levels).

Evidences suggest that activation of nAChRs that contain β2, α4, α6, or α7 subunits mediate the reinforcing and behavioral effects of nicotine (D'Souza and Markou 2011).

Starting from this finding, researchers are developing pharmacological strategies to attenuate nicotine reinforcement and alleviate withdrawal (Fig. 1.6).

1.5 How to Measure Nicotine Dependence

According to what emerges from the scientific literature, the measurement of nicotine dependence assumes a central importance in both the diagnosis and the treatment of tobacco smoking. The most widely approach to measure nicotine dependence was proposed by Fagerstrom in 1978 and after that in several modified version of a Tolerance Questionnaire.

1.5.1 Fagerstrom Tolerance Questionnaire

Fagerstrom Tolerance Questionnaire (FTQ) (Fagerstrom 1978) was presented by the author as a test of "physical dependence to nicotine." FTQ correlates with other measures of nicotine dependence, such as carbon monoxide, nicotine, and cotinine levels.

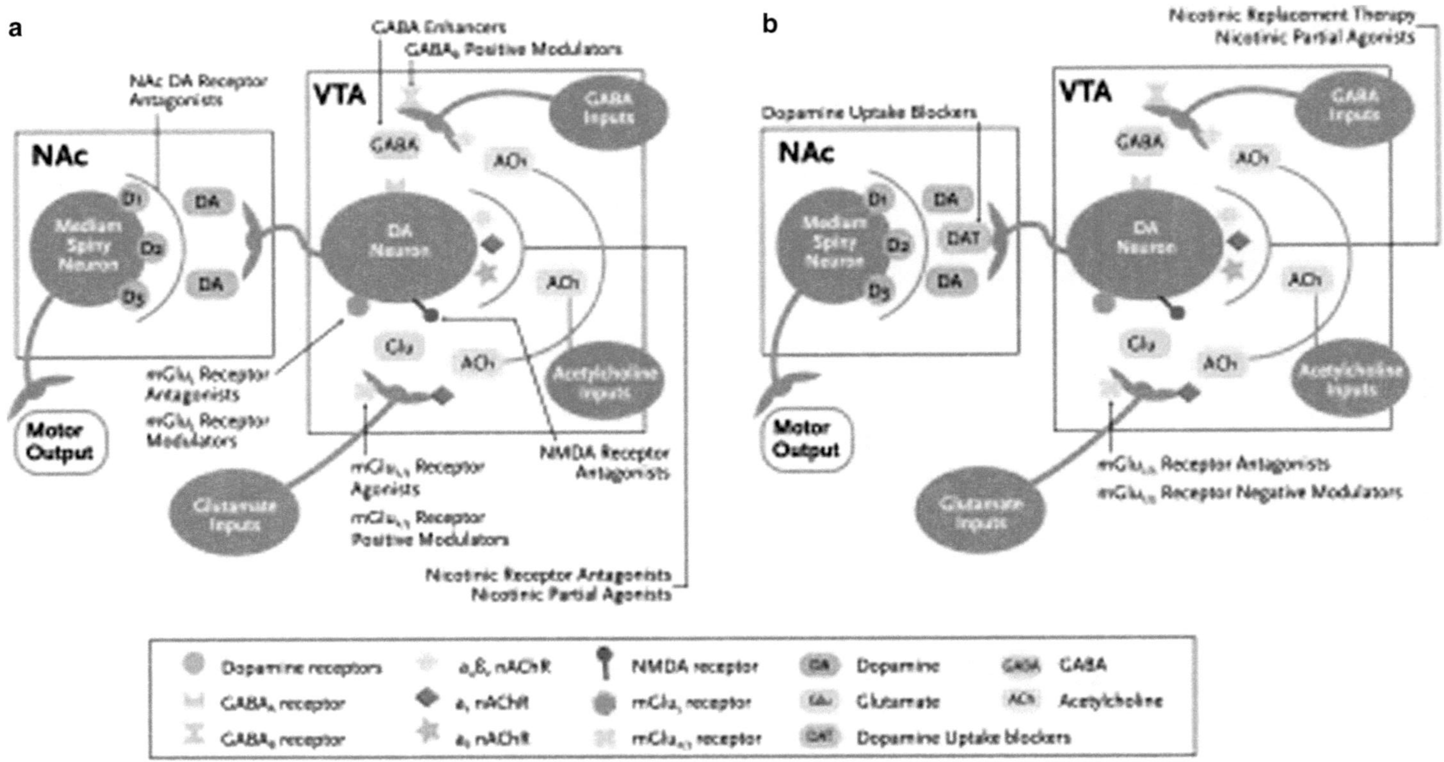

Fig. 1.6 Pharmacological strategies to attenuate nicotine reinforcement and alleviate withdrawal [from D'Souza and Markou (2011)]. (**a**) Potential targets in the mesolimbic reward system can promote smoking cessation by attenuating the reinforcing effects of nicotine. (**b**) Potential targets in the mesolimbic reward system may help to alleviate the negative affective symptoms seen in smokers who quit smoking

Table 1.5 Fagerstrom nicotine tolerance questionnaire

Karl Fagerstrom Nicotine Tolerance Questionnaire	
For each statement, circle the most appropriate number that best describes you	
	Point(s)
1. How many cigarettes do you smoke per day?	
(a) 10 or less	0
(b) 11–20	1
(c) 21–30	2
(d) 31 or more	3
2. How soon after you wake up do you smoke your first cigarette?	
(a) 0–5 min	3
(b) 30 min	2
(c) 31–60 min	1
(d) After 60 min	0
3. Do you find it difficult to refrain from smoking in places where smoking is not allowed (e.g., hospitals, government offices, cinemas, libraries, etc.)?	
(a) Yes	1
(b) No	0
4. Do you smoke more during the first hours after waking than during the rest of the day?	
(a) Yes	1
(b) No	0
5. Which cigarette would you be the most unwilling to give up?	
(a) First in the morning	1
(b) Any of the others	0
6. Do you smoke even when you are very ill?	
(a) Yes	1
(b) No	0
Total Point(s):______	

The items of FTQ, modality for each item and points for each modality are presented in Table 1.5.

The total score of the dependence level is the sum of the score of each item. According to Fagerstrom's interpretation of this scoring, the level of dependence is considered for:

- 0–3 points: low
- 4–6 points: medium
- 7–10 points: high

Low nicotine dependence (score 0–3) indicates a mild physical dependence. In this case the smoker will benefit from professional counseling, and pharmacotherapy is not recommended at initial assessment. In case patient has difficulty in dealing with withdrawal symptoms, further assessment for pharmacotherapy will be carried out to ascertain suitability.

Medium nicotine dependence (score 4–6) indicates a moderate physical dependence. In this case, the smoker requires professional counseling, and a pharmacotherapy could be recommended if patient is assessed to be suitable.

Table 1.6 Items and scoring for Fagerstrom Test for Nicotine Dependence (FTND)

Questions	Answers	Points
1. How soon after you wake up do you smoke your first cigarette?	Within 5 min	3
	6–30 min	2
2. Do you find it difficult to retain from smoking in places where it is forbidden, e.g., in church, at the library, in cinema, etc.?	Yes	1
	No	0
3. Which cigarette would you hate most to give up?	The first one in the morning	1
	All others	0
4. How many cigarettes/day do you smoke?	10 or less	0
	11–20	1
	21–30	2
	31 or more	3
5. Do you smoke more frequently during the first hours after waking than during the rest of the day?	Yes	1
	No	0
6. Do you smoke if you are so ill that you are in bed most of the day?	Yes	1
	No	0

High nicotine dependence (score 7–10) indicates a strong physical dependence. For this kind of smoker a professional counseling is required, as well as pharmacotherapy is useful if patient is assessed to be suitable.

1.5.2 Fagerstrom Test for Nicotine Dependence

The Tolerance Questionnaire receive modification after some years. Fagerstrom himself and a group of collaborators produced a new version, the Fagerstrom Test for Nicotine Dependence (Table 1.6) (FTND) (Heatherton et al. 1991).

As far as the interpretation of this score, Fagerstrom et al. (2000) noted that the scorers are not distributed bimodally (Fig. 1.7), i.e., clearly indicating "dependent" and "nondependent" smokers, suggest a five-level categorization of the nicotine dependence, as following:

- 0–2: very low
- 3–4: low
- 5: medium
- 6–7: high
- 8–10: very high

Pomerlau et al. (1994) found that both the FTQ (in both samples) and the FTND proved to be highly reliable. The validity of the scales, using cotinine, number of years smoked, and the "addictive" factor on the Classification of Smoking by Motives questionnaire as criterion variables, was also supported. No relationship between FTQ score and severity of depression was detected in either sample. Internal consistency was somewhat higher for the FTND than for the FTQ, replicating previous findings in the literature.

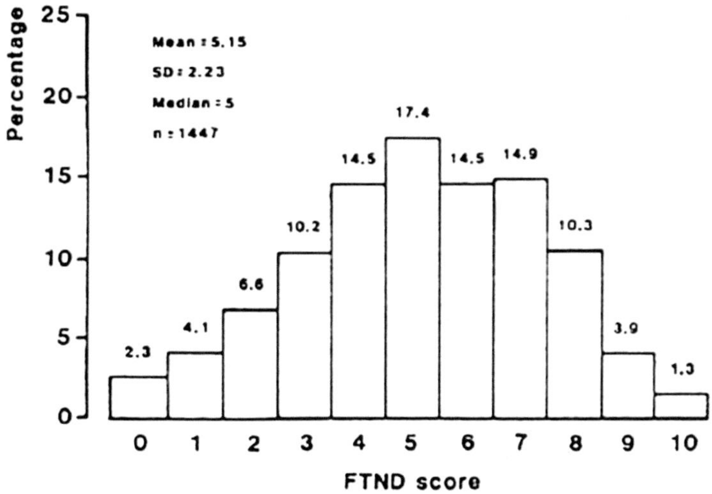

Fig. 1.7 Distribution of FTDN scores (from Fagerstrom, K. O., Heatherton, T. F., & Kozlowski, L. T. (2000). Nicotine addiction and its assessment. *Ear, Nose and Throat Journal, 69*(11), 763–766)

Prokhorov et al. (2000) examined the relationship between a seven-item-modified FTQ and saliva cotinine among 131 adolescent volunteers in a smoking cessation program. As anticipated, the total FTQ score was related to saliva cotinine ($r=0.40$, $p<0.01$), as were six of the seven individual FTQ items ($p<0.05$). Our findings provide preliminary evidence that the modified FTQ scale is valid and applicable to adolescent smokers.

1.6 Motivation to Stop Smoking

To stop smoking is likely to be one of the toughest things that a smoker could do. However, he/she stops with difficulties, and the scientific literature underline that if the motivation to stop is high, the probability to have success increases. In this case, the capability to understand the level of motivation to stop smoking is helpful for both the smoker and the physician that will care.

There are several ways for measuring this motivation. Some of these are very simple, as suggested by West (2004). For most clinical practice, motivation to stop smoking can be assessed in a qualitative way asking simple direct questions about the interest and intentions of the smoker to quit ("do you want to stop smoking for good"; "are you interested in making a serious attempt to stop in the near future?"; "are you interested in receiving help with your quit attempt?").

More complex semiquantitative measures (by means of questions about the degree of desire to stop on a scale from "not at all" to "very much") can also be used by the physician (West 2004).

Table 1.7 Richmond test

Would you like to quit smoking if you could do it easily?	
No	0 points
Yes	1 point
How interested are you to quit smoking?	
Not at all	0 points
A little	1 point
A lot	2 points
Very interested	3 points
Will you try to stop smoking in the following 2 weeks?	
Definitively not	0 points
Perhaps	1 point
Yes	2 points
Definitively yes	3 points
How likely are you to be a nonsmoker in the following 6 months?	
Definitively not	0 points
Perhaps	1 point
Yes	2 points
Definitively yes	3 points

Table 1.8 Mondor motivational questionnaire—score for yes and no answers

	Question	Yes	No
1	I decided to give up spontaneously	2	0
2	I have already given up for more than a week	1	0
3	I don't have any problems at work at the moment	1	0
4	I don't have any family problems at the moment	1	0
5	I want to free myself from my addiction	2	0
6	I do sport or I intend to do sport	1	0
7	I want to be in better physical shape	1	0
8	I want to look after my physical appearance	1	0
9	I am pregnant/my partner is pregnant	1	0
10	I have small children	2	0
11	I am in a good mood at the moment	2	0
12	I usually finish what I start	1	0
13	I am usually calm and relaxed	1	0
14	My weight is usually stable	1	0
15	I want to improve my quality of life	2	0

Finally, two tests were developed for calculating a score of the motivation to stop smoking, the Richmond test and the Mondor Motivational Questionnaire.

The Richmond test (Table 1.7) assesses the motivation to stop smoking in a scale from 0 to 10 points.

Values equal to over eight are indicating a very high level of motivation of stop smoking.

The Mondor Motivational Questionnaire (Table 1.8) is a tool developed in 1994 at the Hospital Henri-Mondor (Paris, France), that measures the level of motivation based on 15 items.

The scoring of the motivation to quit concerns four possibilities of success:

1. It is not the time to quit (<6)
2. Discrete (6–12)
3. Good (12–16)
4. Very good (>16)

1.7 Genetic Determinants of Smoking: An Introduction

Nicotine dependence represents a major public health challenge and is a complex behavior in which both genetic and environmental factors have a role (Greenbaum and Lerer 2009).

The current evidence suggests that the genetic profile is associated with smoking behavior. In fact, data coming from family, adoption and twin studies strongly support the influence of genes on the initiation and persistence of smoking since the late nineties (Sullivan and Kendler 1999). The likelihood to start smoking could be attributed to genetic influences for approximately 60 % (Sullivan and Kendler 1999); nicotine dependence could be due to genetic for about 70 %, being the overlap between genetic determinants of initiation and dependence high (Sullivan and Kendler 1999). Twin studies support also the influence of genetic determinants on smoking cessation and on the efficacy of interventions aimed at quitting smoking (Rossing 1998). Most of the genetic background of smoking behavior is explained because of the involving of dopamine neurotransmission in conditioning tobacco use and tolerance (David and Munafò 2008). Furthermore, smoking is associated with diminished serotonin neurotransmission: indeed, polymorphisms of serotonin transporter gene are potential candidate in studying smoking behavior and cessation.

1.8 Biological Basis

It is universally recognized that addiction to any drug is a complex phenotype influenced by the environment and by more than one gene (Li and Burmeister 2009). Nicotine is an alkaloid (1-methyl-2-(3-pyridyl) pyrrolidine) and is the principal component of tobacco that leads to addiction. It is established that the addiction produced by nicotine is extremely powerful and is at least as strong as addictions to other drugs such as heroin and cocaine. In fact, in February 2000, the Royal College of Physicians (RCP) declared that nicotine can be defined an addictive substance. The RCP report stated as follows: "On present evidence, it is reasonable to conclude that nicotine delivered through tobacco smoke should be regarded as an addictive drug, and tobacco use as the means of self-administration. Cigarettes are highly efficient nicotine delivery devices and are as addictive as drugs such as heroin or cocaine."

When tobacco is smoked, the nicotine in the smoke enters the blood vessels in the lungs and reaches the brain within 10 s of the first puff. Consequently, nicotine binds to receptors located on the cell bodies of neurons in the ventral tegmental area (VTA) and the terminals of these neurons. Normally these receptors bind the neurotransmitter acetylcholine. As nicotine is very similarly structured to acetylcholine, it is able to bind to the acetylcholine receptor.

Nicotine has specific acetylcholine receptors (nAChRs) in the brain and other organs. The stimulation of presynaptic acetylcholine receptors increases transmitter release as well as the metabolism. Similarly to other drugs of abuse, nicotine triggers the dopamine reward system and increases the extracellular level of dopamine in nucleus accumbens (NAc) that has a fundamental role for the reinforcing behavior, stimulant, and dependence properties of nicotine.

Nicotine also acts in the brain on non-dopaminergic structures. In addition, the many actions of nicotine on brain stem cholinergic, GABAergic, noradrenergic, and serotonergic nuclei, could be related to the addiction. Some biological theories show that the neurochemical pathway to nicotine reinforcement is probably related to binding of nicotine to nAChRs containing the b2 subunit, followed by the activation of the mesolimbic dopamine system. This process brings to an initiation of molecular changes that highlight drug addiction. Moreover, some tobacco components contribute to stop both forms of the monoamine oxidase enzymes (MAO A and B). The MAO enzymes are involved in the breakdown of the amine neurotransmitters, like dopamine, that is an important mediator of the reinforcing effects of nicotine determining tobacco dependence (Nisell et al. 1995; Pontieri et al. 1996).

Regarding nicotine addiction, many questions remain and further studies are needed to address this important issue.

From the genetics perspective, even if brain nicotinic acetylcholine receptor (nAChR)-encoding genes are among the most studied genes, because of their biological relevance as binding sites for nicotine, there are several genes that determine who will develop a smoking addiction. These genes code for neurotransmitters involved in the addiction pathways: for how they are produced and metabolized, for the number of receptors that are available and how rapidly nicotine is metabolized by different people (Davies and Soundy 2009).

Table 1.9 shows a list of candidate genes associated with smoking and nicotine addiction.

1.9 Smoking Initiation and Cessation

A literature review performed on PubMed[1] revealed an important amount of publications on genetic determinants of smoking and smoking-related diseases which covers approximately twenty years. Hereby the most important results coming from review

[1] For the literature search the following string was used: (Smoking OR cigarette) AND (cessation or initiation) AND (gene OR genetic OR SNP), Limits Activated: Humans, Meta-Analysis, Review, English, Field: Title/Abstract.

Table 1.9 List of candidate genes associated with smoking and nicotine addiction [modified from Davies and Soundy (2009)]

Candidate gene	Genetic association	Phenotype
Dopaminergic system		
Dopamine receptors, DRD2	Linkage to chromosomal region 11q23	Increased cigarette consumption
DRD4	48 bp VNTR in Exon 3	Habitual smoking, greater craving, Shorter time before first morning cigarette
Dopamine transporter, DAT 1	40 bp VNTR in 3′ UTR	Lower risk of current smoking and starting smoking before age 16, longer periods of abstinence, and increased quitting
Dopamine metabolism, tyrosine hydroxylase (TH)	Linkage to chromosomal region 11.15.5	Habitual smoking
Dopamine β-hydoxylase (DBH)	Linkage to chromosomal region 9q43	Habitual smoking and cigarette consumption
Monoamine oxidase (MAOA)-A	VNTR in promoter region	Higher levels of nicotine dependence and lower risk of smoking
Catechol-*o*-methyl transferase (COMT)	G>A SNP corresponding to Val108/158Met	Protective against smoking in women, protective against nicotine dependence
Serotonergic system		
Serotonin transporter, 5-HTT serotonin metabolism, tryptophan hydroxylase	44 bp insertion/deletion in promoter linkage of chromosomal region 11p15	Association is via genetic effects on personality Habitual smoking
Cholinergic receptors		
CHRNA4 CHRNA7	Alpha-4 subunit variation Polymorphism in intron 2, Linkage to chromosomal region 15q13.1	Lower risk of nicotine dependence in Chinese men Smoking status in schizophrenics Habitual smoking
Nicotine metabolism		
CYP450 2A6 2D	Multiple polymorphisms. CYP2D6	Wide range of enzyme activity affecting metabolism of nicotine to cotinine. Extensive metabolizers of nicotine and heavy smoking

and meta-analysis which specifically addressed the topic of smoking initiation and cessation are discussed.

A recent genome-wide (GW) meta-analysis (The Tobacco and Genetics Consortium 2010) has investigated several single nucleotide polymorphisms (SNPs) associated to smoking initiation and cessation. In particular, eight SNPs of brain-derived neurotrophic factor (BDNF), which belong to the family of neurotrophins that regulate synaptic plasticity and survival of cholinergic and dopaminergic neurons, were found to be associated to smoking initiation, with the variant rs6265 increasing the risk for being regular smoker of 6 % (OR 1.06, 95 % CI 1.04–1.08). As far as smoking cessation is concerned, the SNP rs3025343 of the dopamine

Study name	Statistics for each study				
	Odds ratio	Lower limit	Upper limit	Z-Value	p-Value
Noble 1994	1.849	1.187	2.881	2.719	0.007
Comings 1996	2.716	2.057	3.587	7.044	0.000
Comings 1997	1.580	0.883	2.827	1.542	0.123
Singleton 1998	0.596	0.342	1.037	-1.832	0.067
Spitz 1998 (Control)	2.000	0.521	7.682	1.010	0.313
Spitz 1998 (Lung Cancer)	1.000	0.337	2.965	0.000	1.000
Lerman 1999 (European)	1.207	0.816	1.786	0.942	0.346
Lerman 1999 (Other)	0.926	0.361	2.375	-0.160	0.873
Sabol 1999	1.158	0.968	1.385	1.606	0.108
Costa-Mallen 2000 (Control)	1.184	0.570	2.462	0.453	0.651
Costa-Mallen 2000 (Parkinson)	1.003	0.554	1.816	0.010	0.992
Wu 2000 (African-American)	1.609	0.700	3.699	1.119	0.263
Wu 2000 (Mexican-American)	1.042	0.467	2.324	0.100	0.921
Yoshida 2001	0.370	0.235	0.582	-4.296	0.000
Hamajima 2002	1.063	0.801	1.412	0.424	0.672
Qi 2002 (Control)	1.220	0.765	1.945	0.835	0.403
Qi 2002 (Lung Cancer)	0.930	0.565	1.530	-0.287	0.774
Lee 2003	1.067	0.576	1.978	0.207	0.836
Johnstone 2004b	0.808	0.598	1.093	-1.383	0.167
Timberlake 2007	0.951	0.805	1.124	-0.588	0.556
Munafo 2007	0.985	0.831	1.168	-0.171	0.864
	1.086	1.008	1.169	2.176	0.030

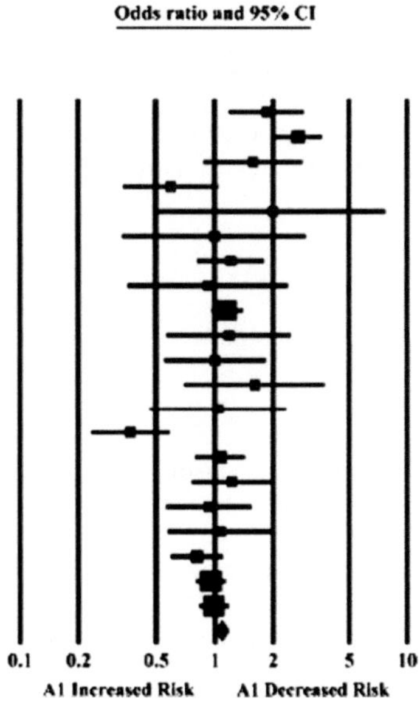

Fig. 1.8 Meta-analysis of association of DRD2 Taq1A1 allele with smoking initiation

β-hydroxylase (DBH), which is involved in the conversion of dopamine to norepinephrine, achieved genome-wide significance being associated to former smoking status (OR 1.12, 95 % CI 1.08–1.18).

Notwithstanding the evidence yielded by GW, twin and adoption studies on the etiology of smoking behavior, replicate reliably has been tested for few candidate genes (Munafò and Johnstone 2008). Among them, the most well known and investigated are as follows: the D2 dopamine receptor (DRD2), the cytochrome P450 (CYP) 2A6 and the enzyme catechol *O*-methyltransferase (COMT).

A systematic review of 28 candidate gene studies of smoking behavior published in 2004 (Munafò et al. 2004) did confirm that DRD2 and CYP2A6 genes are among the most influential in smoking, together with serotonin transporter (5HTT). The meta-analysis showed that DRD2 Taq1A polymorphism is associated to smoking initiation (OR for homozygous wild type vs. heterozygotes and homozygous variant 0.75, 95 % CI 0.65–0.85) even though the result was not more significant using a random effects model. With respect to smoking cessation, the 5HTT LPR polymorphism was associated with reduced risk for successful smoking cessation (OR for homozygous wild type vs. heterozygotes and homozygous variant 1.48, 95 % CI 1.03–2.14) while the presence of a variant CYP2A6 reduced-activity polymorphism allele increased the likelihood of successful smoking cessation (OR for homozygous wild type vs. heterozygotes and homozygous variant 0.67, 95 % CI 0.48–0.95). Similarly, a higher prevalence of the Taq1A allele was demonstrated in smokers by a meta-analysis of 12 case–control studies (OR 1.47, 95 % CI 1.31–1.66) (Li et al. 2004); this result has been confirmed by Mufanò and coll. in 2009 when a significant association was found between the DRD2 Taq1A genotype and the likelihood of being an eversmoker (OR 1.09, 95 % CI 1.01–1.17) (Munafò et al. 2009) (Fig. 1.8).

Study name	Subgroup within study	Statistics for each study				
		Odds ratio	Lower limit	Upper limit	*Z* value	*P* value
Enoch *et al.* [29]	Blank	1.188	0.791	1.785	0.830	0.407
Guo *et al.* [85]	Blank	1.645	1.123	2.411	2.555	0.011
Nedic *et al.* [81]	Blank	1.269	0.960	1.677	1.675	0.094
Omidvar *et al.* [87]	Blank	1.058	0.936	1.196	0.902	0.367
Redden *et al.* [84]	Study1	1.822	1.177	2.822	2.689	0.007
Redden *et al.* [84]	Study2	1.101	0.757	1.603	0.504	0.615
Shiels *et al.* [80]	Blank	1.082	0.973	1.203	1.453	0.146
Tochigi *et al.* [82]	Blank	1.103	0.814	1.496	0.634	0.526
		1.120	1.044	1.201	3.174	0.002

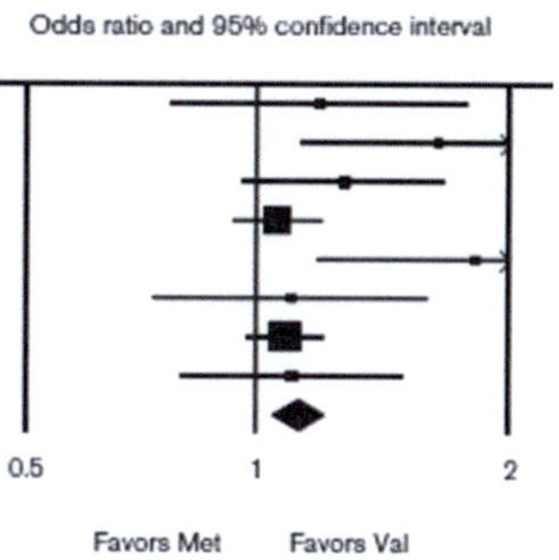

COMT, catechol-O-methyl transferase gene.

Fig. 1.9 Meta-analysis of the association between COMT Val108/158Met polymorphism and smoking

CYP2A6 genetic variations influence nicotine inactivation and smoking behavior too; anyway some evidence suggest that the slow inactivator genotype may increase the risk for nicotine dependence when smoking is initiated during adolescence, whereas it could lower the risk for smoking and the duration and the consumption among adult smokers (Malaiyandi et al. 2005).

Another well-known target in the evaluation of nicotine dependence is the COMT, in particular the Val108/158Met polymorphism in exon 4 at codon 108, in the soluble molecule (rs165688), or codon 158, in the membrane-bound one (rs4680). The rs4680 A (Met) allele of the COMT gene seems to predict the heaviness of smoking but not the likelihood of cessation (Munafò et al. 2011.); furthermore, the COMT Val108/158Met genotype has a small, but significant effect on the risk of smoking with an OR of 1.12 (95 % CI 1.04–1.20) (Fig. 1.9) (Tammimäki and Männistö 2010).

Genetics seems to play an important role also in predicting response to medication; in particular the nicotine-metabolizing enzyme CYP2A6 gene and the low dopamine activity DRD2 have been associated to clinical response to nicotine replacement therapy (NRT) while the bupropion-metabolizing enzyme CYP2B6 and the high dopamine activity DRD2 and COMT genotypes have been associated with greater bupropion efficacy (Sturgess et al. 2011; Quaak et al. 2009; David and Munafò 2008).

Notwithstanding the amount of association and GW association studies on genetic polymorphisms and smoking cessation following NRT and/or bupropion therapy, candidate genes still require additional investigations because of inconsistency (Kortmann et al. 2009). Anyway, there are some exceptions which were analyzed more than twice in different therapeutic schemes (Kortmann et al. 2009).

As far as CYP2A6 is concerned there are evidence that smokers with reduced or null activity alleles are more likely to quit smoking (Gu et al. 2000; Kubota et al. 2006). Similarly smokers with the DRD2 Taq1 A1 allele may benefit from NRT (Johnstone et al. 2004; Yudkin et al. 2004) while homozygous A2/A2 are more likely to benefit from bupropion therapy (David et al. 2003, 2007; Swan et al. 2005).

In a study reporting the results of two transdermal NRT trials, the Patch and Patch in Practice (PiP), the association between 30 candidate gene polymorphisms (SNPs or variable number of tandem repeats (VNTRs)) and smoking cessation have been investigated. The only SNP which has been proved to be significantly associated with abstinence (assessed by self-reporting combined with exhaled carbon monoxide (CO) ≤ 10 ppm and salivary cotinine ≤ 20 ng/ml) was COMT rs4680. Statistical trends were observed for other polymorphisms, such as DRD2 rs6276 and rs6277 and CHRNA rs2273502 (David et al. 2011). COMT rs4680 AA genotype (vs. AG/GG) was associated with greater efficacy of NRT patch (vs. placebo) at 12 weeks in the Patch (Johnstone et al. 2007) and PiP studies (Munafò et al. 2008). Anyhow, the meta-analysis of Tammimäki and Männistö did not show any association between COMT Val108/158Met genotype and the probability of quitting (with or without therapy) (Tammimäki and Männistö 2010).

Other genetic determinants which have been demonstrated to have an association with smoking cessation are those involving genes encoding nicotinic acetylcholine receptor subunits (CHRN) ; in particular, the rs1051730 genetic variant within the CHRN A5-A3-B4 was associated to smoking cessation (Munafò et al. 2011).

References

Brandt, A. M. (2007). *The cigarette century: The rise, fall, and the deadly persistence of the product that defined America*. New York, NY: Basic Books.

Burns, D. M. (1998). Cigar smoking: Overview and current state of the science. In: *Cigars: health effects and trends* (*Smoking and Tobacco Control Monograph 9*) (pp. 1–20). Bethesda, MD: National Cancer Institute.

D'Souza, M. S., & Markou, A. (2011). Neuronal mechanisms underlying development of nicotine dependence: Implications for novel smoking-cessation treatments. *Addiction Science and Clinical Practice, 6*(1), 4–16.

David, S. P., Brown, R. A., Papandonatos, G. D., Kahler, C. W., Lloyd-Richardson, E. E., Munafò, M. R., et al. (2007). Pharmacogenetic clinical trial of sustained-release bupropion for smoking cessation. *Nicotine and Tobacco Research, 9*, 821–833.

David, S. P., Johnstone, E. C., Churchman, M., Aveyard, P., Murphy, M. F., & Munafò, M. R. (2011). Pharmacogenetics of smoking cessation in general practice: Results from the patch II and patch in practice trials. *Nicotine and Tobacco Research, 13*(3), 157–167.

David, S. P., & Munafò, M. R. (2008). Genetic variation in the dopamine pathway and smoking cessation. *Pharmacogenomics, 9*(9), 1307–1321.

David, S. P., Niaura, R., Papandonatos, G. D., Shadel, W. G., Burkholder, G. J., Britt, D. M., et al. (2003). Does the DRD2-Taq1 A polymorphism influence treatment response to bupropion hydrochloride for reduction of the nicotine withdrawal syndrome? *Nicotine and Tobacco Research, 5*, 935–942.

Davies, G. E., & Soundy, T. J. (2009). The genetics of smoking and nicotine addiction. *South Dakota Journal of Medicine*, Spec No:43-9.

Fagerstrom, K. O. (1978). Measuring degree of physical dependence to tobacco smoking with reference to individualization of treatment. *Addictive Behaviors, 3*, 235–241.

Fagerstrom, K. O., Heatherton, T. F., & Kozlowski, L. T. (2000). Nicotine addiction and its assessment. *Ear, Nose, and Throat Journal, 69*(11), 763–766.

Greenbaum, L., & Lerer, B. (2009). Differential contribution of genetic variation in multiple brain nicotinic cholinergic receptors to nicotine dependence: Recent progress and emerging open questions. *Molecular Psychiatry, 14*(10), 912–945.

Gu, D. F., Hinks, L. J., Morton, N. E., & Day, I. N. (2000). The use of long PCR to confirm three common alleles at the CYP2A6 locus and the relationship between genotype and smoking habit. *Annals of Human Genetics, 64*, 383–390.

Heatherton, T. F., Kozlowski, L. T., Frecker, K. C., & Fagerstrom, K. O. (1991). The Fagerstrom test for nicotine dependence: A revision of the Fagerstrom tolerance questionnaire. *British Journal of Addiction, 86*, 1119–1127.

Henningfield, J. E., Miyasato, K., & Jasinski, D. R. (1985). Abuse liability and pharmacodynamic characteristics of intravenous and inhaled nicotine. *The Journal of Pharmacology and Experimental Therapeutics, 234*(1), 1–12.

Henningfield, J. E., & Slade, J. (1998). Tobacco-dependence medications: Public health and regulatory issues. *Food and Drug Law Journal, 53 suppl*, 75–114.

Hoffmann, D., & Hoffmann, I. (2001). The changing cigarette: Chemical studies and bioassays. In: Risks associated with smoking cigarettes with low machine-measured yields of tar and nicotine. Smoking and Tobacco Control Monograph No. 13; NIH Publ. No. 02-5074. Bethesda, MD, *National Cancer Institute*, pp. 159–191.

Hughes, J. R., Gust, S. W., Skoog, K., Keenan, R. M., & Fenwick, J. W. (1991). Symptoms of tobacco withdrawal: A replication and extension. *Archives of General Psychiatry, 48*(1), 52–59.

IARC. (2002, July). *Tobacco smoke and involuntary smoking* (*Monographs on the evaluation of carcinogenic risks to humans*) (Vol .83). Lyon: IARC.

International Agency for Research on Cancer (IARC). (2004). *Tobacco smoke and involuntary smoking (Monographs on the evaluation of carcinogenic risks to humans)* (Vol. 83). Lyon: IARC.

Jha, P., & Chaloupka, F. J. (1999). *Curbing the epidemic: Governments and the economics of tobacco control*. Washington, DC: World Bank.

Johnstone, E. C., Elliot, K. M., David, S. P., Murphy, M. F., Walton, R. T., & Munafò, M. R. (2007). Association of COMT Val108/158Met genotype with smoking cessation in a nicotine replacement therapy randomized trial. *Cancer Epidemiology, Biomarkers and Prevention, 16*, 1065–1069.

Johnstone, E. C., Yudkin, P. L., Hey, K., Roberts, S. J., Welch, S. J., Murphy, M. F., et al. (2004). Genetic variation in dopaminergic pathways and short-term effectiveness of the nicotine patch. *Pharmacogenetics, 14*, 83–90.

Kortmann, G. L., Dobler, C. J., Bizarro, L., & Bau, C. H. (2009). Pharmacogenetics of smoking cessation therapy. *American Journal of Medical Genetics Part B: Neuropsychiatric Genetics, 153B*(1), 17–28.

Kubota, T., Nakajima-Taniguchi, C., Fukuda, T., Funamoto, M., Maeda, M., Tange, E., et al. (2006). CYP2A6 polymorphisms are associated with nicotine dependence and influence withdrawal symptoms in smoking cessation. *The Pharmacogenomics Journal, 6*, 115–119.

Laviolette, S. R., & van der Kooy, D. (2004). The neurobiology of nicotine addiction: Bridging the gap from molecules to behaviour. *Nature Reviews. Neuroscience, 5*(1), 55–65.

Li, M. D., & Burmeister, M. (2009). New insights into the genetics of addiction. *Nature Reviews. Genetics, 10*(4), 225–231.

Li, M. D., Ma, J. Z., & Beuten, J. (2004). Progress in searching for susceptibility loci and genes for smoking-related behaviour. *Clinical Genetics, 66*(5), 382–392.

Loffredo, C. (2006). Hold the hookah: Research warns against trendy tobacco use. Accessed 6th May 2012, http://explore.georgetown.edu/news/?ID=18216

Mackay, J., Eriksen, M., & Shafey, O. (2006). *The tobacco atlas* (2nd ed.). Atlanta, GA: American Cancer Society.

Malaiyandi, V., Sellers, E. M., & Tyndale, R. F. (2005). Implications of CYP2A6 genetic variation for smoking behaviors and nicotine dependence. *Clinical Pharmacology and Therapeutics, 77*(3), 145–158.

Markou, A. (2008). Neurobiology of nicotine dependence. *Philosophical Transactions of the Royal Society of London. Series B, Biological Sciences, 363*(1507), 3159–3168.

Munafò, M., Clark, T., Johnstone, E., Murphy, M., & Walton, R. (2004). The genetic basis for smoking behavior: A systematic review and meta-analysis. *Nicotine and Tobacco Research, 6*(4), 583–597.

Munafò, M. R., & Johnstone, E. C. (2008). Genes and cigarette smoking. *Addiction, 103*(6), 893–904.

Munafò, M. R., Johnstone, E. C., Guo, B., Murphy, M. F., & Aveyard, P. (2008). Association of COMT Val108/158Met genotype with smoking cessation. *Pharmacogenetics and Genomics, 18*, 121–128.

Munafò, M. R., Johnstone, E. C., Walther, D., Uhl, G. R., Murphy, M. F., & Aveyard, P. (2011). CHRNA3 rs1051730 genotype and short-term smoking cessation. *Nicotine and Tobacco Research, 13*(10), 982–988.

Munafò, M. R., Timpson, N. J., David, S. P., Ebrahim, S., & Lawlor, D. A. (2009). Association of the DRD2 gene Taq1A polymorphism and smoking behavior: A meta-analysis and new data. *Nicotine and Tobacco Research, 11*(1), 64–76.

Nisell, M., Nomikos, G. G., & Svensson, T. H. (1995). Nicotine dependence, midbrain dopamine systems and psychiatric disorders. *Pharmacology and Toxicology, 76*, 157–162.

Pitts, J. (2012). *Smoking cessation. What is nicotine withdrawal syndrome?* Accessed May 6, 2012, from http://www.healthguidance.org/entry/11599/1/What-Is-Nicotine-Withdrawal-Syndrome.html

Pollock, D. (1999). *Denial and delay*. London: Action on Smoking and Health.

Pomerleau, C. S., Carton, S. M., Lutzke, M. L., Flessland, K. A., & Pomerleau, O. F. (1994). Reliability of the fagerstromtolerance questionnaire and the fagerstrom test for nicotine dependence. *Addictive Behaviors, 19*(1), 33–39.

Pontieri, F. E., Tanda, G., Orzi, F., & Di Chiara, G. (1996). Effects of nicotine on the nucleus accumbens and similarity to those of addictive drugs. *Nature, 382*, 255–257.

Quaak, M., van Schayck, C. P., Knaapen, A. M., & van Schooten, F. J. (2009). Genetic variation as a predictor of smoking cessation success. A promising preventive and intervention tool for chronic respiratory diseases? *The European Respiratory Journal, 33*(3), 468–480.

Roberts, D. L. (1988). Natural tobacco flavor. *Recent Advances in Tobacco Science, 14*, 49–81.

Rossing, M. A. (1998). Genetic influences on smoking: Candidate genes. *Environmental Health Perspectives, 106*(5), 231–238.

Samet, J. M., & Yoon, S. Y. (2010). Gender, women, and the tobacco epidemic. WHO Library Cataloguing-in-Publication Data.

Slama, K. (2008). Global perspective on tobacco control. Part I. The global state of the tobacco epidemic. *The International Journal of Tuberculosis and Lung Disease, 12*(1), 3–7.

Sturgess, J. E., George, T. P., Kennedy, J. L., Heinz, A., & Müller, D. J. (2011). Pharmacogenetics of alcohol, nicotine and drug addiction treatments. *Addiction Biology, 16*(3), 357–376.

Sullivan, P. F., & Kendler, K. S. (1999). The genetic epidemiology of smoking. *Nicotine and Tobacco Research, 1*(Suppl 2), S51–S57.

Swan, G. E., Valdes, A. M., Ring, H. Z., Khroyan, T. V., Jack, L. M., Ton, C. C., et al. (2005). Dopamine receptor DRD2 genotype and smoking cessation outcome following treatment with bupropion SR. *The Pharmacogenomics Journal, 5*, 21–29.

Tammimäki, A. E., & Männistö, P. T. (2010). Are genetic variants of COMT associated with addiction? *Pharmacogenetics and Genomics, 20*(12), 717–741.

The Tobacco and Genetics Consortium. (2010). Genome-wide meta-analyses identify multiple loci associated with smoking behavior. *Nature Genetics, 42*(5), 441–447.

US Department of Health and Human Services. (2004). *The health consequences of smoking: A report of the surgeon general*. Atlanta, Georgia: US Department of Health and Human Services, Centers for Disease Control and Prevention, National Center for Chronic Disease Prevention and Health Promotion, Office on Smoking and Health.

Ward, M. M., Swan, G. E., & Jack, L. M. (2001). Self-reported abstinence effects in the first month after smoking cessation. *Addictive Behaviors, 26*, 311–327.

West, E. (2004). Assessment of dependence and motivation to stop smoking. *BMJ, 328*, 338–339.

WHO. (2010). In M. S. Jonathan & Y. Soon-Young (Eds.), *Gender, women, and the tobacco epidemic*. WHO Library Cataloguing-in-Publication Data.

Yudkin, P., Munafò, M., Hey, K., Roberts, S., Welch, S., Johnstone, E., et al. (2004). Effectiveness of nicotine patches in relation to genotype in women versus men: Randomized controlled trial. *British Medical Journal, 328*, 989–990.

Chapter 2
State of the Art of Smoking Habits in the World

Giuseppe La Torre and Brigid Unim

Objectives The goal of this chapter is to synthesize available data on incidence and prevalence of global smoking habits by gender, age, and ethnical groups. Summarily, this chapter offers an overview of the actual trend of smoking habits worldwide.

Learning Outcomes

At the end of this chapter the reader will be able to:

- Expand knowledge on the global tobacco epidemic.
- Learn about the parameters that effectively characterize the cigarette epidemic (prevalence, consumption, mortality/morbidity due to smoking).
- Analyze the epidemiological basis of involuntary exposure to tobacco smoke and its different facets (secondhand, thirdhand).
- Learn about remedial actions in approaching the tobacco use.

2.1 Introduction: The Tobacco Epidemic

Tobacco use is the leading preventable cause of premature death and has been reported by the World Health Organization (WHO) as "the single most preventable cause of death in the world today" (WHO Report on the Global Tobacco Epidemic 2008). In fact, tobacco use is responsible each year for nearly six million deaths, including more than 600,000 nonsmokers and causes hundreds of billions of dollars of economic burden worldwide. If current trends continue, tobacco-related

G. La Torre (✉) • B. Unim
Department of Public Health and Infectious Diseases, "Sapienza" University of Rome, Piazzale Aldo Moro 5, Rome 00185, Italy
e-mail: giuseppe.latorre@uniroma1.it; brigidunim@yahoo.it

G. La Torre, *Smoking Prevention and Cessation*, DOI 10.1007/978-1-4614-7046-5_2,

deaths could increase to more than eight million per year by 2030, with 80 % of these premature deaths in low- and middle-income countries where the burden of tobacco-related illness and death is heaviest. The disparity between high- and low-income countries is expected to widen further over the next several decades (WHO Report on the Global Tobacco Epidemic 2011).

The tobacco epidemic continues to expand because of the extreme addictiveness of nicotine, the ongoing industry marketing and population growth in countries where tobacco use is increasing. The World Health Organization Framework Convention on Tobacco Control (WHO FCTC), in the attempt to address the epidemic, provides information about implementation and management of tobacco control programs for all countries in partnership with the United Nations, health development agencies and civil society. Although progress has been made, only 19 countries follow best practice standards. Unfortunately, none of these are low-income countries. In this context, good monitoring of tobacco use and tobacco control policy implementation is critical to understand and reverse the outstanding epidemic (WHO Report on the Global Tobacco Epidemic 2011).

In the past years attempts have been made to model the cigarette epidemic, for example, the four-phase model proposed by Lopez et al. (1994) is based on three major variables (prevalence, consumption, mortality due to smoking) which are responsible for the transition through the various stages. The model shows three to four decade lag between the rise in smoking prevalence and the rise in smoking-attributable mortality. Therefore, for countries in stages I and II it could be dangerous to ignore tobacco as a public health problem because death rates due to smoking are still low (Fig. 2.1).

The constant increment of smoking prevalence will inevitably cause the rise of smoking-attributable mortality in stages III and IV. The explanation is that smoking-attributable mortality is closely related to the smoking patterns 30 or more years previously and not to current prevalence (Lopez et al. 1994).

Tobacco use is heavily socially patterned in developed countries, with prevalence of use being higher in lower income groups compared to higher income groups (Eek et al. 2010; Main et al. 2008). While tobacco use in general, and cigarette use in particular, has declined dramatically in wealthier socioeconomic groups over the last few decades, in the most economically disadvantaged groups, tobacco use prevalence has remained almost unchanged over this period. As a result, tobacco use is one of the largest causes of health disparities between socioeconomic groups (SCENIHR 2010; Gruer et al. 2009).

2.2 Data on Incidence, Prevalence, by Gender, Age Groups, Ethnic Groups

Cigarette smoking is the most common mode of tobacco consumption in many countries; therefore, smoking prevalence is a useful measure of the tobacco epidemic extent. Each country profile includes the most recent available data on the prevalence of tobacco or cigarette smoking by gender, among adults (age 15 years and

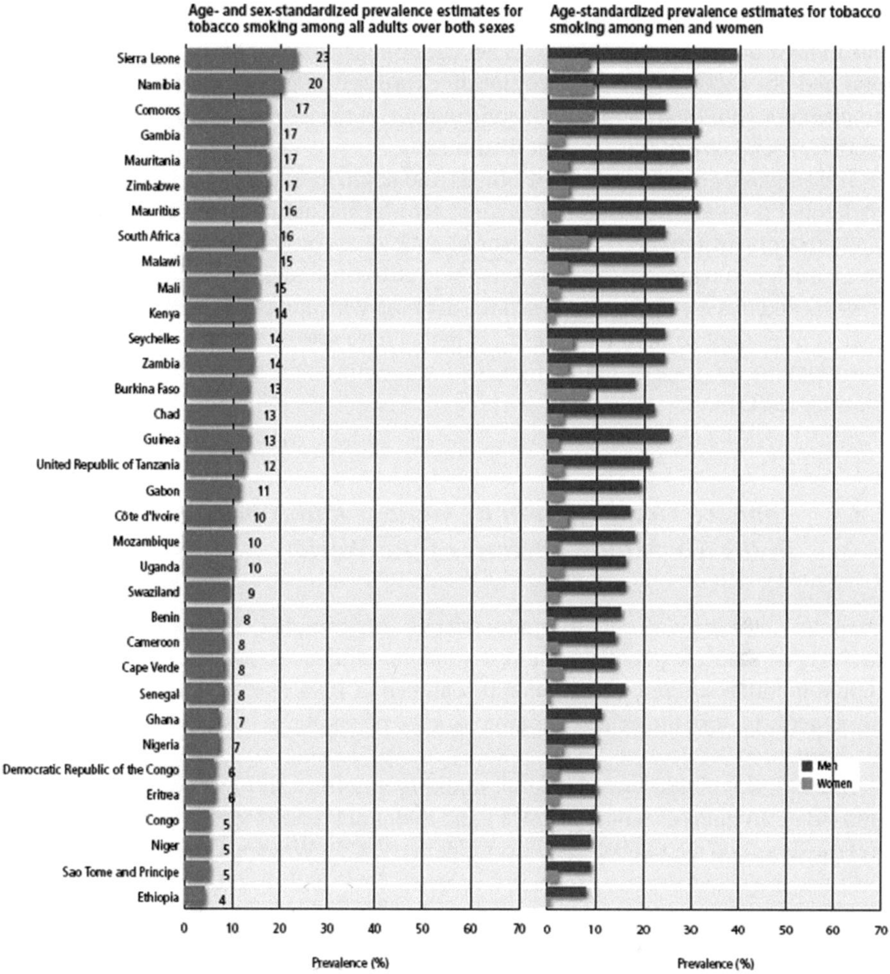

Fig. 2.1 Age and sex standardized prevalence estimates for tobacco smoking in Africa, 2009. From "WHO Report on the Global Tobacco Epidemic (2011)": Appendix vii—graph 7.2.1. Data not reported/not available for Algeria, Angola, Botswana, Burundi, Central African Republic, Equatorial Guinea, Guinea-Bissau, Lesotho, Liberia, Madagascar, Rwanda, and Togo

older), and youth (13–15 years old). Smoking prevalence refers to the proportion (expressed as a percent) of smokers in a study population (Shafey and Guindon 2003).

Smokers can be defined on the basis of the average daily/annual cigarettes consumption or on the basis of the different types of cigarettes. Briefly, smokers can be classified as "heavy smokers" (>20 cigarettes/day), "light smokers" (≤10 CPD), and "medium smokers" (≤5 CPD) (Ekberg-Aronsson et al. 2007).

The epidemiology of tobacco use can be analyzed with direct and indirect indicators. The direct indicator is the estimate of all smokers by gender and age. Other relevant socio-demografic indicators are life expectancy, literacy rates, labor force structure, and human development indexes (The Economist 1997). The indirect indicators, total and per capita tobacco consumption expressed in grams, give an overview of the phenomenon but do not provide information on the identity of smokers (e.g., age, gender), social conditions, and motivations.

Total cigarette consumption is useful as a standard measure of the size of a tobacco market but it does not allow comparisons across time and between countries. A per capita rate of consumption (an indicator of individual consumption) is more appropriate for such comparisons. Dividing total cigarette consumption by the population age 15 years and older is the method used for deriving per capita cigarette consumption.

It is important to note that these estimates may underestimate or overstate true consumption for several reasons such as smuggling and stockpiling (Shafey and Guindon 2003).

2.2.1 Tobacco Consumption by Gender and Adults in the Six Major Regions of the World

Cigarette smoking and nicotine dependence are complex traits arising from the interplay of multiple genetic and environmental influences. Hence, smoking behavior and nicotine addiction have been researched in Behavioral Genetics. In particular, genetic factors are related to two aspects of smoking attitudes: initiation and persistence.

In 2006, the global prevalence of smoking any form of tobacco was higher for men (41.1 %) than for women (8.9 %) and males accounted for 80 % of all smokers (WHO Report on the Global Tobacco Epidemic 2009). Women's smoking prevalence rates are projected to rise, especially in many low- and- middle-income countries where women smoke much less than men. In China, for example, 61 % of men are reported to be current smokers, compared with only 4.2 % of women. Similarly, in Argentina 34 % of men are reported to be current smokers, compared with 23 % of women (WHO Report on the Global Tobacco Epidemic 2008). The reasons of tobacco uptake for women and girls may reflect local beliefs/cultural practices, psychosocial and socioeconomic factors such as body image and peer pressure. For example, some women believe that chewing tobacco can cure toothaches or can be useful during childbirth and that smoking keeps them slim. In the Asian and Pacific countries where smoking has become a symbol of women's liberation, many young women are turning to tobacco as a sign of freedom (WHO: Gender, women, and the tobacco epidemic 2010a).

The social norms that slowed the diffusion of smoking among women are, therefore, diminishing in most parts of the developing world. This is one of the consequences of gender empowerment and economic growth which allow women to freely make choices (Warren et al. 2006).

In high-income countries, including Australia, Canada, the USA, and most countries of Western Europe, women smoke at nearly the same rate as men.

Gender differences in socioeconomic characteristics such as education, employment, and income appear to explain only a small fraction of the difference in smoking prevalence and intensity between males and females even in countries with a high degree of female empowerment (Bauer et al. 2007). In fact, the rise of smoking among women could be attributed not just to social factors and to women's increasing economic resources but also to the tobacco industry's marketing of cigarettes to women as a symbol of emancipation (Amos and Haglund 2000; Nerín 2005).

The main consequences of smoking are heart disease and stroke, chest and lung diseases, and several cancers, especially lung cancer (see Chap. 3). Generally, both sexes fall victim to the morbidity and mortality associated with these diseases, but there is growing evidence that these diseases and effects also have sex-specific elements. For example, women get lung cancers at a lower exposure than men; adenocarcinomas are more prevalent among female smokers than men and may result from gendered smoking behaviors (inhaling more deeply) and/or gendered products that were designed for women (Payne 2001; Samet and Yoon 2001).

Gender targeting can include the development of specific tobacco products and the use of specific additives in these products. For instance, cigarettes with perfumed scents and labeled as "slim" or "light" brands have been marketed to women. This is reflected in evidence that more women than men smoke light and ultralight cigarettes (ONS 2007). Hamilton et al. (2004) found out that advertisements for light cigarettes are perceived to imply that their use is healthier than use of regular cigarettes, partly because consumers wrongly believe that the advertisements must be approved and endorsed by a government agency.

Cigarettes indiscriminately damage and kill most of their users, regardless of their social position or gender. Smokers in all social status have poorer survival than those who never smoked in even the lowest social class; furthermore, smoking by women cancels out their "biological" survival advantage over men (Gruer et al. 2009). It has been observed that among smokers, people from high socioeconomic classes live longer than those from lower socioeconomic classes (see Fig. 2.2).

Another important issue to consider is that there are sex-specific effects on both male and female reproductive systems and capabilities (e.g., erectile dysfunction in men). The effects of smoking during pregnancy are numerous and well documented and include preterm delivery, low-birth-weight infants, and possible long-term effects on child and a propensity to nicotine addiction in later life. Additional female health conditions affected by tobacco use include cervical cancer, bone disease, and enhanced mortality from breast cancer (A Report of the Surgeon General 2010).

Average prevalence rates of smokers vary across the six WHO regions and among gender (see Table 2.1; Figs. 2.1–2.6). For daily smoking among males, the rates varied from 22 % in the African region and the region of the Americas to 46 % in the Western Pacific region. Greater relative differences were observed for females, with rates varying from 2 % in the South-East Asia region to 17 % in the European region.

For current smoking among males, the rates varied from 26 % in the region of the Americas to 47 % in the Western Pacific region. While for females, the rates varied from 2 % in the South-East Asia region to 22 % in the European region. The greatest

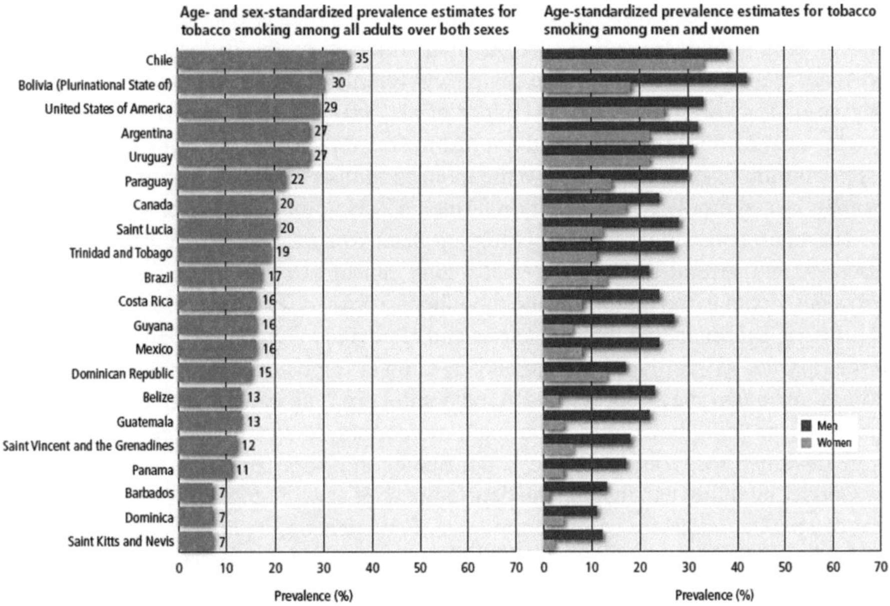

Fig. 2.2 Age and sex standardized prevalence estimates for tobacco smoking in The Americas, 2009. From "WHO Report on the Global Tobacco Epidemic (2011)": Appendix vii—graph 7.2.2. Data not reported/not available for Antigua and Barbuda, Bahamas, Colombia, Cuba, Ecuador, El Salvador, Grenada, Haiti, Honduras, Jamaica, Nicaragua, Peru, Suriname, and Venezuela

difference by gender was observed in the South-East Asia region, with current smoking in males nearly 18 times higher than in females. The smallest difference was observed in the region of the Americas, where the average current smoking rate among males was only 1.6 times higher than among females. Data on former users and never users by gender are also reported in Table 2.1 (WHO Global progress report 2010b).

Cessation activity among smokers is relatively common, for example, more than 40 % of current US smokers report having made a serious attempt to quit in the past 12 months. Unfortunately, only about 3–5 % of smokers maintain abstinence up to 1 year after quitting (Shiffman et al. 2008). Women seem to be less successful at quitting smoking than men since they are more concerned about weight gain and may resume smoking to avoid it. The social and economic status of women smokers is also relevant; in fact, poor and less-educated women are significantly less likely to quit.

Prenatal smoking remains one of the most common preventable causes of poor pregnancy and infant outcomes (US Department of Health 2004). Studies among pregnant women indicate that 82 % want behavioral support and 77 % want self-help materials. In one study, two-thirds of the women declared that if their partner, family, or friends quit smoking, it would be easier for them to quit. In some cultures, tobacco cessation professionals may be involved, while in others, spiritual leaders

Table 2.1 Estimated regional averages for prevalence of smoking and use of smokeless tobacco (%)[a]

	Males						Females					
	Current users		Daily users		Former users	Never users	Current users		Daily users		Former users	Never users
WHO region	Smoking	Smokeless	Smoking	Smokeless	Smoking	Smoking	Smoking	Smokeless	Smoking	Smokeless	Smoking	Smoking
African region	30	NA	22	NA	4	58	7	NA	5	NA	1	94
Region of the Americas	26	1	22	NA	24	49	16	NA	14	NA	13	77
South-East Asia region	35	33	32	33	11	44	2	10	2	10	1	97
European region	42	9	37	5	21	33	22	2	17	1	19	58
Eastern Mediterranean region	31	12	31	10	18	38	5	4	4	3	2	88
Western Pacific region	47	1	46	1	29	34	8	10	7	10	6	84

NA Data not available

[a]Data from "2010 global progress report on the implementation of the WHO Framework Convention on Tobacco Control" (World Health Organization 2010b)

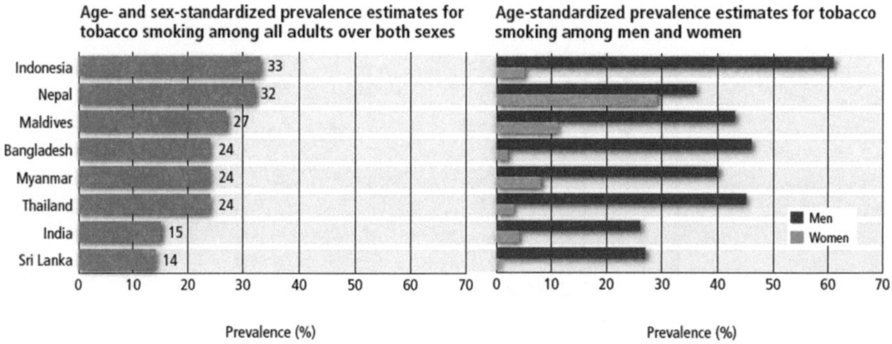

Fig. 2.3 Age and sex standardized prevalence estimates for tobacco smoking in South-East Asia, 2009. From "WHO Report on the Global Tobacco Epidemic (2011)": Appendix vii—graph 7.2.3. Data not reported/not available for Bhutan, Democratic People's Republic of Korea, and Timor-Leste

and faith healers may be consulted. All interventions should be adapted according to subgroups, specific cultures, and different countries (WHO: Gender, women, and the tobacco epidemic 2010a).

Smoking cessation efforts and interventions could be more effective during pregnancy because women know about the adverse effects of smoking on their health and that of a fetus (Fiore et al. 2008). Though, long-term reduction in tobacco exposure during pregnancy can be achieved only by encouraging adolescent girls and young women not to start smoking. Smoking cessation interventions should be continued after delivery to prevent recidivism and partners who smoke should be included in such interventions.

Several studies have confirmed the heritability of smoking initiation, as well as smoking persistence and nicotine dependence (Kendler et al. 1999; Li et al. 2003; Vink et al. 2004; Hamilton et al. 2006; Broms et al. 2007). Differences in heritability coefficients by gender are generally not reported or are minimal, although the study by Hamilton et al. (2006) indicated significantly higher heritability for smoking initiation in males than in females but no significant differences for smoking persistence. In contrast, the meta-analysis carried out by Li et al. (2003) reported higher heritability for smoking initiation in females than in males, while the coefficient for smoking persistence was higher in males.

Summarily, important behavioral indices are similar for women and men such as time to the first cigarette in the morning and the number of cigarettes smoked per day that may represent the most highly heritable symptoms of nicotine dependence for both genders (Lessov et al. 2004).

The heritability of smoking cessation has also been assessed in literature (Xian et al. 2003; Broms et al. 2006; Pergadia et al. 2006). According to Broms et al. (2006) genetic factors are related to the number of cigarettes smoked per day and to smoking cessation but are largely independent of smoking initiation.

See Chap. 7 for more information about the relationship between smoking and genetic factors.

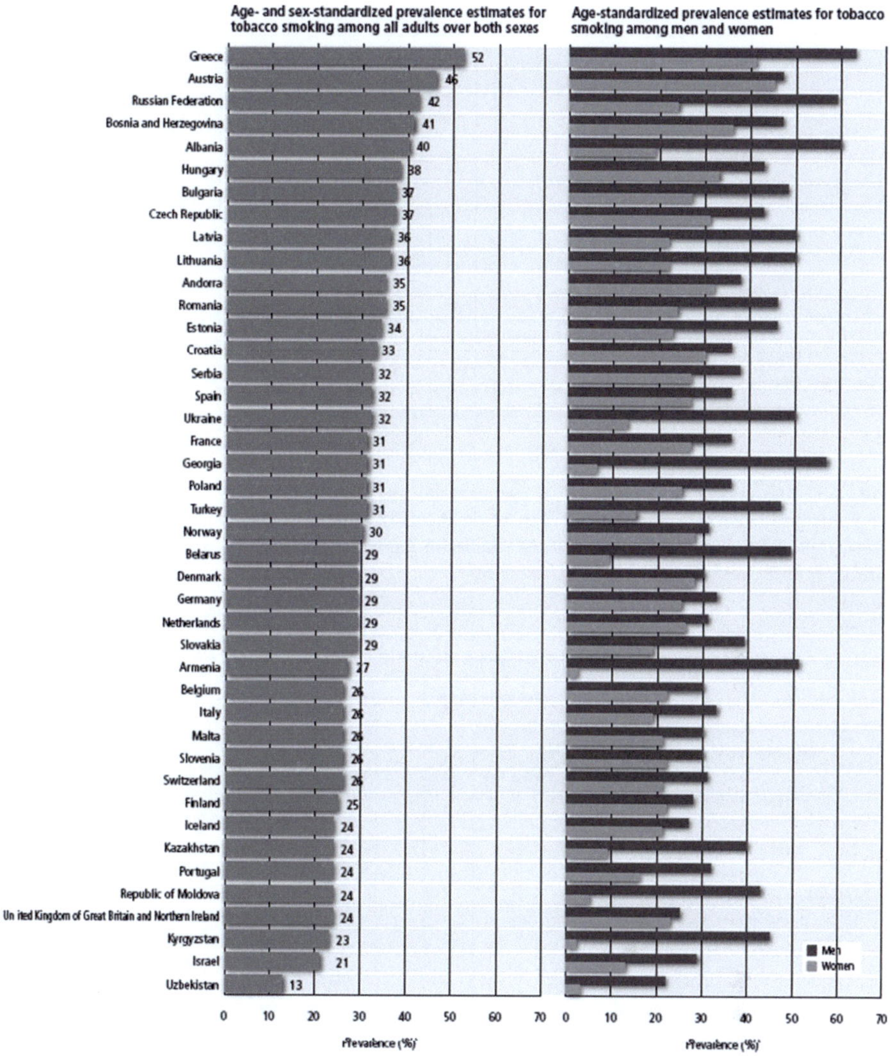

Fig. 2.4 Age and sex standardized prevalence estimates for tobacco smoking in Europe, 2009. From "WHO Report on the Global Tobacco Epidemic (2011)": Appendix vii—graph 7.2.4. Data not reported/not available for Azerbaijan, Cyprus, Ireland, Luxembourg, Monaco, Montenegro, San Marino, Sweden, Tajikistan, The former Yugoslav Republic of Macedonia, and Turkmenistan

2.2.2 *Tobacco Consumption by Adolescents in the Six Major Regions of the World*

Smoking behavior is usually established during adolescence, and this is witnessed by most adult smokers who report that they had their first cigarette or became addicted to nicotine in youth. Adolescent smokers vastly underestimate the

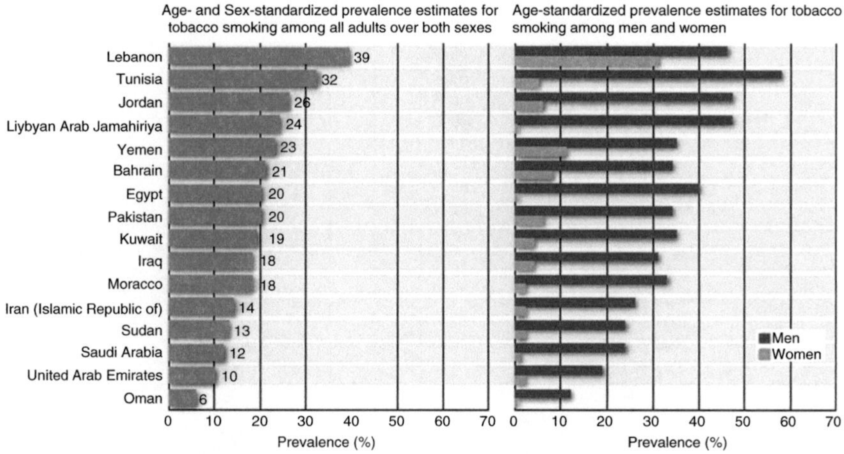

Fig. 2.5 Age and sex standardized prevalence estimates for tobacco smoking in The Eastern Mediterranean, 2009. From "WHO Report on the Global Tobacco Epidemic 2011": Appendix vii—graph 7.2.5. Data not reported/not available for Afghanistan, Djibouti, Qatar, Somalia, Syrian Arab Republic, and West Bank and Gaza Strip

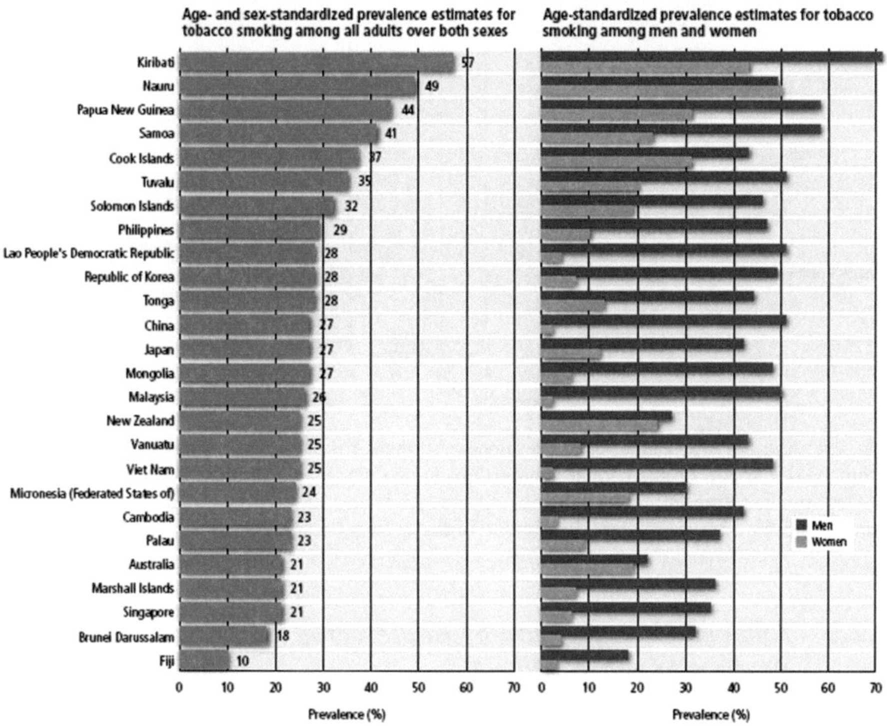

Fig. 2.6 Age and sex standardized prevalence estimates for tobacco smoking in The Western Pacific, 2009. From "WHO Report on the Global Tobacco Epidemic 2011": Appendix vii—graph 7.2.6. Data not reported/not available for Niue

Table 2.2 Estimated regional averages for prevalence of smoking and smokeless tobacco use in youth (%)[a]

WHO region	Boys		Girls	
	Smoking	Smokeless	Smoking	Smokeless
African	20	17	9	11
Americas	18	7	12	5
South-East Asia	7	15	2	7
European	13	8	10	4
Eastern Mediterranean	15	15	7	12
Western Pacific	19	42	9	32

[a]Data refer to current users of tobacco. No comparable data for daily use were available
From "2010 global progress report on the implementation of the WHO Framework Convention on Tobacco Control" (World Health Organization 2010b)

addictive potential of nicotine, hence both occasional and daily smokers think they can quit at any time (Al-Delaimy et al. 2006). Early initiation of cigarette smoking is potentially preventable and can be an important predictor of later substance abuse, such as alcohol (Riala et al. 2004) and illicit drug use (Vega et al. 2006). The uses of tobacco, alcohol, and illicit drugs share common determinants and show a similar potential to induce dependence (McLelland et al. 2000). For this reason, primary prevention in the school setting is believed to be one of the most appropriate strategies to tackle substance use (UNICRI 2003).

The HBSC survey conducted in 2005/2006 presents the key findings on patterns of health among young people aged 11, 13, and 15 years in 41 countries and regions across the WHO European region and North America. The report highlights a general tendency for early onset of cigarette smoking to be more prevalent among boys; this is a significant gender difference in about a third of the countries considered in the study. The survey showed considerable variations between countries in the prevalence of first smoking at age 13 or younger among 15-year-olds: from 9 % (Israel) to 54 % (Estonia). According to gender, the percentages varied from 7 % (Israel) to 49 % (Austria) for girls and from 12 % (Israel) to 65 % (Estonia) for boys. In general, initiation of smoking at age 13 or younger was more likely to be reported by boys mainly in North America and the UK. Family affluence was not strongly associated with early smoking initiation.

Weekly smoking rates were low in all countries at age 11 and increased greatly between ages 13 and 15. Family affluence appeared to be a relatively unimportant factor in weekly smoking for boys. While low affluence was a risk factor in almost half of countries for girls; this pattern was stronger for girls in northern Europe (HBSC 2008).

According to the WHO 2010 global report, the proportion of boys who smoke double than girls among adolescents aged 13–15 (12 % vs. 6 %, respectively). The highest difference between gender is observed in the South-East Asia region (with boys smoking 3.5 times more than girls), followed by the African, Eastern Mediterranean, and Western Pacific regions, where the proportion of girl smokers is approximately half than for boys (see Table 2.2).

Prevalence rates in girls were found less than those for boys also in the region of the Americas and the European region, though with minor variations (WHO Global Progress Report 2010b).

Young people experiment with or begin regular use of tobacco for a variety of reasons, including social and parental norms, advertising, movies and popular media, peer influence, weight control, and curiosity (Baker et al. 2004; Maggi et al. 2007) (see Chap. 4).

The focus of a public health intervention is to prevent or at least delay the onset of such smoking behavior and clinicians should consider delivering tobacco prevention and cessation messages to pediatric patients and their parents. A 2007 national survey of youth tobacco cessation programs in the USA showed a lack of such interventions even in communities most in need: those in which youth smoking prevalence is increasing (Curry et al. 2007).

A similar survey was conducted in seven European countries (Austria, Belgium, Germany, Greece, Italy, Spain, and Sweden) during 2004–2005. The European Drug addiction prevention study (EU-Dap) (Faggiano et al. 2007) is the first European multicenter-randomized trial to evaluate the effectiveness of a school program targeting tobacco, alcohol, and drug use. The survey showed high prevalence of substance abuse, which is actually the predominant health problem in developed countries.

The Global Youth Tobacco Survey (GYTS) is a school-based survey that has been completed in 140 states of the six WHO regions (African, region of the Americas, Eastern Mediterranean, European, South-East Asia, and Western Pacific region) and compares data collected during the period 2000–2007. The findings from the GYTS suggest that interventions targeting tobacco use among youth (e.g., increasing excise taxes, media campaigns, school programs in conjunction with community interventions, and community interventions that decrease minors' access to tobacco) must be broad based, focused on boys and girls, and have components directed toward prevention and cessation. The results also indicate that efforts are needed to reduce the impact of the factors that have the most influence on tobacco use among adolescents, such as secondhand smoke exposure, indirect pro-tobacco advertising, easy access, and availability of tobacco products. In particular, almost 50 % of students who currently smoke cigarettes usually purchased their cigarettes in stores. The rate was highest in the European region (61.7 %) and lowest in the region of the Americas (20.2 %). Students who bought cigarettes in a store (70.5 %) were not refused purchase of cigarettes during the month preceding the survey because of their age. The rate was lowest in the Western Pacific region (47.9 %) and approximately 70 % in the region of the Americas, the European, and Eastern Mediterranean region.

Fortunately, more than half of the students (57.6 %) reported having been taught in school about the dangers of tobacco during the preceding school year; the rate was highest in Western Pacific region (68.8 %) and lowest in Eastern Mediterranean region (47.5 %). If effective programs are not developed and implemented globally, future morbidity and mortality attributed to tobacco probably will increase.

2.2.3 Ethnic Groups

Racial/ethnic differences in age of initiation, duration of smoking, and cigarette consumption have been investigated in literature. Compared to white smokers, African American smokers are usually classified as "light" smokers, smoking 10 or fewer cigarettes per day (Lawrence et al. 2007; Haiman et al. 2006; Trinidad et al. 2009). However, African American smokers are more likely to smoke high-tar and mentholated cigarettes (Allen and Unger 2007; Castro 2004), to inhale more deeply (Patterson et al. 2003), to have a slower rate of nicotine metabolism (Ho et al. 2009a) and show higher levels of cotinine per cigarette smoked (Ho et al. 2009b; Benowitz et al. 2009). Unfortunately, African American smokers are less likely to receive treatment, have poorer treatment outcomes, and suffer a greater share of tobacco-related morbidity and mortality (ACS 2009). The study carried out by Siahpush et al. (2010) highlighted that blacks and American Indians smoked longer (2 and 4 years, respectively) compared to whites, while Hispanics smoked 4 years shorter than whites. The longer smoking duration, access to treatment and treatment outcomes among blacks, with the strong association of smoking duration and lung cancer, can help to explain why blacks are subject to higher lung cancer incidence and mortality rates. It has been demonstrated that lung cancer death rate increases more with each additional year of smoking than with each additional cigarette per day among men, and similar results were observed in women (Flanders et al. 2003).

The risk of heart disease associated with various forms of tobacco use has been documented in individuals from different ethnic groups and regions of the world. The INTERHEART study is a case–control investigation of acute myocardial infarction (AMI) conducted in 52 countries from different continents (Europe, Africa, Asia, Australia, the Middle East Crescent, North and South America) (Teo et al. 2006). The investigation highlighted that the risk of AMI is greater in young than in the old, for both genders. The degree of risk is related to the number of cigarettes smoked; even low levels of smoking (e.g., 5 cigarettes/day) are associated with an appreciable risk of AMI. Thus, current smokers had a greater risk of AMI (OR = 2.95) compared with lifetime nonsmokers.

The risk of AMI is higher among persons who smoked bidis than among nonsmokers in countries where use of this form of tobacco is common. Bidis are small, thin, hand-rolled cigarettes, often consisting of flavored tobacco wrapped in *tendu* or *temburni* leaves. Bidis have a higher concentration of nicotine, tar, and carbon monoxide than conventional cigarettes. They are usually produced in India and other South-East Asian countries (US Public Health Service 2008). The INTERHEART study identified smoking, diabetes, and psychosocial factors as significant risk factors for coronary heart diseases (CHD) particularly among Asian populations (Ajay and Prabhakaran 2010; Teo et al. 2009).

Ethnic differences in the use of tobacco are also present among adolescents worldwide. The Center for Disease and Control (CDC) analyzes data from the national Youth Risk Behavior Survey (YRBS), every 2 years, to evaluate trends in cigarette use among high school students in the USA. Data from 1991 to 2009 show that for cigarette use, rates among high school students began to decline in the late 1990s but the rate of decline slowed during 2003–2009. The findings in this report also evidenced that since 2003 the rate of decline in current cigarette use slowed or leveled off for all racial/ ethnic and sex subgroups except black female students (Institute of Medicine 2007; Nelson et al. 2008). It seems obvious that cigarette smoking rates reflect complex and interrelated individual, social, and environmental factors; but more detailed research is needed to explain such racial/ethnic differences in cigarette use (CDC 2010a).

According to the United Kingdom Census of 2001, 91 % of the English population was from a white ethnic background, the remainder from other ethnic minorities (e.g., 2 % Indian, 1.4 % Pakistani). London is much more diverse, with 29 % of the population belonging to a minority ethnic group (ONS 2003). Health inequalities between the social classes have widened over the last 10 years in the UK. The gap has increased by 4 % and by 11 % among men and women, respectively. Health inequalities are not only apparent between people of different socioeconomic groups; they also exist between different genders and ethnic groups. Smoking remains one of the biggest causes of health inequalities and tobacco smuggling, by offering smokers half-price cigarettes, nullifies the positive impact of political measures such as pricing, taxation policies, and ban of smoking in public places. Beyond doubt, tobacco smuggling has a negative impact on the poor, especially young smokers (House of Commons 2009).

In the UK, white adolescents report high prevalence of initiation and regular use of tobacco, although onset age is not extremely early. Compared to other races, a greater proportion of white teens make the transition from initiation to regular use for both tobacco and alcohol consumption.

In contrast, Asian teens have the lowest prevalence rates for initiation and regular use and the lowest transition rate from first to regular consumption. They also present the highest mean age of initiation of tobacco or alcohol use.

For black adolescents, prevalence of initiation and regular use are lower than for white just as the transition rate between the two forms of use. What looks anomalous in black teens is that the age of first use is younger than for other races/ ethnic groups (Best et al. 2001).

The ethnic differences reported suggest that substance use transitions may be mediated by racial and cultural factors that should be considered in preventive and educational interventions.

Regarding measures of smoking cessation, blacks and Hispanics are less likely to make successful quit attempts than whites according to several studies (Fagan et al. 2007; King et al. 2004).

The goals of Healthy People 2020 are to reduce smoking prevalence among adults to 12 % or less and to increase smoking cessation attempts by adult smokers from 41 to 80 %. Healthy People 2020 is a set of goals and objectives with 10-year targets designed to guide national health promotion and disease prevention efforts to improve the health of all people in the USA. There are also measures designed to eliminate health disparities among racial/ethnic groups by establishing separate targets for different ethnic/ racial communities (US Department of Health and Human Services: Healthy People 2020).

Smoking behaviors (e.g., amount of smoking, years of smoking since initiation, level of nicotine dependence) and type of cigarette smoked (menthol, non-menthol) are also related to the probability of successful cessation, those with high levels of dependence are less likely to quit (Foulds et al. 2006).

Levels of dependence may vary by race/ethnicity; African Americans are more likely to smoke within 30 min of waking than whites (Okuyemi et al. 2003) and whites are more likely to be heavier smokers than Hispanics and blacks (Lawrence et al. 2007; Haiman et al. 2006; Trinidad et al. 2009).

The relationship between using menthol cigarettes and cessation also may vary by race/ethnicity with lower levels of quitting among blacks and Hispanics than among whites (Delnevo et al. 2011); Blacks and women are mostly menthol smokers compared to whites and men (Gardiner 2004).

Racial and ethnic disparities in receiving advice to quit from health care professionals exist; in fact Black and Hispanic smokers are less likely to have been screened for tobacco use and advised to quit by healthcare professionals than white smokers (Cokkinides et al. 2008). Another important barrier to receiving counseling and effective medications is that not all smokers visit a health-care provider each year; young smokers and blacks and Hispanics are less likely to see a physician. A population-based strategy for providing counseling and medications is a toll-free quitline, free tobacco cessation quitlines have been established in all US states since 2006 (Kahende et al. 2011).

Quitlines are cost effective and they increase quit rates among callers by approximately 60 % (Fiore et al. 2008; Tomson et al. 2004). They have the potential to reach large numbers of smokers across all racial/ethnic populations and in recent years more smokers are accessing this service for smoking cessation assistance (Gollust et al. 2008; Borland and Segan 2006).

Prenatal smoking remains one of the most common preventable causes of poor pregnancy and infant outcomes (A Report of the Surgeon General 2004). In the USA, approximately half of female smokers quit when they decide to become pregnant or immediately after they become pregnant, fewer smokers (5–12 %) quit by the last 3 months of pregnancy (Tong et al. 2008). Moreover, two-thirds of women who smoke during the first pregnancy also smoke during the second (A Report of the Surgeon General 2010).

Despite evidence that cessation counseling significantly increases rates of cessation among pregnant smokers, pregnant women who smoke most heavily do not appear to respond to this type of intervention. The US Public Health Service has suggested the need to explore the use of pharmacologic approaches for women who are unable to stop smoking (Fiore et al. 2008)

In the study carried out by Tong et al. (2011), younger women had higher prepregnancy smoking prevalence than older women and in all racial/ethnic groups. They found that approximately 50 % of women aged 18–24 years, or older, of non-Hispanic white, American Indian, or Alaska Native race/ethnicity smoked prepregnancy. Smoking prevalence was lower among Hispanics, non-Hispanic blacks, and Asian/Pacific Islanders.

Smoking cessation services should be integrated into healthcare settings that young women at risk for pregnancy are likely to attend, such as family planning clinics.

Cessation should be encouraged before pregnancy, when the most treatment options, including pharmacotherapy, are available. Services and materials appear to be more effective when they are made age, culturally, racially, and educationally appropriate for the patient. Telephone-based quitlines have also been found to be effective in reaching diverse populations, including pregnant women (Fiore et al. 2008).

More information on this topic can be found on Chap. 3: Smoking-related disease epidemiology.

2.3 Passive Smoking

2.3.1 Secondhand Smoking

Exposure to tobacco smoke in the environment, defined as "passive smoking" or "secondhand smoking" (SHS), is an important cause of mortality and morbidity. SHS is formed from the sidestream smoke emitted into the environment from the smoldering of cigarettes and other tobacco products between puffs and from the mainstream smoke exhaled by the smoker (Oberg et al. 2010). The adverse health effects of SHS were first confirmed in 1980s (A Report of the Surgeon General 2006) and further research in this field has provided the scientific foundation for public health actions aimed at tobacco use prevention, cessation, and protection from SHS exposure.

The relationship between SHS and a variety of health outcomes in children and adults has been examined in the epidemiological and experimental literature. Passive smokers have a significantly increased risk for several diseases such as lung cancer (IARC 2004), respiratory diseases (Murphy 2009), and cardiovascular diseases (A Report of the Surgeon General 2006). The strongest evidence exists in adults for lung cancer, ischemic heart disease, and asthma (new cases). Moreover, 20 mammary carcinogens have been identified in SHS, which have caused detectable genetic damage in women's breasts (California Environmental Protection Agency 2005).

In children SHS causes low birth weight, childhood chronic respiratory symptoms, lower respiratory illness, asthma (new cases and exacerbation), middle-ear infection, reduced pulmonary function, and sudden infant death syndrome (SIDS) (Oberg et al. 2010; Ortega et al. 2010).

There is a clear relationship between the level of SHS exposure and the risk of respiratory complications during anesthesia for children (Drongowski et al. 2003; O'Rourke et al. 2006). In adults, smoking by surgical patients increases their risk for respiratory, cardiac, and wound-related complications, such as wound infections (Warner 2006). Shi and Warner (2011) observed that parents who smoke cigarettes, and are aware of SHS negative health effects, were more likely to make a quit attempt within the past 12 months if their children had surgery within this time, but they were not more likely to succeed in maintaining smoking cessation.

The Surgeon General's report (2006) shows consistently higher risk estimates for lung cancer and SHS in Asian studies, primarily from China, compared to North

American and European studies. Explanations offered for these higher rates include the fact that, in China, more people share smaller residences, so individuals are potentially more exposed. The report also provides higher risk estimates for ischemic heart disease in two developing countries, Argentina and China.

SHS is estimated to have caused about 603,000 premature deaths in 2004. These include 166,000 deaths from lower respiratory infections and 1,100 from asthma in children, 35,800 deaths from asthma, 21,000 deaths from lung cancer, and 379,000 deaths from ischemic heart disease in adults. The global proportion of people exposed to SHS was 41 % of all children (defined as age 0–14 years), 33 % of non-smoking men, and 35 % of nonsmoking women worldwide. Those proportions varied by region according to smoking habits, rural or urban populations, country regulations, and other factors. The highest level of exposure among children, almost 68 %, is found in the Western Pacific region; the lowest level is estimated in Africa, with about 13 % of children living in families with at least one smoking parent. The researchers observed that children under age 5 years were more exposed to respiratory infections in poorer countries, where malnutrition or inadequate health care also may lead to higher disease and mortality rates in children with other health problems that are exacerbated by SHS exposure.

For adults and both gender, the highest exposure was estimated in European region (Belarus, Estonia, Hungary, Kazakhstan, Latvia, Lithuania, Republic of Moldova, the Russian Federation, and Ukraine) with 66 % the population exposed. The lowest regional exposure was estimated in the African region (4–11 %).

The burden of morbidity from SHS exposure, measured by disability-adjusted life years (DALYs), also varied by region and had higher estimates for low-income countries in South-East Asia and the eastern Mediterranean region compared with Europe. Asthma and ischemic heart disease were the most common outcome among adults, while lower respiratory infections were more frequent among children. It was calculated that children overall experienced an estimated 61 % of the disease burden from SHS, in terms of DALYs.

Interestingly, SHS exposure seems to be largely a women's issue: of the 603,000 SHS-related deaths of nonsmokers estimated in 2004, 47 % were among women, compared with 26 % among men, and 28 % among children (Oberg et al. 2010).

Regarding the youth exposure and according to the GYTS, the percentage of never smokers exposed to SHS at home was 46.8 % and ranged from 71.5 % in Europe to 22.6 % in Africa. Furthermore, never smokers exposed to SHS at home, among WHO regions, were 1.4–2.1 times more likely to be susceptible to initiating smoking than those not exposed. The percentage of students exposed to SHS in places other than home was 47.8 % overall and ranged from 79.4 % in Europe to 38.2 % in Africa. By region, never smokers exposed to SHS in places other than home were 1.3–1.8 times more likely to be susceptible to initiating smoking than those not exposed. Data for the analysis were collected in the period 2000–2007 from the six WHO regions (Africa, Americas, Eastern Mediterranean, Europe, South-East Asia, and Western Pacific) and the GYTS is limited to students aged 13–15 years (CDC 2007).

Exposure to SHS imposes economic costs on individuals and the entire society. Economic costs include direct and indirect medical costs and productivity losses. In addition, workplaces where smoking is permitted incur higher renovation and cleaning costs, an increased risk of fire and may experience higher insurance premiums (Ross 2005).

Several studies have examined the costs of smoking at individual country level. The costs of SHS exposure have been evaluated in Australia, Canada, Hong Kong Special Administrative Region (Hong Kong SAR), Ireland, the UK and the USA (Adams 1999). A study estimates that SHS exposure results in over US$ five billion in direct medical costs and in over US$ five billion in indirect medical costs (such as disability, lost wages, and related benefits) annually in the USA (Behan et al. 2005). In Hong Kong SAR, the annual value of direct medical costs, long-term care, and productivity loss due to SHS exposure is estimated to be US$ 156 million (McGhee et al. 2006). Estimates for individual EU Member States ranges from 26€ million in Estonia (Taal et al. 2004) to 17€ billion in Germany (Neubauer 2006). The estimated healthcare costs associated with smoking were highest in high income countries or with large populations such as Germany, Poland, France, and the UK compared to Estonia, Iceland, Finland, Hungary, and Spain (Jarvis et al. 2009).

Scientific evidence has determined that a safe level of exposure to SHS does not exist. Therefore, implementing 100 % smoke-free environments is the only effective way to protect the population from exposure to SHS. Several countries have successfully implemented laws requiring indoor workplaces and public places to be 100 % smoke free. In 2004, Ireland became the first nation to create smoke-free indoor workplaces and public areas with a comprehensive ban that included restaurants, bars, and pubs. Since then, bans have been enacted in other countries: Italy, New Zealand, Niger, Norway, Uganda, United Kingdom (in Northern Ireland, Scotland, and Wales), USA, Canada, etc (World Health Organization 2007).

The prevalence of serum cotinine levels in the nonsmoking population declined significantly from 52.5 % during 1999–2000 to 40 % during 2007–2008 in the USA (CDC 2010b). The declination of SHS is attributable to a number of factors, including increases in the number of local and state laws prohibiting smoking in indoor workplaces and public places, increases in voluntary smoking restrictions in workplaces and homes, and changes in public attitudes regarding social acceptability of smoking near nonsmokers and children; but 88 million nonsmokers aged ≥3 years were still exposed to SHS. The decline was significant for each sex, age, race/ethnicity, and income group except non-Hispanic whites.

The home is the major source of secondhand smoke exposure for children and the persistence of smoking in homes likely are impeding progress toward full protection of children and other nonsmokers. The only way to protect nonsmokers fully is to eliminate smoking in indoor spaces (A report of the Surgeon General 2006).

2.3.2 Thirdhand Smoking

Thirdhand smoking (THS) consists of residual tobacco smoke pollutants that remain on surfaces and in dust after tobacco has been smoked, are re-emitted into the gas phase, or react with oxidants and other compounds in the environment to yield secondary pollutants. The constituents of THS identified include nicotine, 3-ethenylpyridine (3-EP), phenol, cresols, naphthalene, formaldehyde, and tobacco-specific nitrosamines (including some not found in freshly emitted tobacco smoke) (Destaillats et al. 2006; Sleiman et al. 2010).

THS exposure results from the involuntary inhalation, ingestion, or dermal uptake of THS pollutants in the air, in dust, and on surfaces. Although it is important to distinguish SHS from THS because of significant chemical, toxicological, and behavioral differences, SHS and THS are closely related and coexist during the early period of THS formation and in environments in which smoking takes place. The evidence of THS in indoor environments (e.g., cigarette butts, unpleasant odor, smelly clothes), and its aversive impact on nonsmokers is well known and its persistence in residential settings has been demonstrated based on nicotine and 3-EP concentrations in air, dust, and surfaces in the days, weeks, and months after the last smoking has taken place (Destaillats et al., 2006, 2007; Matt et al. 2004, 2008, 2011). Further support comes from quantitative measurements of ultrafine tobacco smoke particles resuspended after their deposition on indoor surfaces, such as tables, bed frames, cabinets, doors, and walls; also in carpets, curtains, pillows, mattresses, and similar materials (Becquemin et al. 2010).

THS exposure is particularly relevant for children and infants living in homes in which adults smoke, even if smoking occurs at times or in rooms when no children are present. It has been estimated that infants and young children are 100 times more sensitive than adults to pollutants in house dust because of their increased respiration relative to body size and immature metabolic capacity (Roberts et al. 2009).

It's important to underline that THS is trapped on the clothes of smokers and nonsmokers who were exposed to SHS. Moreover, THS is detectable on the hands of smokers beyond the environment in which they smoked and smokers may spread THS pollutants to other persons and other objects (e.g., toys, food).

Exposure to constituents of THS may include risks of SHS and active smoking as well as new ones not yet directly associated with tobacco smoke (Matt et al. 2004, 2011). Emphasizing that thirdhand smoke harms the health of children may be an important element in encouraging home smoking bans.

References

A report of the Surgeon General. (2004). *The health consequences of smoking*. Atlanta, GA: US Department of Health and Human Services, Centers for Disease Control and Prevention, National Center for Chronic Disease Prevention and Health Promotion, Office on Smoking and Health.

A Report of the Surgeon General. (2010). *How tobacco smoke causes disease: The biology and behavioral basis for smoking-attributable disease*. U.S. Department of Health and Human Services. Retrieved from http://www.surgeongeneral.gov/library/tobaccosmoke/report/index.html

ACS. (2009). *Cancer facts and figures 2009*. Atlanta: ACS.

Adams, K. (1999). Magnitude of smoking attributable costs, Rollins School of Public Health, Emory University, Atlanta, GA. *Background Paper to the International Consultation on*

Environmental Tobacco Smoke (ETS) and Child Health Geneva, Switzerland (WHO Technical Document WHO/NCD/TFI/99.11).
Ajay, V. S., & Prabhakaran, D. (2010). Coronary heart disease in Indians: Implications of the INTERHEART study. *Indian Journal of Medical Research, 132*(5), 561–566.
Al-Delaimy, W. K., White, M. M., & Pierce, J. P. (2006). Adolescents' perceptions about quitting and nicotine replacement therapy: Findings from the California Tobacco Survey. *The Journal of Adolescent Health, 38*, 465–468.
Allen, B., Jr., & Unger, J. B. (2007). Sociocultural correlates of menthol cigarette smoking among adult African Americans in Los Angeles. *Nicotine and Tobacco Research, 9*, 447–451.
Amos, A., & Haglund, M. (2000). From social taboo to "torch of freedom": The marketing of cigarettes to women. *Tobacco Control, 9*, 3–8.
Baker, T. B., Brandon, T. H., & Chassin, L. (2004). Motivational influences on cigarette smoking. *Annual Review of Psychology, 55*, 463–491.
Bauer, T., Gohlmann, S., & Sinning, M. (2007). Gender differences in smoking behavior. *Health Economics, 16*, 895–909.
Becquemin, M. H., Bertholon, J. F., Bentayeb, M., Attoui, M., Ledur, D., Roy, F., et al. (2010). Third-hand smoking: Indoor measurements of concentration and sizes of cigarette smoke particles after resuspension. *Tobacco Control, 19*, 347–348.
Behan, D., Eriksen, M., & Lin, Y. (2005). *Economic effects of environmental tobacco smoke*. Society of Actuaries. Retrieved from http://www.soa.org/ccm/content/areas-of-practice/lifeinsurance/research/economiceffects-of-environmental-tobacco-smoke-SOA
Benowitz, N. L., Bernert, J. T., Caraballo, R. S., Holiday, D. B., & Wang, J. (2009). Optimal serum cotinine levels for distinguishing cigarette smokers and nonsmokers within different racial/ethnic groups in the United States between 1999 and 2004. *American Journal of Epidemiology, 169*, 236–248.
Best, D., Rawaf, S., Rowley, J., Floyd, K., Manning, V., & Strang, J. (2001). Ethnic and gender differences in drinking and smoking among London adolescents. *Ethnicity and Health, 6*(1), 51–57.
Borland, R., & Segan, C. J. (2006). The potential of quitlines to increase smoking cessation. *Drug and Alcohol Review, 25*, 73–78.
Broms, U., Madden, P. A. F., Heath, A. C., Pergadia, M. L., Shiffman, S., & Kaprio, J. (2007). The nicotine dependence syndrome scale in Finnish smokers. *Drug and Alcohol Dependence, 89*(1), 42–51.
Broms, U., Silventoinen, K., Madden, P. A. F., Heath, A. C., & Kaprio, J. (2006). Genetic architecture of smoking behavior: A study of Finnish adult twins. *Twin Research and Human Genetics, 9*(1), 64–72.
California Environmental Protection Agency. (2005). *Proposed identification of environmental tobacco smoke as a toxic air contaminant, SRP Approved Version. Part B: Health effects*. Retrieved from http://www.arb.ca.gov/toxics/ets/finalreport/finalreport.htm
Castro, F. G. (2004). Physiological, psychological, social, and cultural influences on the use of menthol cigarettes among blacks and Hispanics. *Nicotine and Tobacco Research, 6*(Suppl 1), S29–S41.
Centers for Disease Control and Prevention. (2007). Exposure to secondhand smoke among students aged 13–15 years-worldwide, 2000–2007. *Morbidity and Mortality Weekly Report, 56*(20), 497–500.
Centers for Disease Control and Prevention. (2010a). Cigarette use among high school students-United States, 1991–2009. *Morbidity and Mortality Weekly Report, 59*(26), 797–801.
Centers for Disease Control and Prevention. (2010b). Vital signs: Nonsmokers' exposure to secondhand smoke-United States, 1999–2008. *Morbidity and Mortality Weekly Report, 59*(35), 1141–1146.
Cokkinides, V. E., Halpern, M. T., Barbeau, E. M., Ward, E., & Thun, M. J. (2008). Racial and ethnic disparities in smoking-cessation interventions analysis of the 2005 Nations Health Interview Survey. *American Journal of Preventive Medicine, 34*, 404–412.

Curry, S. J., Emery, S., Sporer, A. K., Mermelstein, R., Flay, B. R., Berbaum, M., et al. (2007). A national survey of tobacco cessation programs for youths. *American Journal of Public Health, 97*, 171–177.

Delnevo, C. D., Gundersen, D. A., Hrywna, M., Echeverria, S. E., & Steinberg, M. B. (2011). Smoking-cessation prevalence among U.S. Smokers of menthol versus non-menthol cigarettes. *American Journal of Preventive Medicine, 41*(4), 357–365.

Destaillats, H., Singer, B. C., & Gundel, L. A. (2007). Evidence of acid–base interactions between amines and model indoor surfaces by ATR-FTIR spectroscopy. *Atmospheric Environment, 41*, 3177–3181.

Destaillats, H., Singer, B. C., Lee, S. K., & Gundel, L. A. (2006). Effect of ozone on nicotine desorption from model surfaces: Evidence for heterogeneous chemistry. *Environmental Science and Technology, 40*, 1799–1805.

Drongowski, R. A., Lee, D., Reynolds, P. I., Malviya, S., Harmon, C. M., Geiger, J., et al. (2003). Increased respiratory symptoms following surgery in children exposed to environmental tobacco smoke. *Paediatric Anaesthesia, 13*, 304–310.

Eek, F., Ostergren, P. O., Diderichsen, F., Rasmussen, N. K., Andersen, I., Moussa, K., et al. (2010). Differences in socioeconomic and gender inequalities in tobacco smoking in Sweden and Denmark; a cross sectional comparison of the equity effect of different public health policies. *BMC Public Health, 10*, 9.

Ekberg-Aronsson, M., Nilsson, P. M., Nilsson, J. A., Lofdahl, C. G., & Lofdahl, K. (2007). Mortality risks among heavy-smokers with special reference to women: A long-term follow-up of an urban population. *European Journal of Epidemiology, 22*, 301–309.

Fagan, P., Augustson, E., Backinger, C., O'Connell, M., Vollinger, R., Kaufman, A., et al. (2007). Quit attempts and intention to quit cigarette smoking among young adults in the United States. *American Journal of Public Health, 97*, 1412–1420.

Faggiano, F., Richardson, C., Bohrn, K., Galanti, M. R., & EU-Dap Study Group. (2007). A cluster randomized controlled trial of school-based prevention of tobacco, alcohol and drug use: The EU-Dap design and study population. *Preventive Medicine, 44*(2), 170–173.

Fiore, M. C., Jaén, C. R., Baker, T. B., Bailey, W. C., Benowitz, N. L., Curry, S. J., et al. (2008). *Treating tobacco use and dependence: 2008 update*. Rockville, MD: U.S. Department of Health and Human Services.

Flanders, W. D., Lally, C. A., Zhu, B. P., Henley, S. J., & Thun, M. J. (2003). Lung cancer mortality in relation to age, duration of smoking, and daily cigarette consumption: Results from cancer prevention study II. *Cancer Research, 63*(19), 6556–6562.

Foulds, J., Gandhi, K. K., Steinberg, M. B., Richardson, D. L., Williams, J. M., Burke, M. V., et al. (2006). Factors associated with quitting smoking at a tobacco dependence treatment clinic. *American Journal of Health Behavior, 30*, 400–441.

Gardiner, P. S. (2004). The African Americanization of menthol cigarette use in the United States. *Nicotine and Tobacco Research, 6*, S55–S65.

Gollust, S. E., Schroeder, S. A., & Warner, K. E. (2008). Helping smokers quit: Understanding the barriers to utilization of smoking cessation services. *The Milbank Quarterly, 84*, 601–627.

Gruer, L., Hart, C. L., Gordon, D. S., & Watt, G. C. (2009). Effect of tobacco smoking on survival of men and women by social position: A 28 year cohort study. *BMJ, 338*, b480.

Haiman, C. A., Stram, D. O., Wilkens, L. R., Pike, M. C., Kolonel, L. N., Henderson, B. E., et al. (2006). Ethnic and racial differences in the smoking-related risk of lung cancer. *The New England Journal of Medicine, 354*, 333–342.

Hamilton, A. S., Lessov-Schlaggar, C. N., Cockburn, M. G., Unger, J. B., Cozen, W., & Mack, T. M. (2006). Gender differences in determinants of smoking initiation and persistence in California twins. *Cancer Epidemiology, Biomarkers and Prevention, 15*(6), 1189–1197.

Hamilton, W. L., Norton, G., Ouellette, T. K., Rhodes, W. M., Kling, R., & Connolly, G. N. (2004). Smokers' Responses to advertisements for regular and light cigarettes and potential reduced-exposure tobacco products. *Nicotine and Tobacco Research, 6*(3), S353–S362.

HBSC international report from the 2005/2006 survey. (2008). *Inequalities in young people's health* (Health Policy for Children and Adolescents, No. 5). Copenhagen, Denmark: WHO Regional Office for Europe. Retrieved from http://www.euro.who.int/__data/assets/pdf_file/0005/53852/E91416.pdf

Healthy People (2010). *U.S. Department of health and human services*. Washington, DC. Retrieved from http://healthypeople.gov/2020/topicsobjectives2020/pdfs/HP2020objectives.pdf

Ho, M. K., Faseru, B., Choi, W. S., Nollen, N. L., Mayo, M. S., Thomas, J. L., et al. (2009a). Utility and relationships of biomarkers of smoking in African-American light smokers. *Cancer Epidemiology, Biomarkers and Prevention, 18*, 3426–3434.

Ho, M. K., Mwenifumbo, J. C., Al Koudsi, N., Okuyemi, K. S., Ahluwalia, J. S., Benowitz, N. L., et al. (2009b). Association of nicotine metabolite ratio and CYP2A6 genotype with smoking cessation treatment in African-American light smokers. *Clinical Pharmacology and Therapeutics, 85*, 635–643.

House of Commons Select Committee on Health. (2009). *Health inequalities* (Vol. 1). London: The Stationery Office (HC 286–1). Retrieved from http://www.publications.parliament.uk/pa/cm200809/cmselect/cmhealth/286/286.pdf

IARC. (2004). Tobacco smoking and involuntary smoking. IARC monofigures on the evaluation of IARC. *Carcinogenic risks to humans* (vol. 83). Lyon: IARC.

Institute of Medicine. (2007). *Ending the tobacco problem: A blueprint for the nation*. Washington, DC: National Academies Press.

Jarvis A, Vincze MP, Falconer B, Garde A, Geber F (2009) A study on liability and the health costs of smoking: Final Report. DG SANCO of the European Commission [contract ref. SANCO/2008/C6/046].

Kahende, J. W., Malarcher, A. M., Teplinskaya, A., & Asman, K. J. (2011). Quit attempt correlates among smokers by race/ethnicity. *International Journal of Environmental Research and Public Health, 8*, 3871–3888.

Kendler, K. S., Neale, M. C., Sullivan, P., Corey, L. A., Gardner, C. O., & Prescott, C. A. (1999). A population-based twin study in women of smoking initiation and nicotine dependence. *Psychological Medicine, 29*(2), 299–308.

King, G., Polednak, A., Bendel, R. B., Vilsaint, M. C., & Nahata, S. B. (2004). Disparities in smoking cessation between African Americans and whites. *American Journal of Public Health, 94*, 1965–1971.

Lawrence, D., Fagan, P., Backinger, C. L., Gibson, J. T., & Hartman, A. (2007). Cigarette smoking patterns among young adults aged 18–24 years in the United States. *Nicotine and Tobacco Research, 9*, 687–697.

Lessov, C. N., Martin, N. G., Statham, D. J., Todorov, A. A., Slutske, W. S., Bucholz, K. K., et al. (2004). Defining nicotine dependence for genetic research: Evidence from Australian twins. *Psychological Medicine, 34*(5), 865–879.

Li, M. D., Ma, J. Z., Cheng, R., Dupont, R. T., Williams, N. J., Crews, K. M., et al. (2003). A genome-wide scan to identify loci for smoking rate in the Framingham Heart Study population. *BMC Genetics, 4*(Suppl 1), S103.

Lopez, A. D., Collishaw, N. E., & Piha, T. (1994). A descriptive model of the cigarette epidemic in developed countries. *Tobacco Control, 3*, 242–247.

Maggi, S., Hertzman, C., & Vaillancourt, T. (2007). Changes in smoking behaviors from late childhood to adolescence: Insights from the Canadian National Longitudinal Survey of Children and Youth. *Health Psychology, 26*, 232–240.

Main, C., Thomas, S., Ogilvie, D., Stirk, L., Petticrew, M., Whitehead, M., et al. (2008). Population tobacco control interventions and their effects on social inequalities in smoking: Placing an equity lens on existing systematic reviews. *BMC Public Health, 8*, 178.

Matt, G. E., Quintana, P. J., Hovell, M. F., Bernert, J. T., Song, S., Novianti, N., et al. (2004). Households contaminated by environmental tobacco smoke: Sources of infant exposures. *Tobacco Control, 13*, 29–37.

Matt, G. E., Quintana, P. J., Hovell, M. F., Chatfield, D., Ma, D. S., Romero, R., et al. (2008). Residual tobacco smoke pollution in used cars for sale: Air, dust, and surfaces. *Nicotine and Tobacco Research, 10*(9), 1467–1475.

Matt, G. E., Quintana, P. J. E., Zakarian, J. M., Fortmann, A. L., Chatfield, D. A., Hoh, E., et al. (2011). When smokers move out and nonsmokers move in: Residential thirdhand smoke pollution and exposure. *Tobacco Control, 20*, e1 [Online 2010].

McGhee, S. M., Ho, L. M., Lapsley, H. M., Chau, J., Cheung, W. L., Ho, S. Y., et al. (2006). Cost of tobacco-related diseases, including passive smoking, in Hong Kong. *Tobacco Control, 15*, 125–130.

McLelland, T., Lewis, D. C., O'Brien, C. P., & Kleber, H. D. (2000). Drug dependence, a chronic medical disease: Implications for treatment, insurance and outcome evaluation. *Journal of the American Medical Association, 284*, 1689–1695.

Murphy, T. D. (2009). *Passive smoking and lung disease*. Medscape Reference 1–4.

Nelson, D. E., Mowery, P., Asman, K., Pederson, L. L., O'Malley, P. M., Malarcher, A., et al. (2008). Long-term trends in adolescent and young adult smoking in the United States: Metapatterns and implications. *American Journal of Public Health, 98*, 905–917.

Nerín, I. (2005). Women and smoking: Fatal attraction. *Archivos de Bronconeumología, 41*, 360–362.

Neubauer, S. (2006). Mortality, morbidity and costs attributable to smoking in Germany: Update and a 10- year comparison. *Tobacco Control, 15*, 464–471.

O'Rourke, J. M., Kalish, L. A., McDaniel, S., & Lyons, B. (2006). The effects of exposure to environmental tobacco smoke on pulmonary function in children undergoing anesthesia for minor surgery. *Paediatric Anaesthesia, 16*, 560–567.

Oberg, M., Woodward, A., Jaakkola, M. S., Peruga, A., & Pruss-Ustun, A. (2010). *Global estimate of the burden of disease from second-hand smoke*. Geneva: World Health Organization.

Okuyemi, K. S., Ahluwalia, J. S., Ebersole-Robinson, M., Catley, D., Mayo, M. S., & Resnicow, K. (2003). Does menthol attenuate the effect of bupropion among African American smokers? *Addiction, 98*, 1387–1393.

ONS. (2003). *KS06 ethnic group: Census 2001, key statistics for local authorities*. London: Office for National Statistics. Retrieved from http://www.bexley.gov.uk/index.aspx?articleid=4527

ONS. (2007). *Results from the General Household Survey (GHS)*. London: Office for National Statistics (ONS), HMSO.

Ortega, G., Castellà, C., Martín-Cantera, C., Ballvé, J. L., Díaz, E., Saez, M., et al. (2010). Passive smoking in babies: The BIBE study (brief intervention in babies: Effectiveness). *BMC Public Health, 10*, 772–782.

Patterson, F., Benowitz, N., Shields, P., Kaufmann, V., Jepson, C., Wileyto, P., et al. (2003). Individual differences in nicotine intake per cigarette. *Cancer Epidemiology, Biomarkers and Prevention, 12*, 468–471.

Payne, S. (2001). "Smoke like a man, die like a man?"—A review of the relationship between gender, sex and lung cancer. *Social Science and Medicine, 53*, 1067–1080.

Pergadia, M. L., Heath, A. C., Martin, N. G., & Madden, P. A. F. (2006). Genetic analyses of DSM-IV nicotine withdrawal in adult twins. *Psychological Medicine, 36*(7), 963–972.

Riala, K., Hakko, H., Isohanni, M., Järvelin, M. R., & Räsänen, P. (2004). Teenage smoking and substance use as predictors of severe alcohol problems in late adolescence and in young adulthood. *Journal of Adolescent Health, 35*, 245–254.

Roberts, J. W., Wallace, L. A., Camann, D. E., Dickey, P., Gilbert, S. G., Lewis, R. G., et al. (2009). Monitoring and reducing exposure of infants to pollutants in house dust. *Reviews of Environmental Contamination and Toxicology, 201*, 1–39.

Ross, H. (2005). Economics of smoke-free policies. In The Smoke Free Europe partnership. *Smoke free Europe makes economic sense. A report on the economic aspects of Smoke free policies*. Retrieved from http://www.ehnheart.org/files/SmokefreeEurope-102853A.pdf

Samet, J. M., & Yoon, S. Y. (Eds.). (2001). *Women and the tobacco epidemic: Challenges for the 21st century*. Geneva: World Health Organization.

SCENIHR. (2010). *Addictiveness and attractiveness of tobacco additives*. Brussels: Scientific Committee on Emerging and Newly Identified Health Risks (SCENIHR). Retrieved from http://ec.europa.eu/health/scientific_committees/emerging/docs/scenihr_o_031.pdf

Shafey, O., & Guindon, G. E. (2003). Monitoring the tobacco epidemic: Past, present, and future. In O. Shafey, S. Dolwick, & G. E. Guindon (Eds.), *Tobacco control country profiles*. Atlanta, GA: American Cancer Society.

Shi, Y., & Warner, D. O. (2011). Pediatric surgery and parental smoking behavior. *Anesthesiology, 115*, 12–17.

Shiffman, S., Brockwell, S. E., Pillitteri, J. L., & Gitchell, J. G. (2008). Use of smoking cessation treatments in the United States. *American Journal of Preventive Medicine, 34*(2), 102–111.

Siahpush, M., Singh, G. K., Jones, P. R., & Timsina, L. R. (2010). Racial/ethnic and socioeconomic variations in duration of smoking: Results from 2003, 2006 and 2007 Tobacco Use Supplement of the Current Population Survey. *Journal of Public Health (Oxford, England), 32*(2), 210–218.

Sleiman, M., Gundel, L. A., Pankow, J. F., Jacob, P., III, Singer, B. C., & Destaillats, H. (2010). Formation of carcinogens indoors by surface-mediated reactions of nicotine with nitrous acid, leading to potential thirdhand smoke hazards. *Proceedings of the National Academy of Sciences, 107*, 6576–6581.

Taal, A., Kiivet, R., & Hu, T. (2004). The economics of tobacco in Estonia. Washington, DC: The International Bank for Reconstruction and Development/The World Bank.

Teo, K. K., Liu, L., Chow, C. K., Wang, X., Islam, S., Jiang, L., et al. (2009). Potentially modifiable risk factors associated with myocardial infarction in China: The INTERHEART China study. *Heart, 95*(22), 1857–1864.

Teo, K. K., Ounpuu, S., Hawken, S., Pandey, M. R., Valentin, V., Hunt, D., et al. (2006). Tobacco use and risk of myocardial infarction in 52 countries in the INTERHEART study: A case–control study. *Lancet, 368*(9536), 647–658.

The Economist. (1997). *Guide to economic indicators: Making sense of economics* (3rd ed.). London: Profile Books.

Tomson, T., Helgason, A., & Gilljam, H. (2004). Quitline in smoking cessation: A cost-effectiveness analysis. *International Journal of Technology Assessment in Health Care, 40*, 469–474.

Tong, V. T., Dietz, P. M., England, L. J., Farr, S. L., Kim, S. Y., D'Angelo, D., Bombard, J. M. (2011). Age and racial/ethnic disparities in prepregnancy smoking among women who delivered live births. *Preventing Chronic Disease 8*(6), A121. Retrieved from http://www.cdc.gov/pcd/issues/2011/nov/11_0018.htm

Tong, V. T., England, L. J., Dietz, P. M., & Asare, L. A. (2008). Smoking patterns and use of cessation interventions during pregnancy. *American Journal of Preventive Medicine, 35*(4), 327–333.

Trinidad, D. R., Perez-Stable, E. J., Emery, S. L., White, M. M., Grana, R. A., & Messer, K. S. (2009). Intermittent and light daily smoking across racial/ethnic groups in the united states. *Nicotine and Tobacco Research, 11*, 203–210.

U.S. Department of Health and Human Services. (2006). *The health consequences of involuntary exposure to tobacco smoke. A Report of the Surgeon General.* Atlanta, GA: Centers for Disease Control and Prevention, Public Health Service. Retrieved from http://tinyurl.com/o9d8r

U.S. Public Health Service Clinical Practice Guideline executive summary. (2008). Treating tobacco use and dependence: 2008 Update. *Respiratory Care, 53*(9), 1217–1222.

UNICRI. (2003). *School-based drug education: A guide for practitioners and the wider community.* Vienna: United Nations Office for Drug Control and Crime Prevention.

US Department of Health and Human Services. (2004). *The health consequences of smoking: A report of the surgeon general.* Atlanta, GA: US Department of Health and Human Services, Centers for Disease Control and Prevention, National Center for Chronic Disease Prevention and Health Promotion, Office on Smoking and Health.

Vega, W. A., Chen, K. W., & Williams, J. (2006). Smoking, drugs, and other behavioural health problems among multiethnic adolescents in the NHSDA. *Addictive Behaviors, 32*(9), 1949–1956.

Vink, J. M., Beem, A. L., Posthuma, D., Neale, M. C., Willemsen, G., Kendler, K. S., et al. (2004). Linkage analysis of smoking initiation and quantity in Dutch sibling pairs. *The Pharmacogenomics Journal, 4*(4), 274–282.

Warner, D. O. (2006). Perioperative abstinence from cigarettes: Physiologic and clinical consequences. *Anesthesiology, 104*, 356–367.

Warren, C. W., Jones, N. R., Eriksen, M. P., & Asma, S. (2006). Patterns of global tobacco use in young people and implications for future chronic disease burden in adults. *Lancet, 367*, 749–753.

WHO Report on the Global Tobacco Epidemic. (2008). *The MPOWER package*. Geneva: World Health Organization.

WHO Report on the Global Tobacco Epidemic. (2009). *Implementing smoke-free environments*. Geneva: World Health Organization.

WHO Report on the Global Tobacco Epidemic. (2011). *Warning about the dangers of tobacco*. Geneva: World Health Organization.

World Health Organization. (2007). Smoke-free inside: Create and enjoy 100% smoke-free environments. Geneva, Switzerland: World Health Organization. Retrieved from http://www.who.int/tobacco/resources/publications/wntd/2007/en/index.html

World Health Organization. (2010). Gender, women, and the tobacco epidemic. Retrieved from http://whqlibdoc.who.int/publications/2010/9789241599511_eng.pdf

World Health Organization. (2010). Global progress report on the implementation of the WHO Framework Convention on Tobacco Control (FCTC/2010.1). Retrieved from http://www.who.int/fctc/reporting/summaryreport.pdf

Xian, H., Scherrer, J. F., Madden, P. A. F., Lyons, M. J., Tsuang, M., True, W. R., et al. (2003). The heritability of failed smoking cessation and nicotine withdrawal in twins who smoked and attempted to quit. *Nicotine and Tobacco Research, 5*(2), 245–254.

Chapter 3
Smoking-Related Diseases Epidemiology

Giuseppe La Torre, Leda Semyonov, and Guglielmo Giraldi

Objectives This section intends to describe the epidemiology of cigarette smoking-related diseases. In particular, this section will discuss cardiovascular and respiratory diseases and few other diseases less frequent but still related to cigarette smoking. For each disease the epidemiology and the scientific evidence will be discussed.

Learning Outcomes

At the end of this chapter the reader will be able to:

– Know the major cardiovascular and respiratory diseases and other deiseases related to cigarette smoking and their epidemiology.

3.1 Introduction

World Health Organization (WHO) affirms that "tobacco use continues to be the leading global cause of preventable death" (World Health Organization 2011).

WHO estimates that in 2005 5.4 million people died due to tobacco use (World Health Organization 2012).

G. La Torre (✉)
Department of Public Health and Infectious Diseases, "Sapienza" University of Rome, Piazzale Aldo Moro 5, Rome 00185, Italy
e-mail: giuseppe.latorre@uniroma1.it

L. Semyonov • G. Giraldi
Section of Hygiene, Department of Public Health and Infectious Diseases, "Sapienza" University of Rome, Piazzale Aldo Moro 5, Rome 00185, Italy
e-mail: ledasemyonov@hotmail.it; guglielmo.giraldi@uniroma1.it

G. La Torre, *Smoking Prevention and Cessation*, DOI 10.1007/978-1-4614-7046-5_3,

Tobacco continues to kill nearly six million people each year, including more than 600,000 nonsmokers who die from passive exposure to tobacco smoke [secondhand smoke (SHS)] (World Health Organization 2011).

If current trends continue, by 2030 tobacco-related deaths are projected to increase to 8.3 million deaths per year worldwide (World Health Organization 2012).

WHO ranks smoking consumption as the first leading causes of the global burden of disease in industrialized countries, using disability-adjusted life years (DALYs) as a combined measure of premature death and disability. Smoking is responsible for 12.2 % of all DALYs (Singer et al. 2011).

In 2008 Centers for Disease Control (CDC) reported that cigarette smoking and exposure to secondhand smoke(SHS) resulted in an estimated 443,000 deaths and 5.1 million years of potential life lost (YPLL) annually in the USA during the period 2000–2004 (Centers for Disease Control and Prevention 2009).

Smoking prevalence is high in Asia, too. China has the largest production and consumption of tobacco worldwide: approximately 67 % of males and 4 % of females aged over 15 years in China are smokers for a total of 350 million smokers (which represents about one-third of all smokers worldwide) and 740 million passive smokers. The number of deaths attributed to tobacco use has reached 1.2 million per year, whereas the death toll is expected to rise to two million annually by 2025. Based on current smoking rates, the predicted deaths attributed to smoking in China will rise to three million in 2050: if the current smoking pattern in China remains unchanged, 100 million men now under 30 years will die from smoking-related diseases (Zhang et al. 2011; Zhang and Cai 2003).

In Europe tobacco is the leading contributor to the disease burden in more than half of the Member States and it is among the three leading contributors in the majority of countries: this issue can be considered a critical international point for public health policy makers (Ficarra et al. 2011).

In Germany one-third of the adult Germans are active smokers, men smoke more frequently than women (34.0 vs. 25.1 %) and annually 110,000–140,000 humans die prematurely because of cigarette smoking (Singer et al. 2011).

In 2010, 21.7 % of Italians (23.9 % of men and 19.7 % of women) described themselves as current smokers. This smoking prevalence is higher than that of several countries including Australia (19.0 %), Sweden (16.0 %), and Finland (21.0 %) (Gallus et al. 2011).

On the basis of data from prospective studies, carried out following population groups over time and collecting standardized information on smoking, it is possible to calculate the risk of death related to smoking and at different levels of exposure (Pearl 1938) (Fig. 3.1).

Several studies show increased risk of having CHD at all levels of cigarette smoking, and increased risks are evident even for persons who smoked fewer than five cigarettes per day (Prescott et al. 2005; Bjartveit and Tverdal 2005).

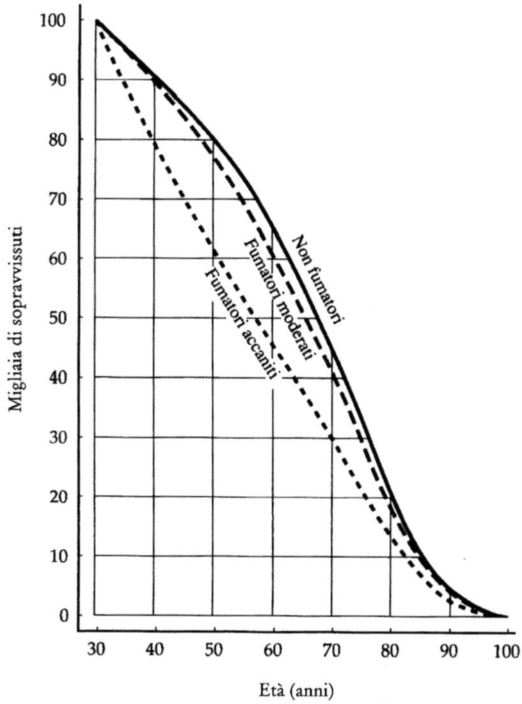

Fig. 3.1 Survival curves for nonsmokers, mild smokers, and heavy smokers (Pearl 1938)

3.2 Cardiovascular Diseases

Main concepts:

- What are the most frequent?
- How does the smoke impact in these diseases?
- Epidemiology of smoking-induced cardiovascular disease (CVD).

Cancer and cardiovascular diseases share risk factors such as smoking, and the onset of both diseases have been suggested to have a common mechanistic basis. Carcinogen–DNA adducts, genetic polymorphisms in carcinogen-detoxifying enzymes glutathione S-transferases (GSTs), and genetic polymorphisms in the vitamin D receptor (VDR) are among the candidates for modifiers of cancer risk (Van Schooten et al. 1998).

Cigarette smoking is a major cause of CVD and has been responsible for approximately 140,000 premature deaths annually from CVD in the USA (U.S. Department of Health and Human Services 2004).

At the international level, in the year 2000, more than one in every ten cardiovascular deaths in the world was attributable to smoking (Ezzati et al. 2005).

Smoking increases the cardiovascular risk, at any level of blood pressure, for coronary heart disease, stroke, and cardiac failure (Kannel and Higgins 1990).

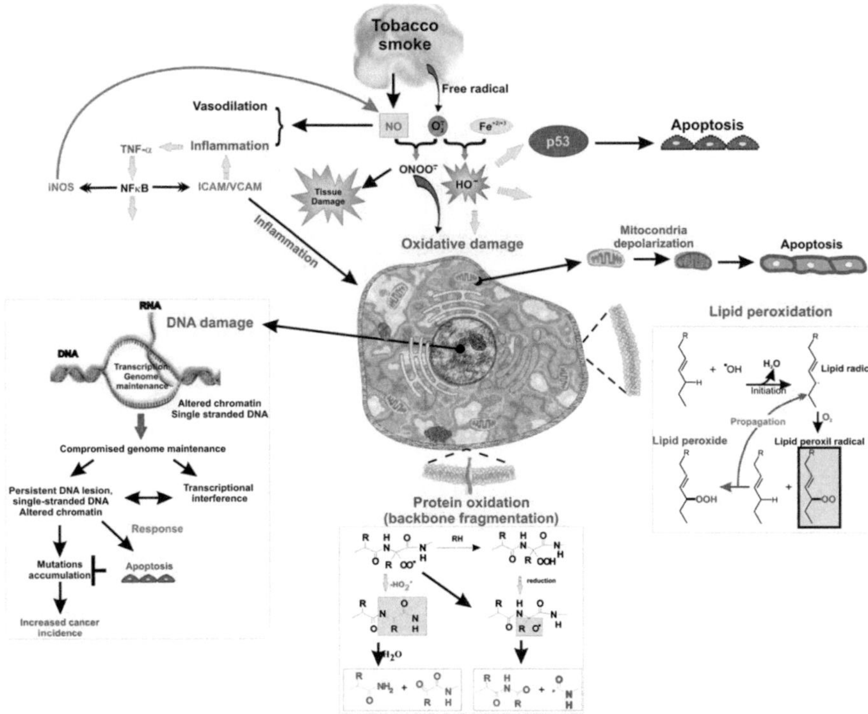

Fig. 3.2 ROS-induced cellular inflammatory response and oxidative damage originated by tobacco combustion: cellular damage and inflammation (Mazzone et al. 2010)

Smoking affects cardiovascular system causing aortic aneurysm, coronary heart diseases, and other arterial diseases including cerebrovascular events. The vascular adverse effects of smoking can be the result of endothelial exposure to reactive oxygen species (ROS): damage to cells occurs as a result of ROS-induced alterations of macromolecules (Mazzone et al. 2010) (Fig. 3.2).

In addition, studies of cigarette smokers showed that the heart tissue contained more DNA adducts than that from nonsmokers or former smokers (Van Schooten et al. 1998). They also demonstrated a linear relationship between DNA adduct levels and daily cigarette smoking. Furthermore, higher DNA adduct levels were associated with a higher degree of coronary artery disease.

The mechanisms by which smoking results in cardiovascular events include the development of atherosclerotic changes: narrowing of the vascular lumen and induction of a hypercoagulable state, which create risk of acute thrombosis. In addition, smoking contributes to development of atherosclerotic plaque and thrombosis (U.S. Department of Health and Human Services 2010) (Fig. 3.3).

Cigarette smoking also influences other cardiovascular risk factors, such as glucose intolerance and low serum levels of high-density lipoprotein cholesterol (HDLc).

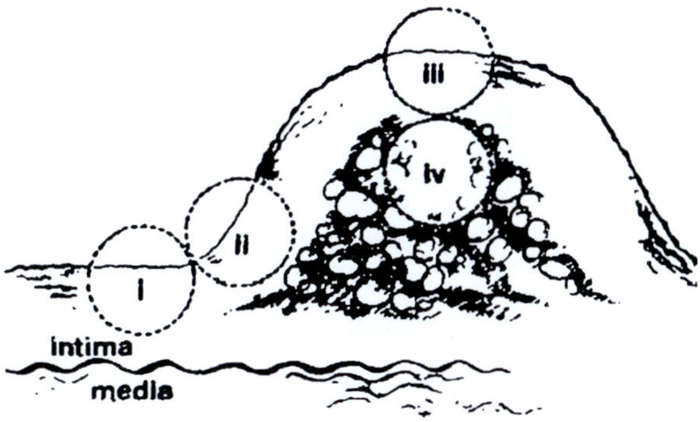

Fig. 3.3 Schematic representation of an atherosclerotic plaque showing the location of the regions where cells were counted: the intima adjacent to the plaque (Region I), the "shoulder" region (II), the fibrous cap (III), and the necrotic core region (IV) (Jonasson et al. 1986)

Tobacco smoking acts as an independent risk factor for CVD, but it also have a multiplicative interaction with the other risk factors, such as high serum levels of lipids, hypertension, diabetes mellitus (U.S. Department of Health and Human Services 2010).

Scientific literature affirms that nonsmokers live many years longer and longer free of cardiovascular disease than smokers (Mamun et al. 2004).

3.2.1 Coronary Heart Disease

Comparing modifiable cardiovascular risk factors, smoking has the strongest impact on cardiovascular mortality. More than 50 % of all premature myocardial infarctions are related to nicotine consumption (Weil et al. 2012).

For each ten cigarettes per day there is an incremental increase in cardiovascular mortality in men (18 %) and in women (31 %) (Kannel and Higgins 1990).

Studies of cigarette smokers showed that the heart tissue contained more DNA adducts than that from nonsmokers or former smokers; they also demonstrated a linear relationship between DNA adduct levels and daily cigarette smoking. Furthermore, higher DNA adduct levels were associated with a higher degree of coronary artery disease (Van Schooten et al. 1998).

Investigators reported that tissue injury induced by oxidative stress, altered serum lipids, increased blood pressure, and endothelial damage were other possible factors in cardiovascular injury from cigarette smoking (Stratton et al. 2001).

In the USA, smoking accounted for 33 % of all deaths from CVD and 20 % of deaths from ischemic heart disease in persons older than 35 years of age (Centers for Disease Control and Prevention 2008).

During 2010, the prevalence of CHD in the USA was greatest among persons aged ≥65 years (19.8 %), followed by those aged 45–64 years (7.1 %), and those aged 18–44 years (1.2 %). CHD prevalence was greater among men (7.8 %) than women (4.6 %). Among racial/ethnic populations, CHD prevalence was greatest among American Indians/Alaska Natives (11.6 %), followed by blacks (6.5 %),

Box 3.1 Epidemiological Definitions (La Torre 2010)

Relative risk (RR)	The probability (risk) of the event occurring in the exposed group divided by the probability of the same event in a not exposed group
Adjusted RR	The relative risk is adjusted for taking into account possible confounding. In epidemiology this refers to a distortion of an association between exposure (E) and disease (D) brought by an extraneous factor (F). To judge if F confound the estimated measure of association, we can use a stratification analysis or a multivariate analysis (regression)
Hazard ratio	The ratio between the predicted hazard for people exposed to a certain factor and that for people not exposed to the factor, with everything else being constant
Attributable fraction	Fraction of the incidence rate of a given disease in the exposed group that is due (attributable) to the exposure

Hispanics (6.1 %), whites (5.8 %), and Asians or Native Hawaiians/Other Pacific Islanders (3.9 %). By race and sex in 2010, the greatest male prevalence were among American Indian/Alaska Natives (14.3 %) and whites (7.7 %), and the greatest females prevalence were among American Indian/Alaska Natives (8.4 %) and blacks (5.9 %) [Centers for Disease Control and Prevention (CDC) 2011].

Prospective mortality studies conducted in the 1960s and 1970s showed a clear increase in CHD mortality with an increase in the number of cigarettes smoked per day, regardless of the actual number (Doll and Peto 1976).

Other studies suggested that risk increased up to at least 40 cigarettes per day (Miettinen et al. 1976; Willett et al. 1987).

A prospective study in Norway screened 23,521 men and 19,201 women, aged 35–49 years, for cardiovascular disease risk factors from 1970s throughout 2002. In both sexes, even smoking 1–4 cigarettes per day was associated with a significantly higher risk of dying from ischaemic heart disease and from all causes and from lung cancer in women. Adjusted RR (95 % CI) in smokers of dying from ischaemic heart disease was 2.74 (95 % CI: 2.07–3.61) in men and 2.94 (95 % CI: 1.75–4.95) in women (Bjartveit and Tverdal 2005) (Box 3.1).

Anyway, the risks of MI and death from CHD are lower among former smokers than among continuing smokers in many studies, including those with data adjusted for levels of other risk factors (Kuller et al. 1991; Frost et al. 1996).

Risks appear to remain slightly elevated for more than a decade even after persons stopped smoking, but in some studies this increased risk was not statistically significant (Kawachi et al. 1993; Jacobs et al. 1999).

Qiao et al. studied the risk of early and late death in relation to smoking and ex-smoking in a cohort of 1,711 Finnish men followed up for 35 years: the hazard ratios for 35-year coronary heart disease mortality were 1.63 (95 % CI: 1.24–2.13) in current smokers and 1.39 (95 % CI: 1.00–1.94) in former smokers.

The risk for 10-year mortality was stronger than for 35-year mortality among both former and current smokers, given the same amount of cigarettes consumed. Smoking increases the risk of premature death in middle-aged men and giving up smoking earlier in life can prevent smoking attributable premature death (Qiao et al. 2000).

As a matter of fact, cigarette smoking has been associated with higher RR of MI (Njølstad et al. 1996) and higher CHD mortality (Thun and Heath 1997)

The absolute increase in risk of CHD from smoking is similar for men and women (U.S. Department of Health and Human Services 2001a).

Data from the Framingham Study have shown a prompt halving of the coronary heart disease risk in those who give up smoking compared to those who continue to smoke, regardless of the duration of the habit Kannel and Higgins 1990. Law and Wald (2003) conducted a meta-analysis of five large studies of smoking and CHD, demonstrating a nonlinear dose–response relationship between the number of cigarettes smoked per day and the RR of disease: data suggested that the effect of cigarette smoking on risk of CHD may have a low threshold and that the dose–response characteristics are less steep at higher doses.

Evidence supports a significant effect of low dose tobacco smoke exposure in causing ischemic heart disease: in experimental studies passive and active smoking have similar effects on platelet aggregation (Malcolm et al. 2003).

The *INTERHEART study* was a standardized case–control investigation of acute MI in 52 countries in Africa, Asia, Australia, the Middle East Crescent, and North and South America. This study showed that tobacco use is one of the most important causes of AMI globally, especially in men. Current smoking was associated with a greater risk of nonfatal AMI (OR 2.95, 95 % CI: 2.77–3.14, $p<0.0001$) compared with never smoking; risk increased by 5.6 % for every additional cigarette smoked. The OR associated with former smoking fell to 1.87 (95 % CI: 1.55–2.24) within 3 years of quitting. A residual excess risk remained 20 or more years after quitting (1.22, 1.09–1.37). Tobacco use should be discouraged to prevent cardiovascular diseases. The odds ratio (OR) for acute MI in smokers was 2.95 for this large multiethnic population compared with lifetime nonsmokers (Koon et al. 2006).

The *International Studies of Infarct Survival* reported that at 30–49 years of age the rates of myocardial infarction in smokers were about five times those in nonsmokers and at ages 50–59 years they were three times those in nonsmokers (Huxley and Woodward 2011).

In a systematic review Skinner and Cooper present information relating to the effectiveness and safety of several interventions concerning the secondary prevention of ischemic cardiac events, including smoking cessation (Skinner and Cooper 2011).

Critchley et al. in a *Cochrane Systematic Review* considered that quitting smoking is associated with a substantial reduction in risk of all-cause mortality among patients with CHD. The pooled crude RR was 0.64 (95 % CI: 0.58–0.71). This 36 % risk reduction appears substantial compared with other secondary preventive therapies such as cholesterol lowering which have received greater attention in recent years. The risk reduction associated with quitting smoking seems consistent regardless of differences between the studies in terms of index cardiac events, age, sex, country, and time period. There was also a reduction in nonfatal myocardial infarctions (crude RR 0.68, 95 % CI: 0.57–0.82) (Critchley and Capewell 2004).

3.2.2 Hypertension

Worldwide, 7.6 million premature deaths (about 13.5 % of the global total) and 92 million DALYs (6.0 % of the global total) were attributed to high blood pressure. About 54 % of stroke and 47 % of ischemic heart disease worldwide were attributable to high blood pressure (Lawes et al. 2008).

Among hypertensive persons, about 39 % of coronary events in men and 68 % in women are attributable to the presence of two or more additional risk factors (O'Donnell and Kannel 2002).

Smoking is reported to increase arterial stiffness. Kim and colleagues examined the acute and chronic effects of smoking on arterial stiffness by measuring brachial-ankle Pulse wave velocity (baPWV), since it is an indicator of arterial stiffness and a marker for vascular damage. Systolic BP was higher in chronic smokers than non-smokers or controls. Acutely, cigarette smoking increased BP, heart rate, and baPWV in chronic smokers and nonsmokers. These effects were more prominent in chronic smokers than in nonsmokers; PWV increased significantly ($p<0.01$): 12.1–17.3 m/s vs. 11.1–12.7 m/s, respectively. These findings suggest that cigarette smoking have deleterious effects on cardiovascular system by stiffening arteries (Kim et al. 2005).

In addition, smoking promote increased sympathetic activity, damage the endothelium, and accelerate atherosclerosis: all these processes important in the physiopathology of hypertension. Studies have shown that even modest smoking rates can cause acute elevations of blood pressure (Halperin et al. 2008).

A Norwegian study showed that stroke cases had increased diastolic (DBP) and systolic blood pressure (SBP); the absolute differences in DBP and SBP between stroke cases and others for never and former smokers vs. daily smokers were DBP, 12.1 mmHg vs. 6.5 mmHg, respectively and SBP, 16.0 mmHg vs. 7.1 mmHg, respectively (Håheim et al. 1996).

The meta-analysis carried out by Xiaofan et al. (2011) emerges that several studies investigated the association between smoking and prehypertension: the pooled OR was 1.13 (95 % CI: 0.93–1.37) and some studies concluded that smoking contributes to hypertension (Kim et al. 2005)

Halperin and colleagues evaluated the relationship between smoking status and incident hypertension in a large cohort of initially healthy middle-aged and older men. Data suggested that cigarette smoking may be a modest but important risk factor for the development of hypertension. Over a median follow-up of 14.5 years, 4,904 men developed hypertension. Compared with never smokers, past smokers and current smokers had corresponding relative risks (RRs) of 1.08 and 1.15 of developing hypertension. The risk for smokers did not differ on number of cigarettes smoked daily. This study showed that smoking is associated with an increased risk of developing hypertension in men, and it remained statistically significant after adjustment for other known hypertension risk factors. Current smokers are at greatest risk of hypertension, whereas former smokers were at an intermediate risk between never and current smokers (Halperin et al. 2008).

Data from the Framingham Study have shown a prompt halving of the coronary heart disease risk in those who give up smoking compared to those who continue to smoke, regardless of the duration of the habit: hypertensives who smoke one pack of cigarettes a day can quickly reduce the risk by 35–40 % by not smoking (Kannel and Higgins 1990).

Smoking tobacco increase the incidence of hypertension. Furthermore, smoking and hypertension together substantially increase the risk of mortality and confer a greater additive risk. Therefore, smoking cessation counseling and treatment should be provided to all hypertensive patients who smoke (Khan et al. 2009).

3.2.3 Cerebro-Vascular Disease

Tobacco smoking causes an estimated 12 % of stroke mortality in low- and middle-income countries (Strong et al. 2007).

A study by De Flora et al. (1997) showed DNA adduct levels in smooth muscle cells (SMCs) of human atherosclerotic lesions to be related to known atherogenic risk factors. Atherogenesis is a degenerative process involving a variety of lesions of the arterial wall. It results from focal intimal thickening formed after endothelian cell injury and uncontrolled proliferation of SMCs, accompanied by the accumulation of extracellular components and by the participation of inflammatory cells. Atherosclerosis is an excessive inflammatory-fibroproliferative response to various forms of insult to the arthery wall.

According to WHO, stroke was the second commonest cause of mortality worldwide in 1990 and the third commonest cause of mortality in more developed countries; it caused about 4.4 million deaths worldwide (Murray and Lopez 1997).

In 1999, the number of deaths due to stroke reached 5.54 million worldwide (World Health Organization 2000).

Annually, 16 million people suffer a stroke worldwide and 5.7 million die from the condition in 2005. Without intervention, the number of global deaths is projected to rise to 6.5 million in 2015 and to 7.8 million in 2030 (Strong et al. 2007).

Stroke is also a major cause of long-term disability and has potentially enormous emotional and socioeconomic implications. By the year 2020, stroke and coronary-artery disease together are expected to be the leading causes of lost healthy life years (Feigin et al. 2003).

Risk of fatal stroke in relation to the amount of cigarette smoking varies between studies.

In the meta-analysis conducted by Shinton and Beevers was found a strong evidence of an excess risk of stroke among cigarette smokers. Data showed a linearly increased risk of smoking with increasing amount. Therefore, stroke should be added to the list of smoking-related diseases (Shinton and Beevers 1989).

The impact of cigarette smoking on stroke incidence was also assessed in the Framingham Heart Study: a cohort of 4,255 men and women aged 36–68 years and free of stroke and transient ischemic attacks were followed-up for 26 years; during this period, 459 strokes occurred. Cigarette smoking appeared to be a significant independent contribution to the risk of stroke generally and brain infarction specifically. The risk of stroke increased as the number of cigarettes smoked increased. The RR of stroke in heavy smokers (>40 cigarettes per day) was twice that of light smokers (<10 cigarettes per day). The risk declined, however, among smokers who had stopped smoking for 2 years and was similar to that of lifetime nonsmokers after 5 years of abstinence from smoking (Wolf et al. 1988).

Higa and Davanipour, in their literature review found a significant dose–response relationship between the amount of cigarettes smoked per day and the relative risk of stroke and that when smoking ceased, the risk of stroke lessened (Higa and Dvanipour 1991).

All smokers, have an increased risk of fatal stroke compared with never smokers. Stroke cases had significantly higher levels of DBP and SBP than other men, but the absolute difference was twice as large for nonsmokers compared with daily smokers. With regard to DBP, the differences were 12.1 mmHg vs. 6.5 mmHg respectively, and for SBP the differences were 16.0 mmHg vs. 7.1 mmHg respectively. Previous smokers had an increased but non-significant risk when compared with never smokers. Fatal cases of stroke were characterized by having increased DBP and SBP. Twice the absolute differences were found among never and previous cigarette smokers compared with daily smokers (Håheim et al. 1996).

Stroke age-specific patterns of stroke mortality were similar to those seen with CHD. The percentage of fatal strokes attributable to cigarette smoking also declined dramatically with age among smokers. In men this fraction fell from 80 % at ages 50–54 years to 31 % at ages ≥80 years; in women it decreased erratically from 87 % at ages 45–49 years to virtually 0 % at ages ≥80 years (Thun et al. 1997).

Haheim et al. in a prospective cohort study on the smoking habits and the risk of fatal stroke in middle aged men, underlined that daily cigarette smoking increased the risk of stroke three and a half times. An amplified risk was also found in relation to cigarette daily consumption. Combined cigarette and pipe or cigar smoking had a higher risk than smoking cigarettes only (Håheim et al. 1996).

In a meta-analysis of data from 32 studies, conducted by Shinton and Beevers, the overall RR for stroke associated with cigarette smoking was 1.5 (95 % CI: 1.4–1.6). The RRs varied with the stroke subtypes: 1.9 for cerebral infarction, 0.7 for cerebral hemorrhage, and 2.9 for subarachnoid hemorrhage. Data reported a dose–response relationship between the number of cigarettes smoked per day and the RR: there exists a higher risk of stroke among former smokers younger than age 75 years than the risk for nonsmokers in the same age group. For all ages combined, RR for former smokers was 1.2 (Shinton and Beevers 1989).

Not only active but also passive smoking and smokeless tobacco products are risk factors for lacunar and atherothrombotic brain infarction and subarachnoid hemorrhage. The risk after smoking cessation for 5–10 years is equal to that faced by a nonsmoker. Support measures to enforce nonsmoking are required in this high-risk population (Hashimoto 2011).

Oono and colleagues in a meta-analysis determined the evidence of a strong, consistent, and dose-dependent association between risk of stroke and SHS exposure. The pooled estimate of risk was 1.25 (95 % CI: 1.12–1.38); the RR increased from 1.16 (95 % CI: 1.06–1.27) for exposure to 5 cigarettes/day to 1.56 (95 % CI: 1.25–1.96) for exposure to 40 cigarettes/day. Results of the study suggested no safe lower limit of exposure (Oono et al. 2011).

3.2.4 Aortic Aneurism

Smoking is the major risk environmental factor for aneurysm formation and resultant death (Hirsch et al. 2006).

Aneurysm can be defined as a permanent and irreversible localized dilatation of a vessel; abdominal aortic aneurysm (AAA), defined as an aortic diameter ≥30 mm (Fanelli et al. 2009).

AAAs cause 1.3 % of all deaths among men aged 65–85 years in developed countries (Sakalihasan et al. 2005).

Aortic aneurysms result in at least 14,000 deaths per year in the USA. This number is likely an underestimation, because approximately 5 % of the 200,000 people who die of sudden death each year may have AAA as the cause (Kent et al. 2010).

The association with smoking is directly related to the number of years of smoking and decreases with the number of years after cessation of smoking (Lederle et al. 1997).

In addition, smoking increases AAA growth and several studies have identified that AAAs appear to expand faster in current smokers (Chang et al. 1997; Lindholt et al. 2001; MacSweeney et al. 1994).

Scientific evidence shows that serum *cotinine*, a nicotine metabolite, is related with aneurysm growth rate: that's why current smokers compared to those who stop smoking have higher aneurysm growth rates. Furthermore, smoking appears to be a more potent risk factor for death from aneurysm than for death from coronary atherosclerosis (Strachan 1991).

A prospective study reported a relationship between cigarette smoking, hypertension, obesity, and physical inactivity and the death rate from aortic aneurysm in the 6 year follow-up of a large population study (Hammond and Garfinkel 1969).

Similarly, the prospective phase of the Honolulu Heart Program showed that high blood pressure, high serum cholesterol, and cigarette smoking were predictors of aortic aneurysms identified at autopsy (Reed et al. 1992).

The CPS-I study provides evidence that the risks of aortic aneurysm are elevated for smokers, both for cigar smokers and cigarette smokers. Risk ratios of aortic aneurysm are shown by the results for the CPS-I data, given by level of cigars/cigarettes per day and by level of inhalation. The overall result is highly significant: 1.76 (1.29–2.35) for primary cigar smokers, 2.82 (1.91–4.00) for secondary cigar smokers, 3.32 (2.34–4.58) for cigar and cigarette smokers, and 4.96 (4.62–5.31) for cigarette only smokers. Among cigar smokers, the RR's for inhalers approach the risks observed for cigarette smokers. The cigarette-only smokers show a strong positive trend both with increasing consumption of cigarettes per day and with increasing levels of inhalation (Burns et al. 1998).

In the Edinburgh Artery Study (Lee et al. 1997), 1,592 men and women aged 55–74 years were followed prospectively over 5 years. After adjustment for age and sex, current and recent ex-cigarette smokers (gave up 5 years ago or less) had over three times the risk of having an increased risk of aortic aneurysm compared with long time ex-smokers and never smokers (OR 3.08, 95 % CI: 1.53 to 6.21, $p<001$); after further adjustment for atherosclerotic disease, the size of the OR was reduced to 2.63 (95 % CI: 1.26 to 5.45, $p<001$). These data suggest the evidence of a direct effect of cigarette smoking on the risk of aortic aneurysm which is independently of atherosclerosis, rather, smoking constituents may promote the destruction of the aortic wall by proteolytic enzymes or copper metabolism and tissue antioxidant levels may be involved (Lee et al. 1997).

More recently, in a study carried out by Brady and colleagues, 1,743 patients were monitored for changes in AAA diameter by ultrasonography over a follow-up of 1.9 years. Data showed that smoking increases AAA growth rates by 15–20 %: current smokers had significantly faster AAA expansion (approximately 0.4 mm/year), and the association between AAA expansion and current smoking persisted after adjustment for potential confounding factors (Brady et al. 2004).

The study conducted by Powell and colleagues, instead, estimated that continued smoking increases the rate of aneurysm growth by 20–25 % (Powell and Greenhalgh 2003).

Besides initial AAA size, only smoking had persisting significance after adjustment of the other significant variables and smoking cessation may inhibit aneurysmal expansion (Lindholt et al. 2001).

Smoking is the major risk factor of developing AAA as well as the risk of rupture. Aneurysm rupture is a medical emergency and risk of aneurysm rupture increases with the history of smoking (Brewster et al. 2003).

Thoracic aortic dissection (TAD) is estimated to occur at a rate of 3–4 cases per 100,000 persons per year and is associated with a high mortality. The incidence of TAD has been increasing over time. Evidence supports that smoking represents a risk factor associated with TAD (LeMaire and Russell 2011).

A comprehensive review by Aggarwal et al. (2011) shows that the risk of AAAs increases dramatically in the presence of some factors such as age older than 60 years, smoking, hypertension, and Caucasian ethnicity. Moreover, smoking has been found to be a major risk factor for aneurysm formation, growth, and rupture.

A retrospective cohort of 3.1 million patients analyzed the effect of smoking history on the risk of AAA: it was higher for current smokers than past smokers, it increased with duration of smoking and quantity of cigarettes smoked per day, and it declined over time after quitting.

The risk attributable to smoking varied over a wide range: the lowest risk was for people who smoked up to a half-pack/day for less than 10 years and quit more than 10 years ago, the highest risk was for current smokers who had been smoking more than 1 pack/day for more than 35 years. The risk score associated with smoking ranged from 1 to 26. These data underline that AAA had a strong positive association with quantity and duration of smoking and an inverse association with the years after smoking cessation (Kent et al. 2010).

3.3 Respiratory Diseases

A recent Indian study was performed to compare the pulmonary function tests among smokers and nonsmokers, to examine the relation of type, quantity, and duration of smoking on the pulmonary function tests. The pulmonary function tests were assessed in 400 male subjects (200 smokers and 200 non smokers): almost all the pulmonary function parameters [expiratory reserve volume (ERV), forced vital capacity (FVC), forced expiratory volume (FEV), functional residual capacity (FRC), residual volume (RV), peak expiratory flow (PEF), slow vital capacity (SVC), and total lung capacity (TLC)] were significantly reduced in smokers; obstructive pulmonary impairment was commonest among smokers (Bano et al. 2011).

Forey and colleagues conducted a systematic review of epidemiological studies relating incidence or prevalence of chronic obstructive pulmonary disease (COPD), chronic bronchitis (CB), and emphysema to smoking. Based on random effects meta-analyses of most-adjusted RR/ORs, estimates seemed to be elevated for ever smoking (COPD 2.89, CI 2.63–3.17, $n=129$ RRs; CB 2.69, 2.50–2.90, $n=114$; emphysema 4.51, 3.38–6.02, $n=28$), current smoking (COPD 3.51, 3.08–3.99; CB 3.41, 3.13–3.72; emphysema 4.87, 2.83–8.41), and ex smoking (COPD 2.35, 2.11–2.63; CB 1.63, 1.50–1.78; emphysema 3.52, 2.51–4.94). For all outcomes RRs are higher when based on mortality. For all outcomes, risk increases with amount smoked and pack–years. Data demonstrate that risk decreases with increasing starting age for COPD and CB and with increasing quitting duration for COPD. Anyway, results confirm the causal relationships with smoking (Forey et al. 2011).

A cross-sectional population-based study conducted by Langhammer examined the prevalence of respiratory symptoms and diseases according to smoking burden. From a total of 65,717 subjects interviewed, 30 % of men and 31 % of women were smokers. Respiratory symptoms increased by smoking burden (pack–years). Smokers reported episodes of wheezing or breathlessness, current asthma, and persistent coughing twice as prevalent as never smokers, and the prevalence increased by smoking burden ($p<0.001$) and the difference between sexes increased by increasing smoking burden and daily cigarette consumption, since women seemed to be more susceptible to the effect of tobacco smoking than men (Langhammer et al. 2000) (Fig. 3.4).

Not only active smoking but even environmental tobacco smoke (ETS) exposure is significantly associated with prevalence of respiratory symptoms such as wheezing, cough, and breathlessness (Gupta et al. 2006).

Furthermore, smoking during pregnancy can negatively affect fetal lung growth and result in development of lung disease (Gilliland et al. 2002).

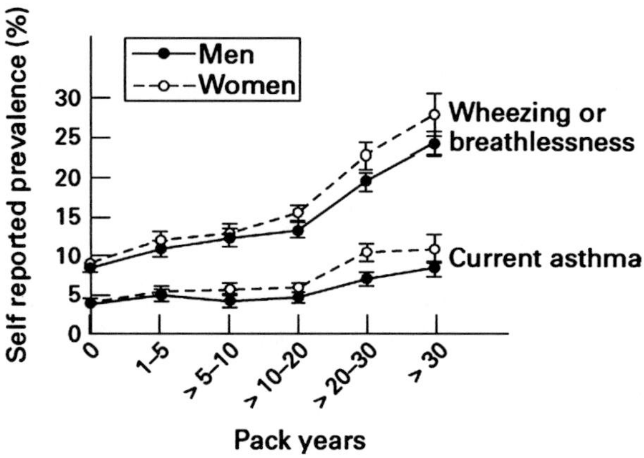

Fig. 3.4 Age-adjusted prevalence (%) of self-reported episodes of wheezing or breathlessness in the past 12 months and current asthma by number of pack–years in men and women (95 % confidence intervals). Nord-Trøndelag, Norway 1997 (Langhammer et al. 2000)

3.3.1 Chronic Obstructive Pulmonary Disease

Smoking is a well-known risk factor for COPD, a group of lung diseases that includes emphysema and chronic bronchitis. Worldwide, COPD affects over 5 % of the adult population and is the fourth leading cause of mortality and the twelfth leading cause of disability; by the year 2020, it is estimated that it will be the third leading cause of death and the fifth leading cause of disability worldwide (Murray and Lopez 1997; Michaud et al. 2001; Mannino et al. 2006).

According to WHO estimates, 65 million people have moderate to severe COPD. More than three million people died of COPD in 2005, which corresponds to 5 % of all deaths globally. Almost 90 % of COPD deaths occur in low- and middle-income countries (World Health Organization 2012).

Oxidative stress produced by the high concentrations of free radicals in tobacco smoke, cytokine release due to inflammation as the body responds to irritant particles such as tobacco smoke in the airway, tobacco smoke, and free radicals impair the activity of antiprotease enzymes such as alpha 1-antitrypsin, allowing protease enzymes to damage the lung are the most important processes causing lung damage. Narrowing of the airways reduces the effectiveness of the lungs: the greatest reduction in air flow occurs during expiration because the pressure in the chest tends to compress rather than expand the airways. A little of the air of the previous breath remains within the lungs when the next breath is started, increasing in the volume of air in the lungs (dynamic hyperinflation). Another factor contributing to shortness of breath in COPD is the loss of the surface area available for the exchange of oxygen and carbon dioxide that leads to low oxygen and high carbon dioxide levels in the body (Calverley and Koulouris 2005).

The primary cause of COPD in the developed world is tobacco smoke (including secondhand or passive exposure) and smoking cessation is the most important intervention in COPD management (Mannino 2002).

WHO estimates that in high-income countries, 73 % of COPD mortality is related to smoking, with 40 % related to smoking in nations of low and middle income (Lopez et al. 2006).

The study of 40-year follow-up on male British doctors delineated the consequences of tobacco smoking. Mortality of COPD was shown to be at least seven times higher in smokers than in nonsmokers (Doll et al. 1994).

As a matter of fact, COPD shows a wide divergence in death rates between smokers and nonsmokers, since and the high proportion of deaths are attributable to cigarettes among smokers. Although the rate difference (RD) consistently increased with age, the rate ratio (RR) oscillated between 8 and 19 in men and between 9.5 and 15 in women. The smoking-attributable fraction (SAF) remained at or above 88 % at all ages in both sexes (Thun et al. 1997).

This relation is highly influenced by genes, because not all smokers go on to develop COPD. However, a much higher proportion of smokers, as much as 50 %, have been developed COPD (Rennard and Vestbo 2006; Lundback et al. 2003).

According to WHO estimates, 65 million people have moderate to severe COPD. More than three million people died of COPD in 2005, which corresponds to 5 % of all deaths globally. Almost 90 % of COPD deaths occur in low- and middle-income countries.

Once, COPD was more common in men, but because of increased tobacco use among women, the disease now affects men and women almost equally (World Health Organization 2012).

During the period 1980–2000, there was an increasing rate of mortality for COPD in the USA for women (from 20.1/100,000 in 1980 to 56.7/100,000 in 2000) compared with the more modest increase in the death rate for men (from 73.0/100,000 in 1980 to 82.6/100,000 in 2000).

For the first time in 2000, the number of women dying from COPD in the USA exceeded the number of men dying from COPD (59,936 vs. 59,118) (Mannino et al. 2002).

In addition, in the U.S. during the year 2000, COPD was responsible for eight million physician office and hospital outpatient visits, 1.5 million emergency department visits, 726,000 hospitalizations, and 119,000 deaths (Mannino et al. 2002).

The prevalence of COPD in individuals between 40 and 80 years of age in Spain is 10.2 % (95 % CI: 9.2–11.1 %), increases with tobacco consumption and was higher in men (15.1 %) than in women (5.6 %). The prevalence of COPD stage II or higher was 4.4 % (95 %CI: 3.8–5.1 %) (Miravitlles et al. 2009).

The European Respiratory Society (ERS) diagnostic criteria for COPD include the following symptoms: coughing, sputum production, and/or dyspnoea, as well as a history of exposure to risk factors for COPD. The diagnosis is confirmed by a post-bronchodilator $FEV_1/FVC < 0.7$ in spirometry, as sign of the airflow limitation that is not fully reversible (Pierson 2006) (Box 3.2).

Nowadays in Japan the prevalence of COPD is 8.6 %. Among the patients who are 40 or more the prevalence of COPD is 8.6–10.3 %. If they have smoking history, the prevalence of COPD is 22 % (Minakata and Ichinose 2011).

Box 3.2 COPD stages (Pierson 2006)

GOLD staging system for COPD severity

Stage	Description	Findings (based on postbronchodilator FEV_1)
0	At risk	Risk factors and chronic symptoms but normal spirometry
I	Mild	FEV_1/FVC ratio <70 % FEV_1 at least 80 % of predicted value May have symptoms
II	Moderate	FEV_1/FVC ratio <70 % FEV_1 50 % to <80 % of predicted value May have chronic symptoms
III	Severe	FEV_1/FVC ratio <70 % FEV_1 30 % to <50 % of predicted value May have chronic symptoms
IV	Very severe	FEV_1/FVC ratio <70 % FEV_1 <30 % of predicted value or FEV_1 <50 % of predicted value plus severe chronic symptoms

GOLD global initiative for chronic obstructive lung disease, *COPD* chronic obstructive pulmonary disease, *FEV_1* forced expiratory volume in one second, *FVC* forced vital capacity

It is estimated that over five million Japanese individuals over the age of 40 years have a diagnosis of COPD: this prevalence seems to be higher than that reported in North America and Europe (Omori et al. 2006)

In Canada, the prevalence rate of COPD was derived from the National Health Survey during the period 1994–1995. Seven-hundred fifty thousand Canadians had chronic bronchitis or emphysema diagnosed by a physician. Prevalence rates were 4.6 % in the age group 55–64 years, 5.0 % in the 65–74 group, and 6.8 % for subjects over 75 years (Lacasse et al. 1999).

Izquierdo et al. (2009) performed a cross-sectional study with 3,935 patients (74.5 % men; mean age, 67 years) in Spain. Of the patients studied, COPD affects old men (more than 50 % were over 65 years of age) and nonemployed men (23 % were employed). 22.7 % of participants continued smoking, especially men (24.4 % of men vs. 18.1 % of women). Nonsmokers had a lower burden than ex-smokers: 2.37 ± 1.15 vs. 2.53 ± 1.23.

A systematic literature search was performed until September 2007 Godtfredsen et al. to examine COPD-related morbidity and mortality in COPD patients in connection with smoking cessation.

Data from the USA and Europe indicate that, even in severe COPD, smoking cessation leads to decreased mortality due to COPD compared with continued smoking (Godtfredsen et al. 2008) (Table 3.1).

Total victims from COPD are projected to increase in the next years if not urgent action is taken to reduce the principal risk factors, especially tobacco use.

Table 3.1 Effects of smoking cessation on all-cause and chronic obstructive pulmonary disease (COPD) mortality (Godtfredsen et al. 2008)

First author [references]	Study	Subjects *n*	Follow-up# years	Mortality outcome	Summary	Comments
Clinically based						
Kanner	USA	140 Utah COPD Pts	7–13	All-cause	+	In a case–control design (sex- and age-matched Pop), 12-year survival probabilities were 86, 79, and 64 % in never, ex-, and current smokers, respectively
Postma	Groningen, NL	129 severe COPD Pts	18	All-cause	+	Pls were stratified according to bronchodilator reversibility; relative survival was higher in both current- and ex-smokers with greater reversibility; within each stratum, mortality was lower in ex- than current smokers
Anthonisen	USA	985 COPD Pts aged 53-68 years	3	All-cause	0	Overall mortality was 23 % (no difference between current and ex-smokers)
Hersh	USA	139 M Severe COPD Pts aged <53 years	8	All-cause	+	Recent smoking status predicted mortality independently of the effects of lifetime smoking intensity; Pls who were ex-smokers at enrolment had better survival than smokers

(continued)

Table 3.1 (continued)

First author [references]	Study	Subjects n	Follow-up[#] years	Mortality outcome	Summary	Comments
Anthonisen	LHS (USA)	5887 M/F smokers with early COPD (FEV_1 55–90 %) aged 35–60 years	5	CV	?	There were 149 deaths during the study, caused largely by lung cancer and CVD; smoking cessation was associated with significant reductions in fatal CVD and coronary artery disease (too few COPD deaths for analysis)
Anthonisen	USA	5887 M/F smokers with early COPD (FEV_1 55–90 %) aged 35–60 years	14.5	All-cause/respiratory	+	After 14.5 years of follow-up, 731 patients had died; all-cause/respiratory MR was significantly lower in the special intervention group than in the usual care group
Population-based						
Doll	UK	6194 F doctors	22	COPD	+	COPD MRs lower in ex- than current smokers [5.0 vs. 10.5–32.0 % (depending on amount smoked)]
Rogot	USA	~200,000 M to US veterans	16	COPD	– to +	COPD MRs higher in ex- than current smokers until 10 years after smoking cessation; thereafter lower MRs in ex- than current smokers (5.2 vs. 12.1 %)

Carstensen	SE	25,129 M	16	COPD	+	COPD MRs lower in ex- than current smokers [1.8 vs. 1.9–5.3 % (depending on amount smoked)]
Marcus	Honolulu Heart Program (USA)	11,136 Japanese-American M aged 45-	20	COPD	– to +	Age-specific COPD MRs calculated at 5-year intervals (1965–1984); after 10 years, MRs were higher in ex- than never and ex-smokers and lower than current smokers
Tockman	USA	36,110 M/F aged 35–84 years from private census Pop, examined in two 6-year periods 884 M with FEV_1 measures (subset of above)		All-cause/COPD	+	M MRs due to both all causes and COPD were greater in ex-than never smokers, but lower than MRs for current smokers ($p<0.05$); this applied to both time periods; same trend for F, but too few COPD deaths in ex-smokers for analysis. Normal FEV_1: OR 1 (never smokers), 1.75 (ex-smokers), 4.80 (current smokers); FEV_1 <65 % pred: OR 3.71 (never smokers), 6.50 (ex-smokers), 17.80 (current smokers)
Kuller	USA	12,866 M from MRRT	10	All-cause	+	Lower all-cause MR in ex-than current smokers

(continued)

Table 3.1 (continued)

First author [references]	Study	Subjects *n*	Follow-up# years	Mortality outcome	Summary	Comments
Lange	DK	14,214 M/F from CCHS	13	COPD	+	Compared to never smokers, RR of COPD mortality in F ex-smokers was 11 (95 % CI: 2.5–53), current smokers 15 (95 % CI: 3.1–65); RR in M ex-smokers was 3.0 (95 % CI: 0.9–10), current smokers 6.4 (95 % CI: 2.0–20)
Tverdal	NO	68,000 M/F aged 35–49 years	13 (mean)	All-cause	+	MRs for ex-smokers were intermediate to rates for never smokers and smokers in both M and F
Ben-Shlomo	UK	19,018 M from Whitehall Study	18	COPD	+	Annual COPD MRs in never, ex-, and current smokers were 0.68, 0.95 and 2.2 per thousand study population
Sunyer	ES	477 M from Barcelona aged >65 years	8	COPD	0	There were similar prevalences of self-reported respiratory illness in ex-and current smokers, and similar annual COPD MRs (6.0 vs. 1.7 per thousand study population in never smokers)

Knuiman	AU	4277 M/F from the Busselton Health Study	20–26	All-cause	–	Per 10 % decrease in FEV_1, HR of all-cause mortality was 1.195 (95 % CI: 1.124–1.2) in ex-smokers and 1.167 (95 % CI: 1.108–1.229) in current smokers compared to never smokers
Engstrom	SE	291 smoking M born 1914	14	CV	0	CV MRs in Current- and ex-smokers similar by FEV_1 decline tertile
Pelkonen	FI	1582 middle-aged M	30	All-cause/COPD	+/–	Compared to current smokers, there was lower total mortality in never smokers, long-term ex-smokers and quitters; RR of COPD mortality in ex-smokers was 2.51 (95 % CI: 0.65–9.70) compared to current smokers.
Godtfredsen	DK	19,732 M/F from 3 Copenhagen Pop 15.5 (mean) studies	15.5 (mean)	All-cause/COPD	+/0	RR of COPD mortality after smoking cessation was 0.77 (95 % CI: 0.44–1.35) compared to current smokers; HR of all-cause mortality was 0.65 (95 % CI: 0.56–0.74); no comparison was made with never smokers

(continued)

Table 3.1 (continued)

First author [references]	Study	Subjects *n*	Follow-up# years	Mortality outcome	Summary	Comments
Mannino	USA	5542 M/F aged 25–74 years from NHANES	22	All-cause	+	HR of all-cause mortality in a multivariate adjusted model was 1.1 in ex-smokers (95 % CI: 0.9–1.4), 1.4 in current smokers (95 % CI: 1.2–1.7)
Doll	UK	34,439 M UK doctors	40, 50	All-cause/COPD	+	COPD MRs in ex-smokers were intermediate between those of never smokers and current smokers; RR of all-cause mortality lower in ex-than current smokers (1.3 vs. 2.2)
Chinese						
Ho	HK	2030 M/F aged ≥0 years	3	All-cause/COPD COPD	0/–	Similar all-cause MRs in ex- and current smokers; higher rate of respiratory mortality in F ex-smokers [RR 2.3 (95 % CI: 1.3–4.0)]
Lam	HK	1268 retired male cadres aged≥60 years	12	COPD	–	RR of COPD mortality 2.13 (95 % CI: 0.55–8.30) in current smokers; 4.10 (95 % CI: 1.18–14.28) in ex-smokers

Hsu	TW	4049 M/F aged≥60 years	7	All-cause/COPD	0	No differences between ex- and current smokers for all-cause or cause-specific mortality; this study does not meet standard quality criteria
Lam	HK	56,167 M/F aged≥65 years	4 (mean)	All-cause/COPD	+/–	RR of all-cause mortality in ex-smokers was 1.39 (95 % CI: 1.23–1.56) in M and 1.43 (95 % CI: 1.25–1.64) in F; rates were significantly higher in current smokers; COPD MRs were higher in ex- than current smokers

NL The Netherlands, *LHS* Lung Health Study, *SE* Sweden, *DK* Denmark, *NO* Norway, *ES* Spain, *AU* Australia, *FI* Finland, *HK* Hong Kong, *TW* Taiwan, *Pt* patient, *M* male, *F* female, FEV_1 forced expiratory volume in one second, *Pop* population, *MRFIT* Multiple Risk Factor Intervention Trial, *CCHS* Copenhagen City Heart Study, *NHANES* National Health and Nutrition Examination Survey, *CV* cardiovascular, *CVD* cardiovascular disease, *MR* mortality rate, *OR* odds ratio, *% pred* % predicted, *RR* relative risk, *CI* confidence interval, *HR* hazard ratio, +: risks lower in ex-smokers than smokers (benefits of quitting), –: risks higher in ex-smokers than smokers, 0: risks similar in ex-smokers and smokers; ?: results not clear. #: after smoking cessation; RR and HR of never smokers (reference group) 51.0.

3.3.2 Chronic Bronchitis

Chronic bronchitis is defined in clinical terms as a cough with sputum production on most days for 3 months of a year, for two consecutive years (Longmore et al. 2004).

During their lifetime, over 40 % of smokers develop chronic bronchitis (CB). It is the earliest manifestation of bronchial susceptibility to cigarette smoke and is associated with an accelerated decline in lung function, risk of developing COPD, and mortality (Pelkonen 2008).

In both sexes cigarette smoking was highly significantly associated with chronic bronchitis (Alderson et al. 1985).

In 1993, in the USA, 14 million (5.4 %) suffered from chronic bronchitis. Data show that the prevalence of CB in the general population had increased compared to 3.3 % in 1970 (Benson and Marano 1994; Wilder 1973)

According to the data of the Italian National Statistics Office (ISTAT) people who died of COPD including asthma in 1994 were 19,704, corresponding to 58 % of 33,787 deaths due to respiratory conditions; 54 % of these deaths were attributable to chronic obstructive respiratory conditions. Chronic bronchitis and pulmonary emphysema were responsible for 15,933 and 1,222 deaths. Chronic obstructive conditions are more frequent in men as compared to women (Viegi et al. 2001).

A French survey was conducted by Huchon et al. to determine the prevalence of chronic bronchitis (CB) in the French adult population and to identify the role of risk factors for CB. This study found a prevalence of 4.1 % for CB (1.7 million), 4.8 % for chronic cough, and 2.8 % for chronic expectoration; these percentages were 2.9 %, 4 %, and 2.3 %, respectively, in individuals without comorbidity. Cigarette smoking appears to be the most important risk factor, being more frequent in males than in females and increasing as the number of years of smoking cumulates; accordingly, in this survey, being a current smoker increases the risk of having CB and the risk rise with increasing numbers of pack–years since daily cigarette consumption was highest among patients with CB.

Prevalence of CB in France is similar in magnitude to that of other industrialized countries. Tobacco smoking increases the frequency of chronic bronchitis symptoms (Fig. 3.5) (Huchon et al. 2002).

The cross-sectional study performed by Desalu determined the prevalence of CB and its association with tobacco smoking among adults aged 35 years in the three selected rural communities in Ekiti state, South West, Nigeria. The prevalence of chronic bronchitis in this study was 5.6 %; 36.4 % of subjects with CB were former smokers. The multivariate logistic regression analysis showed that tobacco smoking (OR = 6.37 95 % C.I 2.12–19.14) had the strongest association with CB (Desalu 2011).

3.3.3 Emphysema

Emphysema is an obstructive airway disorder that occurs either in response to smoking; it is generally incorporated under the broader heading of COPD and is a leading cause of morbidity and mortality worldwide.

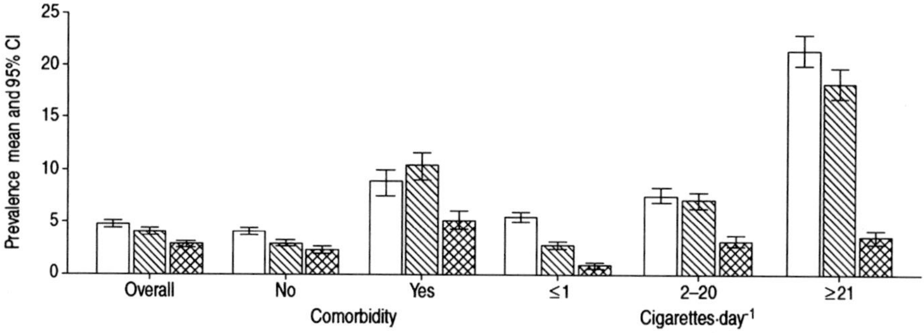

Fig. 3.5 Prevalence of CB according to smoking status and the presence or absence of comorbidity (Huchon et al. 2002)

Emphysema is a condition of the lung characterized by abnormal, permanent enlargement of the air spaces distal to the terminal bronchiole, accompanied by destruction of their walls (American Thoracic Society 1962)

When toxicants, such as cigarette smoke, are breathed into the lungs, the particles become trapped in the alveoli, causing a localized inflammatory response. Chemicals released during the inflammatory response (e.g., elastase) can eventually cause the alveolar septum to disintegrate that leads to significant deformations of the lung architecture that have important functional consequences (Nazari 1998).

Cigarette smoking is particularly associated with the centroacinar form of emphysema.

Smokers had an increased number of transected muscular arteries <200 μm in diameter ($p<0.03$), increased medial smooth muscle ($p<0.02$), and more intimal thickening ($p<0.04$). Hale et al. (1980) state that regular cigarette smoking is significantly associated with morphologic changes in the muscular pulmonary arteries that evolve with small airway disease and emphysema.

Jinno et al. (1994) analyzed retrospectively results of autopsies done on 1,940 men and 1,791 women from 1978 to 1992; emphysema was graded as follows: none (E0), slight (E1), moderate (E2), and severe (E3). Prevalence of each grade of emphysema was: in men, E0: 48.6 %, E1: 31.6 %, E2: 15.8 %, and E3: 4.0 %; in women, E0: 81.6 %, E1: 13.7 %, E2: 3.7 %, and E3: 0.8 %. Evaluating the effects of various risk factors on the severity of emphysema with multiple linear regression analysis, male sex, age, smoking habit, and grade of the anthracosis were independent factors associated to the development of emphysema; especially smoking habit was found to be a strongly contributing factor.

In America, emphysema is the fourth leading cause of death and is a leading cause of morbidity and mortality affecting over 14 million Americans (Copstead and Banasik 2000).

In England and Wales, emphysema is estimated to affect 1.5 million individuals and is the fifth most common cause of death (Health and Safety Executive 2005).

In a study of Japanese subjects undergoing annual health examination, the prevalence of emphysema was 30.5 % in smokers and increased with age. Emphysema was detected in 116 (30.5 %) of 380 current smokers, 19 (14.1 %) of 135 former smokers, and 3 (3.0 %) of 100 never smokers (Omori et al. 2006).

3.3.4 Asthma

Asthma is one the most common chronic diseases in working-age populations and its prevalence continues to increase in western countries. According to WHO estimates, 235 million people suffer from asthma. It is not just a public health problem for high income countries: it occurs in all countries regardless of level of development. Over 80 % of asthma deaths occurs in low and lower middle income countries (World Health Organization 2012).

Tobacco smoke encourages inflammation of the airways by activating the inflammatory cells, altering cell functions, and encouraging proinflammatory mediator release, neurogenic inflammation, and oxidative stress (Floreani and Rennard 1999).

During the second half of the twentieth century, the prevalence, morbidity, and, in some countries, mortality from asthma have increased. The prevalence in the USA and other English-speaking countries is higher than that other countries. Asthma morbidity rates have also risen throughout the world during the last 40 years. Asthma mortality rates declined in the USA during the 1960–1970s but have increased in the past 20 years. This trend contrasts to most of western countries, where asthma mortality rates have been decreasing in the 1990s (Beasley 2002).

Asthma now affects 22 million Americans; approximately 25–35 % of individuals with asthma are current smokers (Stapleton et al. 2011).

A Finnish case–control study assessed the effects of current and past smoking on the development of asthma in adults. The risk of developing asthma was significantly higher among current smokers with an adjusted OR of 1.33 (95 % CI: 1.00–1.77) and with an adjusted OR 1.49 (1.12–1.97) among ex-smokers when compared with never smokers. The risk of asthma was similar in both males and females and increased from occasional smoking to smoking 1–14 cigarettes/day. An increased risk of asthma was also observed among those with lifetime smoking of 1–199 cigarette–years (Piipari et al. 2004).

The study performed by LeSon and Gershwin (LeSon and Gershwin 1996) assessed risk factors for young adult asthmatics who required intubation: active smoking or exposure to SHS were important risk factors for intubation (OR 7.1; 95 % CI: 5.1–9.9).

Smoking or exposure to SHS among asthmatics increase asthma-related morbidity and disease severity and contributes to decline about 18 % in FEV_1 over 10 years (Van der Vaart et al. 2005). Jindal and collegues (Jindal et al. 1994) compared the indices of morbidity and control of asthma in patients exposed to ETS inhalation with asthmatics not exposed. The study underlined that the control of asthma was poor and morbidity greater in patients with asthma exposed to ETS, since exacerbations, missed work, and corticosteroid requirement were larger in the exposed group ($p<0.01$).

The *Epidemiological Study on the Genetics and Environment of Asthma*, carried out in France, found out a strong relation between smoking and asthma severity (Siroux et al. 2000) and evidence exists that the clinical course of the disease is worse in smoking asthmatics than in nonsmoking (Romero Palacios 2004).

A study carried out in Spain found that the evolution of asthma in smoking asthmatics was more aggressive and severe than in nonsmoking asthmatics but no evidence was found of increased incidence of asthma in smokers (Galván Fernández et al. 2000). These results were corroborated in other populations (France), where Siroux and coll. found that smoking increases asthma severity (Siroux et al. 2000).

Evidence has been also found between parental smoking with an increase in the prevalence of asthma and respiratory symptoms in children. Cook and Strachan carried out a meta-analysis and demonstrated an association and a dose-dependent relation between parental smoking and childhood asthma (OR = 1.21; 95 % CI: 1.17–1.31), wheezing (OR=1.24; 95 % CI: 1.27–1.53), and chronic cough (OR=1.4; 95 % CI: 1.27–1.53) (Cook and Strachan 1997).

McCoy's study (McCoy et al. 2006) showed that asthmatic smokers have poor asthma control vs. asthmatic nonsmokers (OR, 1.78; 95 % CI: 1.12–2.85).

An American survey in 2007 revealed that asthmatic current smokers reported more asthma attacks (OR, 1.2; 95 % CI: 1.0–1.4) and more nocturnal asthma symptoms (OR, 2.0; 95 % CI: 1.4–2.7) compared with non smokers (Strine et al. 2007).

A survey of asthmatic patients showed that smoking was significantly and inversely related to long-term control of asthma (OR, 2.6; 95 % CI: 2.0–3.4) (Schatz et al. 2006).

A cross-sectional population-based study in Norway was carried out from 1995 to 1997 to explore the prevalence of reported respiratory symptoms and diseases according to smoking burden. The lowest cumulative prevalence of asthma was reported in the group aged 40–49 (7.9 %) as compared with the groups aged 20–29 (9.3 %, $p<0.001$) and 70–79 (9.6 %, $p<0.001$). "Ever-smoking" women reported current asthma more frequently than "ever-smoking" men (6.4 % vs. 5.7 %, $p=0.005$). The prevalence of current asthma increased with increasing number of cigarettes per day in women, amounting to 10.4 % in those smoking more than 20 cigarettes per day (Langhammer et al. 2000) (Fig. 3.6).

A recent review describes the prevalence and adverse effects of cigarette smoking and SHS in asthmatics in terms of patient outcomes and response to inhaled corticosteroids. In asthmatic smokers disease control is poorer. In addition, maternal exposure increases the frequency and severity of asthma and decreases lung function in children: offspring are 1.8 times more likely to develop asthma and a lifetime history of wheezing (Pattenden et al. 2006).

Smokers have a corticosteroid resistance due to an increased airway mucosal permeability and a decreased histone deacetylase activity: it is clear that cigarette smoking and SHS in asthmatics lead to detrimental effects in patient outcomes and effectiveness of steroid therapy (Stapleton et al. 2011).

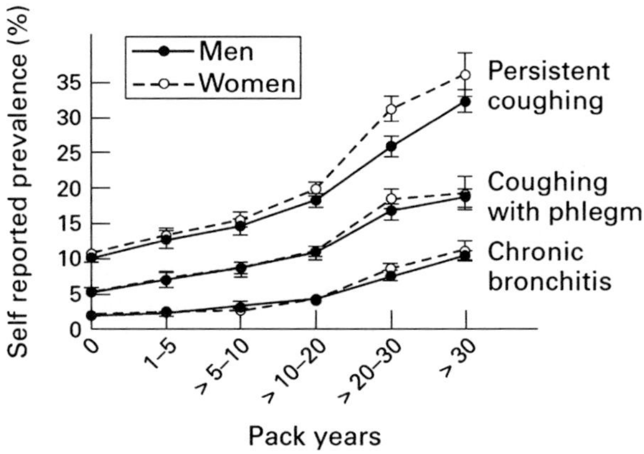

Fig. 3.6 Age–adjusted prevalence of persistent coughing, coughing with phlegm, and chronic bronchitis by number of pack–years in men and women (95 % confidence intervals). Nord-Trøndelag, Norway 1997 (Langhammer et al. 2000)

3.4 Other Diseases

3.4.1 Acne

Acne vulgaris is an inflammatory disease involving the pilosebaceous follicles. Clinically acne is characterized by a typical lesional pleomorphism: the same patient may simultaneously manifest comedones, papules, pustules, nodules, cysts, and scars, deeply impacting on their quality of life and social wellbeing (Mannocci et al. 2010)

Acne vulgaris is considered to be the most common skin disorder in mid-adolescents affecting over 80 % of teenagers in westernized societies and it has a considerable impact on quality of life (Simpson and Cunliffe 2004; Gelmetti et al. 2003; Kerkemeyer 2005).

Several studies have shown that the prevalence of acne varies from 28.9 to 91.3 % in adolescent populations (Purvis et al. 2004; Stathakis et al. 1997; Smithard et al. 2001; Kilkenny et al. 1998).

It affects about 17 million people in the USA, including 85 % or more of adolescents and young adults (Krowchuk and Lucky 2001); it is the fourth most common reason for patients aged 11–21 years to visit a doctor (Ziv et al. 1999) and accounts for 4 % of all visits by patients aged 15–19 years (Stern 1996).

Data gathered from a questionnaire survey in Hong Kong showed that the prevalence of self-reported acne, was 91.3 %: at the time of interview, 52.2 % had acne (Yeung et al. 2002).

A cross-sectional study illustrated that the prevalence of facial acne among the adolescents attending secondary schools in Malaysia was 67.5 %. Facial acne increased with increasing age ($p=0.001$). It was more common among males (71.1 %) than females (64.6 %), $p=0.165$. Males also had a higher prevalence of severe acne ($p=0.001$). In addition, students with severe acne had higher levels of Cardiff Acne Disability Index ($\rho=0.521$) (Hanisah et al. 2009)

Acne vulgaris has a multifactorial pathogenesis, but the contribution of smoking to acne shows contradictory results.

As a matter of fact, some studies have shown that cigarette smoking aggravate acne (Schafer et al. 2001; Green and Sinclair 2001), others did not confirm this association (Jemec et al. 2002) or even showed a protective effect (Klaz et al. 2006; Rombouts et al. 2007).

A large cohort of young men, from 1983 to 2003, investigated the relationship between cigarette smoking and severe acne. Active smokers showed a significantly lower prevalence of severe acne (0.71 %) than nonsmokers (1.01 %) ($p=0.0078$). An inverse dose-dependent relationship between severe acne prevalence and daily cigarette consumption became significant from 21 cigarettes a day (χ^2 and trend test: $p<0.0001$), OR 0.2 (95 % CI: 0.06–0.63) (Klaz et al. 2006).

A cross-sectional study suggested a significant negative association between smoking and inflammatory acne in girls. Smoking, daily cigarette consumption, and duration of smoking appeared to be protective in the development of inflammatory acne in girls (adjusted OR=0.41, 95 % CI:0.13, 0.82) (Rombouts et al. 2007).

On the contrary, according to a cross-sectional study, smoking appears to be a clinically important contributory factor to acne prevalence and severity. Acne was present in 26.8 % of the persons examined, it was more prevalent in men (29.9 %) than women (23.7 %) (OR 1.37, 95 % CI: 1.01–1.87), with peak prevalence between 14 and 29 years ($p<0.001$). According to multiple logistic regression analyses acne prevalence was significantly higher in active smokers (40.8 %, OR 2.04, 95 % CI: 1.40–2.99) as compared with nonsmokers (25.2 %). Moreover, a significant linear relationship between acne prevalence and number of cigarettes smoked daily was obtained (trend test: $p<0.0001$) and a significant dose-dependent relationship between acne severity and daily cigarette consumption was shown by linear regression analysis ($p=0.001$) (Schafer et al. 2001).

A population-based study examined the prevalence of acne among Danish adolescents: 40.7 % for men and 23.8 % for women (OR: 0.46, 95 % CI: 0.24–0.85). The use of tobacco smoking was not significantly associated with acne (OR: 0.54, 95 % CI: 0.17–1.78) (Jemec et al. 2002).

An Iranian study performed by Firooz et al. (2005) did not found an association between acne and cigarette smoking: 4.1 % acne patients and 9.0 % control patients were current smokers (OR=0.43, 95 % CI: 0.22–0.87, $p<0.05$), but after adjustment for sex, this difference was not significant (OR=0.61, 95 % CI: 0.30–1.26, $p>0.05$).

Recently, Mannocci et al. (2010) carried out a systematic review and meta-analysis concerning the association between acne and smoking. The first meta-analysis, including all studies, showed a nonsignificant role of smoke in the development of acne: OR 1.05 (95 % CI: 0.66–1.67) with random effect estimate. The second meta-analyses, including data stratified by gender, showed a OR=0.99 (95 % CI: 0.57–1.73) for males and a OR of 1.45 (95 % CI: 0.08–24.64) for females, using random effect for the heterogeneity in both cases. The third meta-analysis, included studies with a quality score >6 resulted in an estimated OR=0.69 (95 % CI: 0.55–0.85): in this case it was possible to use the fixed effect estimate. The last

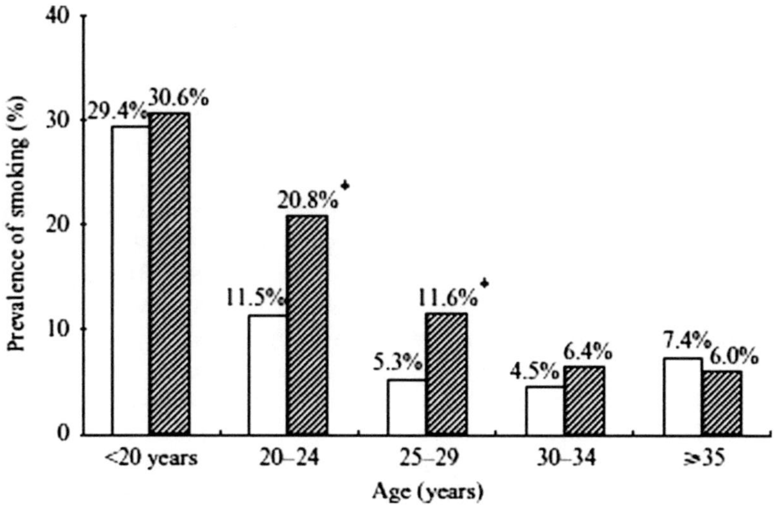

Fig. 3.7 Smoking prevalence according to survey year and maternal age category. *$p<0.01$ between 1990 and 2000 (using χ^2 test). (*Empty bar*) 1990, (*Crossed bar*) 2000 (Takimoto et al. 2005)

meta-analysis, concerning the severity grading, showed a nonsignificant result: OR = 1.09 (95 % CI: 0.61–1.95) using the random effect approach. The first two meta-analyses found no signification association between smoking and the development of acne but the analysis with only good quality studies showed a protective significant effect.

3.4.2 Low Birth Weight

The association between maternal smoking and retarded fetal grow was first time described in 1957 (Simpson 1957).

Despite current knowledge about the negative effects of smoking during pregnancy, it has been estimated that 15–25 % of women smoke during pregnancy and although a minority stop smoking for part of their pregnancy, most of them start again after delivery (Owen and Penn 1999) (Fig. 3.7).

Low birth weight (LBW), <2,500 g, is one of the most reported complications of tobacco smoke in the scientific literature (Kramer 1987).

This condition is related to an increase of perinatal morbidity and mortality, and LBW is, in fact, the second cause of perinatal death after premature birth (De Bernabè et al. 2004).

The number of cigarettes smoked during pregnancy is strictly related increases risk of spontaneous abortion, placenta previa, abruptio placenta, preterm premature rupture of membranes, stillbirth, preterm delivery, and congenital malformations (Polańska and Hanke 2004) (Fig. 3.8).

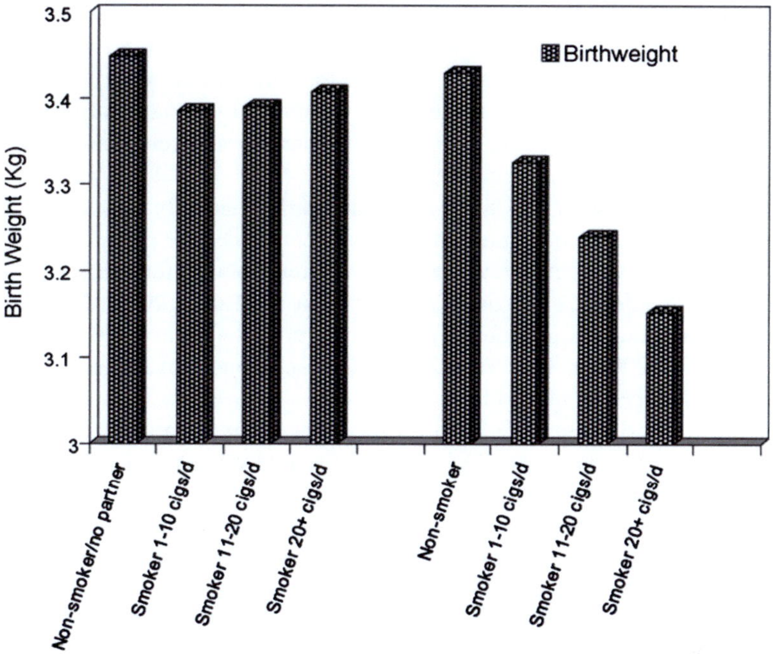

Fig. 3.8 Estimated effects of maternal smoking or exposure to secondhand smoke (by partner's smoking status) on birth weight. Significant trends for effect were observed for both secondhand smoke ($p \leq 0.007$) and active maternal smoking ($p \leq 0.001$) (Ward et al. 2007)

Recent studies also indicate that prenatal exposure to tobacco smoke is a risk factor long-term effects on infants, including respiratory infections, asthma, allergy, childhood cancer, and neurodevelopmental disorders (Polańska and Hanke 2005).

Both maternal and paternal smoking is associated with LBW, and this dose–response relationship seems to be more pronounced among older (30 years) mothers (Windham et al. 2000).

Smokers women have 2–3 times increased risk to deliver an LBW infant with an average decrease in baby's weight of 150–300 g at birth (Vardavas et al. 2010).

Smokers have an increased risk also for a *small for gestational age* (SGA) infant, with a RR ranging from 1.3 to 10.0 (US Department of Health and Human Services, Public Health Service 2001b).

It has been estimated that smoking is responsible for 15 % of all preterm births, 20–30 % of all infants of LBW, and a 150 % increase in overall perinatal mortality. Approximately 15–20 % of women smoke during pregnancy. Cigarette smoking is the most important risk factor in developed countries and is one of the most important and modifiable risk factors of adverse perinatal outcomes (Andres and Day 2000)

The direct effect of smoking on neonatal mortality is weak: maternal smoking appears to have the strongest effect on birth weight through growth retardation and through a shortened gestation. Neonatal mortality among women who smoked during their pregnancy was higher among infants that were between −5 and −1 and between 1 and 5 standard deviation units of the birth weight distribution among smokers. When neonatal mortality rates were examined by gestational age, the mortality curve was higher at every gestational age among smokers than among nonsmokers ($p < 0.001$) (Ananth and Platt 2004).

The prevalence of smoking during pregnancy varies markedly across countries. In many industrialized countries, prevalence rates seems to decline (Cnattingius 2004).

Information on smoking prevalence during pregnancy in the USA is available from the *U.S. Standard Certificate of Live Birth*. In 1989 about 20 % of US pregnant women smoked, but the prevalence decreased from 18.4 % in 1990 to 15.2 % in 2000, 11.4 % in 2002 to 13.8 % in 2005 (U.S. Department of Health and Human Services 2002; Murin et al. 2011).

Smoking during pregnancy is most prevalent among Native Americans and Alaskan natives (20 % in 2000), 16 % of non-Hispanic Whites, 9 % of non-Hispanic Blacks, and 4 % of Hispanics smoke (Martin et al. 2002).

In Sweden, the population-based Swedish Medical Birth Register includes self-reported information about smoking during pregnancy. In 1983, 31 % of Swedish pregnant women smoked; in 1989, 26 % smoked; in 1993, 20 % smoked; in 1997, 15 % smoked; and in 2000, 13 % smoked. Furthermore, 18 % of pregnant women stopped smoking before being registered to antenatal care, 11 % stopped smoking later during pregnancy, and another 6 % stopped smoking temporarily during pregnancy (Cnattingius 2004).

In Canada, cigarette smoking during pregnancy decreased from 31 % in 1992 to 12 % in 2002 (Dodds 1995; Chan et al. 2005).

The same, in Australia, the percentage of women reporting smoking during pregnancy decreased from 23 % in 2001 to 20 % in 2004 (Laws and Hilder 2008).

During the last years, Denmark has experienced a decline in maternal smoking too, from 22 % in 1997 to 16 % in 2005, even if among women younger than 20 years, the prevalence increased from 37 % in 1997 to 43 % in 2005 (Jensen et al. 2008).

Maternal smoking prevalence differs according to several factors, such as age, race, education, and socioeconomic status. Smoking prevalence during pregnancy is influenced by maternal education: in the USA only 2 % of college-educated women reported smoking during pregnancy in 2000, whereas 25 % of nongraduated women smoked (Martin et al. 2002).

The same, in Sweden, 3 % of highly educated women smoked during pregnancy in 1997, compared with 34 % of women with lower education (Cnattingius 2004).

Women who have had previous pregnancies, with low education, who started smoking early in life, heavy smokers, and women exposed to passive smoking at home or at work also are more likely to continue to smoke during pregnancy; in addition, higher smoking rates are reported among younger pregnant women (U.S. Department of Health and Human Services 2001a).

Windham et al. (1999) performed a retrospective study and a review of the literature to examine the relationship between ETS exposure and LBW. The risk of LBW at term was increased (adjusted OR = 1.8, 95 % CI: 0.6–4.8) and SGA (<10th percentile of weight; OR = 1.4, 95 % CI: 0.8–2.5). These results were in the range of the other studies in the literature that had OR from 1.0 to 2.2, the pooled estimate was 1.2 (95 % CI: 1.1–1.3) in nonsmoking women. The pooled estimate of mean birthweight indicated a decrement of 28 g with ETS exposure of nonsmoking women (95 % CI: −41 to −16), with a greater decrement (about 40 g) seen among more homogeneous studies.

Comparing smokers to nonsmokers, the adjusted OR was 2.8 (95 % CI: 1.7–4.6) for LBW and 2.6 (95 %CI: 1.6–4.2) for fetal growth restriction, that corresponded to a 119-g reduction in birth weight, a 0.53-cm reduction in length, and a 0.35-cm reduction in head circumference (Vardavas et al. 2010).

Salmasi et al. (2010) carried out a meta-analysis to determine the effect of ETS on perinatal outcomes. ETS-exposed infants weighed less [weighted mean differences (WMD) −60 g, 95 % CI: −80 to −39 g], with a trend towards (LBW, RR 1.16; 95 % CI: 0.99–1.36), although the duration of gestation and preterm delivery were similar (WMD 0.02 weeks, 95 % CI: −0.09 to 0.12 weeks and RR 1.07; 95 % CI: 0.93–1.22). ETS-exposed infants had longer infant lengths (1.75 cm; 95 % CI: 1.37–2.12 cm), increased risks of congenital anomalies (OR 1.17; 95 % CI: 1.03–1.34) and a trend towards smaller head circumferences (−0.11 cm; 95 % CI: −0.22 to 0.01 cm).

Smoking during pregnancy is the leading cause of adverse maternal and fetal effects, nevertheless women who stopped smoking during pregnancy are at the lower risk for most of those pathologies.

First-trimester quitters reduced their odds of delivering a preterm non-SGA newborn by 31 % (aOR 0.69, 95 % CI: 0.65–0.74), a term SGA newborn by 55 % (aOR 0.45, 95 % CI: 0.42–0.48), and a preterm SGA newborn by 53 % (aOR 0.47, 95 % CI: 0.40–0.55), similar to nonsmokers. Second-trimester quitters also reduced their odds of delivering preterm non-SGA and term SGA newborns but to a lesser magnitude (Polakowski et al. 2009).

3.4.3 *Sudden Infant Death Syndrome*

Sudden infant death syndrome (SIDS) is generally defined as the sudden and unexpected death of an infant <1 year of age, apparently occurring during sleep, that remains unexplained after thorough investigation, such as autopsy and review of circumstances of death and the clinical history (Krous et al. 2004).

SIDS is the most common cause of postneonatal death in developed countries (Anderson and Cook 1997), and it is the third leading cause of all infant mortality in the USA for 2002 (Mathews et al. 2004).

Maternal smoking is one of the major risk factor for SIDS (Martin et al. 2008; Anderson and Cook 1997), since it is responsible for an estimated 1,200–2,200 deaths from SIDS (DiFranza and Lew 1995); assuming a causal association between smoking and SIDS, about one-third of SIDS deaths might have been prevented avoiding maternal smoking in utero (Mitchell and Milerad 2006).

The risk of SIDS among infants of daily smokers is commonly doubled, tripled or more, compared with nonsmokers (MacDorman et al. 1997).

Some authors report evidence that nicotine may affect the ventilatory response to hypoxia, with an impairment of the peripheral autonomic nervous system and an absent adrenomedullary response to hypoxia after nicotine exposure (Anderson and Cook 1997; Slotkin 1998).

Within the past years, the number of deaths attributed SIDS has fallen considerably in the UK (almost 70 % from 1593 in 1988 to 531 in 1992), New Zealand, Australia, the Netherlands, Norway, Denmark, and Ireland (Gilbert 1994).

The rate of SIDS also declined significantly in Canada and the US between the late 1980s and the early 2000s. In the US, this decline is partly due in part to a shift in diagnosis. Deaths from SIDS decreased from 78.4 (95 % CI: 73.4, 83.4) per 100,000 livebirths in 1991–1995 to 48.5 (95 % CI: 44.3, 52.7) in 1996–2000 and to 34.6 (95 % CI: 31.0, 38.3) in 2001–2005 (Gilbert et al. 2012).

The large differences in SIDS rates between race/ethnic groups in the USA have been pointed out; moreover the overall SIDS rate is higher in the USA than in several other developed countries. The adjusted ORs ranged from 1.6 to 2.5 for mothers who smoked 1–9 cigarettes per day during pregnancy and from 2.3 to 3.8 for mothers who smoked ten or more cigarettes. Although birth weight had a strong independent effect on SIDS, the addition of birth weight to the models lowered the odds ratios for maternal smoking only slightly, suggesting that the effect of smoking on SIDS is not mediated through birth weight (MacDorman et al. 1997) (Fig. 3.9).

A systematic review conducted by Anderson and Cook (Anderson and Cook 1997) established that maternal smoking increases the risk of SIDS, and a causal relationship between SIDS and postnatal exposure to tobacco smoke was found.

The risk of SIDS increased with the number of cigarettes smoked by the mother and if both parents smoked (Nicholl and O'Cathain 1992).

A meta-analysis comparing women who smoke during pregnancy with nonsmokers calculated a pooled OR of 2.98 (95 % CI: 2.51–3.54) (DiFranza and Lew 1995).

The effect of postnatal smoking on SIDS risk has been examined predominately in retrospective case–control studies: a review of these studies found consistent evidence for a dose–response effect between maternal smoking and SIDS (Golding 1997; MacDorman et al. 1997).

A case–control analysis performed by Schoendorf and Kiely attempted to separate the effects of prenatal exposure from those of postnatal exposure. The risk of SIDS was increased in infants with only postpartum exposure to tobacco smoke but was even greater with both prenatal and postnatal exposures. Among black infants the OR was 2.4 for passive exposure and 2.9 for combined exposure (maternal smoking during both pregnancy and infancy). Among white infants the OR was 2.2 for passive exposure and 4.1 for combined exposure. After adjustment for demographic risk factors, the odds ratio for SIDS among normal birth weight infants was approximately 2 for passive exposure and 3 for combined exposure for both races. It appears clear that both intrauterine and passive tobacco exposure are associated with an increased risk of SIDS (Schoendorf and Kiely 1992).

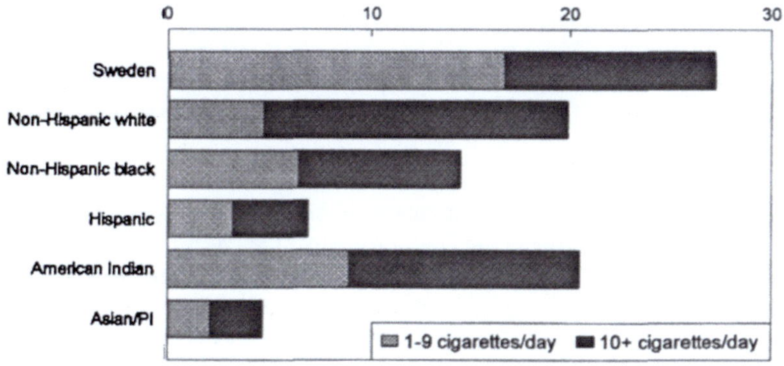

Fig. 3.9 Percentage of mothers who smoked during pregnancy: Sweden, 1983–1992 and total of 45 US states and Washington, DC, 1990–1991. *PI* Pacific Islander (MacDorman et al. 1997)

The large National Maternal and Infant Health Survey in the USA calculated the adjusted OR for both prenatal and postnatal smoking combined was greater (OR=3.10, 95 % CI: 2.27–4.24) than for independent postnatal smoking (OR=1.75,95 % CI: 1.04–2.95) (Schoendorf and Kiely 1992)

3.4.4 Maculopathy

The age-related macular degeneration (AMD) is a multifactorial degenerative disease that affects the macula, that is the portion of the retina responsible for the distinct vision. The AMD occurs when the layer of the retina, responsible for the nutrition of the cones and rods and the disposal of waste products resulting from the metabolism, performs these functions with lower efficacy, due to the aging; consequently the macula deteriorates causing the loss of vision in the central part of the vision field, but leaving peripheral vision intact (Nicolotti et al. 2009).

The clinical and histopathological features of AMD include a relationship with age, the presence of pigmentary disturbances, drusen, thickening of Bruch's membrane, and basal laminar deposits. AMD is an advanced stage of a deteriorative process that takes place in all eyes. The primary lesion in AMD appears to reside in the retinal pigment epithelium (RPE), possibly resulting from its high rate of molecular degradation. These residual bodies (lipofuscin) are remnants of the incomplete degradation of abnormal molecules which have been damaged within the RPE cells or derived from phagocytized rod and cone membranes (Young 1987).

AMD is the leading cause of blindness among people aged 50 years or older in developed countries and the third cause of global blindness. In the USA, it is estimated to affect 16–26 % of people aged 65 years or older (Congdon et al. 2004).

Augood et al. (2006) in the *European Eye Study* (EUREYE) estimated the prevalence of age-related maculopathy in an older population from seven European countries (Norway, Estonia, UK, France, Italy, Greece, and Spain): the prevalence of geographic atrophic AMD was 1.2 % (95 % CI: 0.8–1.7 %) and of neovascular AMD, 2.3 % (95 % CI: 1.7–2.9 %). The prevalence of bilateral AMD was 1.4 % (95 % CI: 1.0–1.8 %). The Italian prevalence of advanced AMD was 3.68 % (CI 95 %: 2:17–5:18).

"Eye Diseases Prevalence Research Group" expected that there will be a substantial increase in the number of patients with AMD by 50 %, from 1.75 million in 2000 to 2.95 million in 2020 in the USA (Tomany et al. 2004).

VanNewkirk et al. (2000) have found a prevalence of neovascular AMD of 0.39 % (CI 95 %: 0:20–0:58) in Australia.

Finally in China, in 2008, Chen et al. (2008) the prevalence of advanced AMD (neovascular and atrophic) of 1.9 % in persons with an age greater than or equal to 65 years.

The literature review performed by Nicolotti et al. (2009) shows a substantial homogeneity of the prevalence and incidence of AMD in different countries of the world: data found in European studies are comparable with those from the American population, as well as those obtained in Australia and China (Nicolotti et al. 2009).

Two studies published on JAMA in 1996 (Christen et al. 1996; Seddon et al. 1996) show that people who smoke more than 20–25 cigarettes a day have a risk which is about 140 times greater than nonsmoking.

Regarding the development of neovascular AMD, smokers seem to have a greater risk of developing pathology, comparing with nonsmokers (Tomany et al. 2004). Men who smoked greater amounts of cigarettes were more likely to develop early age-related maculopathy (OR per 10 pack–years smoked = 1.06, 95 % Cl 1.00–1.13, $p = 0.06$) than men who had smoked less. This association was not observed in women (Klein et al. 1998).

A recent meta-analysis (Cong et al. 2008) shows that smokers or ex-smokers have a statistically significant risk to develop AMD both in case–control studies (OR = 1.76, 95 % CI: 1.56–1.99) and cohort studies (RR = 1.61, 95 % CI: 1:01–2:57); finally, smoking also appears to increase the risk of choroidal neovascularization, with an OR of 1.96 (95 % CI: 1.69–2.27) in case–control studies, while considering the cohort studies an RR of 1.47 (95 % CI: 0.92–2.37) is highlighted.

The Blue Mountains Eye Study highlighted that current smokers had an increased risk of 5-year incident late ARM lesions and that they develop late ARM at a significantly earlier age than never or past smokers. Age-standardized incidence rates for any late ARM lesions were 3.1 %, 1.2 %, and 1.4 %, respectively, among baseline current, past, or never smokers; corresponding age-standardized incidence rates for early ARM were 10.6 %, 8.2 %, and 9.3 %, respectively. The mean age for cases with incident late ARM was 67 years for baseline current smokers, 73 years for past smokers, and 77 years for those who had never smoked ($p = 0.02$). After adjusting for age, current smokers had an increased risk of incident geographic atrophy (age-adjusted RR, 3.6; 95 % CI: 1.1–11.3) and any late ARM lesions (RR, 2.5; 95 % CI: 1.0–6.2) (Mitchell et al. 2002).

3.4.5 Smoking-Related Allergy

An allergy is a hypersensitivity disorder of the immune system, since allergic reactions may take place when a person's immune system reacts to normally harmless substances in the environment (Kay 2000).

An increase in allergic diseases in Western countries has been observed in all epidemiological studies. An adjuvant effect of smoking on IgE antibody production has been observed and it might be due to damage to airways mucosa and supports the mucosal theory of atopy (Zetterstrom et al. 1981).

As a matter of fact, the precise mechanism for the atopy is not known; the risk of sensitization in an individual depends on the degree of exposure to a potential allergen: the greater the exposure the higher is the prevalence of sensitization (Fuiano and Incorvaia 2011).

Smoking is a well-documented risk factor for occupational allergy, possibly by increasing mucosal transport of antigen. The study of TCPA workers showed a statistically significant interaction between smoking and atopy (defined on skin tests with common aeroallergens): 16 % of 31 atopic smokers had IgE antibody against TCPA, 12 % of 111 non-atopic smokers, 8 % of 36 atopic nonsmokers but none of 98 non-atopic nonsmokers (Venables et al. 1988).

Increased atopic sensitisation in smokers might lead to an overrepresentation of allergic diseases among them (Zetterstrom et al. 1981).

Chi et al. (2012) have reported that cigarette smoke extract (CSE) significantly increased IL-6 and IL-8 production in IL-1-activated human mast cell line (HMC-1).

In addition, maternal cigarette smoking can modify aspects of fetal immune function: maternal smoking in pregnancy was associated with significantly higher neonatal T helper type 2 (IL-13 protein) responses to both allergens ovalbumin (OVA) ($p=0.035$) and house dust mite (HDM) ($p=0.01$)] and these effects remained statistically significant after allowing for confounding factors, including the effects of maternal atopy (Noakes et al. 2003).

A Croatian study investigated the impact of active and passive smoking on total and specific serum IgE levels and on incidence of developing allergic diseases. Statistically significant higher prevalence of allergic diseases was found in passive smokers as opposed to nonsmokers ($\chi^2=9.29, p=0.002$) as well as in active smokers compared to nonsmokers ($\chi^2=4.45$, $p=0.034$). The same, total IgE (IU/ml) was significantly higher in passive smokers when compared to nonsmokers ($t=13.039$, $p<0.01$) and in passive smokers as opposed to active smokers as well ($t=4.960$, $p<0.01$). Results of the study indicate that clinical manifestations of allergic diseases are more frequent in smokers (both active and passive) than in nonsmokers (Mlinaric et al. 2011).

A Swedish study was performed to assess the influence of some risk factors for onset of allergic rhinitis and asthma. Onset of asthma was associated with smoking (OR=3.0) and this association is particularly strong among nonatopics (OR=5.7) (Plaschke et al. 2000).

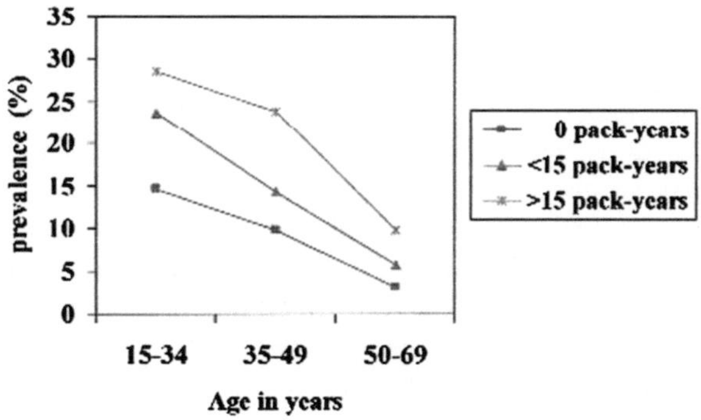

Fig. 3.10 Prevalence of nickel contact allergy by age and smoking among women (Linneberg et al. 2003)

Smoke seems to influence even the development of allergic rhinitis. Allergic rhinitis is common inflammatory disorder of nasal mucosa with a significant impact on quality of life. It can affect 25–35 % of people, depending on the population studied (Weber 2008); despite its high prevalence is often undiagnosed. In the USA, AR results in 3.5 million lost workdays and two million lost schooldays annually (Nathan 2007). Risk factors for allergic rhinitis include heavy maternal smoking during the first year of life (Greiner et al. 2011).

One study of 80 atopic children with wheezy bronchitis showed a significantly increased risk (RR=2) of developing persistent wheezy bronchitis among passive smokers after 4 years (Geller-Bernstein et al. 1987).

A population study in Denmark move up the hypothesis that smoking increases the risk of contact allergy, which is a major public health problem in industrialized countries. Contact allergy (adjusted OR, 1.8; 95 % CI: 1.2–2.9), nickel contact allergy (adjusted OR, 2.7; 95 % CI: 1.4–5.2), and allergic nickel contact dermatitis (adjusted OR, 3.0; 95 % CI: 1.5–6.2) were significantly associated with a smoking history of more than 15 pack–years (Linneberg et al. 2003) (Fig. 3.10).

3.4.6 Early Menopause

Epidemiological literature defines natural menopause when a woman has experienced 12 consecutive months of amenorrhea without an obvious intervening cause, such as exogenous hormone use, dietary deficiencies, or surgical removal of the uterus or ovaries (Harlow and Signorello 2000) (Fig. 3.11).

The overall median age at natural menopause should be 51.4 years; however, Japanese women have a later natural menopause than Caucasian, African-American, Hispanic, or Chinese women (Gold et al. 2001).

Several studies have examined that cigarette smoking has shown to affect menopause onset: the findings support the hypothesis that cigarette smoking is cytotoxic to the ovaries, leading to premature menopause (Harlow and Signorello 2000; Hardy et al. 2000), with smokers frequently reaching menopause as much as 1.5

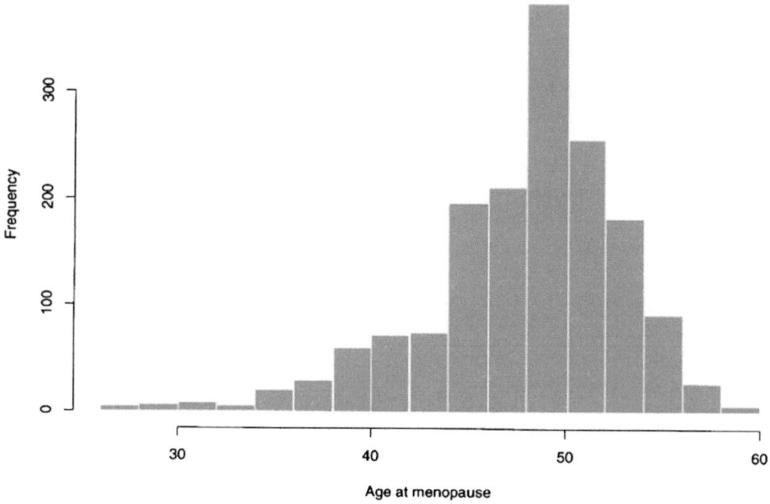

Fig. 3.11 Histogram for the age at natural menopause in 1693 postmenopausal Australian female twins born between 1893 and 1962 (Do, K. A., Broom, B. M., Kuhnert, P., et al. (2000).Genetic analysis of the age at menopause by using estimating equations and Bayesian random effects models. *Statistics in Medicine, 19*(9), 1217–1235)

years sooner than nonsmokers and smokers at greater risk of surgical menopause than nonsmokers.

In the study conducted by Pokoradi et al. (2011), smokers had a mean age at menopause of 45.6 years (SD 6.04 years) while nonsmokers' mean age at menopause was 46.9 years (SD 5.7 years).

The National Survey of Health and Development found that current smoking at age 36 years was associated with significantly increased risk of reaching menopause earlier than nonsmokers (Hardy et al. 2000).

In addition, also, the Massachusetts Women's Health Study found that current smokers reached menopause at a significantly younger age than nonsmokers (McKinlay et al. 1985).

Extensive searching of public literature databases by Sun et al. (2012) found that smoking is a significant independent factor for early age at natural menopause (ANM). Among the studies analyzed, the phenotype of the participants in five studies was classified as early or late ANM ("dichotomous" studies), and odds ratio (OR) was used to evaluate the effect of smoking on early ANM. For the other six studies ("continuous" studies), mean and standard deviation were provided for smoking and nonsmoking samples, and WMD was used as the effect size. The pooled effect was OR=0.74 (95 % CI: 0.60–0.91, $p<0.01$) in the "dichotomous" studies; for the "continuous" ones, the pooled effect estimated by weighted mean difference (WMD) was −1.12 (95 % CI: −1.80 to −0.44, $p=0.04$). After adjustment for heterogeneity, the pooled results were OR=0.67 (95 % CI: 0.61–0.73, $p<0.01$) for "dichotomous" studies and WMD=−0.90 (95 % CI: −1.58 to −0.21, $p=0.01$) for the "continuous" ones.

References

Aggarwal, S., Qamar, A., Sharma, V., Sharma, A. (2011). Abdominal aortic aneurysm: A comprehensive review. *Experimental and Clinical Cardiology, 16*(1), 11–15.

Alderson, M. R., Lee, P. N., & Wang, R. (1985). Risks of lung cancer, chronic bronchitis, ischaemic heart disease, and stroke in relation to type of cigarette smoked. *Journal of Epidemiology and Community Health, 39*(4), 286–293.

American Thoracic Society. (1962). Chronic bronchitis, asthma and pulmonary emphysema: A statement by the committee on diagnostic standards for nontubercoulose respiratory diseases. *American Review of Respiratory Disease, 85*, 762–768.

Ananth, C. V., & Platt, R. W. (2004). Reexamining the effects of gestational age, fetal growth, and maternal smoking on neonatal mortality. *BMC Pregnancy and Childbirth, 4*(1), 22.

Anderson, H. R., & Cook, D. G. (1997). Passive smoking and sudden infant death syndrome: Review of the epidemiological evidence. *Thorax, 52*(11), 1003–1009.

Andres, R. L., & Day, M. C. (2000). Perinatal complications associated with maternal tobacco use. *Seminars in Neonatology, 5*(3), 231–241.

Augood, C. A., Vingerling, J. R., de Jong, P. T., et al. (2006). Prevalence of age-related maculopathy in older Europeans: The European Eye Study (EUREYE). *Archives of Ophthalmology, 124*(4), 529–535.

Bano, R., Ahmad, N., Mahagaonkar, A. M., et al. (2011). Study of lung functions in smokers and non-smokers in rural India. *Indian Journal of Physiology and Pharmacology, 55*(1), 84–88.

Beasley, R. (2002). The burden of asthma with specific reference to the United States. *The Journal of Allergy and Clinical Immunology, 109*(Suppl. 5), S482–S489.

Benson, V., & Marano, M. A. (1994). Current estimate from the National Health Interview Survey, 1993. Vital and Health Statistics—Series 10, No. 190, 1–221

Brady, A. R., Thompson, S. G., Fowkes, F. G., et al. (2004). Abdominal aortic aneurysm expansion risk factors and time intervals for surveillance. *Circulation, 110*, 16–21.

Bjartveit, K., & Tverdal, A. (2005). Health consequences of smoking 1–4 cigarettes per day. *Tobacco Control, 14*(5), 315–320.

Brewster, D. C., Cronenwett, J. L., Hallett, J. W., Jr., et al. (2003). Guidelines for the treatment of abdominal aortic aneurysms. Report of a subcommittee of the joint council of the american association for vascular surgery and society for vascular surgery. *Journal of Vascular Surgery, 37*, 1106–1117.

Burns, D., Cummings, K. M., & Hoffmann, D. (1998). Cigars: Health effects and trends (Smoking and tobacco control Monograph No. 9 (NIH Publication No. 98–4302)). Bethesda, MD: US Department of Health and Human Services, National Institutes of Health, National Cancer Institute.

Calverley, P. M., & Koulouris, N. G. (2005). Flow limitation and dynamic hyperinflation: Key concepts in modern respiratory physiology. *European Respiratory Journal, 25*(1), 186–199.

Centers for Disease Control and Prevention (CDC). (2008). Smoking-attributable mortality, years of potential life lost, and productivity losses—United States, 2000–2004. *MMWR. Morbidity and Mortality Weekly Report, 57*(45), 1226–1228.

Centers for Disease Control and Prevention (CDC). (2009). State-specific smoking-attributable mortality and years of potential life lost—United States, 2000–2004. *MMWR. Morbidity and Mortality Weekly Report, 58*(2), 29–33.

Centers for Disease Control and Prevention (CDC). (2011). Prevalence of coronary heart disease—United States, 2006–2010. *MMWR. Morbidity and Mortality Weekly Report, 60*(40), 1377–1381.

Chan, B., Einarson, A., & Koren, G. (2005). Effectiveness of bupropion for smoking cessation during pregnancy. *Journal of Addictive Diseases, 24*(2), 19–23.

Chang, J. B., Stein, T. A., Liu, J. P., et al. (1997). Risk factors associated with rapid growth of small abdominal aortic aneurysms. *Surgery, 121*, 117–122.

Chen, S. J., Cheng, C. Y., Peng, K. L., et al. (2008). Prevalence and associated risk factors of age-related macular degeneration in an elderly Chinese population in Taiwan: The Shihpai Eye Study. *Investigative Ophthalmology and Visual Science, 49*(7), 3126–3133.

Chi, D. S., Lin, T. C., Hall, K., et al. (2012). Enhanced effects of cigarette smoke extract on inflammatory cytokine expression in IL-1beta-activated human mast cells were inhibited by baicalein via regulation of the NF-kappaB pathway. *Clinical and Molecular Allergy, 10*(1), 3.

Christen, W. G., Glynn, R. J., Manson, J. E., et al. (1996). A prospective study of cigarette smoking and risk of age-related macular degeneration in men. *Journal of the American Medical Association, 276*, 1147–1151.

Cnattingius, S. (2004). The epidemiology of smoking during pregnancy: Smoking prevalence, maternal characteristics, and pregnancy outcomes. *Nicotine and Tobacco Research, 6*(Suppl 2), S125–S140.

Cong, R., Zhou, B., Sun, Q., et al. (2008). Smoking and the risk of age-related macular degeneration: A meta-analysis. *Annals of Epidemiology, 18*(8), 647–656.

Congdon, N., O'Colmain, B., Klaver, C. C., et al. (2004). Causes and prevalence of visual impairment among adults in United States: Eye Diseases Prevalence Research Group. *Archives of Ophthalmology, 122*, 477–485.

Cook, D. G., & Strachan, D. P. (1997). Health effects of passive smoking: 3. Parental smoking and prevalence of respiratory symptoms and asthma in school age children. *Thorax, 52*, 1081–1094.

Copstead, C. L., & Banasik, L. J. (2000). *Pathophysiology biological and behavioural perspectives* (2nd ed.). Philadelphia: Elsevier.

Critchley, J., & Capewell, S. (2004). Smoking cessation for the secondary prevention of coronary heart disease. *Cochrane Database of Systematic Reviews,* (1), CD003041.

De Bernabè, J. V., Soriano, T., Albaladejo, R., et al. (2004). Risk factors for low birth weight: A review. *European Journal of Obstetrics, Gynecology, and Reproductive Biology, 116*, 3–15.

De Flora, S., Izzotti, A., Walsh, A., et al. (1997). Molecular epidemiology of atherosclerosis. *The FASEB Journal, 11*(12), 1021–1031.

Desalu, O. O. (2011). Prevalence of chronic bronchitis and tobacco smoking in some rural communities in Ekiti state, Nigeria. *The Nigerian Postgraduate Medical Journal, 18*(2), 91–97.

DiFranza, J. R., & Lew, R. A. (1995). Effect of maternal cigarette smoking on pregnancy complications and sudden infant death syndrome. *Journal of Family Practice, 40*(4), 385–394.

Dodds, L. (1995). Prevalence of smoking among pregnant women in Nova Scotia from 1988 to 1992. *Canadian Medical Association Journal, 152*(2), 185–190.

Doll, R., & Peto, R. (1976). Mortality in relation to smoking: 20 years' observations on male British doctors. *British Medical Journal, 2*(6051), 1525–1536.

Doll, R., Peto, R., Wheatley, K., et al. (1994). Mortality in relation to smoking: 40 years' observation on male British doctors. *British Medical Journal, 309*, 901–911.

Ezzati, M., Henley, S. J., Thun, M. J., et al. (2005). Role of smoking in global and regional cardiovascular mortality. *Circulation, 112*(4), 489–497.

Fanelli, F. & Dake, M. D. (2009). Standard of practice for the endovascular treatment of thoracic aortic aneurysms and type B dissections. *Cardiovascular and Interventional Radiology, 32*(5), 849–860.

Feigin, V. L., Lawes, C. M., Bennett, D. A., et al. (2003). Stroke epidemiology: a review of population-based studies of incidence, prevalence, and case-fatality in the late 20th century. *Lancet Neurology, 2*(1), 43–53.

Ficarra, M. G., Gualano, M. R., Capizzi, S., et al. (2011). Tobacco use prevalence, knowledge and attitudes among Italian hospital healthcare professionals. *European Journal of Public Health, 21*(1), 29–34.

Firooz, A., Sarhangnejad, R., Davoudi, S. M., et al. (2005). Acne and smoking: Is there a relationship? *BMC Dermatology, 5*, 2.

Floreani, A. A., & Rennard, S. I. (1999). The role of cigarette smoke in the pathogenesis of asthma and as a trigger for acute symptoms. *Current Opinion in Pulmonary Medicine, 5*, 38–46.

Forey, B. A., Thornton, A. J., & Lee, P. N. (2011). Systematic review with meta-analysis of the epidemiological evidence relating smoking to COPD, chronic bronchitis and emphysema. *BMC Pulmonary Medicine, 11*, 36.
Frost, P. H., Davis, B. R., Burlando, A. J., et al. (1996). Coronary heart disease risk factors in men and women aged 60 years and older: Findings from the Systolic Hypertension in the Elderly Program. *Circulation, 94*(1), 26–34.
Fuiano, N., & Incorvaia, C. (2011). The atopy patch test: Is it time to redefine its significance? *Annals of Allergy, Asthma and Immunology, 106*(4), 278–282.
Gallus, S., Muttarak, R., Martinez Sanchez, J. M., et al. (2011). Smoking prevalence and smoking attributable mortality in Italy. *Preventive Medicine, 52*(6), 434–438.
Galván Fernández, C., Suárez López de Vergara, R. G., Oliva Fernández, C., et al. (2000). Patología respiratoria en los jóvenes y hábito tabáquico. *Archivos de Bronconeumología, 36*, 186–190.
Geller-Bernstein, G., Kenett, R., Weisglass, L., et al. (1987). Atopic babies with wheezy bronchitis. *Allergy, 42*, 85–91.
Gelmetti, C. C., Krowchuk, D. P., & Lucky, A. W. (2003). Acne. In L. A. Schachner & S. I. Katz (Eds.), *Pediatric dermatology* (3rd ed., pp. 589–609). Philadelphia: Mosby.
Gilbert, R. (1994). The changing epidemiology of SIDS. *Archives of Disease in Childhood, 70*(5), 445–449.
Gilbert, N. L., Fell, D. B., Joseph, K. S., et al. (2012). Temporal trends in sudden infant death syndrome in Canada from 1991 to 2005: Contribution of changes in cause of death assignment practices and in maternal and infant characteristics. *Paediatric and Perinatal Epidemiology, 26*(2), 124–130.
Gilliland, F. D., Li, Y. F., Dubeau, L., et al. (2002). Effects of glutathione S-transferase M1, maternal smoking during pregnancy, and environmental tobacco smoke on asthma and wheezing in children. *American Journal of Respiratory and Critical Care Medicine, 166*, 457–463.
Godtfredsen, N. S., Lam, T. H., Hansel, T. T., et al. (2008). COPD-related morbidity and mortality after smoking cessation: Status of the evidence. *European Respiratory Journal, 32*, 844–853.
Gold, E. B., Bromberger, J., Crawford, S., et al. (2001). Factors associated with age at natural menopause in a multiethnic sample of midlife women. *American Journal of Epidemiology, 153*(9), 865–874.
Golding, J. (1997). Sudden infant death syndrome and parental smoking—a literature review. *Paediatric and Perinatal Epidemiology, 11*, 67–77.
Green, J., & Sinclair, R. D. (2001). Perception of acne vulgaris in final year medical student written examination answers. *Australian Journal of Dermatology, 42*, 98–101.
Greiner, A. N., Hellings, P. W., Rotiroti, G., et al. (2011). Allergic rhinitis. *Lancet, 378*(9809), 2112–2122.
Gupta, D., Aggarwal, A. N., Chaudhry, K., et al. (2006). Household environmental tobacco smoke exposure, respiratory symptoms and asthma in non-smoker adults: A multicentric population study from India. *The Indian Journal of Chest Diseases and Allied Sciences, 48*(1), 31–36.
Håheim, L. L., Holme, I., Hjermann, I., et al. (1996). Smoking habits and risk of fatal stroke: 18 years follow up of the Oslo study. *Journal of Epidemiology and Community Health, 50*(6), 621–624.
Hale, K. A., Niewoehner, D. E., & Cosio, M. G. (1980). Morphologic changes in the muscular pulmonary arteries: Relationship to cigarette smoking, airway disease, and emphysema. *American Review of Respiratory Disease, 122*(2), 273–278.
Halperin, R. O., Gaziano, J. M., & Sesso, H. D. (2008). Smoking and the risk of incident hypertension in middle-aged and older men. *American Journal of Hypertension, 21*(2), 148–152.
Hammond, E. C., & Garfinkel, L. (1969). Coronary heart disease, stroke, and aortic aneurysm. Factors in the etiology. *Archives of Environmental Health, 19*, 167–182.
Hanisah, A., Omar, K., & Shah, S. A. (2009). Prevalence of acne and its impact on the quality of life in school-aged adolescents in Malaysia. *Journal of Primary Health Care, 1*(1), 20–25.
Hardy, R., Kuh, D., & Wadsworth, M. (2000). Smoking, body mass index, socioeconomic status and the age at menopause by using estimating equations and Bayesian random effects models. *Statistics in Medicine, 19*, 1217–1235.

Harlow, B. L., & Signorello, L. B. (2000). Factors associated with early menopause. *Maturitas, 35*, 3–9.
Hashimoto, Y. (2011). Smoking and stroke. *Brain and Nerve, 63*(5), 483–490.
Health and Safety Executive. (2005). *Occupational respiratory diseases: Work-related chronic obstructive respiratory disease—intervention and evaluation plans draft document*. London: Health and Safety Executive.
Higa, M., & Dvanipour, Z. (1991). Smoking and stroke. *Neuroepidemiology, 10*, 211–222.
Hirsch, A. T., Haskal, Z. J., Hertzer, N. R., et al. (2006). ACC/AHA 2005 Practice Guidelines for the management of patients with peripheral arterial disease (lower extremity, renal, mesenteric, and abdominal aortic): A collaborative report from the American Association for Vascular Surgery/Society for Vascular Surgery, Society for Cardiovascular Angiography and Interventions, Society for Vascular Medicine and Biology, Society of Interventional Radiology, and the ACC/AHA Task Force on Practice Guidelines (Writing Committee to Develop Guidelines for the Management of Patients With Peripheral Arterial Disease): Endorsed by the American Association of Cardiovascular and Pulmonary Rehabilitation; National Heart, Lung, and Blood Institute; Society for Vascular Nursing; Trans-Atlantic Inter-Society Consensus; and Vascular Disease Foundation. *Circulation, 113*, e463–e654.
Huchon, G. J., Vergnenègre, A., Neukirch, F., et al. (2002). Chronic bronchitis among French adults: High prevalence and underdiagnosis. *European Respiratory Journal, 20*(4), 806–812.
Huxley, R. R., & Woodward, M. (2011). Cigarette smoking as a risk factor for coronary heart disease in women compared with men: A systematic review and meta-analysis of prospective cohort studies. *Lancet, 378*(9799), 1297–1305.
Izquierdo, J. L., Barcina, C., Jiménez, J., et al. (2009). Study of the burden on patients with chronic obstructive pulmonary disease. *International Journal of Clinical Practice, 63*(1), 87–97.
Jacobs, E. J., Thun, M. J., Apicella, L. F. (1999). Cigar smoking and death from coronary heart disease in a prospective study of US men. *Archives of Internal Medicine, 159*(20), 2413–2418.
Jemec, G. B. E., Linneberg, A., Nielsen, N. H., et al. (2002). Have oral contraceptives reduced the prevalence of acne? a population-based study of acne vulgaris, tobacco smoking and oral contraceptives. *Dermatology, 204*, 179–184.
Jensen, D. M., Korsholm, L., Ovesen, P., et al. (2008). Adverse pregnancy outcome in women with mild glucose intolerance: Is there a clinically meaningful threshold value for glucose? *Acta Obstetricia et Gynecologica Scandinavica, 87*(1), 59–62.
Jindal, S. K., Gupta, D., & Singh, A. (1994). Indices of morbidity and control of asthma in adult patients exposed to environmental tobacco smoke. *Chest, 106*, 746–749.
Jinno, S., Kida, K., & Ootsubo, K. (1994). Epidemiology of emphysema: Analysis by autopsy in a series of elderly patients. *Nihon Kyōbu Shikkan Gakkai zasshi, 32*(Suppl), 193–199.
Jonasson, L., Holm, J., Skalli, O., et al. (1986). Regional accumulations of T cells, macrophages, and smooth muscle cells in the human atherosclerotic plaque. *Arteriosclerosis, 6*(2), 131–138.
Kannel, W. B., & Higgins, M. (1990). Smoking and hypertension as predictors of cardiovascular risk in population studies. *Journal of Hypertension. Supplement, 8*(5), S3–S8.
Kawachi, I., Colditz, G. A., Stampfer, M. J., et al. (1993). Smoking cessation in relation to total mortality rates in women: A prospective cohort study. *Annals of Internal Medicine, 119*(10), 992–1000.
Kay, A. B. (2000). Overview of 'allergy and allergic diseases: With a view to the future'. *British Medical Bulletin, 56*(4), 843–864.
Kent, K. C., Zwolak, R. M., Egorova, N. N., et al. (2010). Analysis of risk factors for abdominal aortic aneurysm in a cohort of more than 3 million individuals. *Journal of Vascular Surgery, 52*(3), 539–548.
Kerkemeyer, K. (2005). Acne vulgaris. *Plastic Surgical Nursing, 25*, 31–35.
Khan, N. A., Hemmelgarn, B., Herman, R. J., et al. (2009). Canadian hypertension education program. The,Canadian hypertension education program recommendations for the management of hypertension: Part 2-therapy. *Canadian Journal of Cardiology, 25*(5), 287–298.
Kilkenny, M., Merlin, K., Plunkett, A., et al. (1998). The prevalence of common skin conditions in Australian school students: 3. Acne vulgaris. *British Journal of Dermatology, 139*, 840–845.

Kim, J. W., Park, C. G., Hong, S. J., et al. (2005). Acute and chronic effects of cigarette smoking on arterial stiffness. *Blood Pressure, 14*(2), 80–85.

Klaz, I., Kochba, I., Shohat, T., et al. (2006). Severe acne vulgaris and tobacco smoking in young men. *Journal of Investigative Dermatology, 126*(8), 1749–1752.

Klein, R., Klein, B. E., & Moss, S. E. (1998). Relation of smoking to the incidence of age-related maculopathy. The Beaver Dam Eye Study. *American Journal of Epidemiology, 147*(2), 103–110.

Koon, K. T., Stephanie, O., Steven, H., et al. (2006). Tobacco use and risk of myocardial infarction in 52 countries in the INTERHEART study: A case-control study. *Lancet, 368*, 647–658.

Kramer, M. S. (1987). Determinants of low birth weight: Methodological assessment and meta-analysis. *Bulletin of the World Health Organization, 65*(5), 663.

Krous, H. F., Beckwith, J. B., Byard, R. W., et al. (2004). Sudden infant death syndrome and unclassified sudden infant deaths: A definitional and diagnostic approach. *Pediatrics, 114*, 234–238.

Krowchuk, D. P., & Lucky, A. W. (2001). Managing adolescent acne. *Adolescent Medicine, 12*(2), vii, 355–374.

Kuller, L. H., Ockene, J. K., Meilahn, E., et al. (1991). Cigarette smoking and mortality. *Preventive Medicine, 20*(5), 638–654.

Lacasse, Y., Brooks, D., & Goldstein, R. S. (1999). Trends in the epidemiology of COPD in canada, 1980 to 1995. COPD and Rehabilitation Committee of the Canadian Thoracic Society. *Chest, 116*, 306–313.

Langhammer, A., Johnsen, R., Holmen, J., et al. (2000). Cigarette smoking gives more respiratory symptoms among women than among men. The Nord-Trondelag Health Study (HUNT). *Journal of Epidemiology and Community Health, 54*(12), 917–922.

La Torre, G. (2010). Applied epidemiology and biostatistics. Torino: SEEd.

Law, M. R., & Wald, N. J. (2003). Environmental tobacco smoke and ischemic heart disease. *Progress in Cardiovascular Diseases, 46*(1), 31–38.

Lawes, C. M., Vander Hoorn, S., & Rodgers, A. (2008). Global burden of blood-pressure-related disease, 2001. *Lancet, 371*(9623), 1513–1518.

Laws, P., & Hilder, L. (2008). *Australia's mothers and babies 2006. Perinatal statistics series no 22*. Sydney: AIHW National Perinatal Statistics Unit: 2006.

Lederle, F. A., Johnson, G. R., Wilson, S. E., et al. (1997). Prevalence and associations of abdominal aortic aneurysm detected through screening. *Annals of Internal Medicine, 126*, 441–449.

Lee, A. J., Fowkes, F. G., Carson, M. N., et al. (1997). Smoking, atherosclerosis and risk of abdominal aortic aneurysm. *European Heart Journal, 18*, 671–676.

LeMaire, S. A., & Russell, L. (2011). Epidemiology of thoracic aortic dissection. *Nature Reviews Cardiology, 8*(2), 103–113.

LeSon, S., & Gershwin, M. E. (1996). Risk factors for asthmatic patients requiring intubation. III. Observations in young adults. *Journal of Asthma, 33*, 27–35.

Lindholt, J. S., Heegaard, N. H., Vammen, S., et al. (2001). Smoking, but not lipids, lipoprotein(a) and antibodies against oxidised LDL, is correlated to the expansion of abdominal aortic aneurysms. *European Journal of Vascular and Endovascular Surgery, 21*, 51–56.

Linneberg, A., Nielsen, N. H., Menné, T., et al. (2003). Smoking might be a risk factor for contact allergy. *The Journal of Allergy and Clinical Immunology, 111*, 980–984.

Longmore, J. M., Wilkinson, I., & Supraj, R. R. (2004). *Oxford handbook of clinical medicine* (pp. 188–189). Oxford, Oxfordshire: Oxford University Press.

Lopez, A. D., Mathers, C. D., Ezzati, M., et al. (2006). *Measuring the global burden of disease and risk factors, 1990–2001. Source Global burden of disease and risk factors, Chap. 1.* Washington, DC: World Bank.

Lundback, B., Lindberg, A., Lindstrom, M., et al. (2003). Not 15 but 50 % of smokers develop COPD? Report from the Obstructive Lung Disease in Northern Sweden Studies. *Respiratory Medicine, 97*, 115–122.

MacDorman, M. F., Cnattingius, S., Hoffman, H. J., et al. (1997). Sudden infant death syndrome and smoking in the United States and Sweden. *American Journal of Epidemiology, 146*(3), 249–257.

MacSweeney, S. T., Ellis, M., Worrell, P. C., et al. (1994). Smoking and growth rate of small abdominal aortic aneurysms. *Lancet, 344*, 651–652.

Malcolm, J., Meggison, H., & Sigal, R. (2003). Prevention of cardiovascular events in diabetes. *Clinical Evidence, 26*(4), 422–426.

Mamun, A. A., Peeters, A., Barendregt, J., et al. (2004). Smoking decreases the duration of life lived with and without cardiovascular disease: a life course analysis of the Framingham Heart Study. *European Heart Journal, 25*(5), 409–415.

Mannino, D. M. (2002). COPD: Epidemiology, prevalence, morbidity and mortality, and disease heterogeneity. *Chest, 121*(Suppl. 5), 121S–126S.

Mannino, D. M., Homa, D. M., Akinbami, L. J., et al. (2002). Chronic obstructive pulmonary disease surveillance–United States, 1971–2000. *MMWR Surveillance Summaries, 51*, 1–16.

Mannino, D. M., Watt, G., Hole, D., et al. (2006). The natural history of chronic obstructive pulmonary disease. *European Respiratory Journal, 27*, 627–643.

Mannocci, A., Semyonov, L., Saulle, R., et al. (2010). Evaluation of the association between acne and smoking: Systematic review and meta-analysis of cross-sectional studies. *Italian Journal of Publich Health, 7*(3), 256–261.

Martin, J. A., Hamilton, B. E., Ventura, S. J., et al. (2002). Epidemiology of smoking M. M. Births: Final data for 2000. *National Vital Statistics Reports, 50*(5), 1–104.

Martin, J. A., Kung, H. C., Mathews, T. J., et al. (2008). Annual summary of vital statistics: 2006. *Pediatrics, 121*(4), 788–801.

Mathews, T. J., Menacker, F., & MacDorman, M. F. (2004). Infant mortality statistics from the 2002 period: Linked birth/infant death data set. *National Vital Statistics Reports, 53*(10), 1–29.

Mazzone, P., Tierney, W., Hossain, M., et al. (2010). Pathophysiological impact of cigarette smoke exposure on the cerebrovascular system with a focus on the blood-brain barrier: Expanding the awareness of smoking toxicity in an underappreciated area. *International Journal of Environmental Research and Public Health, 7*(12), 4111–4126.

McCoy, K., Shade, D. M., Irvin, C. G., et al. (2006). Predicting episodes of poor asthma control in treated patients with asthma. *The Journal of Allergy and Clinical Immunology, 118*, 1226–1233.

McKinlay, S. M., Bifano, N. L., & McKinlay, J. B. (1985). Smoking and age at menopause in women. *Annals of Internal Medicine, 103*, 350–356.

Michaud, C. M., Murray, C. J., & Bloom, B. R. (2001). Burden of disease—Implications for future research. *Journal of the American Medical Association, 285*, 535–539.

Miettinen, O. S., Neff, R. K., & Jick, H. (1976). Cigarette-smoking and nonfatal myocardial infarction: Rate ratio in relation to age, sex and predisposing conditions. *American Journal of Epidemiology, 103*(1), 30–36.

Minakata, Y., & Ichinose, M. (2011). Epidemiology of COPD in Japan. *Nihon Rinsho, 69*(10), 1721–1726.

Miravitlles, M., Soriano, J. B., García-Río, F., et al. (2009). Prevalence of COPD in Spain: Impact of undiagnosed COPD on quality of life and daily life activities. *Thorax, 64*(10), 863–868.

Mitchell, E. A., & Milerad, J. (2006). Smoking and the sudden infant death syndrome. *Reviews on Environmental Health, 21*(2), 81–103.

Mitchell, P., Wang, J. J., Smith, W., et al. (2002). Smoking and the 5-year incidence of age-related maculopathy: The Blue Mountains Eye Study. *Archives of Ophthalmology, 120*(10), 1357–1363.

Mlinaric, A., Popovic Grle, S., Nadalin, S., et al. (2011). Passive smoking and respiratory allergies in adolescents. *European Review for Medical and Pharmacological Sciences, 15*(8), 973–977.

Murin, S., Rafii, R., & Bilello, K. (2011). Smoking and smoking cessation in pregnancy. *Clinics in Chest Medicine, 32*(1), 75–91.

Murray, C. J., & Lopez, A. D. (1997). Global mortality, disability, and the contribution of risk factors: Global Burden of Disease Study. *Lancet, 349*(9063), 1436–1442.

Nathan, R. A. (2007). The burden of allergic rhinitis. *Allergy and Asthma Proceedings, 28*(1), 3–9.

Nazari, S. (1998). The surgical physiopathology of essential pulmonary emphysema and volume-reduction intervention. *Minerva Chirurgica, 53*(11), 899–918.

Nicholl, J. P., & O'Cathain, A. (1992). Antenatal smoking, postnatal passive smoking and the sudden infant death syndrome. In D. Poswillo & E. Alberman (Eds.), *Effects of smoking on the fetus, neonate and child* (pp. 138–149). Oxford: Oxford Universitv Press.

Nicolotti, N., La Torre, G., & Gualano, M. R. et al. (2009). Epidemiologia della degenerazione maculare senile (AMD). *Italian Journal of Public Health, 6*(2) Suppl. 3

Njølstad, I., Arnesen, E., & Lund-Larsen, P. G. (1996). Smoking, serum lipids, blood pressure, and sex differences in myocardial infarction: A 12-year follow-up of the Finnmark Study. *Circulation, 93*(3), 450–456.

Noakes, P. S., Holt, P. G., & Prescott, S. L. (2003). Maternal smoking in pregnancy alters neonatal cytokine responses. *Allergy, 58*, 1053–1058.

O'Donnell, C. J., & Kannel, W. B. (2002). Epidemiologic appraisal of hypertension as a coronary risk factor in the elderly. *The American Journal of Geriatric Cardiology, 11*(2), 86–92.

Omori, H., Nakashima, R., Otsuka, N., et al. (2006). Emphysema detected by lung cancer screening with low-dose spiral CT: Prevalence, and correlation with smoking habits and pulmonary function in Japanese male subjects. *Respirology, 11*(2), 205–210.

Oono, I. P., Mackay, D. F., & Pell, J. P. (2011). Meta-analysis of the association between secondhand smoke exposure and stroke. *Journal of Public Health (Oxford, England), 33*(4), 496–502.

Owen, L., & Penn, G. (1999). *Smoking and pregnancy: A survey of knowledge attitudes and behaviour, 1992–1999*. London: Health Development Agency.

Pattenden, S., Antova, T., Neuberger, M., et al. (2006). Parental smoking and children's respiratory health: Independent effects of prenatal and postnatal exposure. *Tobacco Control, 15*, 294–301.

Pearl, R. (1938). Tobacco smoking and longevity. *Science, 87*, 216–217.

Pelkonen, M. (2008). Smoking: Relationship to chronic bronchitis, chronic obstructive pulmonary disease and mortality. *Current Opinion in Pulmonary Medicine, 14*(2), 105–109.

Pierson, D. J. (2006). Clinical practice guidelines for chronic obstructive pulmonary disease: A review and comparison of current resources. *Respiratory Care, 51*(3), 277–288.

Piipari, R., Jaakkola, J. J. K., Jaakkola, N., et al. (2004). Smoking and asthma in adults. *European Respiratory Journal, 24*, 734–739.

Plaschke, P. P., Janson, C., Norrman, E., et al. (2000). Onset and remission of allergic rhinitis and asthma and the relationship with atopic sensitization and smoking. *American Journal of Respiratory and Critical Care Medicine, 162*(3 Pt 1), 920–924.

Pokoradi, A. J., Iversen, L., & Hannaford, P. C. (2011). Factors associated with age of onset and type of menopause in a cohort of UK women. *American Journal of Obstetrics and Gynecology, 205*(1), 34.e1–34.e13.

Polakowski, L. L., Akinbami, L. J., & Mendola, P. (2009). Prenratal smoking cessation and the risk of delivering preterm and small-for-gestational-age newborns. *Obstetrics and Gynecology, 114*(2 Pt 1), 318–325.

Polańska, K., & Hanke, W. (2004). Effect of smoking during pregnancy on maternal condition and birth outcome–overview of epidemiologic studies. *Przegl Epidemiologiczny, 58*(4), 683–691.

Polańska, K., & Hanke, W. (2005). Influence of smoking during pregnancy on children's health—overview of epidemiologic studies. *Przegl Epidemiologiczny, 59*(1), 117–123.

Powell, J. T., & Greenhalgh, R. M. (2003). Clinical practice. Small abdominal aortic aneurysms. *New England Jouranl of Medicine, 348*, 1895–1901.

Prescott, E., Scharling, H., Osler, M., et al. (2005). Importance of light smoking and inhalation habits on risk of myocardial infarction and all cause mortality: A 22 year follow up of 12,149 men and women in the Copenhagen City Heart Study. *Journal of Epidemiology and Community Health, 56*(9), 702–706.

Purvis, D., Robinson, E., & Watson, P. (2004). Acne prevalence in secondary school students and their perceived difficulty in accessing acne treatment. *The New Zealand Medical Journal, 117*, U1018.

Qiao, Q., Tervahauta, M., Nissinen, A., et al. (2000). Mortality from all causes and from coronary heart disease related to smoking and changes in smoking during a 35-year follow-up of middle-aged Finnish men. *European Heart Journal, 21*(19), 1621–1626.

Reed, D., Reed, C., Stemmermann, G., et al. (1992). Are aortic aneurysms caused by atherosclerosis? *Circulation, 85*, 205–211.
Rennard, S. I., & Vestbo, J. (2006). COPD: The dangerous underestimate of 15%. *Lancet, 367*, 1216–1219.
Rombouts, S., Nijsten, T., & Lambert, J. (2007). Cigarette smoking and acne in adolescents: Results from a cross-sectional study. *Journal of the European Academy of Dermatology and Venereology, 21*(3), 326–333.
Romero Palacios, P. J. (2004). Asthma and tobacco smoke. *Archivos de Bronconeumología, 40*(9), 414–418.
Sakalihasan, N., Limet, R., & Defawe, O. D. (2005). Abdominal aortic aneurysm. *Lancet, 365*(9470), 1577–1589.
Salmasi, G., Grady, R., Jones, J., et al. (2010). Environmental tobacco smoke exposure and perinatal outcomes: A systematic review and meta-analyses. *Acta Obstetricia et Gynecologica Scandinavica, 89*(4), 423–441.
Schafer, T., Niehnaus, A., Vieluf, D., et al. (2001). Epidemiology of acne in the general population: The risk of smoking. *British Journal of Dermatology, 145*, 100–104.
Schatz, M., Zeiger, R. S., Vollmer, W. M., et al. (2006). Determinants of future long-term asthma control. *The Journal of Allergy and Clinical Immunology, 118*, 1048–1053.
Schoendorf, K. C., & Kiely, J. L. (1992). Relationship of sudden infant death syndrome to maternal smoking during and after pregnancy. *Pediatrics, 90*(6), 905–908.
Seddon, J. M., Willett, W. C., Speizer, F. E., et al. (1996). A prospective study of cigarette smoking and age-related macular degeneration in women. *Journal of the American Medical Association, 276*(14), 1141–1146.
Shinton, R., & Beevers, G. (1989). Meta-analysis of relation between cigarette smoking and stroke. *BMJ, 298*, 789–794.
Simpson, W. J. (1957). A preliminary report on cigarette smoking and the incidence of prematurity. *American Journal of Obstetrics and Gynecology, 73*(4), 807–815.
Simpson, N. B., & Cunliffe, W. J. (2004). Disorders of sebaceous glands. In T. Burns, S. Breathnach, N. Cox, & C. Griffiths (Eds.), *Rook's textbook of dermatology* (7th ed., pp. 43.1–43.75). Oxford: Blackwell Publishing.
Singer, M. V., Feick, P., & Gerloff, A. (2011). Alcohol and smoking. *Digestive Diseases, 29*(2), 177–183.
Siroux, V., Pin, I., Oryszczyn, M. P., et al. (2000). Relationships of active smoking and asthma severity in the EGEA study. Epidemiological study on the Genetics and Environment of Asthma. *European Respiratory Journal, 15*, 470–477.
Skinner, J. S., & Cooper, A. (2011). Secondary prevention of ischemic cardiac events. *Clinical Evidence (Online)*, pii, 0206.
Slotkin, T. A. (1998). Fetal nicotine or cocaine exposure: Which one is worse? *Journal of Pharmacology and Experimental Therapeutics, 285*(3), 931–945.
Smithard, A., Glazebrook, C., & Williams, H. C. (2001). Acne prevalence, knowledge about acne and psychological morbidity in midadolescents: A community-based study. *British Journal of Dermatology, 145*, 274–279.
Stapleton, M., Howard-Thompson, A., George, C., et al. (2011). Smoking and asthma. *Journal of the American Board of Family Medicine, 24*, 313–322.
Stathakis, V., Kilkenny, M., & Marks, R. (1997). Descriptive epidemiology of acne vulgaris in the community. *Australian Journal of Dermatology, 38*, 115–125.
Stern, R. S. (1996). Acne therapy. Medication use and sources of care in office-based practice. *Archives of Dermatology, 132*, 776–780.
Strachan, D. P. (1991). Predictors of death from aortic aneurysm among middle-aged men: The Whitehall study. *British Journal of Surgery, 78*, 401–404.
Stratton, K., Shetty, P., Wallace, R., et al. (2001). Clearing the smoke: The science base for tobacco harm reduction—executive summary. *Tobacco Control, 10*, 189–195.

Strine, T. W., Balluz, L. S., & Ford, E. S. (2007). The associations between smoking, physical inactivity, obesity, and asthma severity in the general US population. *The Journal of Asthma, 44*, 651–658.

Strong, K., Mathers, C., & Bonita, R. (2007). Preventing stroke: Saving lives around the world. *Lancet Neurology, 6*, 182–187.

Sun, L., Tan, L., Yang, F., et al. (2012). Meta-analysis suggests that smoking is associated with an increased risk of early natural menopause. *Menopause, 19*(2), 126–132.

Takimoto, H., Yokoyama, T., Yoshiike, N., et al. (2005). Increase in low-birth-weight infants in Japan and associated risk factors, 1980–2000. Journal of obstetric and gynaecology research, *31*(4), 314–322.

Thun, M. J., & Heath, C. W. Jr. (1997). Changes in mortality from smoking in two American Cancer Society prospective studies since 1959. *Preventive Medicine, 26*(4), 422–426.

Tomany, S. C., Wang, J. J., Van Leeuwen, R., et al. (2004). Risk factors for incident age-related macular degeneration: Pooled findings from 3 continents. *Ophthalmology, 111*(7), 1280–1287.

U.S. Department of Health and Human Services. (2001a). *Women and smoking: A report of the surgeon general* (pp. 272–307). Rockville, MD: U.S. Department of Health and Human Services, Public Health Service, Office of the Surgeon General.

U.S. Department of Health and Human Services. (2001b). Patterns of tobacco use among women and girls. In *Women and smoking: A report of the surgeon general* (pp. 19–176). Rockville, MD: U.S. Department of Health and Human Services, Centers for Disease Control and Prevention, National Center for Chronic Disease Prevention and Health Promotion, Office of Smoking and Health.

U.S. Department of Health and Human Services. (2002). *Health, United States, 2002, with chartbooks on trends in the health of Americans* (DHHS Publication No. 1232). Hyattsville, MD: U.S. Department of Health and Human Services, Centers for Disease Control and Prevention, National Center for Health Statistics.

U.S. Department of Health and Human Services. (2004). *The health consequences of smoking: A report of the surgeon general*. Atlanta: U.S. Department of Health and Human Services, Centers for Disease Control and Prevention, National Center for Chronic Disease Prevention and Health Promotion, Office on Smoking and Health.

U.S. Department of Health and Human Services. (2010). *How tobacco smoke causes disease: The biology and behavioral basis for smoking-attributable disease. A report of the surgeon general*. Rockville, MD: Public Health Service Office of the Surgeon General.

Van der Vaart, H., Postma, D. S., et al. (2005). Acute effects of cigarette smoking on inflammation in healthy intermittent smokers. *Respiratory Research, 6*, 22.

Van Schooten, F. J., Hirvonen, A., Maas, L. M., et al. (1998). Putative susceptibility markers of coronary artery disease: Association between VDR genotype, smoking, and aromatic DNA adduct levels in human right atrial tissue. *The FASEB Journal, 12*(13), 1409–1417.

VanNewkirk, M. R., Nanjan, M. B., Wang, J. J., et al. (2000). The prevalence of age-related maculopathy: The visual impairment project. *Ophthalmology, 107*(8), 1593–1600.

Vardavas, C. I., Chatzi, L., Patelarou, E., et al. (2010). Smoking and smoking cessation during early pregnancy and its effect on adverse pregnancy outcomes and fetal growth. *European Journal of Pediatrics, 169*(6), 741–748.

Venables, K. M., Upton, J. L., Hawkins, E. R., et al. (1988). Smoking, atopy, and laboratory animal allergy. *British Journal of Industrial Medicine, 45*, 667–671.

Viegi, A., Scognamiglio, S., Baldacci, F., et al. (2001). Epidemiology of chronic obstructive pulmonary disease (COPD). *Respiration, 68*, 4–19.

Ward, C., Lewis, S., Coleman, T. (2007). Prevalence of maternal smoking and environmental tobacco smoke exposure during pregnancy and impact on birth weight: retrospective study using Millennium Cohort. *BMC Public Health, 7*, 81.

Weber, R. W. (2008). Allergic rhinitis. *Primary Care, 35*(1), 1–10.

Weil, J., Stritzke, J., & Schunkert, H. (2012). Risk factor "smoking": Smoking cessation in patients with cardiovascular diseases. *Internist (Berlin), 53*(1), 45–50.

Wilder, C. S. (1973). Prevalence of selected chronic respiratory conditions: United States, 1970. *Vital and health statistics, 10*(84), 1–49.
Willett, W. C., Green, A., Stampfer, M. J., et al. (1987). Relative and absolute excess risks of coronary heart disease among women who smoke cigarettes. *The New England Journal of Medicine, 317*(21), 1303–1309.
Windham, G. C., Eaton, A., & Hopkins, B. (1999). Evidence for an association between environmental tobacco smoke exposure and birthweight: A meta-analysis and new data. *Paediatric and Perinatal Epidemiology, 13*(1), 35–57.
Windham, G. C., Hopkins, B., Fenster, L., et al. (2000). Prenatal active or passive tobacco smoke exposure and the risk of preterm delivery or low birth weight. *Epidemiology, 11*(4), 427–433.
Wolf, P. A., D'Agostino, R. B., Kannel, W. B., et al. (1988). Cigarette smoking as a risk factor for stroke. The Framingham Study. *Journal of the American Medical Association, 259*(7), 1025–1029.
World Health Organization. (2000). *The world health report 2000—Health systems: Improving performance*. Geneva: World Health Organization.
World Health Organization. (2011). *Chronic respiratory diseases*. Burden. Accessed April 27, 2012, from http://www.who.int/respiratory/copd/burden/en
World Health Organization. Accessed February 16, 2012, from http://www.who.int/mediacentre/factsheets/fs297/en/
Xiaofan, G., Liling, Z., Xingang, Z., et al. (2011). A meta-analysis of the epidemiology, risk factors, and predictors of progression. *Texas Heart Institute Journal, 38*(6), 643–652.
Yeung, C. K., Teo, L. H., Xiang, L. H., et al. (2002). A community-based epidemiological study of acne vulgaris in Hong Kong adolescents. *Acta Dermato-Venereologica, 82*(2), 104–107.
Young, R. W. (1987). Pathophysiology of age-related macular degeneration. *Survey of Ophthalmology, 31*, 291–306.
Zetterstrom, K., Osterman, L., Machado, S., et al. (1981). Another smoking hazard: Raised serum IgE concentration and increased risk of occupational allergy. *British Medical Journal (Clinical Research Ed.), 283*(6301), 1215–1217.
Zhang, H., & Cai, B. (2003). Tobacco and lung health in China. *Respirology, 8*, 17–21.
Zhang, J., Ou, J. X., & Bai, C. X. (2011). Tobacco smoking in China: Prevalence, disease burden, challenges and future strategies. *Respirology, 16*(8), 1165–1172.
Ziv, A., Boulet, J. R., & Slap, G. B. (1999). Utilization of physician offices by adolescents in the United States. *Pediatrics, 104*, 35–42.

Chapter 4
Smoking-Related Cancer Epidemiology

Giuseppe La Torre, Guglielmo Giraldi, and Leda Semyonov

Objectives This section intends to describe the epidemiology of cigarette smoking-related cancers. For each disease, the epidemiology and the scientific evidence will be discussed.

Learning Outcomes

At the end of this chapter the reader will be able to:

– Know the main smoking-related cancers and their epidemiology

4.1 Introduction

In 1926, Lane-Clayton conducted the first case–control study assessing the etiology of breast cancer (Lane-Clayton 1926).

As more and more evidence accumulated indicating tobacco as the major cause of lung cancer and a number of other diseases, the tobacco industry claimed that there was no proof that the tobacco was responsible for causing these diseases. The battle continued for years, and Bradford Hill subsequently published a series of criteria to be considered when making a judgment of whether a given "exposure" was truly a cause of a given disease. These are now commonly referred to as "Hill's Criteria" for causal inference (Doll and Hill 1950) (Fig. 4.1).

G. La Torre (✉) • G. Giraldi • L. Semyonov
Department of Public Health and Infectious Diseases, "Sapienza" University of Rome, Piazzale Aldo Moro 5, Rome 00185, Italy
e-mail: giuseppe.latorre@uniroma1.it; guglielmo.giraldi@uniroma1.it; ledasemyonov@hotmail.it

G. La Torre, *Smoking Prevention and Cessation*, DOI 10.1007/978-1-4614-7046-5_4,

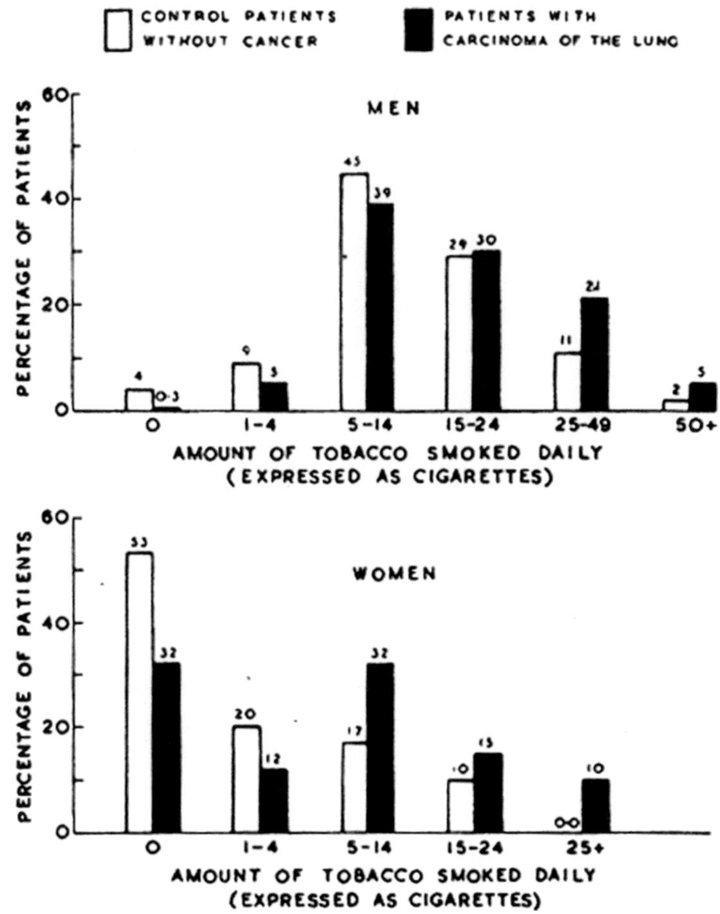

Fig. 4.1 Percentage of patients smoking different amounts of tobacco daily (Doll and Hill 1950)

In 1985, under the auspice of the International Agency for Research on Cancer (IARC) an international Working Group of experts recognized a causal relationship between tobacco smoking and cancer of the lung, oral cavity, pharynx, larynx, pancreas, urinary bladder, renal pelvis, and urethra (Tobacco Smoking 1986).

The association was primarily based on worldwide epidemiological studies. Recently, in a revised Monograph on Tobacco Smoke and Involuntary Smoking (IARC 2004), the IARC added cancers of the nasal cavities and nasal sinuses, the esophagus, stomach, liver, kidney (renal-cell carcinoma), uterine cervix, and bone marrow (myeloid leukemia) to the list of smoking-related cancers.

In a stately study of English in the long term, Doll et al. followed 34,439 male British doctors. Information about their smoking habits was obtained in 1951, and periodically thereafter, cause-specific mortality was monitored for 50 years. The excess mortality associated with smoking chiefly involved vascular, neoplastic, and respiratory diseases that can be caused by smoking.

Longevity has been improving rapidly for nonsmokers but not for men who continued smoking cigarettes. Cessation at age 50 halved the hazard, while cessation at 30 avoided almost all of it.

On average, cigarette smokers die about 10 years younger than nonsmokers. Stopping at age 60, 50, 40, or 30 gains, respectively, about 3, 6, 9, or 10 years of life expectancy (Doll et al. 2004).

Jacobs et al. (1999) collected data on 16 cohorts from seven different populations of Europe, Asia, and the USA showing that the devastating effect of smoking on health is independent of the state of residence and that the differences observed between countries are to be found in the first place differences in smoking habits.

In the same way, even light smoking, that is a small amount of cigarettes, significantly increases the risk of dying from smoking-related diseases (Bjartveit and Tverdal 2005).

In addition, smokers are responsible for the increased incidence of tobacco-related diseases in nonsmokers exposed to secondhand tobacco smoke. Lifelong nonsmoking spouses of smokers who smoke at home had a significant and consistent 20–30 % increase in lung cancer risk. Similarly, never smokers exposed to secondhand tobacco smoke at the workplace have a 16–19 % increase in risk to develop lung cancer (Sasco et al. 2004).

The highest rate of male smokers is in South Korea (68 %), the highest rate of female smokers is in Denmark (37 %); a third of women smoke in developed countries and 1/8 in developing countries. The majority of smokers are found in developing countries (Peto et al. 2006).

Tobacco-attributable mortality is projected to increase from 3.0 million deaths in 1990 to 8.4 million deaths in 2020 (Murray and Lopez 1997). If current trends will continue, 80 % of premature deaths related to tobacco will be among people living in low- and middle-income countries. Over the course of the twenty-first century, tobacco use could kill a billion people or more unless urgent action is taken (World Health Organization 2011).

The vast scientific literature on smoking and health contains few large studies with direct estimates of long-term mortality by smoking habits. A population-based cohort study performed in Norway enrolled 24,505 women and 25,034 men who were born between 1925 and 1941. Rates of smoking-associated lung cancer were similar in women and men, while lower cardiovascular mortality rates in women explained most of the difference in smoking-associated all-cause mortality between men and women. Despite similar rates for lung cancer death, women who smoked had lower mortality rates in middle age than men with similar smoking histories due to fewer cardiovascular deaths in women (Vollset et al. 2006).

4.2 Cancers: Main Smoking-Related Cancers

Tobacco smoking is the main cause of cancer-related death worldwide and it is responsible for 1.8 million cancer deaths per year; it causes about 25 % of all cancers in men and 4 % in women and approximately 16 % of cancers in developed countries and 10 % in less developed countries (Stewart and Kleihues 2003) (Fig. 4.2).

Cigarette smoke contains about 4,000 chemical agents, including over 60 substances that are known to cause cancer in humans (carcinogens). In addition, many of these substances, such as carbon monoxide, tar, arsenic, and lead, are poisonous and toxic to the human body. Nicotine is a drug that is naturally present in the tobacco plant and is primarily responsible for a person's addiction to tobacco products, including cigarettes. During smoking, nicotine is absorbed quickly into the bloodstream and travels to the brain in a matter of seconds (U.S. Department of Health and Human Services 1988).

As a matter of fact, smoking is currently responsible for a third of all cancer deaths in Western countries. The earlier in life a person starts smoking, the greater will be his risk to develop a cancer in older age. The risk of smokers to develop lung, urinary, oral, esophagus, larynx, and pancreas cancer increased three to fivefold compared to nonsmoker, while nasopharynx, stomach, liver, kidney, uterine cervix cancer, and myeloid leukemia show a 1.5- to 2-fold increased risk (Sasco et al. 2004).

Since 1920s evidence of the association between cigarette smoking and cancer was observed and by the 1950s a causal relationship with lung cancer was established (Levin et al. 1950).

During the last decades the International Agency for Research on Cancer (IARC) have recognized a causal relationship between tobacco smoking and cancer of the lung, oral cavity, pharynx, larynx, pancreas, urinary bladder, renal pelvis, urethra, cancers of the nasal cavities and nasal sinuses, esophagus, stomach, liver, kidney (renal-cell carcinoma), uterine cervix, and bone marrow (myeloid leukemia) (IARC 2004).

In developing regions, 67 % of smoking-attributable cancer deaths were between the ages of 30 and 69 compared to 52 % in industrialized regions (Ezzati et al. 2005).

The risk of tobacco smoking depends on cumulative exposure to carcinogens in tobacco smoke; therefore, it varies with the amount smoked, duration of smoking, the type of cigarette smoked, and time since cessation (in ex-smokers).

For both sexes, between 43 and 60 % of cancers of the upper aerodigestive tract (esophagus, larynx, and oral cavity) are attributable to tobacco (Boyle et al. 2003).

In the UK it has been estimated that 36,102 (22.8 % of the total) cancers in men and 23,722 (15.2 % of the total) in women in 2010 are attributable to smoking tobacco (Parkin 2011).

According to several population surveys in Italy, the prevalence of male smokers reached a maximum (almost 80 %) in the 1920–1930 birth cohorts and decreased to 60 % among males born in the 1940–1950s. In that period, the mean number of cigarettes per day increased while the age of starting smoking decreased; in addition, the market trend changed from unfiltered black tobacco to filtered low-tar cigarettes and this trend reflects the decreasing incidence and mortality of both larynx

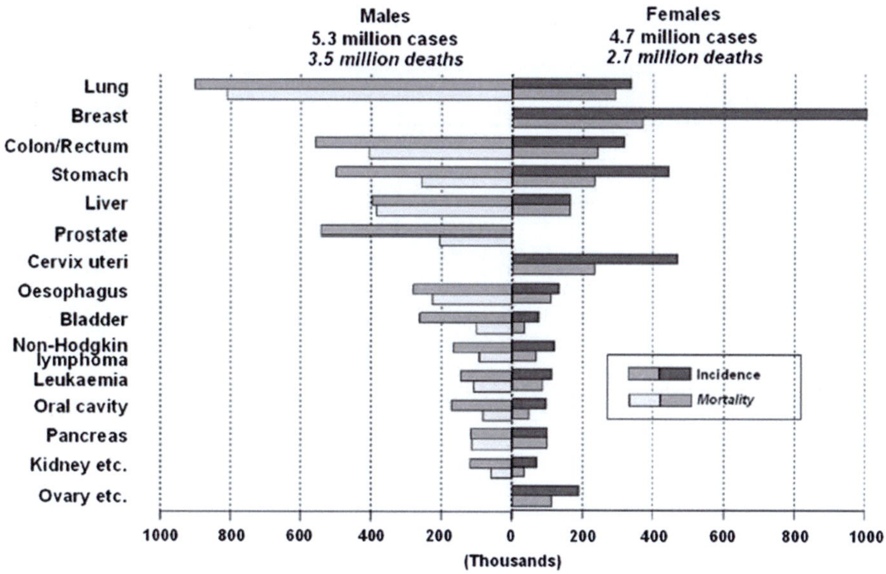

Fig. 4.2 Estimated new cases and deaths worldwide, by sex, in 2000 (Parkin 2004)

and lung cancer in young male cohorts and the persistent increase of both cancers in older males. The prevalence of female smokers increased from 10 % in the 1920s birth cohorts to over 30 % among women born in the late 1940s; this is reflected by an increase in respiratory cancer mortality which, however, is still lower than the mortality for males (Berrino 1992).

A systematic meta-analysis of observational studies from 1961 to 2003 was performed to quantify the risk for 13 cancer sites, recognized to be smoking-related by the International Agency for Research on Cancer (IARC), and to analyze the risk variation for each site. The highest pooled RR for current smokers was for lung cancer (RR=8.96; 95 % CI: 6.73–12.11) and the risk of lung cancer increases by 7 % for each additional cigarette smoked per day (RR=1.07; 95 % CI: 1.06–1.08) and it appears to be slightly higher in women (RR=1.08; 95 % CI: 1.07–1.10) than in men (RR=1.07; 95 % CI: 1.05–1.08) ($p<0.001$). Then, laryngeal (RR=6.98; 95 % CI: 3.14–15.52) and pharyngeal (RR=6.76; 95 % CI: 2.86–15.98) cancers presented the highest relative risks for current smokers, followed by upper digestive tract, oral cancers, stomach, pancreas, cancer of the nasal cavity, lower urinary tract, kidney, cancer of the cervix uteri, liver, myeloid leukemia. Pooled relative risk for former smokers was highest for stomach cancer (RR=1.31; 95 % CI: 1.17–1.46) followed by pancreatic cancer, cancer of the nasal cavity, lower urinary tract cancer, kidney cancer, cancer of the cervix uteri, for liver cancer, and myeloid leukemia (Gandini et al. 2008) (Table 4.1).

For most of these associations a dose–response effect of tobacco use on cancer risk is evident, as is a decline in risk on cessation of tobacco use.

Table 4.1 Pooled RRs by cancer site and type of exposure to cigarette smoking (Gandini et al. 2008)

Cancer site ICD 10	Smoking status	RR[a] (95 % CI)	No. of studies	*p*-Value heterogeneity	I^2%
Upper digestive tract C10–15	Current	3.57 (2.63, 4.84)	11	0.010	53
	Former	1.18 (0.73, 1.91)	14	<0.001	84
Oral cavity C10	Current	3.43 (2.37, 4.94)	12	0.001	65
	Former	1.40 (0.99, 2.00)	9	0.098	40
Pharynx C14	Current	6.76 (2.86, 16.0)	7	<0.001	85
	Former	2.28 (0.95, 5.50)	3	0.034	71
Esophagus C15	Current	2.50 (2.00, 3.13)	22	<0.001	81
	Former	2.03 (1.77, 2.33)	21	0.175	20
Stomach C16	Current	1.64 (1.37, 1.95)	32	<0.001	75
	Former	1.31 (1.17, 1.46)	33	<0.001	51
Liver C22	Current	1.56 (1.29, 1.87)	24	<0.001	69
	Former	1.49 (1.06, 2.10)	12	0.009	53
Pancreas C25	Current	1.70 (1.51, 1.91)	18	0.038	37
	Former	1.18 (1.04, 1.33)	22	0.172	24
Nasal-sinuses, C11	Current	1.95 (1.31, 2.91)	10	<0.001	68
Nasopharynx, C30–31	Former	1.39 (1.08, 1.79)	6	0.830	0
Larynx C32	Current	6.98 (3.14, 15.5)	10	<0.001	89
	Former	4.65 (3.35, 6.45)	3	0.550	0
Lung C34	Current	8.96 (6.73, 12.1)	21	<0.001	75
	Former	3.85 (2.77, 5.34)	20	<0.001	51
Cervix C53	Current	1.83 (1.51, 2.21)	23	<0.001	77
	Former	1.26 (1.11, 1.42)	22	0.645	0
Kidney C64	Current	1.52 (1.33, 1.74)	14	0.031	39
	Former	1.25 (1.14, 1.37)	12	0.001	59
Lower urinary tract C65–67	Current	2.77 (2.17, 3.54)	21	<0.001	76
	Former	1.72 (1.46, 2.04)	15	<0.001	63
Myeloid leukemia C92	Current	1.09 (0.70, 1.70)	4	0.183	36
	Former	1.27 (0.28, 5.83)	3	0.030	66

[a]Reference category "Never smokers"; I^2 represents the percentage of total variation across studies that is attributable to heterogeneity rather than to chance

In addition, even secondhand tobacco smoke have its own carcinogenicity, since the risk of developing smoking-related cancers increases with increasing the exposure to passive smoke.

4.3 Lung Cancer

At the beginning of the twentieth century, lung cancer has become the most common, in terms of incidence and mortality, nonskin malignancy worldwide (Parkin et al. 1999) (Fig. 4.3).

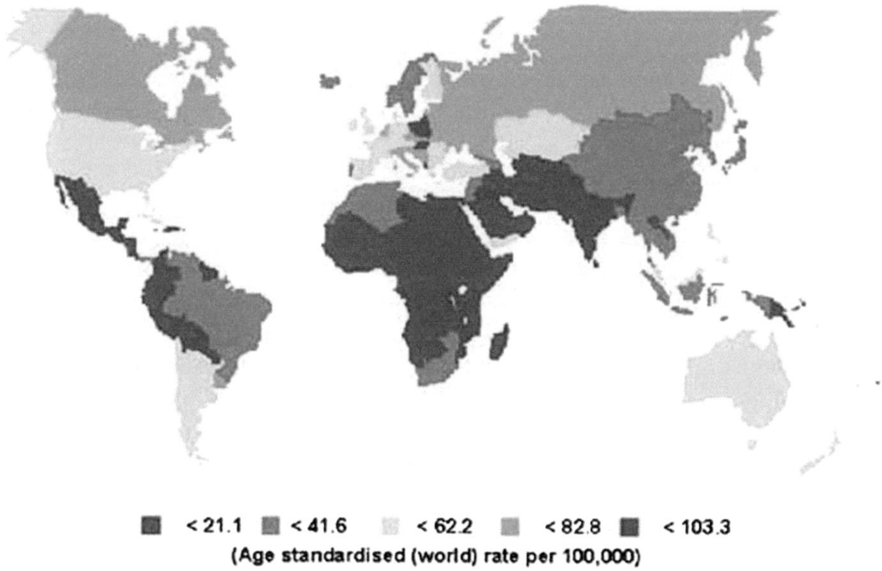

Fig. 4.3 Incidence of lung cancer in males (Parkin 2004)

Lung cancer was the most commonly diagnosed cancer and the leading cause of cancer death in males in 2008 worldwide. It was the fourth most commonly diagnosed cancer among females and the second leading cause of cancer death. Lung cancer accounts for 13 % (1.6 million) of the total cases and 18 % (1.4 million) of the deaths in 2008 (Jemal et al. 2011); 772,000 new cases each year in men (18 % of all nonskin cancers) and 265,000 new cases among women (7 %), 42 % of which occur in developing countries (Kuper et al. 2002).

The highest lung cancer incidence rates for males, are found in East–South Europe, North America, Eastern Asia, Micronesia, and Polynesia. In females, the highest lung cancer incidence rates are found in North America, Northern Europe, and Australia/New Zealand. Despite their lower prevalence of smoking (<4 % adult smokers), Chinese females have higher lung cancer rates (21.3/100,000) than those in certain European countries such as Germany (16.4) and Italy (11.4), with an adult smoking prevalence of about 20 % (Mackay et al. 2006).

Ninety one percentage of all lung cancers in men and 69 % in women are attributable to cigarette smoking (Sasco et al. 2004).

In 1950s, it has been demonstrated that lung cancer is causatively associated with cigarette smoking.

Although cigarette consumption has gradually decreased in the USA, lung cancer death rate amounts 74.9/100,000/year among males and 28.5/100,000/year among females. However, in the younger cohorts, the lung cancer death rate is decreasing in both sexes (Wynder and Muscat 1995).

According to WHO, in 2008 there were 1.37 million deaths from lung cancer worldwide and tobacco use is the most important risk factor causing 71 % of global lung cancer deaths. Lung cancer kills more people than any other cancer and this trend is expected to continue (World Health Organization 2012).

Almost 90 % of lung cancers in men and 83 % in women are estimated to be caused by smoking. Current smokers are 15 times more likely to die from lung cancer than nonsmokers. Risk of developing lung cancer is affected by level of consumption and duration of smoking.

Doll and Peto, analyzing the data of the British doctors prospective study, concluded that lung cancer risk raises in proportion to the square of the number of cigarettes smoked per day and to the fourth or fifth power of the duration of smoking (Doll et al. 2004, 2005)

Death rates from lung cancer increase dramatically with age (between ages 45 and 74 years), especially in male smokers while rates remained essentially constant in lifelong never smokers. The RR is biphasic, first increasing (in men) and later decreasing (in both sexes). The RR in men increased from 7 (at ages 45–49) to 39 (at ages 55–59) and then decreased to 13.8 (at age 80 and older). In women, the RR decreased from 22.1 (at ages 45–49) to 7.3 (at age 80 and older) (Thun et al. 1997).

Eighty six percentage of the total cases of lung cancer in the UK in 2010 were due to exposure to tobacco smoke, of which 97.4 % are due to current or past active smoking. 87 % of male cases are due to tobacco exposure (of which 97.7 % were due to smoking), and 84 % of cases for women (of which 96.2 % were due to smoking). In total, 60,837 cancer cases (19.4 % of all new cancer cases) are attributable to tobacco: 36,537 (23.0 %) in men and 24,300 (15.6 %) in women (Parkin 2011).

Compared with nonsmokers, those who smoke between 1 and 14 cigarettes a day have eight times the risk of dying from lung cancer and those who smoke 25 or more cigarettes a day have 25 times the risk. However, risk is more dependent on duration of smoking than consumption: smoking one pack of cigarettes a day for 40 years is more hazardous than smoking two packs a day for 20 years (Lubin et al. 2006, 2007).

Smoking cessation has very significant health benefits: a lifelong male smoker has a cumulative risk of 15.9 % for dying from lung cancer by age 75. For men who cease smoking at ages 60, 50, 40, and 30 years, their cumulative risk of dying from lung cancer decreases to 9.9 %, 6.0 %, 3.0 %, and 1.7 %, respectively (Fig. 4.4) (Peto et al. 2000).

The substantial decrease in lung cancer risk occurs 5–15 years after cessation (Thun et al. 1997).

People who stop smoking, avoids most of their risk of lung cancer, and stopping before middle age avoids more than 90 % of the risk attributable to tobacco (Peto et al. 2000).

Age at the start of regular tobacco smoking is also important. There is evidence that starting to smoke at a young age carries additional risks of lung damage: starting before age 15 have a four- to fivefold higher risk of lung cancer than starting at age 25 or later (IARC International Agency for Research on Cancer 1986; Wiencke et al. 1999).

Tobacco smoking induces all major histological types of lung cancer, but the strongest associations are with squamous cell and small cell carcinoma: the RR for adenocarcinoma are four- to fivefold lower than for other histological types (Lubin et al. 1984).

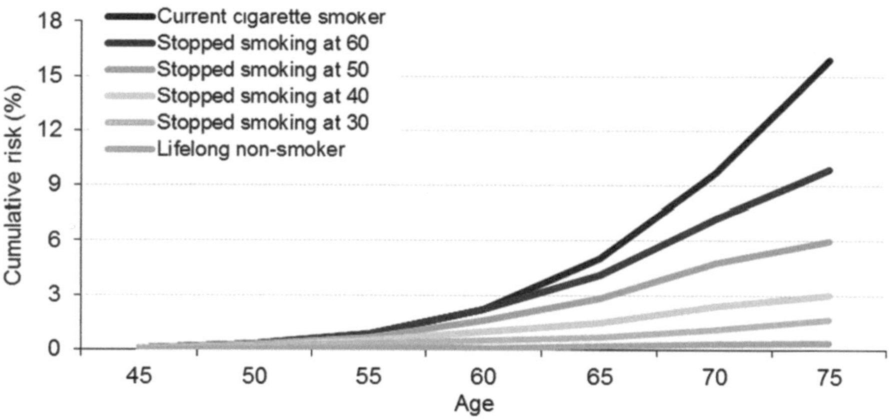

Fig. 4.4 Effects of stopping smoking at various ages on the cumulative risk (%) of death from lung cancer by age 75 for men (Peto et al. 2000)

Over the last two decades in the USA and Europe squamous cell carcinoma has become less common and adenocarcinoma more frequent, and this maybe reflects changes in patterns of tobacco consumption (Levi et al. 1997).

Nonsmokers exposed to environmental tobacco smoke (ETS) have an increased risk of lung cancer. The carcinogenicity of secondhand tobacco smoke is based on the fact that people exposed to secondhand tobacco smoke at home had 20–30 % increased lung cancer risk; similarly, never smokers exposed at the workplace have a 16–19 % increased risk (Sasco et al. 2004).

Meta-analyses have shown that exposure to ETS at home or at work among nonsmokers increases risk by about a quarter, heavy exposure doubles risk (Taylor et al. 2007; Stayner et al. 2007).

Two percentage of lung cancer cases in nonsmoking men and 10.1 % in women would be due to their current partner's smoke as well as 8 % of cases in never-smoking men and 9 % in women would be due to workplace exposure to ETS (Parkin 2011).

Taylor et al. performed a meta-analyses to review the epidemiological evidence for the association between passive smoking and lung cancer. The pooled RR for never-smoking women exposed to ETS from spouses was 1.29 (95 % CI: 1.17–1.43): this statistically significant result indicates an increased risk of approximately 30 % for nonsmoking women exposed to spousal ETS.

Since 1992 the RR has been greater than 1.25. For western industrialized countries the RR for never-smoking women exposed to ETS compared with unexposed never-smoking women, was 1.21 (95 % CI: 1.10–1.33) (Taylor et al. 2001).

Compared with adults, children may be more susceptible to secondhand smoke. Daily exposure for many hours to environmental tobacco smoke exposure during childhood showed an association with lung cancer, mainly among those who had never smoked.

Case–control studies have confirmed the link with exposure to ETS in childhood, showing that risk increases 47–125 %. The European Prospective Investigation into

Cancer and Nutrition (EPIC) has shown that heavy exposure to ETS (daily for many hours) in childhood increases risk of lung cancer by almost four times (OR, 3.63; 95 % CI: 1.19–11.11); the association between childhood secondhand smoke exposure and lung cancer risk has been also confirmed in several studies such as the Mayo Clinic study (OR, 1.47; 95 % CI: 1.00–2.15), and the meta-analysis conducted in the Surgeon General's report (OR, 0.93; 95 % CI: 0.81–1.07) in US studies (Vineis et al. 2005; Olivo-Marston et al. 2009).

As already discussed, it appears clear that the most important and cost-effective management for lung cancer is smoking cessation.

4.4 Cancer of the Larynx

The carcinogenic effect of smoking on laryngeal cancer is well established; though light-inhalation smoking is lower risk than deeper inhalation, carcinogenic effect is confirmed even also for merely puffing on smoking products (Ramroth et al. 2011). 140,000 new cases of laryngeal cancer occurred worldwide in 1990, 120,000 of which were among men (Parkin et al. 1999). Male incidence is particularly high in Southern and Central Europe (the highest mortality rates in the world for laryngeal cancer in men are in Hungary, Poland, Slovakia, and Romania), South America, and amongst Blacks in the USA, while it is low in South-east Asia and Central Africa (Parkin et al. 1997).

From 1978 to 1982, the respective age-adjusted morbidity rate for men in Spain was 17.2/100,000, in Italy 16.2/100,000, in France 12.6/100,000, and in Poland 11.4/100,000. In 1996 in Poland the morbidity rate had reached 13.9/100,000 for men (Bień et al. 2008).

Several studies have shown a dose–response relationship for intensity and duration of smoking, since the odds ratios for current smokers range widely from about 3–20; the risk decreases in past smokers compared to current smokers, although the number of years of quitting needed to have a significant reduction in risk compared with current smokers range from 6–9 to 20 or more (Bosetti et al. 2006; Hashibe et al. 2007; Talamini et al. 2002; Austin et al.1996; Kuper et al. 2002).

A recent study showed that people who stopped smoking before the age of 35 or 20 or more years ago did not have a significantly higher risk of developing upper aerodigestive tract cancer than never smokers (Bosetti et al. 2006).

Moreover, smoking unfiltered high-tar cigarettes leads to a stronger risk (Baron et al. 1996).

A case–control study on larynx and hypopharynx cancer carried out in different European countries (Italy, Spain, Switzerland, France) shows the effect of tobacco is similar for all sites of larynx and the risk associated with ever smoking is of the order of 10. For all sites the risk decreases after quitting (RR = 0.3 after 10 years); exclusive use of filter cigarettes is protective (RR = 0.5 relative to smokers of plain cigarettes only) as is exclusive use of blond tobacco (RR = 0.5 relative to smokers of black tobacco only). Inhalation increases the risk of endolaryngeal cancer but not that of hypopharynx or epilarynx. The RR for exposure to both alcohol and tobacco are consistent with a multiplicative model (Tuyns et al. 1988).

Also cigar and pipe smoking has been associated with a tenfold increased risk of cancer of the larynx and hypopharynx combined (Lee et al. 2009).

Some studies show that risks associated with smoking are twice as high or more for tumors of the supraglottis than glottis (De Stefani et al. 2004; Menvielle et al. 2004; Dosemeci et al. 1997).

According to a large population-based case–control study in Southern Europe, over 90 % of the incidence of laryngeal cancer could be prevented by avoiding smoking and alcohol consumption; most of the risk is attributable to tobacco smoking, including passive smoking (Berrino and Crosignani 1992).

A population-based case–control study in Germany, found a clear dose–response relationship not only for deep inhalers but also for those puffing on a cigarette; anyway, changing inhalation habits could be considered as a first step to reducing the risk of developing laryngeal cancer (Ramroth et al. 2011).

4.5 Cancer of the Esophagus

There are two main histological types of esophageal cancer: squamous cell carcinoma (SCC) and adenocarcinoma (AC). In the upper two-thirds the most common histology is SCC: in the lower third AC; tobacco consumption increases the risk of both SCC and AC, although the effect is stronger for SCC (Vizcaino et al. 2002) (Fig. 4.5).

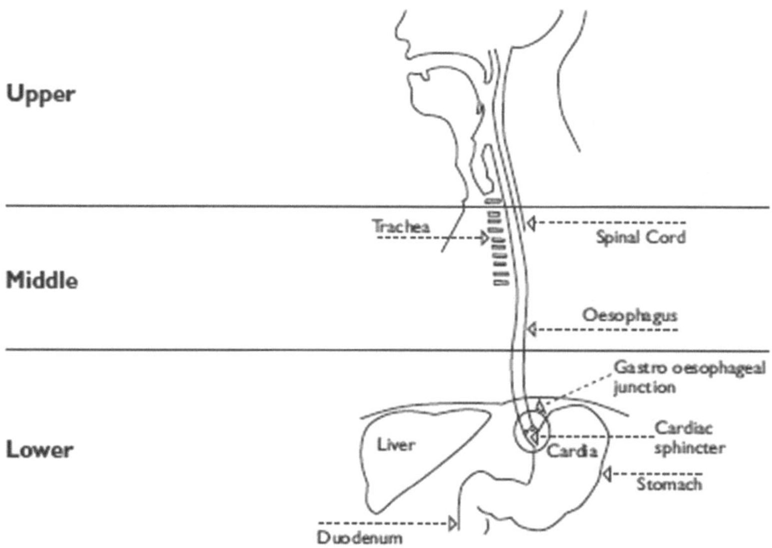

Fig. 4.5 Diagram of esophagus

Worldwide, an estimated 462,000 new cases of esophageal cancer occurred in 2002. About 80–85 % of cases are diagnosed in developing countries where it is the fourth most common cancer in men (Parkin et al. 2005a, b).

The area with the highest reported incidence for esophageal cancer ranges from eastern Turkey through north-eastern Iran, northern Afghanistan, and southern Russia to northern China and also south-east Africa, south America, and parts of Europe have high rates (Parkin 2004; Castellsague et al. 2000).

In Iran, rates are more than 200 per 100,000 and the male/female ratio is 0.8:1.0 (Hormozdiari et al. 1975a, b).

In China, rates per 100,000 are 184 for men and 123 for women compared with 8.4 for English men and 3.5 for English women (Parkin et al. 2002).

In the United Kingdom (UK), esophageal cancer is the fifth most common cause of cancer death in men and women combined with more than 7,000 deaths annually. Incidence rates in the UK are significantly higher than the EU average; during the last 25 years incidence rates for esophageal cancer have increased in Britain. UK men have the third highest rates after French and Hungarian men while UK women have the highest incidence, more than ten times higher than Greek women (IARC 2004). The British male incidence rates rose from 8.8 per 100,000 in 1975 to 14.1 in 2001 while female rates rose from 4.8 to 5.8. In particular, a recent analysis recorded the highest incidence for esophageal cancer in Scotland, North West England, and north Wales. Especially in Scotland the male rates also show a substantial increase from 11.3 per 100,000 population in 1975 to 17.2 in 2001 and women from 6.3 in 1979 to 8.7 in 1996 but have decreased to 6.8 in 2001 (ISD Online 2004; Quinn et al. 2005).

The association between tobacco smoking and cancer of the esophagus was already clear in 1985 (IARC 1986).

Smoking cigarettes, cigars, or pipes or by chewing tobacco increases the risk of esophageal cancer. The RR of esophageal cancer among cigar smokers is similar to that for cigarette smokers. The higher rates for higher numbers of cigars per day or with deeper inhalation confirms a dose–response effect (Burns et al. 1998).

A recent pooled analysis of European studies showing a fourfold risk increased for esophageal cancer among current smokers (Lee et al. 2009).

Smoking increases the risk of both squamous cell carcinoma (SCC) and adenocarcinoma (AC), although the effect is stronger for SCC: a cohort study shows that current smokers have a ninefold risk increase for esophageal SCC and a fourfold risk increase for esophageal AC (Sharp et al. 2001).

In addition, alcohol increases the effect of tobacco consumption (even if they can also act independently). They are the main risk factors for SCC of the esophagus in western countries: heavy smoking and drinking increased the risk by 20-fold for SCC (Zambon et al. 2000).

The quantity of cigarettes smoked and the duration of smoking are directly related to risk and the risk declines on smoking cessation (wipes 10 or more years after giving up) (Zambon et al. 2000) although the study performed by Freedman et al. (2007) shows that the risk of both tumor types remain three times higher than never smokers among ex-smokers who gave up 10 or more years previously.

From a case–control study in India emerged that the strongest risk factor for esophageal cancers was tobacco smoking, with OR of 2.83 (95 % CI: 2.18–3.66) in current smokers (Znaor et al. 2003).

4.6 Lower Urinary Tract

A systematic review quantified the impact of different smoking characteristics (status, amount, duration, cessation, and age at first exposure) on urinary tract cancer. Smoking status and increased amount and duration of smoking were associated with a strong increased risk of urinary tract cancer. Smoking cessation and age at first exposure were negatively associated with the risk of urinary tract cancer. The age- and gender-adjusted pooled ORs for current and former smokers compared with nonsmokers were 3.33 (95 % CI: 2.63–4.21) and 1.98 (CI: 1.72–2.29), respectively. Results suggest that current smokers have about threefold higher risk of urinary tract cancer than nonsmokers. In Europe, approximately half of urinary tract cancer cases among males and one-third of cases among females might be attributable to cigarette smoking (Zeegers et al. 2000).

4.6.1 Bladder Cancer

Bladder cancer is categorized as "*non-muscle invasive bladder cancer*" or "*muscle invasive bladder cancer*." Histological classification is based on the architecture and degree of differentiation. *Papillary urothelial neoplasms* of low malignant potential have a very low risk for malignant transformation; low and high grade papillary urothelial carcinoma (UC) and carcinoma in situ (CIS) are malignancies. Staging is based on the 2002 TNM Classification of Malignant Tumors. Ta, T1, and CIS are categorized as non-muscle invasive bladder cancer or "superficial" bladder cancer and is stratified into low, intermediate, and high risk groups. Primary bladder cancers include *transitional cell carcinoma* (TCC), *adenocarcinoma*, *neuroendocrine*, or *mesenchymal* tumors (Arianayagam et al. 2011).

Cancer of the bladder is the ninth most common cause of cancer worldwide (357,000 cases in 2002) and the 13th most numerous cause of death from cancer (145,000 deaths). Rates in males are 3–4 times those in females. Incidence rates are high in many southern and eastern European countries, Africa, Middle East and North America. Egypt has the highest mortality, more than three times greater than in Europe and eight times greater in the USA (Parkin et al. 2008).

During the last two decades, bladder cancer mortality has shown downward trends in several western European countries but is still increasing in some eastern European countries (Pelucchi et al. 2006).

Generally, trends are related to prevalence of known risk factors, especially exposure to tobacco.

Smoking cigarettes is the principal preventable risk factor for bladder cancer in both men and women. Current smokers have 2–6 times the risk of never smokers of developing bladder cancer, with the highest risks for people smoking for the longest or smoking a large amount of cigarettes per day. Two-thirds of bladder cancer cases in men and a third in women are caused by cigarette smoking in Europe. Smoking cessation reduces risk, but risk in ex-smokers remains higher than never smokers for more than 20 years (Brennan et al. 2000, 2001).

The risk of bladder cancer in former smokers decreases at a rate of up to 40 % in the first 4 years after cessation; in addition, continued tobacco use after the diagnosis of cancer has been associated with an increased risk of treatment-related complications, tumor recurrence, second primary malignancies, and morbidity and mortality (Guzzo et al. 2012).

The precise mechanism by which cigarette smoking induces bladder cancer is unclear. Studies show that risk varies by type of tobacco, with a higher risk for black "air-cured" than blond "flue-cured" tobacco (Samanic et al. 2006)

Smokers of black tobacco have higher levels of aromatic amines in their urine than smokers of blond tobacco (Malaveille et al. 1989). These aromatic amines are urothelial carcinogens and the ability to detoxify them is compromised in people who are "slow acetylators" and it is suggested that these people are at higher risk than "fast acetylators" (Marcus et al. 2000)

It has also been suggested that high fruit consumption may reduce the effect of smoking on developing bladder cancer (Kellen et al. 2006).

Even the exposure to environmental tobacco smoke (ETS) during childhood increased the risk of bladder cancer by almost 40 % (Bjerregaard et al. 2006). Supporting this theory, the evidence of a significant increase in risk of bladder cancer in those whose mothers had lung cancer, but no increased risk for paternal lung cancer: the authors interpreted this as evidence that exposure to tobacco carcinogens in utero or while breastfeeding may lead to bladder cancer in later life (Hemminki et al. 2006).

Several European studies estimated that the proportion of cancers of the urinary bladder attributable to tobacco smoking are in average 30 % in ever-smoking women and 66 % in ever-smoking men (Brennan et al. 2000, 2001).

Gandini et al. (2008) estimated that the pooled risk for current smokers among men was greater for cancer of the bladder (RR 5 2.80; 95 % CI: 2.01–3.92) than for cancer of the kidney (RR 5 1.59; 95 % CI: 1.32–1.91). For bladder cancer, this pooled estimate is slightly lower than that of a pooled-analysis (Puente et al. 2006) of 14 case–control studies performed by Puente et al. (RR for current smokers 5 3.89, 95 % CI: 3.53–4.29 for men and RR=3.55, 95 % CI: 3.06–4.10 for women) but similar to that of a previous meta-analysis of 23 case–control and cohort studies (RR=2.57; 95 % CI: 2.20–3.00, for men and women combined) (Zeegers et al. 2000).

4.6.2 *Kidney Cancer*

The two most common types of kidney cancer are renal cell carcinoma (RCC) and urothelial cell carcinoma (UCC) of the renal pelvis. Less common types of kidney cancer include squamous cell carcinoma, juxtaglomerular cell tumor (reninoma), angiomyolipoma, renal oncocytoma, Bellini duct carcinoma, clear-cell sarcoma of the kidney, mesoblastic nephroma, Wilms' tumor (which occurs in children under the age of 5), and mixed epithelial stromal tumor (Ferlay et al. 2007).

In 2002, 208,000 new cases (1.9 % of the world total) and 102,000 deaths of kidney cancer occurred. Kidney cancer is a disease of high-income countries, since the highest rates are in North America, Australia/New Zealand, and western, eastern, and northern Europe, but are low in Africa, Asia (except Japanese males), and the Pacific (Parkin et al. 2005a, b).

In 1988–1992, kidney cancer incidence rates were highest in France (16.1/100,000 man–years and 7.3/100,000 woman–years) and lowest in India (2.0 and 0.9, respectively). Between 1973–1977 and 1988–1992, incidence rates rose among men and women in all regions and ethnic groups; the largest percentage increase for men was in Japan (171 %) and for women in Italy (107 %) (Mathew et al. 2002).

Kidney cancers account for 2–3 % of all adult malignancies in the UK. Men are predominantly affected by renal cancer with an average age at diagnosis of 64 years (Lewis et al. 2012).

Renal and pelvic cancer is the third most commonly diagnosed urinary cancer in USA, accounting for about 3 % of all cancer cases. It is estimated that 30,800 new cases of renal and pelvic cancer may be diagnosed in Americans in 2001 and almost 40 % deaths (Greeenlee et al. 2001).

In the USA, from 1975 to 1995, there were 31,105 invasive cancers of the kidney and 4,985 cancers of the renal pelvis diagnosed; the age-adjusted incidence rates for white men, white women, black men, and black women were, respectively, 9.6, 4.4, 11.1, and 4.9 per 100,000 person–years. The corresponding rates for renal pelvis cancer were 1.5, 0.7, 0.8, and 0.5 per 100,000 person–years. Renal cell cancer incidence rates increased progressively during this lapse of time, by 2.3 % annually among white men, 3.1 % among white women, 3.9 % among black men, and 4.3 % among black women (Chow et al. 1999). 64,770 new cases and 13,570 deaths from kidney (renal cell and renal pelvis) cancer in the USA have been estimated in 2012 (http://www.cancer.gov/cancertopics/types/kidney. Last accessed April 23, 2012).

Epidemiological evidence shows that cigarette smoking is the major risk factor for renal cell carcinoma and cancer of the renal pelvis (IARC 2002).

On average, current smokers have a 50 % increase in risk of kidney cancer (Gandini et al. 2008). The IARC cancer mortality database indicates approximately 20,000 kidney cancer deaths attributable to smoking (US Department of Health and Human Services 2004) and it has been estimated that 24–32 % of renal cell cancer cases in men and 9–16 % in women can be related to smoking (Setiawan et al. 2007; McLaughlin et al. 1995)

Case–control studies have found that smoking doubles the risk and risk increases with the duration of smoking and number of cigarettes smoked per day (Doll 1996).

People who smoke more than 20 cigarettes per day increase their risk by 60–100 % compared to nonsmokers. Former smokers have a 25 % higher risk of kidney cancer, while the risk for cancer of the renal pelvis is more than threefold time higher in current smokers (Hunt et al. 2005; McLaughlin et al. 1992).

Some studies reported that long-term quitters (>15 years) have a 15–25 % reduced risk compared with current smokers (Kuper et al. 2002), but others have not found a clear dose–response effect (Doll et al. 1994).

4.7 Pancreatic Cancer

Even if pancreatic cancer has been increasing in incidence over the past 40 years, it still has a relative low incidence (it ranks 13th), but despite that, its mortality rates are high, responsible for 227,000 deaths per year, and is the eighth most common cause of cancer death (Lowenfels and Maisonneuve 2006; IARC 2004).

Pancreatic cancer is one of the most aggressive tumors: the 5-year survival rate is <5 % and a mortality rate is almost 100 % (MacLeod et al. 2006).

The most common type of pancreatic cancer (95 % of the total) is the adenocarcinoma (tumors exhibiting glandular architecture on light microscopy) arising within the exocrine component of the pancreas, while neuroendocrine tumors arise from islet cells (Ghaneh et al. 2008).

The sex ratio is close to one. 61 % of cases and deaths occur in developed countries, where incidence and mortality rates are 7–9 per 100,000 in men and 4.5–6 per 100,000 in women, with lower rates in developing countries (but this probably reflects lower diagnostic capacity rather than etiology). Among developing countries, the highest rates are observed in Central and South America (Parkin et al. 2005a, b).

Incidence rates vary in different countries implying that environmental factors are important. Of these factors, smoking is the most well-documented etiologic agent (Lowenfels and Maisonneuve 2006).

Smoking has been recognized as a cause of pancreatic cancer with an approximate two- to fourfold increased risk (Chiu et al. 2001).

An increased risk of pancreatic cancer was found for current cigarette smokers compared with never smokers (HR = 1.71, 95 % CI: 1.36–2.15), and risk increased with greater intensity and pack–years (Vrieling et al. 2009).

In the UK, smoking is estimated to cause up to 20 % of pancreatic cancers (Iodice et al. 2008). A British study reported that ex-smokers were 1.4 times more likely to die of pancreatic cancer compared with never smoked. Current smokers of less than 25 cigarettes a day had 1.8 times the risk of death and smokers of 25 or more cigarettes a day were at 3.1 times the risk of never smokers (Doll et al. 1994).

A recent meta-analysis showed that smoking could be responsible for about 75 % increase in the risk of pancreatic cancer and that the risk increases with the number of cigarettes smoked and the duration. The risk of pancreatic cancer was estimated to be 1.74 (95 % confidence interval [CI]: 1.61–1.87) for current smokers and 1.2 (95 % CI: 1.11–1.29) for former ones; the study also showed an increase in pancreatic cancer risk for pipe and/or cigar smokers (Iodice et al. 2008).

Studies have reported a positive trend with number of years of smoking among men but not women; in addition, smokers are diagnosed on average 10 years younger than nonsmokers (Coughlin et al. 2000; Lowenfels and Maisonneuve 2004; Gold and Goldin 1998).

Recent results from the European Prospective Investigation into Cancer and Nutrition (EPIC) showed that former cigarette smokers who quit for <5 years were at increased risk of pancreatic cancer (HR = 1.78, 95 % CI: 1.23–2.56), but risk was comparable to never smokers after quitting for 5 years or more (Vrieling et al. 2009) but some other studies have reported that it takes 10–20 years after cessation for risk to return to the level of a never smoker (Coughlin et al. 2000; Bonelli et al. 2003; Lowenfels and Maisonneuve 2004; Lynch et al. 2009; Heinen et al. 2010).

La Torre et al. performed a meta-analysis of observational studies on association between cigarette smoking and pancreatic cancer. Six cohort studies and 24 case–control studies were selected, with median quality scores of 8 and 10, respectively. Pooled case–control studies' OR and cohort studies' risk ratio were, respectively, 1.45 (95 % CI: 1.33–1.57) and 1.78 (95 % CI: 1.64–1.92). After stratifying for quality scoring, high-quality-scored case–control studies yielded an OR of 1.38 (95 % CI: 1.27–1.49), whereas the others gave an OR of 1.52 (95 % CI: 1.34–1.73). The results of meta-analysis for cohort studies showed a risk ratio of 1.74 (95 % CI: 1.61–1.90) and of 2.10 (95 % CI: 1.64–2.67), respectively, for high- and low-quality score studies. The results obtained shows a significant excess risk of pancreatic cancer associated with cigarette smoking habit of nearly 80 % for cohort studies and nearly 50 % for case–control studies. RR varies from a minimum of 1.60 (95 % CI: 0.95–2.60) to a maximum of 3.81 (95 % CI: 2.08–7.00) for cohort studies and OR ranging from a minimum of 0.98 (95 % CI: 0.77–1.24) to a maximum of 3.25 (95 % CI: 1.94–5.44) for case–control studies; none of the studies selected showed a significant protective effect of smoking. The estimation of the association greatly relies on the studies' quality, showing an increased risk of 74 % and 110 % for cohort studies and of 38 % and 52 % for case–control studies: low-quality studies seem to overestimate the risk (La Torre et al. 2009b).

Risk for pancreatic cancer is increased almost threefold also among cigar smokers who inhaled their smoke, particularly those who smoke higher number of cigars per day but not for cigar smokers overall (Shapiro et al. 2000).

Furthermore pancreatic cancer risk is increased among never smokers daily exposed to ETS (for many hours) during childhood (HR = 2.61, 95 % CI: 0.96–7.10) and exposed to ETS at home and/or work (HR = 1.54, 95 % CI: 1.00–2.39): both active cigarette smoking, as well as exposure to ETS, is associated with increased risk of pancreatic cancer (Vrieling et al. 2009).

4.8 Stomach Cancer

Stomach cancer is the fourth most frequent cancer worldwide: 989,600 new cases (8.7 % of the total) and it is the second most frequent cause of death from cancer with 738,000 deaths (10.4 % of cancer deaths). Over 70 % of new cases and deaths occur in developing countries. Generally, stomach cancer rates are about twice as high in males as in females (Jemal et al. 2011).

Almost 90 % of stomach cancers are adenocarcinomas, originating from glandular epithelium of the gastric mucosa. Histologically, there are two major types of gastric adenocarcinoma: intestinal type or diffuse type (Lauren classification). Intestinal type adenocarcinoma tumor cells describe irregular tubular structures, pluristratification with multiple lumens and reduced stroma. Diffuse type adenocarcinoma tumor cells (mucinous, colloid, linitis plastica, leather-bottle stomach) are discohesive and secrete mucus producing large pools of mucus/colloid and is poorly differentiated. About 5 % of gastric malignancies are lymphomas (MALTomas, or MALT lymphoma); carcinoid and stromal tumors may also occur (Paterson et al. 2006).

Most of cases occur in developing countries. Incidence rates are highest in Japan Korea, China, Eastern Europe, Central and South America. Incidence rates are low in Southern Asia, North-East Africa, North America, Australia, and New Zealand (Parkin 2004) (Fig. 4.6).

Among European countries, the 5-year survival rate varies from 10 to 20 %. In the last two decades, its incidence has gradually decreased in both developing and developed countries, but the risk appears clearly related to strong environmental component (La Torre et al. 2009a, b).

Beyond *Helicobacter pylori* infection, an important cause of stomach cancer is tobacco smoking: smokers have a 50–60 % increased risk of stomach cancer, as compared to nonsmokers; this could explain that the recent decline in smoking prevalence in men from developed countries may account for part of the fall in gastric cancer rates (Bertuccio et al. 2009; Boyle et al. 2003).

Although tobacco smoking has not been considered the major risk factor for gastric cancer, a large number of epidemiological studies reported information on this association. In total, over 80,000 cases of gastric cancer (11 % of all estimated cases) may be attributed to tobacco smoking each year worldwide (Trédaniel et al. 1997).

It has been estimated that 11 % of men and 4 % of women in developing countries and 17 % men and 11 % women in developed countries who have stomach cancer are related to smoking habit (Boyle et al. 2003).

Trédaniel et al. (1997) carried out a meta-analysis to estimate the association between gastric cancer risk and tobacco smoking. Results suggest a risk among smokers of 1.5–1.6 as compared to nonsmokers. The RR was higher in men (1.59) than in women (1.11). Several studies examined the dose–response too.

A more recent quantitative meta-analysis found a statistically significant result for the association between ever-smoking status and gastric cancer risk (OR = 1.48; 95 % CI: 1.28–1.71; $p<0.00001$). The meta-analysis also showed a 69 % increase in the risk of gastric cancer for current smokers compared to never smokers (OR = 1.69; 95 % CI: 1.35–2.11; $p<0.00001$). Considering only high quality

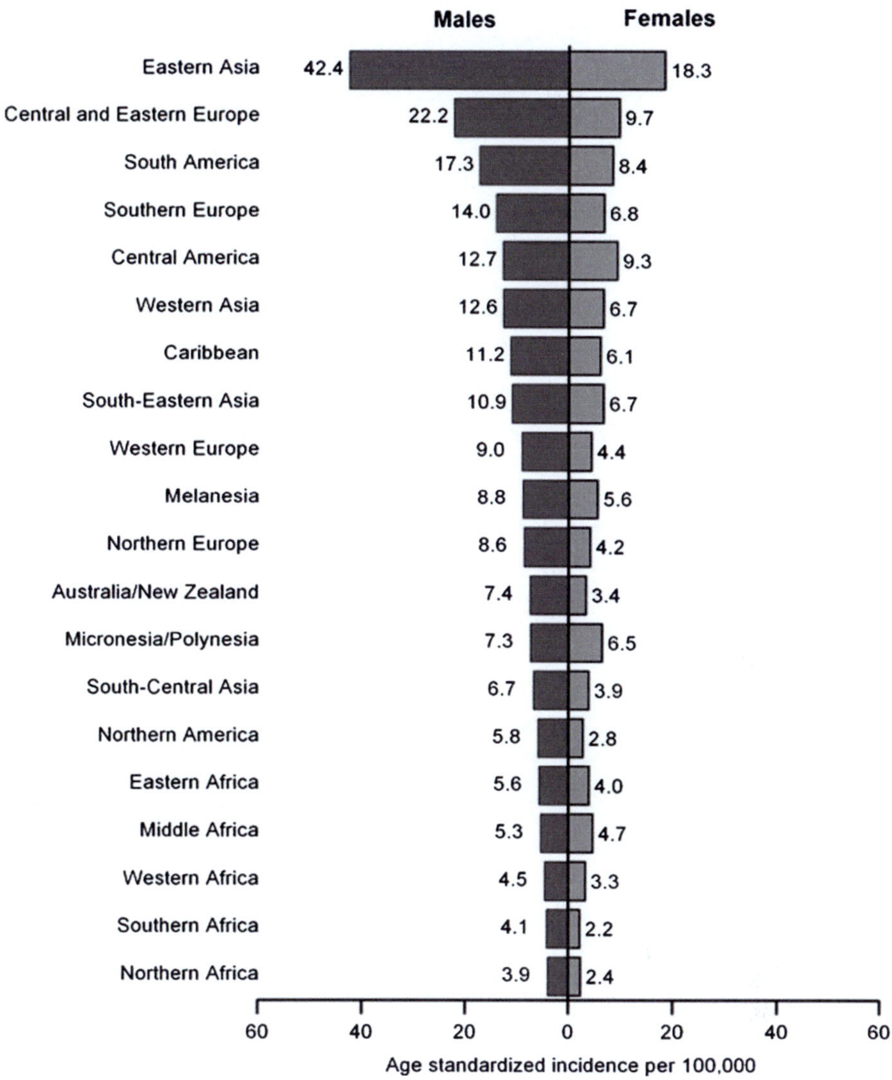

Fig. 4.6 Age-standardized stomach cancer incidence rates by sex and world area (Ferlay et al. 2010)

studies, the OR increased by 43 % for gastric cancer risk in ever smokers (OR = 1.43; 95 % CI: 1.24–1.66; $p < 0.00001$) and by 57 % in current smokers (OR = 1.57; 95 % CI: 1.24–2.01). Taking into account separately Caucasians and Asian studies, we found for ever smokers an OR of 1.46 (95 % CI: 1.25–1.70; $p < 0.00001$) and an OR of 1.47 (95 % CI: 1.13–1.91; $p < 0.00001$), respectively.

Furthermore, considering the two different types of gastric cancer separately, was found for noncardia gastric cancer an OR of 1.32 (95 % CI: 1.11–1.57; $p = 0.30$) for ever smokers and an OR of 2.04 (95 % CI: 1.66–2.50; $p = 0.10$) for current smokers. For cardia gastric cancer, was found an OR of 1.47 (95 % CI: 1.15–1.87; $p=0.73$) for ever smokers and an OR of 2.05 (95 % CI: 1.50–2.81; $p=0.84$) for current smokers (La Torre et al. 2009a).

Data obtained from a Russian case–control study showed that smoking increases the risk of developing gastric cancer in men, but not in women. In men a dose–response relationship between mean number of cigarettes smoked per day ($p=0.03$), pack–years of cigarettes smoked ($p=0.01$), duration of smoking ($p=0.08$), and the risk of cancer of gastric cardia was observed. The risk of gastric cancer associated with smoking varied according to *H. pylori* infection status since it was significantly increased among *H. pylori*-infected men (OR = 2.3, CI = 1.1–4.7) (Zaridze et al. 2000).

This result suggests that smoking may increase the carcinogenic effect of *H. pylori*.

A pooled analysis of two population-based prospective cohort studies in rural northern Japan (Koizumi et al. 2004) was performed to examine the association between cigarette smoking and the risk of gastric cancer. The pooled multivariate RRs (95 % CI) for current smokers and past smokers were 1.84 (1.39–2.43) and 1.77 (1.29–2.43), respectively. A linear increase in risk associated with the higher number of cigarettes smoked per day was observed: the pooled multivariate RRs (95 % CIs) for current smokers who smoked 1–19, 20–24, and >25 cigarettes per day were 1.41 (1.00–1.98), 1.98 (1.45–2.71), and 2.15 (1.53–3.02), respectively. A linear increase in risk associated with pack–years of smoking was also found: the pooled multivariate RRs (95 % CIs) for <25, 25–39, and >40 pack–years of smoking in comparison to never smokers were 1.55 (1.07–2.25), 2.20 (1.56–3.11), and 2.26 (1.61–3.18), respectively. For past smokers, a significant increase in risk remained for up to 14 years after cessation: the pooled multivariate RRs (95 % CIs) for past smokers who had quit <5, 5–14, and >15 years previously compared to subjects who had never smoked were 1.72 (1.12–2.64), 2.08 (1.41–3.07), and 1.31 (0.77–2.21), respectively.

A systematic review provided solid evidence to classify smoking as the most important behavioral risk factor for gastric cancer, addressing the magnitude of the association for different levels of exposure, and cancer locations. Comparing current smokers with never smokers: the pooled RR estimates were 1.62 in males (95 % CI: 1.50–1.75) and 1.20 in females (95 % CI: 1.01–1.43); the RR increased from 1.3 for the lowest consumptions to 1.7 for the smoking of approximately 30 cigarettes per day in the trend estimation analysis; in addition, smoking was significantly associated with both cardia (RR = 1.87; 95 % CI: 1.31–2.67) and non-cardia (RR = 1.60; 95 % CI: 1.41–1.80) cancers (Ladeiras-Lopes et al. 2008).

4.9 Breast Cancer

Breast cancer is the most frequently diagnosed cancer and the leading cause of cancer death in females worldwide, accounting for 23 % (1.38 million) of the total cancer cases and 14 % (458,400) of the total cancer deaths in 2008. About 50 % of

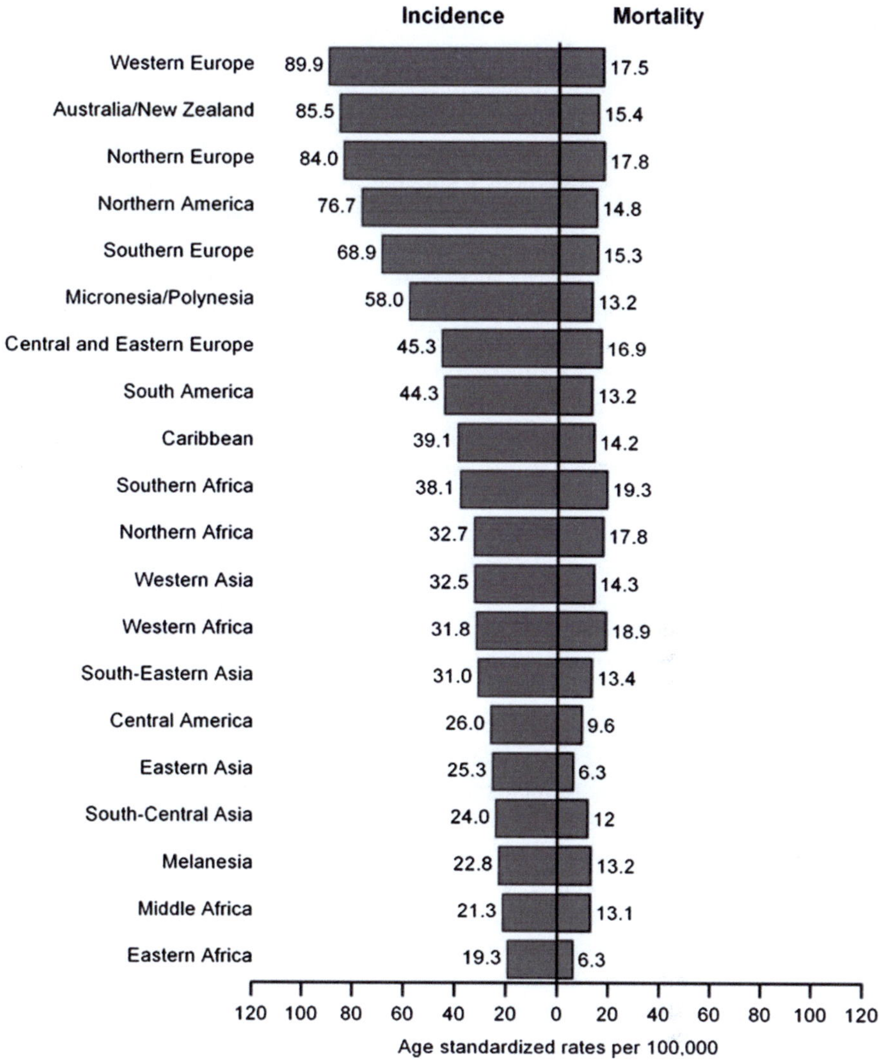

Fig. 4.7 Age-standardized breast cancer incidence and mortality rates by world area (Ferlay et al. 2010)

the cases and 60 % of the deaths occur in economically developing countries. Incidence rates are high in Western and Northern Europe, Australia/New Zealand, and North America; intermediate in South America, the Caribbean, and Northern Africa; and low in sub-Saharan Africa and Asia females (Jemal et al. 2011) (Fig. 4.7).

The familial tendency to develop the hereditary breast cancer is due to the BRCA mutations that confer a lifetime risk of breast cancer of between 60 and 85 %. Some mutations associated with cancer, such as p53, BRCA1, and BRCA2, occur in mechanisms to correct errors in DNA. These mutations are either inherited or acquired after birth. Presumably, they allow further mutations, which allow uncontrolled division, lack of attachment, and metastasis to distant organs (Dunning et al. 1999).

Most breast cancers are classified as ductal or lobular carcinoma and derived from the epithelium lining the ducts or lobules. Carcinoma in situ is growth of low grade cancerous or precancerous cells without invasion of the surrounding tissue. In contrast, invasive carcinoma does not confine itself to the initial tissue compartment (Hartmann et al. 1999).

During the past 25 years, breast cancer death rates have been decreasing in North America and several European countries as a result of early detection and improved treatment (Jemal et al. 2010), while in many African and Asian countries incidence and mortality rates have been rising (Parkin et al. 2005a, b).

Despite Japan is a low-risk country, it is now the fourth leading cause of cancer death among Japanese women: the incidence and mortality of breast cancer have increased over the past three decades with incidence rates of 17.0 per 100,000 in 1975 compared with 44.4 in 2005 (Matsuda et al. 2011; Shin et al. 2010).

On the opposite, mortality rates in the UK and US have been declining since the early 1990s, maybe attributable to improvements in screening and treatment (Jatoi and Miller 2003).

Geographical distribution and trends in cancer incidence and mortality highlight the influence of environmental factors and lifestyle in cancer etiology (Iwasaki and Tsugane 2011).

A prospective cohort study (Luo et al. 2011) examined the association between smoking and risk of invasive breast cancer among postmenopausal women. The risk was elevated by 9 % among former smokers HR = 1.09 (95 % CI 1.02–1.17) and by 16 % among current smokers HR = 1.16 (1.00–1.34). Significantly higher risk was found in active smokers with high intensity and duration of smoking, who started smoking in the teenage years. The highest breast cancer risk was found among women who had smoked for ≥50 years HR 1.35 (1.03–1.77) compared with all nonsmokers, HR 1.45 (1.06–1.98) compared with nonsmokers with no exposure to passive smoking. Furthermore, an increased risk persisted for up to 20 years after smoking cessation. There was also a suggestion of an association between passive smoking and increased risk of breast cancer: among nonsmokers women, those with ≥10 years' exposure in childhood, ≥20 years' exposure as an adult at home, and ≥10 years' exposure as an adult at work to passive smoking had a 32 % excess risk of breast cancer compared with those who had never been exposed to passive smoking HR 1.32 (1.04–1.67).

The Japan Public Health Center-based Prospective (JPHC) study found that both active and passive smoking are associated with an increased risk of breast cancer among premenopausal women. Adjusted HR (95 % CI) for ever smokers were 3.9 (1.5–9.9) and 1.1 (0.5–2.5) in pre and postmenopausal women, respectively. In never-active smokers, the adjusted HR (95 % CI) for passive smoking was 2.6 (1.3–5.2) in premenopausal women and 0.6 (0.4–1.0) in postmenopausal women (Hanaoka et al. 2005).

With regard to passive smoking, in 2007 a meta-analysis showed that it was associated with a 60–70 % increased risk for breast cancer among younger, primarily premenopausal women who had never smoked. The analysis of case–control studies which included all major sources of lifetime passive smoke exposure (combined childhood residential, adult residential and occupational), showed the pooled RR of 1.91 (95 % CI: 1.53, 2.39). The estimated summary RR was 1.06 (95 % CI: 0.96, 1.17) for those studies with more limited exposure assessment: the cohort and case–control studies yielded summary estimates of 1.02 and 1.14, respectively. The pooled RR got from the analysis of the studies reporting risk for breast cancer in premenopausal women was 1.68 (95 % CI: 1.31, 2.15) (Miller et al. 2007).

On the contrary, the meta-analysis conducted by Pirie et al. found no association between secondhand smoke and breast cancer in studies that collected information on exposure prior to the development of breast cancer (Pirie et al. 2008).

A large prospective cohort study suggest that active smoking especially smoking before first birth may be associated with a modest increase in the risk of BC. It has been estimated a HR of breast cancer (BC) of 1.06 % (95 % CI 1.01 %–1.11 %) for ever smokers compared to never smokers. BC incidence was linked with higher quantity of current ($p=0.02$) and past smoking ($p=0.003$), younger age of initiation ($p=0.01$), longer duration ($p=0.01$) and more pack–years (PKY) of smoking ($p=0.005$). Premenopausal smoking was associated with a slightly higher incidence of BC (HR = 1.11, 95 % CI 1.07–1.15 for increase of every 20 PKY) especially smoking before first birth (HR = 1.18, 95 % CI 1.10–1.27 for increase of every 20-PKY) (Xue et al. 2011).

Data obtained from the Canadian National Breast Screening Study (NBSS) showed that breast cancer risk was associated with the duration (40 years) RR = 1.50 (95 % CI: 1.19, 1.89), intensity (40 cigarettes per day) RR = 1.20 (95 % CI: 1.00, 1.44), cumulative exposure (40 pack–years) RR = 1.17 (95 % CI: 1.02, 1.34), and latency of cigarette smoking (40 years since beginning of smoking) RR = 1.28 (95 % CI: 1.06, 1.55), as well as smoking initiation before a first full-term pregnancy (among parous women, more than 5 years of smoking) RR = 1.13 (95 % CI: 1.01–1.25). These results strongly suggest that cigarette smoking plays an important role in breast cancer etiology, particularly when started early in life and for long durations (Cui et al. 2006; Collishaw et al. 2009).

In 2004, the International Agency for Research on Cancer (IARC) supported the "lack of carcinogenicity of tobacco smoking in humans for cancers of the female breast" (International Agency for Research on Cancer 2004a, b). However, several studies since 2002 have observed an increased risk associated with a long duration and/or high number of pack–years of smoking (Xue et al. 2011; Hanaoka et al. 2005; Luo et al. 2011).

A meta-analysis found a significant interaction between smoking, *N-acetyltransferase* 2 (NAT2) genotype, and risk of breast cancer: higher pack–years were associated with an increased risk among women with the NAT2 slow genotype but not among rapid acetylators (Ambrosone et al. 2008)

References

Ambrosone, C. B., Kropp, S., Yang, J., Yao, S., Shields, P. G., & Chang-Claude, J. (2008). Cigarette smoking, N-acetyltransferase 2 genotypes, and breast cancer risk: Pooled analysis and meta-analysis. *Cancer Epidemiology, Biomarkers & Prevention, 17*(1), 15–26.

Arianayagam, R., Arianayagam, M., & Rashid, P. (2011). Bladder cancer–current management. *Australian Family Physician, 40*(4), 209–213.

Austin, D. F., & Reynolds, P. (1996). Laryngeal cancer. In D. Schottenfeld & J. F. Fraumeni Jr. (Eds.), *Cancer epidemiology and prevention* (2nd ed., pp. 619–636). New York, NY: Oxford University Press.

Baron, J. A., & Rohan, T. E. (1996). Tobacco. In D. Schottenfeld & J. F. Fraumeni Jr. (Eds.), *Cancer epidemiology and prevention* (2nd ed., pp. 269–289). New York, NY: Oxford University Press.

Berrino, F., & Crosignani, P. (1992). Epidemiology of malignant tumors of the larynx and lung. *Annali dell'Istituto Superiore di Sanità, 28*(1), 107–120.

Bertuccio, P., Chatenoud, L., Levi, F., et al. (2009). Recent patterns in gastric cancer: A global overview. *International Journal of Cancer, 125*(3), 666–673.

Bień, S., Kamiński, B., Zyłka, S., et al. (2008). Evolution of the epidemiology and clinical characteristics of larynx and hypopharynx carcinoma in Poland from 1991 to 2001. *European Archives of Oto-Rhino-Laryngology, 265*(Suppl 1), S39–S46.

Bjartveit, K., & Tverdal, A. (2005). Health consequences of smoking 1–4 cigarettes per day. *Tobacco Control, 14*, 315–320.

Bjerregaard, B. K., Raaschou-Nielsen, O., Sørensen, M., et al. (2006). Tobacco smoke and bladder cancer-in the European prospective investigation into cancer and nutrition. *International Journal of Cancer, 119*(10), 2412–2416.

Bonelli, L., Aste, H., Bovo, P., et al. (2003). Exocrine pancreatic cancer, cigarette smoking and diabetes mellitus: a case control study in northern Italy. *Pancreas, 27*(2), 143–149.

Bosetti, C., Garavello, W., Gallus, S., & La Vecchia, C. (2006). Effects of smoking cessation on the risk of laryngeal cancer: An overview of published studies. *Oral Oncology, 42*(9), 866–872.

Boyle, P., Autier, P., Bartelink, H., et al. (2003). European code against cancer and scientific justification: Third version (2003). *Annals of Oncology, 14*, 973–1005.

Brennan, P., Bogillot, O., Cordier, S., et al. (2000). Cigarette smoking and bladder cancer in men: A pooled analysis of 11 casecontrol studies. *International Journal of Cancer, 86*, 289–294.

Brennan, P., Bogillot, O., Greiser, E., et al. (2001). The contribution of cigarette smoking to bladder cancer in women (pooled European data). *Cancer Causes and Control, 12*, 411–417.

Burns, D., Cummings, K. M., & Hoffmann, D. (1998). *Cigars: Health effects and trends* (Smoking and tobacco control Monograph No. 9 (NIH Publication No. 98–4302)). Bethesda, MD: US Department of Health and Human Services, National Institutes of Health, National Cancer Institute.

Castellsagué, X., Muñoz, N., De Stefani, E., Victora, C. G., Castelletto, R., & Rolón, P. A. (2000). Influence of mate drinking, hot beverages and diet on oesophageal cancer risk in South America. *International Journal of Cancer, 88*, 658–664.

Chiu, B. C., Lynch, C. F., Cerhan, J. R., & Cantor, K. P. (2001). Cigarette smoking and risk of bladder, pancreas, kidney and colorectal cancers in Iowa. *Annals of Epidemiology, 11*, 28–37.

Chow, W. H., Devesa, S. S., Warren, J. L., & Fraumeni, J. F., Jr. (1999). Rising incidence of renal cell cancer in the United States. *Journal of the American Medical Association, 281*, 1628–1631.

Collishaw, N. E., Boyd, N. F., Cantor, K. P., et al. (2009). *Canadian expert panel on tobacco smoke and breast cancer risk* (OTRU special report series). Toronto, Canada: Ontario Tobacco Research Unit.

Coughlin, S. S., Calle, E. E., Patel, A. V., & Thun, M. J. (2000). Predictors of pancreatic cancer mortality among a large cohort of United States adults. *Cancer Causes & Control, 11*(10), 915–923.

Cui, Y., Miller, A. B., & Rohan, T. E. (2006). Cigarette smoking and breast cancer risk: Update of a prospective cohort study. *Breast Cancer Research and Treatment, 100*(3), 293–299.

De Stefani, E., Boffetta, P., Deneo-Pellegrini, H., et al. (2004). Supraglottic and glottic carcinomas: Epidemiologically distinct entities? *International Journal of Cancer, 112*(6), 1065–1071.

Doll, R. (1996). Cancers weakly related to smoking. *British Medical Bulletin, 52*, 35–49.

Doll, R., & Hill, A. B. (1950). Smoking and carcinoma of the lung: Preliminary report. *British Medical Journal, 2*(4682), 739–748.

Doll, R., Peto, R., Boreham, J., & Sutherland, I. (2004). Mortality in relation to smoking: 50 years' observations on male British doctors. *British Medical Journal, 328*(7455), 1519.

Doll, R., Peto, R., Boreham, J., & Sutherland, I. (2005). Mortality from cancer in relation to smoking: 50 years observations on British doctors. *British Journal of Cancer, 92*(3), 426–429.

Doll, R., Peto, R., Wheatley, K., Gray, R., & Sutherland, I. (1994). Mortality in relation to smoking: 40 years' observation on male British doctors. *British Medical Journal, 309*(6959), 901–911.

Dosemeci, M., Gokmen, I., Unsal, M., Hayes, R. B., & Blair, A. (1997). Tobacco, alcohol use, and risks of laryngeal and lung cancer by subsite and histologic type in Turkey. *Cancer Causes & Control, 8*(5), 729–737.

Dunning, A. M., Healey, C. S., Pharoah, P. D., Teare, M. D., Ponder, B. A., & Easton, D. F. (1999). A systematic review of genetic polymorphisms and breast cancer risk. *Cancer Epidemiology, Biomarkers & Prevention, 8*(10), 843–854.

Ezzati, M., Henley, S. J., Lopez, A. D., & Thun, M. J. (2005). Role of smoking in global and regional cardiovascular mortality. *Circulation, 112*(4), 489–497.

Ferlay, J., Autier, P., Boniol, M., Heanue, M., Colombet, M., & Boyle, P. (2007). Estimates of the cancer incidence and mortality in Europe in 2006. *Annals of Oncology, 18*(3), 581–592.

Ferlay, J., Shin, H. R., Bray, F., Forman, D., Mathers, C., & Parkin, D. M. (2010). *GLOBOCAN 2008 v1.2, Cancer incidence and mortality worldwide: IARC CancerBase No. 10 [Internet]*. Lyon, France: International Agency for Research on Cancer. http://globocan.iarc.fr.

Freedman, N. D., Abnet, C. C., Leitzmann, M. F., et al. (2007). A prospective study of tobacco, alcohol, and the risk of oesophageal and gastric cancer subtypes. *American Journal of Epidemiology, 165*(12), 1424–1433.

Gandini Botteri, E., Iodice, S., et al. (2008). Tobacco smoking and cancer: A meta-analysis. *International Journal of Cancer, 122*(1), 155–164.

Ghaneh, P., Costello, E., & Neoptolemos, J. P. (2008). Biology and management of pancreatic cancer. *Postgraduate Medicine Journal, 84*(995), 478–497.

Gold, E. B., & Goldin, S. B. (1998). Epidemiology and risk factors for pancreatic cancer. *Surgical Oncology Clinics of North America, 7*, 67–91.

Greeenlee, R., Hill-Harmon, M. B., Murray, T., et al. (2001). Cancer statistics, 2001. *CA: A Cancer Journal for Clinicians, 51*, 15.

Guzzo, T. J., Hockenberry, M. S., Mucksavage, P., Bivalacqua, T. J., & Schoenberg, M. P. (2012). Smoking knowledge assessment and cessation trends in patients with bladder cancer presenting to a tertiary referral center. *Urology, 79*(1), 166–171.

Hanaoka, T., Yamamoto, S., Sobue, T., et al. (2005). Active and passive smoking and breast cancer risk in middle-aged Japanese women. *International Journal of Cancer, 114*, 317–322.

Hartmann, L. C., Schaid, D. J., Woods, J. E., et al. (1999). Efficacy of bilateral prophylactic mastectomy in women with a family history of breast cancer. *The New England Journal of Medicine, 340*(2), 77–84.

Hashibe, M., Boffetta, P., Zaridze, D., et al. (2007). Contribution of tobacco and alcohol to the high rates of squamous cell carcinoma of the supraglottis and glottis in Central Europe. *American Journal of Epidemiology, 165*(7), 814–820.

Heinen, M. M., Verhage, B. A., Goldbohm, R. A., & van den Brandt, P. A. (2010). Active and passive smoking and the risk of pancreatic cancer in the Netherlands Cohort Study. *Cancer Epidemiology, Biomarkers & Prevention, 19*(6), 1612–1622.

Hemminki, K., & Chen, B. (2006). Parental lung cancer as predictor of cancer risks in offspring: Clues about multiple routes of harmful influence? *International Journal of Cancer, 118*(3), 744–748.

Hormozdiari, H., Day, N. E., Aramesh, B., & Mahboubi, E. (1975a). Dietary factors and oesophageal cancer in the Caspian Littoral of Iran. *Cancer Research, 35*, 3493–3498.

Hormozdiari, H., Day, N. E., Aramesh, B. et al. (1975b). Dietary factors and oesophageal cancer in the Caspian Littoral of Iran. *Cancer Research 35*:3493–8. Accessed April 23, 2012, from http://www.cancer.gov/cancertopics/types/kidney

Hunt, J. D., van der Hel, O. L., McMillan, G. P., Boffetta, P., & Brennan, P. (2005). Renal cell carcinoma in relation to cigarette smoking: Meta-analysis of 24 studies. *International Journal of Cancer, 114*(1), 101–108.

IARC. (2002). *Monograph on the Evaluation of Carcinogenic Risk to Humans* vol. 82. Lyon, France.

IARC. (2004). Group on the evaluation of carcinogenic risks to humans. Tobacco smoke and involuntary smoking. *IARC Working Group on the Evaluation of Carcinogenic Risks to Humans, 83*, 1–1438.

IARC. (1986). Tobacco smoking. IARC Monogr Eval Carcinog Risk Chem Hum, vol. 38. Lyon, France.

Iodice, S., Gandini, S., Maisonneuve, P., & Lowenfels, A. B. (2008). Tobacco and the risk of pancreatic cancer: A review and meta-analysis. *Langenbeck's Archives of Surgery, 393*, 535–545.

Iwasaki, M., & Tsugane, S. (2011). Risk factors for breast cancer: Epidemiological evidence from Japanese studies. *Cancer Science, 102*(9), 1607–1614.

Jacobs, D. R., Jr., Adachi, H., Mulder, I., et al. (1999). Cigarette smoking and mortality risk: Twenty-five-year follow-up of the seven countries study. *Archives of Internal Medicine, 159*(7), 733–740.

Jatoi, I., & Miller, A. B. (2003). Why is breast-cancer mortality declining? *The Lancet Oncology, 4*, 251–254.

Jemal, A., Bray, F., Center, M. M., Ferlay, J., Ward, E., & Forman, D. (2011). Global cancer statistics. *CA: A Cancer Journal for Clinicians, 61*(2), 69–90.

Jemal, A., Center, M. M., DeSantis, C., & Ward, E. M. (2010). Global patterns of cancer incidence and mortality rates and trends. *Cancer Epidemiology, Biomarkers & Prevention, 19*, 1893–1907.

Kellen, E., Zeegers, M., Paulussen, A., Van Dongen, M., & Buntinx, F. (2006). Fruit consumption reduces the effect of smoking on bladder cancer risk. The Belgian case control study on bladder cancer. *International Journal of Cancer, 118*(10), 2572–2578.

Koizumi, Y., Tsubono, Y., Nakaya, N., Kuriyama, S., et al. (2004). Cigarette smoking and the risk of gastric cancer: A pooled analysis of two prospective studies in Japan. *International Journal of Cancer, 112*, 1049–1055.

Kuper, H., Boffetta, P., & Adami, O. (2002). Tobacco use and cancer causation: Association by tumour type. *Journal of Internal Medicine, 252*, 206–224. Blackwell Science.

La Torre, G., Chiaradia, G., Gianfagna, F., et al. (2009a). Smoking status and gastric cancer risk: An updated meta-analysis of case–control studies published in the past ten years. *Tumori, 95*, 13–22.

La Torre, G., de Waure, C., Specchia, M. L., et al. (2009b). Does quality of observational studies affect the results of a meta-analysis?: The case of cigarette smoking and pancreatic cancer. *Pancreas, 38*(3), 241–247.

Ladeiras-Lopes, R., Pereira, A. K., Nogueira, A., et al. (2008). Smoking and gastric cancer: Systematic review and meta-analysis of cohort studies. *Cancer Causes and Control, 19*(7), 689–701.

Lane-Claypon, J. E. (1926). *A further report on cancer of the breast, with special reference to its associated antecedent conditions* (Vol. 32). London: HMSO.

Lee, Y. C., Marron, M., Benhamou, S., et al. (2009). Active and involuntary tobacco smoking and upper aerodigestive tract cancer risks in a multicenter case–control study. *Cancer Epidemiology, Biomarkers and Prevention, 18*(12), 3353–3361.

Levi, F., Franceschi, S., La Vecchia, C., Randimbison, L., & Te, V. C. (1997). Lung carcinoma trends by histologic type in Vaud and Neuchatel, Switzerland, 1974–94. *Cancer, 79*, 906–914.

Levin, M. L., Goldstein, H., & Gerhardt, P. R. (1950). Cancer and tobacco smoking: A preliminary report. *Journal of the American Medical Association, 143*, 336–338.

Lewis, G., & Maxwell, A. P. (2012). Early diagnosis improves survival in kidney cancer. *The Practitioner, 256*(1748), 13–16. 2.

Lowenfels, A. B., & Maisonneuve, P. (2004). Epidemiology and prevention of pancreatic cancer. *Japanese Journal of Clinical Oncology, 34*, 238–244.

Lowenfels, A. B., & Maisonneuve, P. (2006). Epidemiology and risk factors for pancreatic cancer. *Best Practice and Research. Clinical Gastroenterology, 20*(2), 197–209.

Lubin, J. H., Blot, W. J., Berrino, F., et al. (1984). Patterns of lung cancer risk according to type of cigarette smoked. *International Journal of Cancer, 33*, 569–576.

Lubin, J. H., & Caporaso, N. (2006). Cigarette smoking and lung cancer: Modeling total exposure and intensity. *Cancer Epidemiology, Biomarkers and Prevention, 15*(3), 517–523.

Lubin, J. H., Caporaso, N., Wichmann, H. E., et al. (2007). Cigarette smoking and cancer risk: Modeling total exposure and intensity. *American Journal of Epidemiology, 166*(4), 479–489.

Luo, J., Margolis, K. L., Wactawski-Wende, J., et al. (2011). Association of active and passive smoking with risk of breast cancer among postmenopausal women: A prospective cohort study. *British Medical Journal, 342*, d1016.

Lynch, S. M. (2009). Cigarette smoking and pancreatic cancer: A pooled analysis from the pancreatic cancer cohort consortium. *American Journal of Epidemiology, 170*(4), 403–413.

Mackay, J., Eriksen, M., & Shafey, O. (2006). *The tobacco atlas* (2nd ed.). Atlanta, GA: American Cancer Society.

MacLeod, S. L., & Chowdhury, P. (2006). The genetics of nicotine dependence: Relationship to pancreatic cancer. *World Journal of Gastroenterology, 12*(46), 7433–7439.

Malaveille, C., Vineis, P., Estéve, J., et al. (1989). Levels of mutagens in the urine of smokers of black and blond tobacco correlate with their risk of bladder cancer. *Carcinogenesis, 10*(3), 577–586.

Marcus, P. M., Hayes, R. B., Vineis, P., et al. (2000). Cigarette smoking, *N*-acetyltransferase 2 acetylation status, and bladder cancer risk: A case-series meta-analysis of a gene-environment interaction. *Cancer Epidemiology, Biomarkers and Prevention, 9*(5), 461–467.

Mathew, A., Devesa, S. S., Fraumeni, J. F., Jr., & Chow, W. H. (2002). Global increases in kidney cancer incidence, 1973–1992. *European Journal of Cancer Prevention, 11*(2), 171–178.

Matsuda, T., Marugame, T., Kamo, K., et al. (2011). Cancer incidence and incidence rates in Japan in 2005: Based on data from 12 population-based cancer registries in the monitoring of cancer incidence in Japan (MCIJ) project. *Japanese Journal of Clinical Oncology, 41*, 139–147.

McLaughlin, J. K., Lindblad, P., Mellemgaard, A., et al. (1995). International renal-cell cancer study. I. *International Journal of Cancer, 60*(2), 194–198.

McLaughlin, J. K., Silverman, D. T., Hsing, A. W., et al. (1992). Cigarette smoking and cancers of the renal pelvis and ureter. *Cancer Research, 52*, 254–257.

Menvielle, G., Luce, D., Goldberg, P., Bugel, I., & Leclerc, A. (2004). Smoking, alcohol drinking and cancer risk for various sites of the larynx and hypopharynx. A case–control study in France. *European Journal of Cancer Prevention, 13*(3), 165–172.

Miller, M. D., Marty, M. A., Broadwin, R., et al. (2007). The association between exposure to environmental tobacco smoke and breast cancer: A review by the California environmental protection agency. *Preventive Medicine, 44*, 93–106.

Murray, C. J., & Lopez, A. D. (1997). Alternative projections of mortality and disability by cause 1990–2020: Global burden of disease study. *The Lancet, 349*(9064), 1498–1504.

Olivo-Marston, S. E., Yang, P., Mechanic, L. E., et al. (2009). Childhood exposure to secondhand smoke and functional mannose binding lectin polymorphisms are associated with increased lung cancer risk. *Cancer Epidemiology, Biomarkers and Prevention, 18*(12), 3375–3383.

ISD Online (2004). Cancer incidence and mortality data: Information and statistics division, NHS Scotland.

Parkin, D. M. (2004). International variation. *Oncogene, 23*, 6329–6340.

Parkin, D. M. (2008). The global burden of urinary bladder cancer. *Scandinavian Journal of Urology and Nephrology. Supplementum, 218*, 12–20.

Parkin, D. M. (2011). Tobacco-attributable cancer burden in the UK in 2010. *British Journal of Cancer, 105*(S2), S6–S13.

Parkin, D. M., Pisani, P., & Ferlay, J. (1999). Global cancer statistics. *CA: A Cancer Journal for Clinicians, 49*, 33–64.

Parkin, D. M., Whelan, S. L., Ferlay, J., et al. (1997). *Cancer incidence in five continents VII (IARC. Scientific Publications no 143)*. Lyon, France: IARC.

Parkin, D. M., Whelan, S. L., Ferlay, J., et al. (2002). *Cancer Incidence in five continents Volume VIII. IARC Scientific Publications* (Vol. 155). Lyon, France: IARC Press.

Parkin, D. M., Bray, F., Ferlay, J., & Pisani, P. (2005a). Global cancer statistics, 2002. *CA: A Cancer Journal for Clinicians, 55*, 74–108.

Parkin, D. M., Whelan, S., Ferlay, J., et al. (2005b). *Cancer incidence in five continents I to VIII. Cancer base No. 7.* Lyon, France: IARC Press.

Paterson, H. M., McCole, D., & Auld, C. D. (2006). Impact of open-access endoscopy on detection of early oesophageal and gastric cancer 1994–2003: Population-based study. *Endoscopy, 38*(5), 503–507.

Pelucchi, C., Bosetti, C., Negri, E., Malvezzi, M., & La Vecchia, C. (2006). Mechanisms of disease: The epidemiology of bladder cancer. *Nature Clinical Practice Urology, 3*(6), 327–340.

Peto, R., Darby, S., Deo, H., Silcocks, P., Whitley, E., & Doll, R. (2000). Smoking, smoking cessation, and lung cancer in the UK since 1950: Combination of national statistics with two case–control studies. *BMJ, 321*(7257), 323–329.

Peto, R., Lopez, A. D., Boreham, J., et al. (2006). *Mortality from smoking in developed countries: 1950–2000* (2nd ed.). Oxford: Oxford University Press.

Pirie, K., Beral, V., Peto, R., et al. (2008). Passive smoking and breast cancer in never smokers: Prospective study and meta-analysis. *International Jounal of Epidemiology, 37*, 1069–1079.

Puente, D., Hartge, P., Greiser, E., Cantor, K. P., King, W. D., González, C. A., et al. (2006). A pooled analysis of bladder cancer case–control studies evaluating smoking in men and women. *Cancer Causes Control, 17*, 71–9.

Quinn, M. W. H., Cooper, N., & Rowan, S. (2005). *Cancer atlas of the United Kingdom and Ireland 1991–2000. Studies on medical and population subjects* (Vol. 68). New York, NY: Palgrave Macmillan.

Ramroth, H., Dietz, A., & Becher, H. (2011). Intensity and inhalation of smoking in the aetiology of laryngeal cancer. *International Journal of Environmental Research and Public Health, 8*(4), 976–984.

Samanic, C., Kogevinas, M., Dosemeci, M., et al. (2006). Smoking and bladder cancer in Spain: Effects of tobacco type, timing, environmental tobacco smoke, and gender. *Cancer Epidemiology, Biomarkers and Prevention, 15*(7), 1348–1354.

Sasco, A. J., Secretan, M. B., & Straif, K. (2004). Tobacco smoking and cancer: A brief review of recent epidemiological evidence. *Lung Cancer, 45*(Suppl 2), S3–S9.

Setiawan, V. W., Stram, D. O., Nomura, A. M., Kolonel, L. N., & Henderson, B. E. (2007). Risk Factors for Renal Cell Cancer: The Multiethnic Cohort. *American Journal of Epidemiology, 166*(8), 932–940.

Shapiro, J. A., Jacobs, E. J., & Thun, M. J. (2000). Cigar smoking in men and risk of death from tobacco-related cancers. *Journal of the National Cancer Institute, 92*, 333–337.

Sharp, L., Chilvers, C. E., Cheng, K. K., et al. (2001). Risk factors for squamous cell carcinoma of the oesophagus in women: A case–control study. *British Journal of Cancer, 85*, 1667–1670.

Shin, H. R., Boniol, M., Joubert, C., et al. (2010). Secular trends in breast cancer mortality in five East Asian populations: Hong Kong, Japan, Korea, Singapore and Taiwan. *Cancer Science, 101*, 1241–1246.

Stayner, L., Bena, J., & Sasco, A. J. (2007). Lung cancer risk and workplace exposure to environmental tobacco smoke. *American Journal of Public Health, 97*(3), 545–551.
Stewart, B. W., & Kleihues, P. (2003). *World cancer report*. Lyon, France: IARC Press.
Talamini, R., Bosetti, C., La Vecchia, C., et al. (2002). Combined effect of tobacco and alcohol on laryngeal cancer risk: A case–control study. *Cancer Causes and Control, 13*(10), 957–964.
Taylor, R., Cumming, R., Woodward, A., & Black, M. (2001). Passive smoking and lung cancer: A cumulative meta-analysis. *Australian and New Zealand Journal of Public Health, 25*(3), 203–211.
Taylor, R., Najafi, F., & Dobson, A. (2007). Meta-analysis of studies of passive smoking and lung cancer: effects of study type and continent. *International Journal of Epidemiology, 36*(5), 1048–1059.
Thun, M. J., Myers, D. G., Day-Lally, C. et al. (1997). Age and the exposure-response relationships between cigarette smoking and premature death in Cancer Prevention Study II. In: Changes in cigarette-related disease risks and their implications for prevention and control. Smoking and Tobacco Control Monograph No. 8. Citied: http://cancercontrol.cancer.gov/tcrb/monographs/8/index.html
Tobacco Smoking (1986). *IARC monographs on the evaluation of the carcinogenic risk of chemicals to humans* (Vol. 38, pp. 35–394).
Trédaniel, J., Boffetta, P., Buiatti, E., Saracci, R., & Hirsch, A. (1997). Tobacco smoking and gastric cancer: Review and meta-analysis. *International Journal of Cancer, 72*(4), 565–573.
Tuyns, A. J., Esteve, J., Raymond, L., et al. (1988). Cancer of the larynx/hypopharynx, tobacco and alcohol: IARC international case–control study in Turin and Varese (Italy), Zaragoza and Navarra (Spain), Geneva (Switzerland) and Calvados (France). *International Journal of Cancer, 41*, 483–491.
U.S. Department of Health and Human Services. (1988). *Nicotine addiction: A report of the surgeon general*. Rockville, MD: U.S. Department of Health and Human Services, Public Health Service, Centers for Disease Control, Center for Health Promotion and Education, Office on Smoking and Health.
Vineis, P., Airoldi, L., Veglia, F., et al. (2005). Environmental tobacco smoke and risk of respiratory cancer and chronic obstructive pulmonary disease in former smokers and never smokers in the EPIC prospective study. *British Medical Journal, 330*(7486), 277.
Vizcaino, A. P., Moreno, V., Lambert, R., & Parkin, D. M. (2002). Time trends incidence of both major histologic types of esophageal carcinomas in selected countries, 1973–1995. *International Journal of Cancer, 99*, 860–868.
Vollset, S. E., Tverdal, A., & Gjessing, H. K. (2006). Smoking and deaths between 40 and 70 years of age in women and men. *Annals of Internal Medicine, 144*(6), 381–389.
Vrieling, A., Bueno-de-Mesquita, H. B., Boshuizen, H. C., et al. (2009). Cigarette smoking, environmental tobacco smoke exposure and pancreatic cancer risk in the European prospective investigation into cancer and nutrition. *International Journal of Cancer, 126*(10), 2394–2403.
Wiencke, J. K., Thurston, S. W., Kelsey, K. T., et al. (1999). Early age at smoking initiation and tobacco carcinogen DNA damage in the lung. *Journal of the National Cancer Institute, 91*(7), 614–619.
World Health Organization. (2011). *Report on the global tobacco epidemic, 2011: Warning about the dangers of tobacco*. Cited on April 27, 2012, http://www.who.int/tobacco/global_report/2011/en/
World Health Organization. (2012). Accessed February 16, 2012, from http://www.who.int/mediacentre/factsheets/fs297/en/
Wynder, E. L., & Muscat, J. E. (1995). The changing epidemiology of smoking and lung cancer histology. *Environmental Health Perspectives, 103*(Suppl 8), 143–148.
Xue, F., Willett, W. C., Rosner, B. A., Hankison, S. E., & Michels, K. B. (2011). Cigarette smoking and the incidence of breast cancer. *Archives of Internal Medicine, 171*(2), 125–133.
Zambon, P., Talamini, R., La Vecchia, C., et al. (2000). Smoking, type of alcoholic beverage and squamous-cell oesophageal cancer in Northern Italy. *International Journal of Cancer, 86*, 144–149.

Zaridze, D., Borisova, E., Maximovitch, D., & Chkhikvadze, V. (2000). Alcohol consumption, smoking and risk of gastric cancer: Case–control study from Moscow, Russia. *Cancer Causes & Control, 11*, 363–371.

Zeegers, M. P., Tan, F. E., Dorant, E., & van Den Brandt, P. A. (2000). The impact of characteristics of cigarette smoking on urinary tract cancer risk: A meta-analysis of epidemiologic studies. *Cancer, 89*(3), 630–639.

Znaor, A., Brennan, P., Gajalakshmi, V., et al. (2003). Independent and combined effects of tobacco smoking, chewing and alcohol drinking on the risk of oral, pharyngeal and oesophageal cancers in Indian men. *International Journal of Cancer, 105*(5), 681–686.

Chapter 5
Classical Determinants of Smoking Initiation

Giuseppe La Torre and Domitilla Di Thiene

Objectives The aim of this chapter is the description of sociodemographical and personal characteristics described as on smoking initiation determinants. The importance of these aspects is highlighted by scientific evidence. The knowledge of initiation determinants allowed the choice of public health interventions. Moreover, a better understanding of these factors will permit future decisions.

Learning Outcomes

By the end of this chapter the reader will be able to:

- Recognize the role of the family, particularly the parents one.
- Recognize the role of the peer, particularly in the socialization dynamics.
- Recognize the role of the society, particularly in the socioeconomic aspects.
- Recognize the personal characteristics involved, particularly in the behavior psychology overview.

5.1 Introduction

It is well recognized that social pressure coming from peers or older siblings can be considered a prime factor for initial experimentation of the smoking habits (Leventhal and Cleary 1980). On the other hand, smoking can be also considered as a means through which one can adopt a behavior for dealing with stress. Moreover, according to Anda and Collegues (1999) a very strong association between smoking and adverse childhood experiences does exist. Among these

G. La Torre (✉) • D. Di Thiene
Department of Public Health and Infectious Diseases, "Sapienza" University of Rome, Piazzale Aldo Moro 5, Rome 00185, Italy
e-mail: giuseppe.latorre@uniroma1.it

G. La Torre, *Smoking Prevention and Cessation*, DOI 10.1007/978-1-4614-7046-5_5,

experiences we need to include issues such as emotional, physical or sexual abuse, parental separation, and parental substance abuse.

Another issue we need to take into account is that reasons for smoking initiation can differ across cultures, even if some factors represent have an established association with tobacco smoking. Smoking habits among parents, siblings, and friend are strongly associated with an individual's smoking status (de Vries et al. 2003; Kokkevi et al. 2007). Di Franza and Colleagues (2006) performed a review in order to study if a causal link between exposure to tobacco promotion and the initiation of tobacco use by children does exist. They found that tobacco promotion is the cause of children's initiation of tobacco use through different modalities:

1. Children are exposed to tobacco promotion before the initiation of tobacco use.
2. The exposure increases the risk for tobacco use initiation.
3. A dose–response direct relationship exists.
4. The increased risk is robust; observed with different methods, in different settings and populations.
5. There are plausible mechanisms from the scientific point of view whereby promotion could influence tobacco use initiation.

But also low socioeconomic status and low educational level have been recognized as factors associated with smoking (Reijneveld 1998; Dragano et al. 2007).

Finally, recent research has focused on weight issues in the decision to smoke initiation and progression of this habit, especially among women. Honjo and Siegel (2003) revealed that the level of perceived importance of being thin among young female adolescents predicts future smoking initiation. In a prospective cohort study they found that girls who valued thinness most/somewhat strongly had a higher odds of becoming established smokers, if compared to the girls who valued thinness least strongly. Weiss and Colleagues (2007) found that, among students in Los Angeles County, weight concern is significantly associated with increased risk for smoking. Nevertheless, ethnic disparities do exist, since Hispanic students are more likely to report having tried smoking, while Asian-American and African-American students are significantly less likely to report having tried smoking if compared to White students.

According to 1994 Surgeon General's Report on preventing Tobacco Use among young people (Preventing Tobacco Use among Young People: A Report of the Surgeon General U.S. Department of Health and Human Services, 1994), there are four major psychosocial risk factors that have to be taken into account in the association to smoking initiation, i.e., sociodemographic, environmental, behavioral, and personal factors (Table 5.1).

Moreover, according to Brannon and Feist (1992) smoking initiation is strongly associated to (Fig. 5.1):

(a) The perception of smoking
(b) Social pressure
(c) Adverse life events
(d) Personal resources

Table 5.1 Psychosocial risk factors in the initiation of tobacco use among adolescents

Sociodemographic factors
Low socioeconomic status
Developmental stage
Environmental factors
Accessibility
Advertising
Parental use
Sibling use
Peer use
Normative expectations
Social support
Behavioral factors
Academic achievement
Other problem behaviors
Constructive behaviors
Behavioral skills
Intentions
Experimentation
Personal factors
Functional meanings
Subjective expected utility
Self-esteem/self-image
Self-efficacy
Personality factors
Psychological well-being

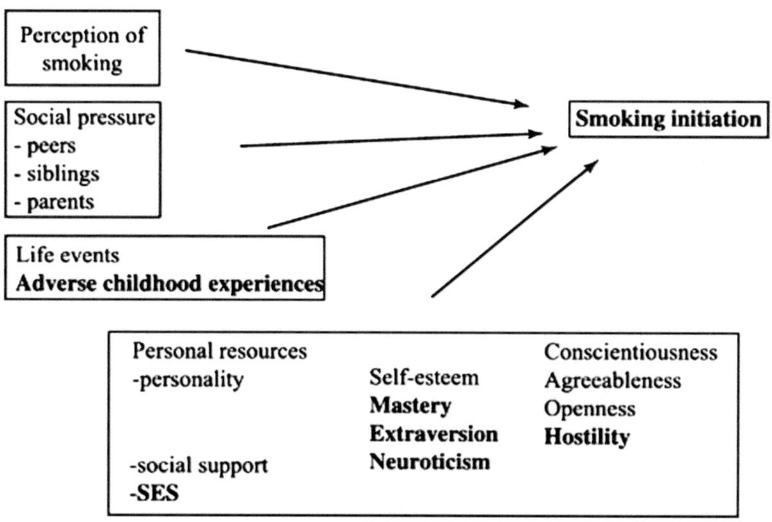

Fig. 5.1 Factors associated with smoking initiation, according to Brannon and Feist (1992)

So, considering these last two papers, we would like to face with these classical determinants of smoking initiation: (1) the family; (2) the peer; (3) the society; and (4) personal characteristics.

5.2 The Role of the Family

The family unit is the primary source of transmission of basic social, cultural, genetic, and biological factors that may underlie individual differences in smoking Avenevoli and Merikangas (2003). Parental smoking may influence childhood or adult smoking status through social, biological, and genetic pathways. Socially, parental smoking might normalize smoking, increase access to cigarettes, and model tobacco use for offspring (Paul et al. 2008).

Parental smoking was associated with a significantly higher risk of smoking initiation in adolescent offspring. In addition, the likelihood of offspring smoking initiation increased with the number of smoking parents and the duration of exposure to parental smoking, suggesting a dose–response relationship between parental smoking and offspring smoking. There is evidence to suggest that specific parental/familial characteristics can serve as protective factors to decrease youths' vulnerability to smoking. One mechanism by which parents can protect their children from smoking and other undesired behaviors is to discourage their association with friends who engage in these behaviors, provide bad examples, and otherwise exert negative socializing influences. Several studies have demonstrated that parent influence on adolescent smoking occurs indirectly by preventing friendship formation with smoking peers (Avenevoli and Merikangas 2003; Simons-Morton and Farhat 2010), moderating the effects of friend influence (Dielman et al. 1993), or moderating affiliation with smoking peers (Engels and van der Vorst 2003).

Interestingly, adolescents living with smoking fathers were more than three times as likely to initiate smoking; in contrast, nonresident fathers' smoking had no effect on the risk of their offspring's initiation (Gilman et al. 2009).

A recent systematic review (Leonardi-Bee et al. 2011) shows how parental and sibling smoking is a strong and significant determinant of the risk of smoking uptake by children. In the 58 studies included in the meta-analyses, the relative odds of uptake of smoking in children were increased significantly if at least one parent smoked (OR 1.72, 95 % CI 1.59–1.86), more so by smoking by the mother (OR 2.19, 95 % CI 1.73–2.79) than the father (OR 1.66, 95 % CI 1.42–1.94). The risk if both parents smoked increased almost three time (OR 2.73, 95 % CI 2.28–3.28). Similar results are present also by smoking of a sibling 2.30 (95 % CI 1.85–2.86) and smoking by any household member, 1.92 (95 % CI 1.70–2.16).

The Childhood Determinants of Adult Health (CDAH) study, a 20-year follow-up of 8,498 participants in the 1985 Australian Schools Health and Fitness Survey (ASHFS) shows that all levels of smoking experimentation in childhood, but particularly greater experimentation among older children, increased the risk of being a daily smoker 20 years later (Paul et al. 2008). In authors opinion, the finding that parental smoking was associated with adult current smoking, but not childhood experimentation, is consistent with the hypothesis that genes are involved in nicotine dependence. The influence on adult smoking could occur also in a prenatal phase; animal studies have suggested an association between prenatal nicotine exposure and subsequent offspring sensitivity to nicotine. To explore the association between maternal smoking during pregnancy and subsequent offspring smoking, while controlling for other risk factors associated with likelihood of smoking, such as parental smoking after birth, Roberts and colleagues examined two British cohorts, with data of about 13,000 births and offspring (Roberts et al. 2005). The data support an association between maternal smoking during pregnancy and an increased risk of offspring smoking later in life among female offspring but not among male offspring.

Those findings appear similar with the results of a recent study where girls prenatally exposed to maternal tobacco use had a two- to threefold increased odds of experiencing a high number of withdrawal symptoms (OR = 2.83, 95 % CI 1.68–4.87), craving for tobacco (OR = 2.04, 95 % CI 1.28–3.32) and heavy tobacco use (OR = 1.93, 95 % CI 1.30–2.86) (Rydell et al. 2012). These associations were weaker among boys and did not reach formal statistical significance.

A comprehensive review of the literature Avenevoli and Merikangas (2003) examines 87 studies and reveals that findings show weak and inconsistent associations between parent and adolescent smoking. However the review underlines that methods are limited by a lack of standardized instruments, failure to measure important confounding and mediating factors, reliance on cross-sectional designs, and the use of inconsistent definitions of tobacco-related behavior and assessment procedures.

5.3 The Peer

There is a considerable body of empirical research that has identified adolescent peer relationships as a primary factor involved in adolescent cigarette smoking.

A recent study (McVicar 2011) exploits a rich source of individual level, school-based, survey data on adolescent substance use across countries, utilizing the 2007 European Schools Survey Project on Alcohol and Other Drugs. The results were estimated for 75,000 individuals across 26 European countries to provide peer effects between classmates in adolescent smoking using the same methods in each case. The results suggest statistically significant peer effects in almost all cases. These peer effects estimates are large: on average across countries, the probability that a "typical" adolescent smokes increases by between 0.31 and 0.38 percentage points for a one percentage point increase in the proportion of classmates that smoke. Peer effects appear larger in magnitude for heavier smokers than for lighter smokers and effects are larger for intra-gender peer groups than for inter-gender peer groups: boys smoking behavior is most associated with the smoking behaviour of other boys in the class, and vice versa, with the relevant marginal effects being 0.203 (boy peers on boys), 0.058 (girl peers on boys), 0.055 (boy peers on girls), and 0.243 (girl peers on girls), with all effects statistically significant at 99 %.

The magnitude of the peer effects found here varies across countries, ranging from around one fifth for Belgium to around one half for the Netherlands.

In their comprehensive review of the literature, Avenevoli and Merikangas (2003) conclude that the relationship between peer smoking and adolescent smoking is robust, with research providing overwhelming evidence to suggest that the smoking of peers is tied more strongly to adolescent smoking than to the smoking behavior of siblings or parents.

Moreover, five factors robustly predicted quitting across studies in which the factor was investigated: not having friends who smoke, not having intentions to smoke in the future, resisting peer pressure to smoke, being older at first use of cigarette, and having negative beliefs about smoking (Cengelli et al. 2012)

Best friends appear to provide the greatest peer influence on adolescent smoking; peer groups (close friends) provide independent influence, but their influence may also interact with that of the best friend. Crowd affiliation is another friendship dimension that appears in limited research to be associated with adolescent substance use (Simons-Morton and Farhat 2010)

The adolescent could be influenced to smoke by his friends in order to be more like them (peer socialization, that includes peer pressure), or he is selecting friends based on their smoking status. Selection and socialization processes could have both influence as smoking determinants:

5.3.1 Peer Socialization

Peer socialization is the effect of existing social relationships on the formation of social norms. With socialization, the group accepts an adolescent based on shared characteristics (Simons-Morton and Farhat 2010). Behaviors of the others is adopted to be accepted (Evans et al. 2006). Peer pressure is a form of a peer socialization and suggests that adolescents directly persuade their friends to conform to their behavior, but socialization is mainly a normative process and not one of overt peer pressure. However, peer pressure is only one aspect of socialization, although there is evidence that adolescents do offer their friends cigarettes and that smoking is typically initiated in the context of peers (Kirke 2004; Lucas and Lloyd 1999; Robinson et al. 2006). In surveys, youth report that overt peer pressure is not a factor for their smoking but report that they sometimes experience internal pressure to smoke in the presence of other adolescents who are smoking, evidence for the influence of perceived social norms rather than overt peer pressure. In this vein, the decision to try cigarettes has been tied to youths' attempts to avoid potential exclusion by peers, to gain social approval, to facilitate social interactions and to achieve a sense of autonomy or independence (Nichter et al. 1997). These findings suggest that perceived social norms exert a socializing effect. Social norms need only be perceived to influence behavior, are not necessary legal issues or other. Behaviors are learned through the observation of others engaged in a behavior and subsequent modeling of this behavior. Interestingly, it has been previously demonstrated that the prevalence of smoking among adolescents is perceived higher than the reality, by the adolescent of the group (Bauman and Ennett 1996;

Iannotti et al. 1996), which may be due to several possible factors: adolescents may psychologically project their own smoking behavior onto others, thereby overestimating smoking prevalence (Miller et al. 2000) or adolescents may also develop a false consensus that one's attitudes and behavior are normative when they are not. Moreover, youth tend to report that in their decision-making regarding tobacco use, peer pressure is not a factor (Kobus 2003). According whit (Simons-Morton and Farhat 2010), it seems that socialization occurs mainly through indirect pressure to conform to actual or perceived social norms. Although direct and overt peer pressure almost certainly operates, there is substantially less empirical evidence of its importance compared with the indirect influence on social norms.

5.3.2 Peer Selection

Ostensible characteristics, such as sex and race, and those that facilitate physical proximity, such as age and grade in school, have been found to serve as a primary filter for friendship selection and group formation (Kobus 2003). Later, selection occurs when an individual seeks or affiliates with a friend or group with shared attitudes, behaviors, or other characteristics (i.e., smoking adolescents choosing smoking peers as friends). When some members of a peer group begin smoking or experimenting with other substances, other members of the peer group can respond by dropping out of the group (deselection); conforming to the new group norm (socialization), risking group disapproval; or living with the dissonance between their norms and the group's (Simons-Morton and Farhat 2010). In social settings, such as schools, it is easy to observe congregation of those who are similar and separation of different. Selection may be abstract and internal, when a person affiliates with others by identifying with them or with what they represent rather than affiliating on the basis of observable behaviors. For example, adolescents may identify with groups according to musical preferences, reputation, or interests (Ter Bogt et al. 2006). Such affiliations may be highly transient among adolescents. Selection also involves actual affiliation and, within the limits of their social network, people gravitate toward individuals or groups who share their interests and values and provide a supportive context for their own views and behavior. Adolescents who are interested in smoking, for example, may select as friends adolescents with similar interests in smoking (Ennett and Bauman 1994), although smoking may be just one manifestation of a constellation of social norms leading to social selection.

5.4 The Society

Social influence is the effect others have on individual and group attitudes and behavior (Berkman 2000).

The social environment undoubtedly plays a critical role in determining how innate biological factors that are involved in nicotine dependency actually get expressed at the population level.

The great diversity in tobacco use behaviors observed in studies population-wide basis both between countries and within countries over time demonstrates that biology alone cannot fully explain these variations (WHO 2008). As an example, the progressive limitation to where people can smoke in industrialized countries has contributed to the social marginalization of smoking as an accepted behavior (Cummings et al. 2009).

The importance of the social environment in influencing trends in tobacco use behaviors was illustrated nicely in a recent study that monitored the smoking habits of 12,067 people over a 30-year period as part of the Framingham Heart Study (Christakis and Fowler 2008). In this study, trends in smoking behavior were strongly linked to an individual's social ties. Smokers whose social network included an increasing share of nonsmokers or former smokers were much more likely to stop smoking over time, whereas those whose social ties were mainly among smokers continued to smoke.

The gender is one of the first determinant in smoking initiation. Worldwide it is estimated that men smoke nearly five times as much as women, but the ratios of female-to-male smoking prevalence rates vary dramatically across countries. In high-income countries, including Australia, Canada, the USA, and most countries of Western Europe, women smoke at nearly the same rate as men. However, in many low- and middle-income countries women smoke much less than men. In China, for example, 61 % of men are reported to be current smokers compared with only 4.2 % of women. While rates of smoking among men in many high income European nations have fallen steadily in recent years, rates of smoking among women have risen, remained steady, or fallen only slightly (Hitchman and Fong 2011).

Socioeconomic status (SES) has also been found to be a strong predictor of tobacco use status (Jarvis and Wardle 1999; Siahpush et al. 2006a, b). The association is so strong that smoking is regarded as a marker for deprivation, and one can identify disadvantaged groups by simply observing their smoking prevalence (Jarvis 1994). Not only are social inequalities in smoking prevalence pervasive, but they also have been widening in many countries, such as USA and the UK, over the past few decades (Jarvis and Wardle 1999; Siahpush et al. 2006a, b).

The mechanism of the link between SES and cessation has not been adequately explored. Nicotine dependency, self-efficacy, and intention to quit are strong predictors of the propensity to quit and/or successful cessation, and research has shown that lower SES is associated with higher levels of nicotine dependency, having low self-efficacy to quit, and having no intention to quit across four different countries (i.e., the USA, Canada, the UK, and Australia) (Siahpush et al. 2006a, b, 2007). Higher levels of dependency among lower-SES groups may be due to the association of social disadvantage with financial and psychological stress.

The complex and ravaging interrelationship between tobacco use and social determinants of health is explored in "Equity, social determinants and public health programmes," a 300-page report released by the World Health Organization

(WHO 2010) where smoking uptake is strongly associated with family background and socioeconomic and educational status, with adolescents from lower socioeconomic backgrounds most at risk. Low parental income and low parental educational status are independently associated with higher adolescent smoking rates, and the association becomes stronger as socioeconomic status declines.

The social gradient is widely recognized, and has been used by tobacco industry too. A study of USA has sought to explore whether and how the tobacco industry considers social class and gender in its efforts to market cigarettes in the USA. The results show how companies have heavily targeted the socially disadvantaged, including working class young women. They focused on the virile core, that is "younger, more male, less well educated and includes fewer blacks." Regarding female core, a 1989 document of a tobacco company cited in the article reported "an 18–24 year old female who…primarily exhibits traditionally "masculine" character traits…independent, streetwise, somewhat tough, yet approachable… Her aspirations are very short term in focus… The … smoker is fairly downscale with a high school education or less and generally has an "unskilled" job… she will not smoke a product her boyfriend or male "buddies" find unacceptable… she is not professionally ambitious."

Recent research has conceptualized smoking epidemic variations in the age, educational, and gender patterns in smoking behaviour (Huisman et al. 2005). It has been noted that those variations fit very well into the conceptual framework of the diffusion of innovation in societies (Rogers and Shoemaker 1971): higher socioeconomic groups lead the way and lower socioeconomic groups follow. Following this rationale, smoking prevalence rises and declines first within the population groups that are at the forefront of initiation, and at the same time most sensitive to messages regarding the risks of tobacco. In the last stage, smoking is likely to become restricted to the groups who adopted it relatively late in the diffusion process. As long as prevalence has not completed its decline at the bottom of the social scale, the association between social position and tobacco will remain very strong, and possibly grow stronger over time. Many European countries have reached the last stage of this epidemic model and therefore display persistent or widening socioeconomic differences in relation to smoking, with nevertheless a declining prevalence of smoking in the population as a whole (Huisman et al. 2005; Legleye et al. 2011). The differences in the timing of the cigarette epidemic across the nations may correspond to age, gender, and education patterns of smoking.

Cigarette prices are more consistently a significant determinant of youth smoking initiation, especially for disadvantaged people. The most cost-effective strategies are population-wide public policies, like bans on advertising, promotion, and sponsorship of tobacco products; tobacco tax and price increases; forbidding smoking in all public and workplaces; and requiring large, clear and visible graphic health messages on tobacco packaging. All of these measures are outlined in the WHO Framework Convention on Tobacco Control (WHO).

5.5 Personal Characteristics

A large number of studies have examined the relationships between personality traits and cigarette smoking variables. Although the personality differences between smokers and nonsmokers are usually small, they are important considering the large number of people who smoke. Even a small contribution of personality research may enhance knowledge of smoking behavior and have a clinical impact through the improvement of smoking prevention and cessation programs (Terracciano and Costa 2004).

In the last century psychoanalytic theories have great influence and nicotine dependence has been read in this view too. In a famous 1972 document, William L. Dunn 1972, principal scientist and leader of "smoker psychology" programs at Philip Morris, explain reasons to smoke, and among others wrote: "for oral gratification in the psychoanalytic sense." Later, in the same paragraph he added: "I might mention one other explanation, not because anybody believes it but as an example of how distorted one's reasoning can become when under the influence of psychoanalytic theory. Smoking, according to this argument, is the consequence of pulmonary eroticism. Translated, this means the lungs have become sexualized and smoking is but another form of the sexual act" (http://www.tobaccodocuments.org).

In the past decades interpretations on smoking behavior have continued by behavior psychology, especially of genetic of personality such as Hans Eysenck. The controversial psychologist (he was criticized, among others things, for secret funding by Tobacco industry), he described two personalities dimensions, Extraversions and Neuroticism, and later added Psychoticism. On these dimensions he developed different scales, still utilized. Introversion involves directing attention on inner experiences, while extraversion relates to focusing attention outward on other people and the environment. So, a person high in introversion might be quiet and reserved, while an individual high in extraversion might be sociable and outgoing. This dimension of Eysenck's trait theory is related to moodiness versus even-temperedness. Neuroticism refers to an individual's tendency to become upset or emotional, while stability refers to the tendency to remain emotionally constant Extraverts, according to Eysenck's theory, are chronically under-aroused and bored and are therefore in need of external stimulation to bring them up to an optimal level of performance. Introverts, on the other hand, are chronically over-aroused and jittery and are therefore in need of peace and quiet to bring them up to an optimal level of performance. Neurotic people, who have low activation thresholds, and unable to inhibit or control their emotional reactions, experience negative affect (fight-or-flight) in the face of very minor stressors—they are easily nervous or upset (Eysenck 1983). According to Eysenck, genetically determined differences in physiological functioning make some people more vulnerable to behavioral conditioning. The finding that smokers demonstrate elevated levels of extraversion compared with nonsmokers is consistent with both the possibility that increased sociability is associated with increased likelihood of smoking and the possibility that increased dopaminergic activity, which is hypothesized to constitute the neurobiological substrate of extraversion, is associated with increased likelihood of smoking (Munafò and Black 2007).

Smokers have a higher prevalence of alcohol and drug dependence, depression, and anxiety disorders than nonsmokers, particularly if the dependence is severe (Degenhardt and Hall 2001; Kandel et al. 2001). Also, cigarette smoking is an independent risk factor of suicidality in many studies (Bronisch et al. 2008; Ostacher et al. 2009). Although depression (or a depressive state) has been associated with smoking, our study shows that the depressive temperament is less prone to smoking than unstable externalized temperaments (Bisol et al. 2010).

Current smokers were found to score significantly higher than never smokers on Neuroticism and significantly lower on Agreeableness and Conscientiousness. Tobacco users have been described as more risk-taking, impulsive, interpersonally aggressive, and with higher novelty seeking, extraversion, disinhibition, sensation seeking, neuroticism, and monotony avoidance relative to nonsmokers (Vollrath and Torgersen 2008; Dinn et al. 2004; Rondina et al. 2007; Munafò et al. 2007).

A recent cross-sectional study evaluated the associations of smoking status and heaviness of smoking with emotional and affective temperament dimensions in a large population with high risk for psychiatric disorders. Regarding emotional temperament, externalized emotional temperament traits such as fear, poor control, and high anger were associated with smoking status, in agreement with other studies (Rondina et al. 2007; Munafò et al. 2007; Bisol et al. 2010).

References

Anda, R. F., Croft, J. B., Felitti, V. J., Nordenberg, D., Giles, W. H., Williamson, D. F., et al. (1999). Adverse childhood experiences and smoking during adolescence and adulthood. *JAMA, 282*, 1652–1658.

Avenevoli, S., & Merikangas, K. R. (2003). Familial influences on adolescent smoking. *Addiction, 98*(Suppl 1), 1–20.

Bauman, K. E., & Ennett, S. T. (1996). On the importance of peer influence for adolescent drug use: Commonly neglected considerations. *Addiction, 91*, 185–198.

Berkman, L. F. (2000). Social support, social networks, social cohesion and health. *Social Work in Health Care, 31*, 3–14.

Bisol, L. W., Soldado, F., & Albuquerque, C. (2010). Emotional and affective temperaments and cigarette smoking in a large sample. *Journal of Affective Disorders, 127*, 89–95.

Brannon, L., & Feist, J. (1992). *Health Psychology. An introduction to behavior and health* (2nd ed.). California: Wadsworth Publishing Company.

Bronisch, T., Höfler, M. L., & Lieb, R. (2008). Smoking predicts suicidality: Findings from a prospective community study. *Journal of Affective Disorders, 108*(1–2), 135–145.

Cengelli, S., O'Loughlin, J., Lauzon, B., & Cornuz, J. (2012). A systematic review of longitudinal population-based studies on the predictors of smoking cessation in adolescent and young adult smokers. *Tobacco Control, 21*(3), 355–362.

Christakis, N. A., & Fowler, J. H. (2008). The collective dynamics of smoking in a large social network. *The New England Journal of Medicine, 358*, 2249–2258.

Cummings, K. M., Fong, G. T., & Borland, R. (2009). Environmental influences on tobacco use: Evidence from societal and community influences on tobacco use and dependence. *Annual Review of Clinical Psychology, 5*, 433–458.

Degenhardt, L., & Hall, W. (2001). The relationship between tobacco use, substance-use disorders and mental health: Results from the National Survey of Mental Health and Well-being. *Nicotine & Tobacco Research, 3*(3), 225–234.

de Vries, H., Engels, R., Kremers, S., Wetzels, J., & Mudde, A. (2003). Parents' and friends' smoking status as predictors of smoking onset: Findings from six European countries. *Health Education Research, 18*, 627–636.

Dielman, T. E., Butchart, A. T., & Shope, J. T. (1993). Structural equation model tests of patterns of family interaction, peer alcohol use, and intrapersonal predictors of adolescent alcohol use and misuse. *Journal of Drug Education, 23*, 273–316.

DiFranza JR, Wellman RJ, Sargent JD, Weitzman M, Hipple BJ, Winickoff JP, for the Tobacco Consortium CfCHRotAAoP. (2006). Tobacco promotion and the initiation of tobacco use: Assessing the evidence for causality. *Pediatrics, 117*, e1237–e1248.

Dinn, W. M., Aycicegi, A., & Harris, C. L. (2004). Cigarette smoking in a student sample: Neurocognitive and clinical correlates. *Addictive Behaviors, 29*(1), 107–126.

Dragano, N., Bobak, M., Wege, N., Peasey, A., Verde, P., Kubinova, R., Weyers, S., Moebus, S., Mohlenkamp, S., Stang, A., Erbel, R., Jockel, K. H., Siegrist, J., & Pikhart, H. (2007). Neighbourhood socioeconomic status and cardiovascular risk factors: A multilevel analysis of nine cities in the Czech Republic and Germany. *BMC Public Health, 7*, 255.

Dunn, W. L. (1972). *Motives and incentives in cigarette smoking. Anne Landman's collection.* Available at http://tobaccodocuments.org/landman/2024273959-3975.html

Engels, R., & van der Vorst, H. (2003). The roles of parents in adolescent and peer alcohol consumption. *The Netherlands journal of sociology, 39*, 53–68.

Ennett, S. T., & Bauman, K. E. (1994). The contribution of influence and selection to adolescent peer group homogeneity: The case of adolescent cigarette smoking. *Journal of Personality and Social Psychology, 67*, 653–663.

Evans, W. D., Powers, A., Hersey, J., & Renaud, J. (2006). The influence of social environment and social image on adolescent smoking. *Health Psychology, 25*, 26–33.

Eysenck, H. J. (1983). Smoking, personality and reasons for smoking. *Psychological Medicine, 13*, 447–448.

Gilman, S. E., Rende, R., Boergers, J., Abrams, D.B., Buka, S.L., Clark, M.A. et al. (2009). Parental smoking and adolescent smoking initiation: An intergenerational perspective on tobacco control. *Pediatrics, 123*, e274–e281.

Hitchman, S. C., & Fong, G. T. (2011). Gender empowerment and female-to-male smoking prevalence ratios. *Bulletin of the World Health Organization, 89*, 195–202.

Honjo, K., & Siegel, M. (2003). Perceived importance of being thin and smoking initiation among young girls. *Tobacco Control, 12*, 289–295.

Huisman, M., Kunst, A., & Mackenbach, K. (2005). Educational inequalities in smoking among men and women aged 16 years and older in 11 European countries. *Tobacco Control, 14*, 106–113.

Iannotti, R. J., Bush, P. J., & Weinfurt, K. P. (1996). Perception of friends' use of alcohol, cigarettes, and marijuana among urban schoolchildren: A longitudinal analysis. *Addictive Behaviors, 21*, 615–632.

Jarvis, M. J. (1994). A profile of tobacco smoking. *Addiction, 89*, 1371–1376.

Jarvis, M. J., & Wardle, J. (1999). Social patterning of individual health behaviors: the case of cigarette smoking. In M. Marmot & R. G. Wilkinson (Eds.), *Social determinants of health* (pp. 240–255). London: Oxford University Press.

Kandel, D. B., Huang, F. Y., & Davies, M. (2001). Comorbidity between patterns of substance use dependence and psychiatric syndromes. *Drug and Alcohol Dependence, 64*(2), 233–241.

Kirke, D. M. (2004). Chain reactions in adolescents' cigarette, alcohol, and drug use: Similarity through peer influence or the patterning of ties in peer networks. *Social Networks, 26*, 3–28.

Kobus, K. (2003). Peers and adolescent smoking. *Addiction, 98*(Suppl. 1), 37–55.

Kokkevi, A., Richardson, C., Florescu, S., Kuzman, M., & Stergar, E. (2007). Psychosocial correlates of substance use in adolescence: A cross-national study in six European countries. *Drug and Alcohol Dependence, 86*, 67–74.

Legleye, S., Khlat, M., Beck, F., & Peretti-Watel, P. (2011). Widening inequalities in smoking initiation and cessation patterns: a cohort and gender analysis in France. *Drug and Alcohol Dependence, 117*, 233–241.
Leonardi-Bee, J., Jere, M. L., & Britton, J. (2011). Exposure to parental and sibling smoking and the risk of smoking uptake in childhood and adolescence: A systematic review and meta-analysis. *Thorax, 66*, 847–855.
Leventhal, H., & Cleary, P. D. (1980). The smoking problem: A review of the research and theory in behavioral risk modification. *Psychological Bulletin, 88*, 370–405.
Lucas, L., & Lloyd, B. (1999). Starting smoking: Girls' explanations of the influence of peers. *Journal of Adolescence, 22*, 647–655.
McVicar, D. (2011). Estimates of peer effects in adolescent smoking across twenty six European Countries. *Social Science and Medicine, 73*(8), 1186–1193.
Miller, D. T., Monin, B., & Prentice, D. A. (2000). Pluralistic ignorance and inconsistency between private attitudes and public behaviors. In D. J. Terry & M. A. Hogg (Eds.), *Attitudes, behavior and social context: The role of norms and group membership* (pp. 95–114). Mahway, NJ: Erlbaum Associates.
Munafò, M. R., & Black, S. (2007). Personality and smoking status, a longitudinal analysis. *Nicotine and Tobacco Research, 9*, 397–404.
Munafò, M. R., Zetteler, J. I., & Clark, T. G. (2007). Personality and smoking status, a metaanalysis. *Nicotine and Tobacco Research, 9*, 405–413.
Nichter, M., Nichter, M., Vuckovic, N., Quintero, G., & Ritenbaugh, C. (1997). Smoking experimentation and initiation among adolescent girls: Qualitative and quantitative findings. *Tobacco Control, 6*, 285–295.
Ostacher, M. J., Lebeau, R. T., Perlis, R. H., Nierenberg, A. A., Lund, H. G., Moshier, S. J., et al. (2009). Cigarette smoking is associated with suicidality in bipolar disorder. *Bipolar Disorders, 11*(7), 766–771.
Paul, S. L., Blizzard, L., Patton, G. C., Dwyer, T., & Venn, A. (2008). Parental smoking and smoking experimentation in childhood increase the risk of being a smoker 20 years later: The Childhood determinants of adult health study. *Addiction, 103*(5), 846–853.
Preventing tobacco use among young people. A report of the Surgeon General. Executive summary (1994). *MMWR Recommendations and Report 1, 43*(RR-4), 1–10.
Reijneveld, S. A. (1998). The impact of individual and area characteristics on urban socioeconomic differences in health and smoking. *International Journal of Epidemiology, 27*, 33–40.
Roberts, K., Munafo, M., Rodriguez, D., Drury, M., Murphy, M. & Neale, R. (2005). Longitudinal analysis of the effect of prenatal nicotine exposure on subsequent smoking behavior of offspring. *Nicotine and Tobacco Research, 7*, 801–808.
Robinson, L. A., Murray, D. M., Alfano, C. M., Zbikowski, S. M., Blitstein, J. L., & Klesges, R. C. (2006). Ethnic differences in predictors of adolescent smoking onset and escalation: A longitudinal study from 7th to 12th grade. *Nicotine & Tobacco Research, 8*, 297–307.
Rogers, E., & Shoemaker, F. (1971). *Communication of innovations: A cross-cultural approach*. London: Collier Macmilan.
Rondina Rde, C., Gorayeb, R., & Botelho, C. (2007). Psychological characteristics associated with tobacco smoking behavior. *Jornal Brasileiro de Pneumologia, 33*(5), 592–601.
Rydell, M., Cnattingius, S., Granath, F., Magnusson, C., & Galanti, M. R. (2012). Prenatal exposure to tobacco and future nicotine dependence: Population-based cohort study. *The British Journal of Psychiatry, 200*, 202–209.
Siahpush, M., McNeill, A., Borland, R., & Fong, G. T. (2006a). Socioeconomic variations in nicotine dependence, self efficacy, and intention to quit across four countries: Findings from the International Tobacco Control (ITC) Four Country Survey. *Tobacco Control, 15*, iii71–iii75.
Siahpush, M., McNeill, A., Hammond, D., & Fong, G. T. (2006b). Socioeconomic and country variations in knowledge of health risks of tobacco smoking and toxic constituents of smoke: Results from the 2002 International Tobacco Control (ITC) Four Country Survey. *Tobacco Control, 15*, iii65–iii70.

Simons-Morton, B., & Farhat, T. (2010). Recent findings on peer group influences on adolescent smoking. *Journal of Primary Prevention, 31*, 191–208.

Ter Bogt, T. F., Engels, R. C., & Dubas, J. S. (2006). Party people: Personality and MDMA use of house party visitors. *Addictive Behaviors, 31*, 1240–1244.

Terracciano, A., & Costa, T. P., Jr. (2004). Smoking and the five-factor model of personality. *Addiction, 99*, 472–481.

Vollrath, M. E., & Torgersen, S. (2008). Personality types and risky health behaviors in Norwegian students. *Scandinavian Journal of Psychology, 49*(3), 287–292.

Weiss, J. W., Merrill, V., & Gritz, E. R. (2007). Ethnic variation in the association between weight concern and adolescent smoking. *Addictive Behaviors, 32*, 2311–2316.

WHO. (2010). *Why is tobacco a public health priority?* Geneva, World Health Organization. http://www.who.int/tobacco/ health_priority/en/index.html

World Health Organization. (2008). *WHO report on the global tobacco epidemic: The MPOWER package*. Geneva: World Health Organisation.

Chapter 6
Smoking Prevention in the Communities

Giuseppe La Torre and Flavia Kheiraoui

Objectives The goal of this chapter is to synthesize available data on incidence and prevalence of smoking at school. Summarily, this chapter offers an overview of the actual trend of smoking habits among adolescents.

Moreover, a synthesis of available information of smoking at workplace will be given.

Learning Outcomes

By the end of this chapter the reader will be able to:

- Expand his/her knowledge on the tobacco epidemic at school and at the workplace.
- Evaluate the evidence-based recommendations and guidelines that define remedial actions in approaching the tobacco abuse.
- Analyse the epidemiological basis of smoking among adolescents and workers and its different facets.
- Evaluate the evidence-based recommendations and guidelines that define remedial actions in approaching the tobacco abuse at school.

G. La Torre (✉)
Department of Public Health and Infectious Diseases, "Sapienza" University of Rome, Piazzale Aldo Moro 5, Rome 00185, Italy
e-mail: giuseppe.latorre@uniroma1.it

F. Kheiraoui
Institute of Hygiene, Catholic University of the Sacred Heart, Largo Francesco Vito, 1, Rome 00168, Italy
e-mail: flavia.kheiraoui@rm.unicatt.it

G. La Torre, *Smoking Prevention and Cessation*, DOI 10.1007/978-1-4614-7046-5_6,

6.1 Smoking Prevention at School: Introduction

Tobacco use is addictive and is responsible for more than 20 % of deaths in the industrialized countries. Despite this, every day that many children and adolescents do not understand the real nature of tobacco addiction and are unaware of, or at least underestimate, the health consequences relating to tobacco use (Centers for Disease Control and Prevention 1989).

Each day, nearly 4,000 kids in the United States try their first cigarette and an additional 1,000 kids under 18 years of age become new regular, daily smokers. That's nearly 400,000 new underage daily smokers in this country each year SAMHSA, HHS (2011).

In Europe the prevalence of smoking among adolescents and young adults ranges 23–47 % in males and 18–46 % in females (Steptoe et al. 2002). Moreover, individuals who start smoking early in their life have much more difficulty quitting, and are more likely to become heavy smokers and to develop smoking-related diseases (Taioli and Wynder 1991). A systematic review of controlled trials of adolescent smoking cessation (Garrison et al. 2003) has shown that there is, on the one hand, very limited evidence demonstrating efficacy of smoking cessation interventions in adolescents, and, on the other hand, no evidence of the long-term effectiveness of these interventions. Another issue we must take into consideration in this field is passive smoking (environmental passive smoking, ETS), that is responsible in children and adolescents for the onset of respiratory morbidity and increased bronchial responsiveness (Rizzi et al. 2004; Jang et al. 2004), chronic ear infections (National Cancer Institute 1999), and a higher risk of developing atopic eczema (Kramer et al. 2004).

There is evidence that if adolescents think they are less vulnerable to smoking-related health risks, then they have a higher probability of starting to smoke (Kropp and Halpern-Felsher 2004). Many studies have shown that almost all smokers smoked their first cigarette as a teenager. In that way it would be logical that making it more difficult for teenagers to obtain cigarettes would be helpful in educating the probability that a child/adolescent would become a smoker.

Schools are in a uniquely powerful position to play a major role in reducing the serious problem of smoking and other tobacco use by kids. Children spend almost a third of their waking time in school and much of the peer pressure kids feel regarding whether or not to smoke occurs in school (Jackson 1997; Banks et al. 1981).

Moreover, the vast majority of all smokers begin before leaving high school (SAMHSA 2007).

A national survey in 2010 found that 7.1 % of eighth graders, 13.6 % of tenth graders, and 19.2 % of 12th graders had smoked in the past month (Johnston et al. 2010).

6.2 Data on Incidence and Prevalence Among Adolescents

Smoking behaviour is usually established during adolescence, most adult smokers report that they had their first cigarette or became addicted to nicotine in youth. For this reason primary prevention in the school setting is believed to be one of the most appropriate strategies to tackle substance use (UNICRI 2003).

The meta-analysis from Fichtenberg and Glantz (2002) demonstrated that interventions relating to the access of the young to cigarettes are not associated with consistent positive effects on smoking prevalence among the young. Moreover, we must consider that earlier-onset tobacco smokers might have a modestly higher probability of expressing dependence features within 2 years of smoking onset compared with later onset smokers (Storr et al. 2004).

According to the WHO 2010 global report, the proportion of boys who smoke doubles that of girls among adolescents aged 13–15 (12 % vs. 6 %, respectively). The highest difference between gender is observed in the South-East Asia Region (with boys smoking 3.5 times more than girls), followed by the African, Eastern Mediterranean and Western Pacific Regions, where the proportion of girl smokers is approximately half of what it is for boys. Prevalence rates in girls were found less than those for boys also in the Region of the Americas and the European Region, though with minor variations (WHO 2010 Global Progress Report).

Young people experiment with or begin regular use of tobacco for a variety of reasons, including social and parental norms, advertising, movies and popular media, peer influence, weight control, and curiosity (Baker et al. 2004; Maggi et al. 2007).

6.3 Smoking Prevention Interventions at School

In the field of smoking prevention an important role could be played by school-based interventions designed to deter students from smoking, and this type of intervention is increasingly being implemented. School is the ideal setting for providing smoking prevention programmes to all children and adolescents, and this could be an ethical imperative (National Cancer Institute 1990).

A Systematic review on this issue demonstrated that in order to achieve a higher level of effectiveness it is widely recognized that smoking prevention programmes should have the following components: sustained application, booster sessions over several years; reinforcement in the community; involvement of parents and the mass media; programming smoking prevention activities within a more comprehensive school health promotion programme (La Torre et al. 2005). In Tables 6.1 and 6.2 the principal findings from this systematic review are presented.

There is evidence that the most efficacious preventive approach is based on developing and reinforcing refusal skills for dealing with the social pressures to smoke, and many researchers believe it is fundamental to start smoking prevention programmes at elementary schools. Nevertheless, most studies have focused on smoking prevention programmes in adolescent populations, while there are very few studies on interventions in children (Best et al. 1988; Rasmussen et al. 2002). School-based tobacco prevention education programmes focused on skills training approaches have proven effective in increasing the age of starting the smoking habit, according to several independent studies. A summary of the findings of these studies demonstrates positive outcomes across programmes that vary in format, scope, and delivery method (Centers for Disease Control and prevention 1994). Since the

Table 6.1 Selection criteria of the systematic reviews investigating the effectiveness of smoking prevention programmes in children and adolescents (from La Torre et al. 2005)

References	Selection criteria
Tobler (1986)	Type of programme: assisting young people in developing attitudes, values, behavior and skills, using: (a) positive peer influence; (b) peer teaching; (c) peer counselling, helping and facilitating; (d) peer participations in addition to refusal skills; (e) social and life skills Participants: students from 6th to 12th grade
Rundall and Bruvold (1988)	Type of programme: (a) school-based tobacco prevention programmes identifying the social influences that promote tobacco use among the young: (b) programmes that teach skills to resist such influences
Bangert-Drowns (1988)	Type of programme: (a) involving peers; (b) delivered by adults (lectures, group discussion) Type of interventions: (a) knowledge only; (b) affective education only; (c) mixed interventions Other: programmes with or without volunteer participants
Bruvold (1993)	Type of programme: those involving teaching the skills to resist social pressures to use tobacco Studies concerned with the short- and long-term consequences of using tobacco
Rooney and Murray (1996)	Type of programme: school-based smoking prevention programmes based on peer or social-type programmes Studies published between 1974 and 1991
Thomas (2002)	Type of programme: (a) those providing information; (b) those using social influences approaches; (c) those facing social competence; (d) those including interventions beyond the school into the community. Studies in which individual students, classes, schools, or school districts were randomized to the intervention or control groups and followed for at least 6 months Participants: Children (aged 5–12 years) or adolescents (aged 13–18 years) in the school setting Interventions: Classroom programmes or curricula aimed at deterring the use of tobacco Other: included programmes with a drug or alcohol focus if outcomes for tobacco use were reported
Hwang et al. (2004)	Type of programme: (a) social influence modality; (b) cognitive behavior modality; (c) life skills modality Randomized controlled trials published between 1978 and 1997 School-based or school/community-combined smoking programmes aimed at mainstream students in the US Participants: students from 6th to 12th grade Interventions: programmes with psychological theory-based approaches to tobacco use

end of the 1980s, several quantitative systematic reviews have been conducted. Review of the scientific literature regarding school-based smoking prevention programmes demonstrated that this type of intervention is effective if methodologically rigorous. Programmes based only on information are typically ineffective. Educational programmes vary in format, scope, delivery methods, and community

Table 6.2 Main results of the systematic reviews investigating the effectiveness of smoking prevention programmes in children and adolescents (from La Torre et al. 2005)

References	Number of studies evaluated	Main results
Tobler (1986)	143	Peer programmes were found to show a definite superiority in terms of magnitude of the effect size obtained on all outcome measures (knowledge, attitudes, use, skills, and behavior). Peer programmes showed a high effect size for alcohol, soft drugs and hard drugs, as well as for cigarette use
Rundall and Bruvold (1988)	47	Innovative interventions relying on social reinforcement, social norms, and developmental behavioural models were more effective than traditional "awareness" programmes designed to inform adolescents about the health risks associated with tobacco use
Bangert-Drowns (1988)	33	Typical substance abuse education had the most positive effects on knowledge and attitudes, but was unsuccessful in changing drug-using behaviours of students. Attitudinal effects were significantly higher when peers were instructional leaders and when group discussion was part of the instructional mode
Bruvold (1993)	94	Behavioural effect sizes were largest for interventions with a social reinforcement orientation, moderate for interventions with either a developmental or a social norm orientation, and small for interventions with the traditional orientation
Rooney and Murray (1996)		The average effect of peer or social-type programmes is likely to be quite limited in magnitude, and the reduction in smoking may be only 0.10 standard deviation units, or perhaps 5 %, and under optimal conditions, the reduction in smoking may be only 0.50–0.75 standard deviation units, or perhaps 20–30 %
Thomas (2002)	75	Among 15 high quality studies, 8 showed some positive effect of intervention on smoking prevalence, and 7 failed to detect an effect on smoking prevalence
Hwang et al. (2004)	65	Knowledge had the highest effect sizes in the short term but rapidly decreased after 1 year The behavioural effect was the most meaningful, being persistent over 3 years. Adolescent smoking reduction rates were increased by using either cognitive behavior or life skills programme modalities, and/or a school/community-incorporated program setting

setting, and show differences in smoking prevalence between intervention and non intervention groups: the mean difference between groups receiving and those not receiving an intervention (schools or classrooms) went from 5 % to 60 %, with a duration of 1–4 years.

There are some essential elements of smoking prevention interventions; these include:

1. Information about social influences including media, peer, and parents.
2. Information about short-term physiological effects of tobacco use.
3. Training in refusal skills. It is evident that school programmes designed to prevent tobacco use in children and adolescents could become one of the most effective strategies available to reduce tobacco use in all the world, especially if the programmes involve communities.

These programmes should encourage target individuals (children and adolescents) who have not yet experimented with tobacco and give them the ability to continue their abstinence.

As suggested by Centers for Disease Control and Prevention (2000), it is also important that, in order to model a tobacco-free environment, schools should rigorously enforce policies to protect children from the hazards of tobacco smoke at school. Only in that way schools will be able to reduce the opportunities for young people to experiment with tobacco on the school premises. In order to achieve the greatest effectiveness, school-based programmes should target youngers before they initiate tobacco use.

The involvement of sociological and psychological theories appears to be fundamental in smoking prevention programmes. The first intervention based on these theories was developed by Evans (1976) who underlined the sociological communication model. After that first attempt, several approaches were used. Many of those relied on the fact that intervention directed at prevention of smoking in children and adolescents should involve careful assessment of primary behavioral, normative and control beliefs held by the target group and then moving forward with educational exercises specifically designed to significantly modify beliefs and attitudes, norms and perceived controls they produce, as suggested by Ayzen and Fishbein (1980).

Typically a smoking prevention programme is designed as a school-based intervention focused on deterring students from using tobacco. The curriculum may consist of different levels of instruction, but at least the following items should be present (La Torre et al. 2004):

1. Health facts and the effects of smoking.
2. Analysis of the mechanisms that lead children and adolescent to start smoking.
3. Refusal skills training for dealing with the social pressures to smoke.

In the intervention, the effects of smoking over the short term, more than the long term, need to be emphasized. Students should be allowed to clarify their opinions with regard to the use of tobacco, and peer-led discussions and skill practice activities should be encouraged. A prevention programme based on cognitive and behavioral aspects underlines psychosocial themes, including relational stress within the peer group or family, that can influence and perpetuate the attitude toward tobacco smoking. The main aim is to develop the capacity of children to refuse the offer of a cigarette from peers and to maintain a conversation to firmly sustain their refusal position.

6.4 Community Interventions

A promising field of research in this area is represented by the assessment of community intervention. Sowden et al. (2003) reported that there is some support for the effectiveness of community interventions in helping prevent the uptake of smoking in young people.

They assessed the effectiveness of multicomponent community interventions compared to no intervention or to single component or school-based programmes only.

As shown in the Control of Adolescent Smoking (CAS) Study, a project developed in eight European countries, with the aim of investigating the relationships between national tobacco policies, school smoking policies and adolescent smoking, there are significantly lower prevalence rates in smoke-free schools (Griesbach et al. 2002; Wold et al. 2004). To achieve greater effectiveness, Raczynski and Di Clemente (1997) recognized that a smoking prevention programme should contain sustained treatment, reinforcement of the treatment within the community, involving parents and the mass media; and programming smoking prevention activities within a more comprehensive school health promotion programme.

Wang et al. (2001) demonstrated that a school-based tobacco-use prevention programme, designed to prevent tobacco use among high school students, was highly cost-effective, if compared with other prevention interventions. Such results have to be taken into serious consideration by policy makers and programme planners.

6.5 Evidence-Based Recommendations and Guidelines

The Center for Diseases Control (CDC) guidelines on preventing tobacco use among the young summarize school-based strategies most likely to be effective (Centers for Disease Control and Prevention 1994). These guidelines were drawn up by the CDC in collaboration with experts from 29 national, federal and voluntary agencies, and with other leading authorities in the field of tobacco-use prevention with the aim of helping school personnel implement effective tobacco-use prevention programmes. These interesting guidelines are based on an indepth review of research, theory, and current practice in the area of school-based tobacco-use prevention.

The CDC guidelines offer the following seven strategies that are effective in preventing tobacco use among the young:

1. Develop and enforce a school policy on tobacco use.
2. Provide instruction about the short- and long-term negative physiological and social consequences of tobacco use, social influences on tobacco use, peer norms regarding tobacco use, and refusal skills.
3. Provide tobacco-use prevention education in kindergarten through 12th grade.
4. Provide programme-specific training for teachers.
5. Involve parents or families in supporting school-based programmes to prevent tobacco use.
6. Support cessation efforts among students and all school staff who use tobacco.
7. Assess the tobacco-use prevention programme at regular intervals.

It is remarkable that school-based programmes to prevent tobacco use could contribute preventing the use of illicit drugs, especially if such programmes are also designed to prevent the use of these substances (Errecart et al. 1991). Tobacco is one of the most commonly available and widely used drugs, and its use can be considered the most widespread drug dependency. Many studies have shown that the use of other drugs is often preceded by the use of tobacco or alcohol. Even though the vast majority of young persons who use tobacco do not use illicit drugs, Yamaguchi and Kandel underline that when further drug involvement does occur it is typically sequential—from tobacco or alcohol to marijuana, and from marijuana to other illicit drugs or psychoactive prescription drugs (Yamaguchi and Kandel 1984). A recent report by Hansen on preventing drug abuse suggests that approaches effective in preventing tobacco use can also help prevent the use of alcohol and other drugs (Hansen 1992).

6.6 Smoking Prevention in the Workplace: Introduction

Smoking is a major cause for concern within a workplace. It can have a direct impact on both smokers and non-smokers, and ultimately employers. In addition, most employers now have a legal responsibility to ensure that people do not smoke in the workplace.

Exposure to environmental tobacco or secondhand smoke in the workplace is an important contemporary issue. The workplace is an important source of smoking exposure. Occupational exposure has been linked with important chronic health effects including lung cancer, cardiovascular disease, impaired lung function, and COPD (U.S. Department of Health and Human Services 2006).

In economically developed countries, adults spend the majority of their time indoors. Consequently, pollution of the indoor environment has substantive effects on health. In households and workplaces that allow smoking, second hand smoking exposure is often the major source of indoor pollution. After the home, the workplace is the major source of involuntary exposure to tobacco smoke for most adults

(Jefferis et al. 2009; Pirkle et al. 2006). In certain workplaces, employees are exposed to very high levels of second hand smoking (Siegel and Skeer 2003). For example bar and tavern workers, in particular, are exposed to high ambient levels of second hand smoking, up to 4–6 times higher than in other workplaces (Siegel 1993).To prevent the adverse health effects of passive smoking, the workplace remains a high priority for smoke-free legislation.

Other factors determining the prevalence of workplace passive smoking exposure include the type of workplace (higher levels of exposure in office than non-office workplaces) and the workplace smoking policy (Hammond et al. 1995). The lowest levels of second hand smoking exposure are found in workplaces that completely ban smoking, intermediate levels in those that restrict smoking, and highest levels in those that allow smoking.

6.7 Data on Incidence and Prevalence Among Workers

According to International Agency Research Cancer (IARC), the exposed workers had all together 42 million exposures (1.3 mean exposures for each exposed worker). The second most common exposure was environmental tobacco smoke (ETS) (7.5 million workers exposed at least 75 % of working time). The World Health Organization estimates that in the world approximately 700 millions are exposed to second-hand smoke. Exposure to ETS in the workplace has become a major public and occupational health issue in the recent years (Borland et al. 1992; Parrott et al. 2000; Woodward 1991). Strong evidence identify ETS as one of the most important contaminants of indoor air and as a major health hazard in the working environment.

In the United Kingdom smoking at work is likely to be responsible for the deaths of more than two employed people per working day (617 deaths/year).

Workplace has been established as a major source of exposure to the tobacco smoke (Jamrozik 2005; Moussa et al. 2004). Some occupational groups experience higher levels of ETS than others due to the greater density of smokers at work.

6.8 Workplace Interventions for Smoking Cessation

Smoking at workplaces is a real health hazard in the indoor environment. There are no safe levels of exposure, and employers have to provide a safe environment for their employees. There are many benefits of providing a smoke-free workplace. In addition to meeting the legal obligations and eliminating the risk of prosecution for non-compliance in relation to enclosed workplaces, a smoke-free policy can reducing levels of smoking among employees and helping to reduce some illnesses and conditions (such as cardiovascular disease and respiratory diseases) that are important causes of sickness absence. This will result in improved productivity and

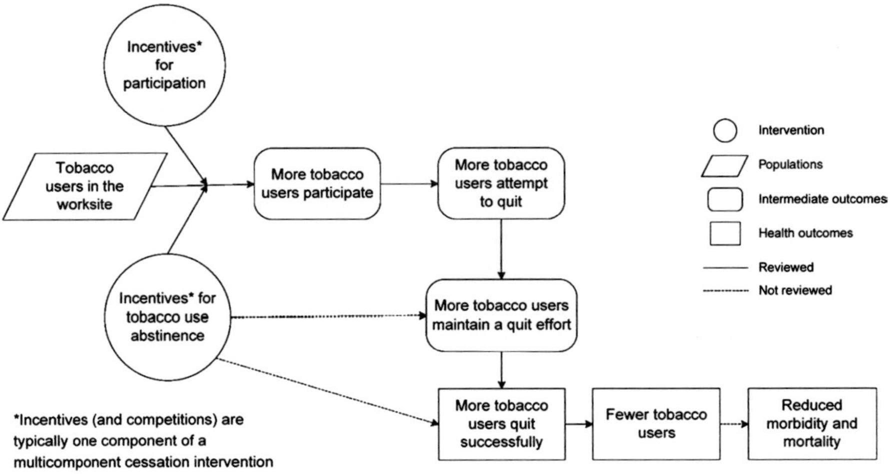

Fig. 6.1 Analytic framework of the effect of incentives and competitions on reducing tobacco use among workers (from Leeks et al. 2010)

also less costs for employers (Halpern et al. 2001; Winstanley et al. 1995). There are several reasons for employers to support smoking cessation in the workplace: improved employee health; increased productivity; reduced costs; enhanced job satisfaction; better corporate image. Computer technology and psychological theory can be combined to produce effective individualized self-help smoking cessation materials and to disseminate them at the population level, in particular using Internet o social networks.

Moreover, as underlined by Leeks and colleagues (2010), there is evidence of effectiveness in increasing the number of workers who quit using tobacco of worksite-based incentives (i.e., entrance in a lottery as reward for a 10-day abstinence) and competitions if these are combined with additional interventions. In this context, incentives and competitions, alone or as part of a coordinated program (Fig. 6.1), can contribute among workers to:

1. Increase or improve motivations to quit.
2. Increase or improve action to quit.
3. Increase or improve maintenance of an effort to quit.

Interventions designed to motivate the cessation efforts of tobacco users are also important options for health promotion in most community settings, including worksites. Employee populations use tobacco products because many adults spend the majority of their day in a workplace environment, so worksites are viable places to conduct health promotion activities.

The worksite provides a number of advantages as a setting for health promotion interventions, including:

1. Accessibility to a large and rather stable population, which provides the potential for achieving intervention exposure.

2. The potential for adequate or enhanced promotion, recruitment, and participation in comparison to non-worksite environments.
3. The potential for reinforcing social support networks and peer influences among co-workers.

Incentives and competitions to reduce tobacco use represent one intervention option for consideration by worksite health promotion programs. In addition, participation might prompt the individual to make use of new or existing cessation support resources offered within the workplace, through the workplace, or in the community (Cahill et al. 2008; Smedslund et al. 2004). For a designated population (at a worksite or within a workforce), effectiveness of incentives or competitions within a cessation program would be demonstrated by a reduction in the number of baseline smokers who continue to use tobacco (for example fewer tobacco product users) (Cahill and Perera 2008).

6.9 Smoking-Free Workplace Legislation

In recent years, smoking has been banned in public places in several countries.

Prohibition of smoking at workplaces has been shown to lead to lower levels of smoking by individuals and an increase in rates of quitting tobacco use. Therefore, a comprehensive smoke-free policy at the workplace can have a strong and positive influence on the behaviour of smoking workers, since they are less exposed to ETS at work, their attempts to quit smoking will be supported, and the general perception of smoking is changing (Broder et al. 1993; Stillman et al. 1990). Smoke-free workplace legislation is highly effective for reducing passive smoke exposure. These laws are expected to improve respiratory health, prevent chronic disease, and extend lifespan.

The WHO guidelines of 2006 support the Member States of the WHO European Region in strengthening protection from exposure to tobacco smoke at the workplace (WHO 2006).

Many state and local governments in U.S. passed the laws prohibiting smoking in public places as well as requiring private workplaces to be non smoking area.

Several studies results suggest that anti-smoking legislation appears to play an important role in decreasing second hand smoking exposure. Overall, smoking bans appear most effective in decreasing exposure to second hand smoking in public places. They also appear to increase the prevalence of complete smoking restrictions at work. But they appear to have additional benefits by decreasing the percentage of current smokers and decreasing exposures to second S in private settings (Farrelly et al. 1999; Millar 1998).

For example, when the legislation mandating smoke-free bars and taverns was enacted, several bartenders reported a substantial reduction in workplace smoking exposure, so prohibition of workplace smoking has effectively reduced employee ETS exposure. Smoke-free workplaces have been associated from many authors with decreased personal cigarette consumption, public smoking, and self-reported ETS exposure.

6.10 Smoke-Free Legislation

Smokefree policies consist in rules and regulations that prohibit smoking in indoor workspaces and designated public areas. These policies can be applied to private or public sector. In the first sector a complete ban on tobacco use on worksite property or restrict smoking to designated outdoor locations, while in the public sector smokefree standards are established for all or for designated indoor workplaces and public areas (Hopkins et al. 2010).

There is evidence that smoke-free policies have an important impact on public health (Fig. 6.2), since they have an effect on:

(a) Reducing or eliminating the exposure to second-hand smoke.
(b) Decreasing the prevalence of smokers.
(c) Encouraging smokers to quit or preventing the initiation of smoking.
(d) Reducing cigarettes consumption among smokers.

According to WHO, in16 countries (comprising only 5 % of the world's population), a comprehensive national smoke-free law does exist, with high compliance in many of these countries (WHO 2008). The first country in the world that created and enjoyed smoke-free indoor workplaces and public places (including restaurants, bars and pubs) was Ireland (March 2004), followed by Norway (June 2004), Italy and Uruguay (2005), and by many cities in all the world. Moreover, we must remember that most people in Canada, Australia and the United States have state or local smokefree legislation.

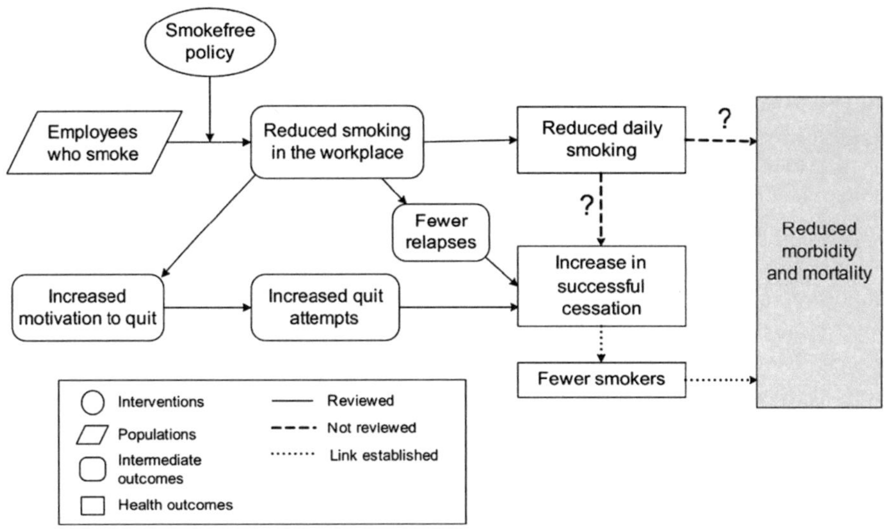

Fig. 6.2 Analytic framework of the pathways through which smokefree policy interventions are hypothesized to affect intermediate and health outcomes (from Hopkins et al. 2010). *Question mark* indicates that the relationship/link is not well reviewed/established

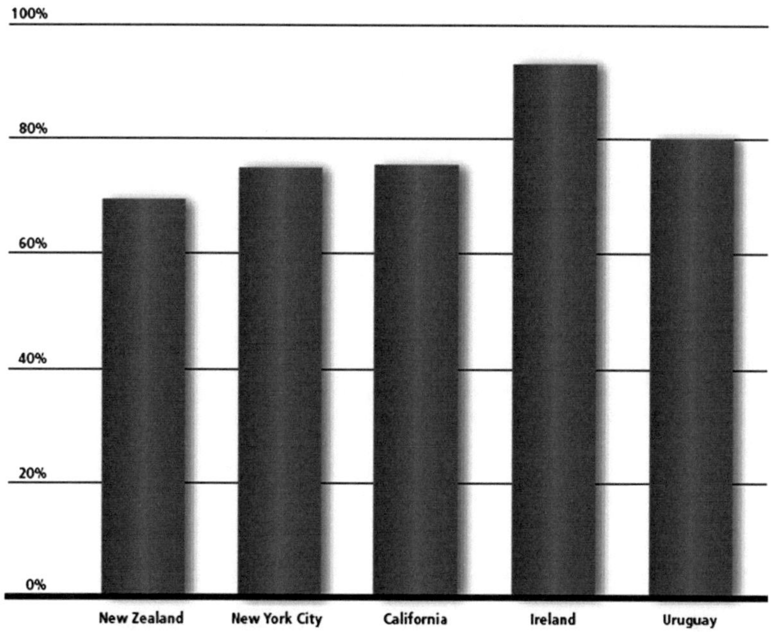

Fig. 6.3 Support for comprehensive smoking bans in bars and restaurants after implementation

The success and popularity of smoke-free legislation in countries that have adopted it contradict false claims by the tobacco industry that these laws are unworkable and costly to businesses (WHO 2008).

The support for smoking bans (Fig. 6.3) was very high. Moreover, there is also evidence from a review of the literature on the economic effects of smoke-free environments around the world that no study had a negative economic impact, giving on the other hand a neutral or positive impact on businesses (Scollo et al. 2003).

References

Ayzen, I., & Fishbein, M. (1980). *Understanding attitudes and predicting social behaviour*. Englewood Cliffs: Prentice-Hall.

Baker, T. B., Brandon, T. H., & Chassin, L. (2004). Motivational influences on cigarette smoking. *Annual Review of Psychology, 55*, 463–491.

Bangert-Drowns, R. L. (1988). The effects of school-based substance abuse education—a meta-analysis. *Journal of Drug Education, 18*, 243–264.

Banks, M., et al. (1981). Adolescent attitudes to smoking: Their influence on behavior. *International Journal of Health Education, 24*(1), 39–44.

Best, J. A., Thomson, S. J., Santi, S. M., Smith, E., & Brown, K. S. (1988). Preventing cigarette smoking among school children. *Annual Review of Public Health, 9*, 161–201.

Borland, R., Pierce, J. P., Burns, D. M., Gilpin, E., Johnson, M., & Bal, D. (1992). Protection from environmental tobacco smoke in California: The case for a smoke-free workplace. *Journal of the American Medical Association, 268*(6), 749–752.

Broder, I., Pilger, C., & Correy, P. (1993). Environment and well-being before and following smoking ban in office buildings. *Canadian Journal of Public Health, 84*, 254–258.

Bruvold, W. H. (1993). A meta-analysis of adolescent smoking prevention programs. *American Journal of Public Health, 83*(6), 872–880.

Cahill, K., Moher, M., & Lancaster, T. (2008). Workplace interventions for smoking cessation. *Cochrane Database of Systematic Reviews, 8*(4).

Cahill, K., & Perera, R. (2008). Competitions and incentives for smoking cessation. *Cochrane Database of Systematic Reviews, 16*(3).

Centers for Disease Control and Prevention. (1989). *Reducing the health consequences of smoking: 25 years of progress. A report of the Surgeon General* (DHHS publication no. (CDC) 89-8411). Atlanta: US Department of Health and Human Services, Centers for Disease Control and Prevention.

Centers for Disease Control and Prevention. (1994). Guidelines for school health programs to prevent tobacco use and addiction. *MMWR Recommendations and Reports, 43*(RR-2), 1–18.

Centers for Disease Control and Prevention. (2000). *Reducing tobacco use. A report of the Surgeon General*. Atlanta: US Department of Health and Human Services, Centers for Disease Control and Prevention.

Errecart, M. T., Walberg, H. J., Ross, J. G., Gold, R. S., Fiedler, J. L., & Kolbe, L. J. (1991). Effectiveness of teenage health teaching modules. *The Journal of School Health, 61*(1), 19–42.

Evans, R. I. (1976). Smoking in children: Developing a social psychological strategy of deterrence. *Preventive Medicine, 5*, 122–127.

Farrelly, M. C., Evans, W. N., & Sfekas, A. E. (1999). The impact of workplace smoking bans: Results from a national survey. *Tobacco Control, 8*(3), 272–277.

Fichtenberg, C. M., & Glantz, S. A. (2002). Youth access interventions do not affect youth smoking. *Pediatrics, 109*(6), 1088–1092.

Garrison, M. M., Christakis, D. A., Ebel, B. E., Wiehe, S. E., & Rivara, F. P. (2003). Smoking cessation interventions for adolescents: A systematic review. *American Journal of Preventive Medicine, 25*(4), 363–367.

Griesbach, D., Inchley, J., & Currie, C. (2002). More than words? The status and impact of smoking policies in Scottish schools. *Health Promotion International, 17*(1), 31–41.

Halpern, M., Shikiar, R., Rentz, A., & Khan, Z. (2001). Impact of smoking status on workplace absenteeism and productivity. *Tobacco Control, 10*, 233–238.

Hammond, S. K., Sorensen, G., Youngstrom, R., & Ockene, J. K. (1995). Occupational exposure to environmental tobacco smoke. *Journal of the American Medical Association, 274*, 956–960.

Hansen, W. B. (1992). School-based substance abuse prevention: A review of the state of the art in curriculum. *Health Education Research, 7*(3), 403–430.

Hopkins, D. P., Razi, S., Leeks, K. D., Priya Kalra, G., Chattopadhyay, S. K., Soler, R. E., et al. (2010). Smokefree policies to reduce tobacco use. A systematic review. *American Journal of Preventive Medicine, 38*(2 Suppl), S275–S289.

Hwang, M. S., Yeagley, K. L., & Petosa, R. (2004). A meta-analysis of adolescent psychosocial smoking prevention programs published between 1978 and 1997 in the United States. *Health Education & Behavior, 31*(6), 702–719.

Jackson, C. (1997). Initial and experimental stages of tobacco and alcohol use during late childhood: Relation to peer, parent, and personal risk factors. *Addictive Behaviors, 22*(5), 685–698.

Jamrozik, K. (2005). Estimate of deaths attributable to passive smoking among UK adults: Database analysis. *BMJ, 330*(7495), 812–815.

Jang, A. S., Choi, I. S., Lee, S., Nam, H. S., Kweon, S. S., Son, M. H., et al. (2004). The effect of passive smoking on asthma symptoms, atopy, and airway hyperresponsiveness in schoolchildren. *Journal of Korean Medical Science, 19*(2), 214–217.

Jefferis, B. J., Thomson, A. G., Lennon, L. T., et al. (2009). Changes in environmental tobacco smoke (ETS) exposure over a 20-year period: Cross-sectional and longitudinal analyses. *Addiction, 104*, 496–503.

Johnston, L. D., O'Malley, P. M., Bachman, J. G., & Schulenberg, J. E. (2010). *Monitoring the Future National Survey Results on Drug Use, 1975-2010, "Smoking stops declining and shows signs of increasing among younger teens."* Ann Arbor, MI: University of Michigan News Service. http://www.monitoringthefuture.org/data/10data.html#2010data-cigs

Kramer, U., Lemmen, C. H., Behrendt, H., Link, E., Schafer, T., Gostomzyk, J., et al. (2004). The effect of environmental tobacco smoke on eczema and allergic sensitization in children. *British Journal of Dermatology, 150*(1), 111–118.

Kropp, R. Y., & Halpern-Felsher, B. L. (2004). Adolescents' Beliefs about the risks involved in smoking "light" cigarettes. *Pediatrics, 114*(4), 445–451.

La Torre, G., Chiaradia, G., & Ricciardi, G. (2005). School-based smoking prevention in children and adolescents: Review of the scientific literature. *Journal of Public Health, 13*, 285–290.

La Torre, G., Moretti, C., Capitano, D., Alonzi, M. T., Ferrara, M., Gentile, A., et al. (2004). La prevenzione del tabagismo: Risultati di uno studio controllato randomizzato in adolescenti scolarizzati in Cassino. *Rivista Italiana di Medicina dell'Adolescenza, 2*(3), 36–40.

Leeks, K. D., Hopkins, D. P., Soler, R. E., Aten, A., Chattopadhyay, S. K., & Task Force on Community Preventive Services. (2010). Worksite-based incentives and competitions to reduce tobacco use. A systematic review. *American Journal of Preventive Medicine, 38*(2 Suppl), S263–S274.

Maggi, S., Hertzman, C., & Vaillancourt, T. (2007). Changes in smoking behaviors from late childhood to adolescence: insights from the Canadian National Longitudinal Survey of Children and Youth. *Health Psychology, 26*, 232–240.

Millar, W. J. (1998). Evaluation of the impact of smoking restrictions in a government work setting. *Canadian Journal of Public Health, 79*, 379–382.

Moussa, K. M., Lindström, M., & Östergren, P. O. (2004). Socioeconomic and demographic differences in exposure to environmental tobacco smoke at work: The Scania Public Health Survey 2000. *Scandinavian Journal of Public Health, 32*(3), 194–202.

National Cancer Institute. (1990). *School programs to prevent smoking: The national cancer institute guide to strategies that succeed.* Rockville, MD: US Department of Health and Human Services, Public Health Service, National Institutes of Health, National Cancer Institute.

National Cancer Institute. (1999). *Health effects of exposure to environmental tobacco smoke: The report of the California Environmental Protection Agency*. Bethesda, MD: US Department of Health and Human Services, National Institutes of Health, National Cancer Institute.

Parrott, S., Godfrey, C., & Raw, M. (2000). Costs of employee smoking in the workplace in Scotland. *Tobacco Control, 9*(2), 187–192.

Pirkle, J. L., Bernert, J. T., Caudill, S. P., et al. (2006). Trends in the exposure of nonsmokers in the U.S. population to secondhand smoke: 1988–2002. *Environmental Health Perspectives, 114*, 853–858.

Raczynski, J. M., & Di Clemente, R. J. (1997). *Handbook of health promotion and disease prevention*. New York, NY: Plenum.

Rasmussen, M., Damsgaard, M. T., Due, P., & Holstein, B. E. (2002). Boys and girls smoking within the Danish elementary school classes: A group-level analysis. *Scandinavian Journal of Public Health, 30*, 62–69.

Rizzi, M., Sergi, M., Andreoli, A., Pecis, M., Bruschi, C., & Fanfulla, F. (2004). Environmental tobacco smoke may induce early lung damage in healthy male adolescents. *Chest, 125*(4), 1387–1393.

Rooney, B. L., & Murray, D. M. (1996). A meta-analysis of smoking prevention programs after adjustment for errors in the unit of analysis. *Health Education Quarterly, 23*(1), 48–64.

Rundall, T. G., & Bruvold, W. H. (1988). Meta-analysis of school-based smoking and alcohol use prevention programs. *Health Education Quarterly, 15*(3), 317–334.

Scollo, M., Lal, A., Hyland, A., & Glantz, S. (2003). Review of the quality of studies on the economic effects of smoke-free policies on the hospitality industry. *Tobacco Control, 12*(1), 13–20.

Siegel, M. (1993). Involuntary smoking in the restaurant workplace: A review of employee exposure and health effects. *Journal of the American Medical Association, 270*, 490–493.

Siegel, M., & Skeer, M. (2003). Exposure to secondhand smoke and excess lung cancer mortality risk among workers in the '5 B's': Bars, bowling alleys, billiard halls, betting establishments, and bingo parlours. *Tobacco Control, 12*, 333–338.

Smedslund, G., Fisher, K. J., Boles, S. M., & Lichtenstein, E. (2004). The effectiveness of workplace smoking cessation programmes: A meta-analysis of recent studies. *Tobacco Control, 13*(2).

Sowden, A., Arblaster, L., Stead, L. (2003). Community interventions for preventing smoking in young people. *Cochrane Database Systematic Review* (1):CD001291.

Steptoe, A., Wardle, J., Cui, W., Baban, A., Glass, K., Pelzer, K., et al. (2002). An international comparison of tobacco smoking, beliefs and risk awareness in university students from 23 countries. *Addiction, 97*, 1561–1571.

Stillman, F. A., Becker, D. M., Swank, R. T., et al. (1990). Ending smoking at the Johns Hopkins medical institutions. *Journal of the American Medical Association, 264*, 1565–1569.

Storr, C. L., Zhou, H., Liang, K. Y., & Anthony, J. C. (2004). Empirically derived latent classes of tobacco dependence syndromes observed in recent-onset tobacco smokers: Epidemiological evidence from a national probability sample survey. *Nicotine and Tobacco Research, 6*(3), 533–545.

Substance Abuse and Mental Health Services Administration (SAMHSA), HHS. (2011). *Results from the 2010 National Survey on Drug Use and Health, NSDUH: Summary of National Findings*. http://oas.samhsa.gov/NSDUH/2k10NSDUH/tabs/Sect4peTabs10to11.pdf

Substance Abuse and Mental Health Services Administration (SAMHSA), HHS, Calculated based on data in National Household Survey on Drug Use and Health, 2007.

Taioli, E., & Wynder, E. (1991). Effect of the age at which smoking begins on frequency of smoking in adulthood. *New England Journal of Medicine, 325*, 968–969.

Thomas, R. (2002). School-based programmes for preventing smoking. *Cochrane Database of Systematic Reviews, 4*, CD001293.

Tobler, N. S. (1986). Meta-analysis of 143 adolescent drug prevention programs: Quantitative outcome results of program participants compared to a control or comparison group. *Journal of Drug Issues, 16*, 537–567.

U.S. Department of Health and Human Services. (2006). *The health consequences of involuntary exposure to tobacco smoke: A report of the Surgeon General*. Atlanta, Georgia: U.S. Department of Health and Human Services, Centers for Disease Control and Prevention, Coordinating Center for Health Promotion, National Center for Chronic Disease Prevention and Health Promotion, Office on Smoking and Health.

UNICRI. (2003). *School-Based Drug Education: a guide for practitioners and the wider community*. United Nations Office for Drug Control and Crime Prevention.

Wang, L. Y., Crossett, L. S., Lowry, R., Sussman, S., & Dent, C. W. (2001). Cost-effectiveness of a school-based tobacco-use prevention program. *Archives of Pediatrics and Adolescent Medicine, 155*(9), 1043–1050.

WHO. (2008). *WHO report on the global tobacco epidemic: The MPOWER package*. Geneva, Switzerland: World Health Organization.

WHO Legislating for smoke-free workplaces 2006 (http://www.euro.who.int/__data/assets/pdf_file/0004/68116/E88864.pdf)

Winstanley, M., Woodward, S., & Walker, N. (1995). *Tobacco in Australia: Facts and issues 1995* (2nd ed.). Melbourne: Victorian Smoking and Health Program.

Wold, B., Torsheim, T., Currie, C., & Roberts, C. (2004). National and school policies on restrictions of teacher smoking: A multilevel analysis of student exposure to teacher smoking in seven European countries. *Health Education Research, 19*(3), 217–226.

Woodward, A. (1991). Is passive smoking in the workplace hazardous to health? *Scandinavian Journal of Work, Environment and Health, 17*(5), 293–301.

World Health Organization. (2010). *2010 global progress report on the implementation of the WHO Framework Convention on Tobacco Control (FCTC/2010.1)*. Retrieved from http://www.who.int/fctc/reporting/summaryreport.pdf

Yamaguchi, K., & Kandel, D. (1984). Patterns of drug use from adolescence to young adulthood. II. Sequences of progression. *American Journal of Public Health, 74*, 668–672.

Chapter 7
Smoking Prevention Through Mass Media Campaigns

Giuseppe La Torre, Ferruccio Pelone, Marta Marino, and Antonio Giulio De Belvis

Objectives The goal of this chapter is to describe the role of health communication in preventing smoking habits providing the reader with useful insight toward the theoretical and empirical underpinning of mass media campaigns. At the end of this chapter you will be able to address the tobacco prevention mass media campaigns core issues (e.g., theoretical framework and basic knowledge) and summarizing both the up-to-date scientific evidence and institutional reports.

Learning Outcomes

By the end of this chapter the reader will be able to:

- Evaluate the evidence-based recommendations and guidelines that define remedial actions in approaching the tobacco abuse at school.
- Learn the theory underlying the phenomenon "smoking prevention "by means of public health and preventive community interventions.
- Identify the differences between the main preventive strategies on preventing smoking initiation in terms of setting, outcomes, and target populations.
- Evaluate the most effective strategies according to the intervention type (i.e., school based, workplace, mass media, health authority) and its by-handle aim (i.e., policy maker, academic researcher).

G. La Torre (✉)
Department of Public Health and Infectious Diseases, "Sapienza" University of Rome, Piazzale Aldo Moro 5, Rome 00185, Italy
e-mail: giuseppe.latorre@uniroma1.it

F. Pelone • M. Marino • A.G. De Belvis
Institute of Hygiene - Department of Public Health, Faculty of Medicine, Università Cattolica del Sacro Cuore, Largo Francesco Vito 1, Rome 00168, Italy

G. La Torre, *Smoking Prevention and Cessation*, DOI 10.1007/978-1-4614-7046-5_7,

7.1 Mass Media Campaigns

7.1.1 Mass Media Campaigns Definition

Mass media campaigns (Box 7.1) can be defined as a tool to transfer information, concepts, and ideas to large populations through the routine use of existing media, including newspaper, television, or Internet (Rice and Atkin 2009). Since the 1950s, they have played an important role in achieving public health goals worldwide (Wakefield et al. 2010). Public health media campaigns are used to expose specific audiences to messages in order to shape desirable behavioral outcomes (e.g., producing positive changes and preventing negative changes in health-related behaviors) within a specific time period (National Cancer Institute 2008; Atkin and Salmon 2010).

Box 7.1 Mass Media Definition

Mass media refers collectively to all media technologies—whether written, broadcast, or spoken—that reach a large audience (Oxford English Dictionary 2011). Until recent times, mass media was clearly defined and consisted of eight industries: books, newspapers, magazines, radio, movies, television, and the Internet.

We can define all the media as communication channels that reach a large audience and we can divide the various types into three broad categories*:

- *Broadcast media* (also known as digital or electronic media), is any media in which information is transmitted electronically and consists of television, radio, movies, and Internet. According to the broadest definition, broadcast media is any communication channel that can be broadcast over airwaves, sound waves, or through the Internet.
- *Print media* uses a physical object as a means of sending information, such as newspapers, magazines, books, leaflets, and pamphlets.
- *Outdoor media* encompasses a wide range of "out-of-home" media in which information is aimed at reaching consumers where they live, work, play drive, shop, and commute. Outdoor communication is associated with billboards, signs, placards placed inside and outside of commercial buildings/objects like shops/buses, blimps, and skywriting.

---

*Mass media From Wikipedia, the free encyclopedia 2011.

7.1.2 *The Use of Mass Media Campaigns in Public Health*

The results of mass media for promoting social change have increasingly become important for public health (Randolph and Viswanath 2004). Communicating about health through mass media is complex, however, and challenges professionals in diverse disciplines (Strasburger et al. 2010). Government leaders, policy-makers, health and media professionals, and sociologists involved in public health delivery process have all recognized the high potential of mass media campaigning to foster preventive and health promotion strategies. Mass media has the potential to reach a large proportion of the population, particularly groups that may be difficult to access through more traditional approaches and is a relatively inexpensive way of exposing the population to information regarding their health (Kremers et al. 2004; Brinn et al. 2010).

Health-related media campaigns have three important functions: they fulfill a valuable role in distributing information to fill health knowledge gaps differentially distributed in the population; they help to keep health issues on the political agenda; finally mass media can help in raising an individual's awareness about health issues (Wellings and Macdowall 2000).

Mass media campaigns have long been a tool for promoting public health. Snyder and Hamilton (2002) conducted the first meta-analysis of the US health mass media campaign literature (Snyder and Hamilton 2002). Overall, they found, in percentage terms, the average campaign changed the behavior of about 8 % of the population in the expected, positive direction. In addition, Snyder and Hamilton (2002) found that (1) success varied with different behaviors, with seatbelt, oral health, and alcohol campaigns being the most successful; (2) greater effects were found for campaigns focused on adoption of new behaviors as compared with prevention or cessation of problem behaviors; and (3) greater effects were found in campaigns with greater reach/exposure.

A second meta-analysis of mass media campaigns appeared in the drug abuse prevention literature and was conducted by Derzon and Lipsey (2002). Noar (2006) reviewed the literature on public health media campaigns to summarize how design principles were considered in developing the communication strategies (Table 7.1), showing that the past 10 years of campaign research have not resulted in new campaign design principles (Derzon and Lipsey 2002; Noar 2006).

Using mass media can be counterproductive if the channels used are not audience-appropriate, or if the message being delivered is too emotional, fear arousing, or controversial. Undesirable side effects can usually be avoided through proper formative research, knowledge of the audience, experience in linking media channels to audiences, and message testing (Fischer et al. 2011; Noar 2006). Health media campaigns are characterized by several elements, which constitute the input variables of their communication models and, additionally, determine their success (Atkin and Rice 2012; Noar 2006):

Table 7.1 Summary of major principles of effective campaign designs applied to health mass media campaigns

Designing principles	Description	Discussion
Formative research	Formative research is extremely important to the design and implementation of a successful mass media campaign. Such research can enable campaign planners to truly understand their target audience in terms of the problem behavior at hand, their message preferences, and the most promising channels through which they can be reached	Few studies, however, reported using formative research to select campaign channels
Use of theory	Use of theory as a guide to campaigns may be vital to campaign success. Theory can serve as a conceptual foundation for a campaign and can suggest important determinants upon which campaign messages might focus	Health mass media campaigns over the past 10 years have taken greater advantage of a variety of theories, and this is a positive development
Audience segmentation	The ultimate purpose of segmentation is to create homogeneous groups whose message preferences are similar to one another so that campaign messages can be designed to be maximally effective with the target audience (Atkin 2001; Slater 1996)	Each of these projects resulted in an effective campaign, suggesting that the segmentation and subsequent message targeting was successful
Message design and targeting	Use a message design approach that is targeted to and likely to be effective with the audience segment; develop novel and creative messages; design messages that will spark interpersonal discussions and may persuade individuals important to the target audience (e.g., influencers)	An obvious implication for message designers is to find ways to encourage dialogue about the health issue among members of the target audience. Such an approach may be different from creating messages to influence individuals directly, and some message design approaches may lend themselves well to such an orientation (e.g., entertainment education)

(continued)

Table 7.1 (continued)

Designing principles	Description	Discussion
Channel selection	Independently of the campaign's message, they cannot be effective without being placed in channels with great potential to reach the target audience	Synergy among campaign components can likely increase exposure and may increase the impact of a campaign (Derzon and Lipsey 2002)
Process evaluation and message exposure	Process evaluation is concerned with the monitoring and collection of data on fidelity and implementation of campaign activities (e.g., Valente 2001). Such data can improve the execution of campaigns and can inform campaign planners as to why certain outcomes of a campaign were or were not achieved	This may be related to the fact that these campaign articles spent most of their time focused on outcome evaluation and had little space to devote to process data: Both reach and frequency have been found to be important to campaign success (Derzon and Lipsey 2002; Snyder and Hamilton 2002), and because 95 % of an audience was reached does not mean that the frequency of exposure was enough to influence them

- Target audience (e.g., subpopulation groups or general population).
- Characteristics of the message (e.g., emotional appeal, content, and format).
- Design of the message (e.g., organization, style, contents tone, and frequency).
- Dissemination strategy and channel characteristics (e.g., in terms reach, economy, or accessibility).

These elements, which are central to most mass media campaigns, will be briefly discussed here with a focus on health communication.

7.1.3 Identifying the Target Audience

Targeting the media campaign to specific subpopulations—rather than the general population, is necessary to determine which people will be object of the communication strategy, and the outcome behavior that it will engender. Identifying the audience in terms of its demographic characteristics, predispositions, personality traits, and social contexts is likely to have a significant advantage: (1) message efficiency can be improved if subsets of the audience are prioritized according to their centrality in attaining the campaign's objectives as well as receptivity to being influenced; (2) effectiveness can be increased if message content, form, style, and channels are tailored to the attributes and abilities of subgroups. Therefore, such preliminary steps enable campaign designers to inform the overall communication strategy in terms of messages characteristics (e.g., emotional appeal, source, contents, and format) and dissemination strategy (e.g., channel type, frequency, or duration).

7.1.4 Characteristics of the Message: Design, Contents, Emotional Appeal, and Source

Once groups are segmented and it is clear who the target audience is, campaigners have to develop proper and effective messages in order to maximize impact in terms of the individual's behavior/attitude change and desirable social outcomes. According to Atkins and Rice (2012; Noar 2006), four components need to be considered when designing effective campaign messages:

- Strategic approach (e.g., messages aimed to prevent negative changes in health-related behaviors or to promote positive attitudes and healthy lifestyle).
- Content (e.g., informational versus persuasive messages).
- Emotional appeal (e.g., a planner could opt three ways to design a health-related ad message for persuading its target audience he could emphasize: (1) The physical health treats—such as the illness, the death; (2) the negative consequences—social rejection, or (3) the positive incentives—social acceptance to adopt the advocated behavior).
- Format, design, implementation, and "source".

7.1.5 Dissemination Strategy and Channel Characteristics

To be effectively disseminated, campaign messages need to be delivered through channels with high potential to reach the target audience (Salmon and Atkin 2003). There is great diversity in the choice of the channels and methods that campaigners have used in disseminating their messages. Although channels should be selected depending on the usage patterns of target audiences, the nature of the message, and the constraints of available resources, few mass media campaigns have used media only; rather, most campaigns have used a number of varied channels (Noar 2006). Salmon and Atkins (2003) proposed a number of features to assess pros and cons of the alternative mediated communication channels. Table 7.2 reports some of the more relevant features for health-related mass media campaigns.

Hereafter follows a summary of the major print, broadcast, and outdoor media channels, in regard to their main advantages and drawbacks (Breslow 2002):

- *Television*. Television is a powerful medium for appealing to mass audiences—it reaches people regardless of age, sex, income, or educational level. Public health authorities have expressed concern about the indirect influence of television in promoting false norms about acts of violence, drinking, smoking, and sexual behavior (Blackburn et al. 2011; Wahi et al. 2011).
- *Radio*. Radio also reaches mass and diverse audiences. The specialization of radio stations by listener age, taste, and even gender permits more selectivity in reaching audience segments. Since placement and production costs are less for radio than for TV, radio is able to convey public health messages in greater detail. Thus, radio is sometimes considered to be more efficient (Kreps and Neuhauser 2010).

Table 7.2 Features of health-related mass media campaigns

Reach	Proportion of population exposed to the message
Specializability	Narrowcasting to specific subgroups or tailoring to individuals
Depth	Channel capacity for conveying detailed and complex content
Credibility	Believability of material conveyed
Agenda setting	Potency of channel for raising salience priority of issues
Accessibility	Ease of placing messages in channel
Economy	Low cost for producing and disseminating stimuli

- *Internet*. The advent of the World Wide Web and the massive increase in Internet users offers public health personnel enormous opportunities and challenges. Unlike TV or radio, which are available in nearly all households, Internet access requires some technical skill, as well as the resources to purchase hardware and Internet subscription services (Kreps and Neuhauser 2010).
- *Newspapers* permit a level of detail in health reporting not feasible with broadcast media. Whereas one can miss a television broadcast about breast cancer, and thus lose its entire message, one can read the same (and more detailed) message in a newspaper at one's choice of time and venue. Although newspapers permit consumers flexibility concerning what is read, and when, they do have a brief shelf life.
- *Magazines* have several strengths, including audience selectivity, reproduction quality, prestige, and reader loyalty.
- *Outdoor media*. For people who regularly pass by billboards or use public transportation, these media may provide repeated exposure to messages.

7.2 Mass Media Campaigns in Smoking Prevention Strategies

To be successful, media campaigns for preventing tobacco use, as with any health media campaign, should be designed keeping in mind the following six main elements:

- The use of *formative research* to let campaigners discover the key target audience and accordingly pretest health communication strategy in terms of effectiveness and efficiency.
- The use of *theory* as a conceptual foundation of the communication strategy, indeed to identify the critical determinants upon which campaign messages might focus, in terms of their contents, tone, and format.
- The use of *audience segmentation* as a tool to define the target of the communication strategy, in terms of groups and subgroups of population.
- The development of *message design*, in regard to its *contents*, *format*, and *tone*.
- The *channel selection*.
- Finally the application of an *evaluation process* to assess the level of audience exposure to the campaign message, in addition to the degree of awareness to the message contents.

In 2006, based on the evidence—both scientific and empirical– from nine countries (i.e., Australia, Canada, England, Finland, the Netherlands, Norway, Poland, Scotland, and USA), the Center for Disease Control and prevention (CDC) produced a report to effectively design youth tobacco prevention mass media campaigns. According to the aforementioned elements, which are central to most mass media campaigns, a briefly report the CDC recommendations will be given, with a focus on health communication (Schar et al. 2006).

7.2.1 Formative Research, Theory and Evaluation

Media campaign developers should apply formative research and theory as a means for identifying the relevant audience on which they wish to target the communication strategy in order to develop proper message content, format, and emotional features. Then, formative research could be used to assess how the health communication strategy is going in terms of effectiveness and efficiency (e.g., Is the ad message enough clear and persuasive for the target audience? Are the tone, format and contents of the message effective in terms of expected outcomes?). Using theory is likely to make the overall mass media tobacco control campaigns successful, by providing planners with important feedback as to what degree the various ad components are working—such as the selected channels, the size and makeup of the target audience, the level of audience exposure (in terms of reach and frequency), allowing adjustments to be made while the campaign is in progress.

7.2.2 Audience Segmentation

In designing youth tobacco prevention ads, designers should develop age-targeted messages to enhance the effectiveness of the ad. Both mass media campaigns targeted on youth audiences only and those directed at both adults and youth have been successful in changing youth attitudes and behaviors. Research indicates that youth-targeted tobacco control programs are successful in developing awareness and changing attitudes and behaviors associated with tobacco use. However, other research indicates that campaigns targeted to the general population can also reduce smoking among youth.

7.2.3 Message Appeal, Contents, Format, and Tone

Success is more likely when campaign designers "[…] (1) include media campaigns with strong negative emotional appeal that produce, for example, a sense of loss, disgust, or fear; (2) introduce persuasive new information or new perspectives about health risks to smokers and nonsmokers (3) and, use personal-testimony or graphic-depiction formats that youth find emotionally engaging but not authoritarian [...] (Schar et al. 2006).

7.2.4 Channel Selection and Message Placement

The health communication strategy will be effective only if the target audience is adequately exposed to the message over a sufficient length of time. In other words, to be effective, the messages must be placed through media channels widely viewed by the target audience, and they should be enough frequent in order to reach, influence, and change attitudes and health behavior in the audience. Effective mass media campaigns for preventing tobacco use in adolescents should maintain a strong presence in broadcast media (e.g., TV, Internet, radio, etc.) to achieve their strategic goals; additionally, mass media designers have recognized the importance of their use to increase the impact of other community interventions.

Evaluation process, in regard to the evaluation process, youth tobacco prevention mass media campaigns are more likely to be effective when they include a formative process and outcome evaluation plan. Incorporating such evaluation plans will allow managers to monitor and collect data during the planning and the implementation of campaigns, therefore letting them adjust the execution of campaigns in progress, or understand why the expected goals were or were not achieved.

7.3 Overview of the Theoretical Approaches of Tobacco Control Mass Media Campaigns

Health communication plays an important role in promoting prevention and improving public health. Mass media campaigns are widely used—both in developed and developing countries—to target communities of large populations to messages focused on the prevention of various risk factors (e.g., use of tobacco, alcohol and illicit drugs, physical inactivity, and detrimental eating habits) and the adoption of healthy lifestyles and behaviors (Valente and Schuster 2002). The outcomes of such campaigns are determined by the concurrent availability of many factors that are, in turn, the required services and products, community-based programs and policies that support behavioral change (Wakefield et al. 2010).

Analyzing the theoretical underpinnings "behavioral change research" fosters the comprehension of how communication strategies can be used for promoting health. The use of theory can be seen as a tool (Institute of Medicine 2002; Noar 2006):

- To develop an effective program and message design according to the behavioral changes needed to encourage individuals to adopt healthy lifestyles.
- To ensure that health communication guides the individuals to the expected outcomes, in terms of attitude/belief/behavior change.

Table 7.3 Input–output persuasion model

		Conceptual framework to evaluation	
		First generation of health campaign research	Second generation of health campaign research
Expectancy value theories of attitude and behavior change	Yes	• Input–output persuasion model • Health beliefs model	• Theory of reasoned action (theory of planned behavior) • Integrative model of behavior • Transtheoretical model (or state of changes)
	No		• Social learning (cognitive) theory • Social influence, social comparisons, and convergence theories • Dual process model of attitude and persuasion

- To estimate how much impact can be expected from a health media campaign, in terms of sample size, target audience, and consumer media behaviors.

Since the first tobacco control campaigns have been placed in the USA in 1964 (U.S. Department of Health, Education, and Welfare, 1964), mass media campaigns have increasingly been an important tool for preventing tobacco use and fostering tobacco control (Logan 2004). As a result, the tobacco-related communication literature is extensive and provides us with a broad spectrum of theoretical approaches. They can be distinguished along two key features (Table 7.3):

- Whether they posit that individuals have control of their choices and that people make their choices only based on the information available to them (i.e., expectancy value theories of attitude and behavior change) or not.
- According to their conceptual approaches in evaluating consumer media attitude/behavior changes and the resulting health outcomes, the National Cancer Institute proposed to classify the different theories—as regards their conceptual evaluation approach, into two generations: first generation and second generation health campaign research (National Cancer Institute 1991).

Early mass media campaigns tended to be based on persuasion models which in turn were based on the assumption that young people lacked information about the negative effects of smoking and if that gap of information was filled they would then make rational decisions about smoking. These approaches designed mass media campaigns to prevent tobacco use in adolescents are under the category of the rational model, including the "input–output persuasion model" and the "health beliefs model." These two approaches born, respectively in 1969 and 1974, share a common theoretical underpinning, that is, the assumption that individuals strive to maximize the perceived benefits and minimize the perceived costs associated with performing a behavior. To prevent smoking initiation in adolescents, such communication models (in general the expectancy-value theories of behavior change), try to enforce the individual's perception of the risk of smoking tobacco, the negative aspects of a smoking addiction, as well as the positive benefits of not smoking (e.g., personal and societal costs) (National Cancer Institute 2008).

Such tobacco-related communication theories have been overcome by a second generation of health campaign research (in the 1980s), which evaluate the outcome of socio-psychological factors and individual skills in addition to cognitive, attitudinal, and motivational factors (Logan 2004). Within the second generation mass media research, we can distinguish between theories based on expectancy-value theories of behavior change (i.e., theory of reasoned action, integrative model of behavior, and transtheoretical model, or state of changes) and other theories of behavior change (Social learning–cognitive–theory, Social influence, social comparisons and convergence theories, dual process model of attitude and persuasion).

Over time, other theoretical frameworks have been advanced to improve the effectiveness of mass media campaigns for preventing the use of tobacco in nonsmokers, such as the developmentally oriented affective and the social norms approach. Campaigns following the first approach were based on the idea that information should be aimed at fostering self-esteem in nonsmokers to improve their decision-making skills, without a specific focus on smoking information. The focus of the social norms approach was on increasing self-esteem and reducing alienation in nonsmokers too, often by means of active participation in activities (Institute of Medicine 2002; National Cancer Institute 2008). We will describe following the most prominent theories on media research with a focus to tobacco use prevention.

7.3.1 Input–Output Persuasion Model

Formulated by William McGuire in 1969, the input–output persuasion model suggests that to be influenced by a message, an audience must be exposed to it, pay attention to, understand it, and develop a cognitive or affective response. Five steps will determine how successful a persuasion program is in effecting an individual's change (see Fig. 7.1) (McGuire 1969).

7.3.2 Health Beliefs Model

The "Health Beliefs" model (Becker 1974), one of the most dominant health-related behavioral change models, suggests that individuals are likely to be influenced by a message (IOM 2002):

- If they feel at risk of becoming affected by the disease or condition;
- Or if they believe that the benefits of taking the recommended action outweigh the perceived barriers (or costs) of performing the preventive action.

The HBM assumes that self-destructive behavior, as, for example, smoking occurs when individuals do not have adequate information about the health risks posed by their behavior, the consequences of their behavior, or fail to understand that avoiding the behavior will reduce health risks (NCI 2008).

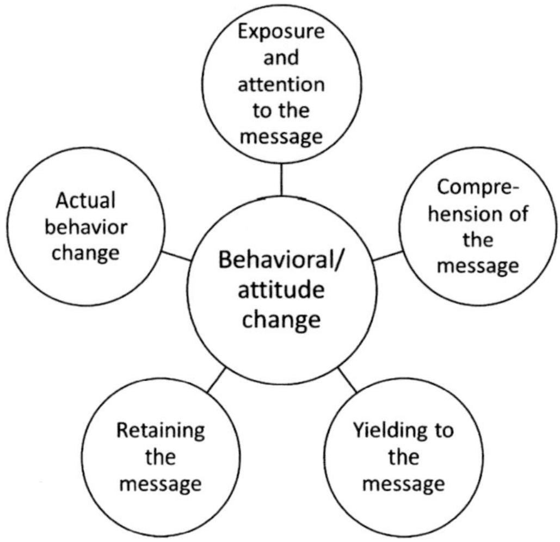

Fig. 7.1 Input–output persuasion model

7.3.3 *Theory of Reasoned Action (Theory of Planned Behavior)*

Advanced in 1980 (Ajzen and Fishbein 1980), the theory of reasoned action assumes that health behavior choices are the result of a process of reasoning and are based on the information available to the individual who is making the behavioral choice. According to this theory, an individual's intention to act is the single best predictor of behavior.

This intention to perform a determined behavior is shaped by one or the combination of three components (Fig. 7.2):

1. Individual's attitude toward performing the behavior (e.g., belief that taking up smoking will lead to certain outcomes and the expected value of the outcome).
2. Perceived social norms toward performing the behavior (e.g., belief that a specific member of the community thinks that one should or should not take up smoking cigarettes).
3. Motivations to comply (the degree to which, in general, one wants to do what the referent thinks one should perform).

Mass media campaigns should influence the strengths of a belief that drives behavior. For different groups of people, different consequences of performing the behavior may be salient and may be held with different belief strengths. Therefore, the attitudes, social norms, and motivation driving the behavior for one group (e.g., teens) may differ considerably for another group (e.g., adults, elderly), and as a result, communication messages should vary accordingly.

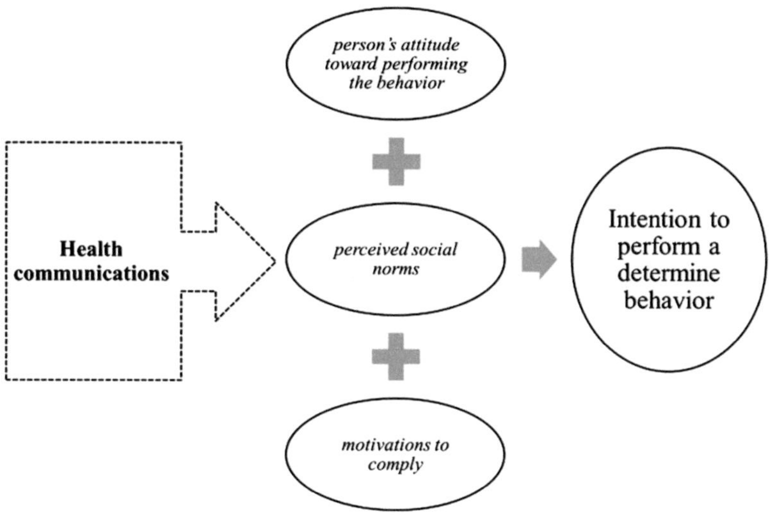

Fig. 7.2 Theory of reasoned action

7.3.4 Integrative Model of Behavior Change

The integrative model of behavior (Cappella et al. 2001) has been proposed as a development of the theory of reasoned action, based on the assumption that there are only a finite number of determinants that lead to behavior change (National Cancer Institute 2008). According to the integrative model, media messages should primarily target those beliefs that are strongly associated with behavioral intentions and determined by formative research. Formative research plays an important role within the integrative model; it has to be used to effectively understand the target audience in terms of beliefs to be addressed and the most appropriate communication strategy. The integrative model incorporates the construct of self-efficacy, or, in other words, the feeling of self-trust an individual has in performing a recommended action. In the integrative model, an individual's intentions to perform a behavior, in turn, are determined by attitudes toward the behavior, the perceived norms concerning the behavior, and self-efficacy in performing the behavior.

7.3.5 Transtheoretical Model (or State of Changes)

Born in the late 1990s, the state of changes theory posits that behavior change is a process that occurs in stages (Prochaska and Velicer 1997). This concept means that people need different information and face different behavior problems while in different stages.

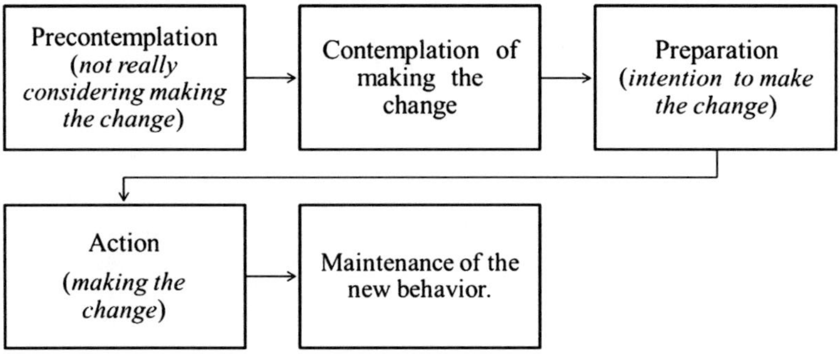

Fig. 7.3 Transtheoretical model

According to the IOM this approach supplemented the "Health Beliefs" theory; in fact it evaluates individual and psychological states more specifically (IOM 2002). The psychological process believed to result in subsequent attitude and behavior changes goes through the stages as shown in Fig. 7.3.

7.3.6 Social Learning (Cognitive) Theory (Bandura 1977)

Social learning (cognitive) theory describes the importance of symbolic learning. One of the core methods for acquiring knowledge and skills, according to this theory, is by learning through observation and imitation of others (Cleary et al. 1988). That is, adolescents "learn" about smoking and the positive and negative consequences of smoking by watching peers and adults smoke. The social learning theory identifies four components that play a key role to determine behavioral change (NCI 2008):

- First, an information component is needed to increase awareness and knowledge and to convince people that they have the ability to change behavior.
- Second, a motivational component is needed to develop social and self-regulatory skills to practice the new behavior.
- A third component enhances the development of social and self-regulatory skills (through the promotion of self efficacy).
- A Fourth component develops or engages social supports for the individual making the change.

7.4 Mass Media Campaigns: Overview of Scientific Evidence

7.4.1 Overview of Scientific Literature

Several and different socio-demographic, behavioral, environmental, and personal factors associated with smoking onset were identified and deeply described in recent years (Tyas et al. 1997).

The peer group, in particular, has been identified to play an important role. As we described above, a key theoretical perspective used to explain the association between peer smoking and adolescents' smoking is the "social influences" or Social learning theory approach, frequently adopted in schools-based health prevention programs and used as a basis for designing programs delivered by the mass media.

The mass media (TV, radio, newspapers, and others) have progressively been used as a way of delivering health messages (Brinn et al. 2010).

In 2004 Kremers debated in his review that smoking prevention should aim at influencing the image of nonsmoking (e.g., their identity) by using mass media interventions and restrictive policies. Mass media can potentially reach a large amount of the population and above all groups that more traditional approaches may not access: on average, they are an inexpensive way of exposing the population to information concerning their health and they can probably modify the knowledge or attitudes of a large size of the community simultaneously (Redman et al. 1990).

Mass media are also identified as particularly appropriate for delivering anti-smoking messages to young people, exposed to and greatly interested in the media (US DHHS 1994). In 1988 Worden estimated young people to spend nearly 12,000 h in formal education and almost twice as many hours watching TV (22,000 h) (Worden et al. 1988), while Davies evaluated a young person to have spent more time being entertained by the media than doing any other activity except sleeping by the age of 18 years (Davies 1993). TV and other mass media can influence young peoples' perceptions of what the real world and acceptable social behavior are and help to convey important and believable messages about the behaviors it describes (Strasburger 1995).

7.4.2 *Effectiveness, Opportunities, and Shortcomings of Mass Media Campaigns in Preventing Smoking Initiation*

The social learning theory approach has also been used as a basis for programs delivered by the mass media and frequently adopted in schools-based health prevention programs. Mass media campaigns, by presenting positive role models, would influence behavior in order to reject smoking in those situations where it is encouraged. In order to develop an effective prevention program it is necessary that the target audience pays attention to the model developing the capacity to respond to social pressure and to accept alternative behaviors and the programs based on social learning theory help this by addressing the motivations behind smoking and providing options for alternative behavior.

There is some not strong evidence that mass media can prevent the uptake of smoking in young people but this is in contrast to those theories assuming that young people lack information about the negative effects of smoking and that they would decide not to smoke if that information gap was filled. In the course of time, literature reviews assessed the effectiveness of mass media campaigns in influencing smoking behavior in young people. However, those reviews included several types of intervention such as schools-based programs or community initiatives, without including all relevant studies in any one area (Michell 1994; US DHHS 1994; Reid et al. 1995; Reid 1996; Stead et al. 1996; Silver 2001; Friend and Levy 2002; Farrelly et al. 2003). Overall, these reviews reported different results on the mass media effectiveness, above all for smaller community-level campaigns.

On the other hand, the potential to influence youth smoking rates has been demonstrated: other reviews of the literature concentrated exclusively on the mass media, focusing on smoking cessation with adult smokers (Flay 1987a) and concluding that mass media campaigns can reduce smoking rates, particularly when they are intense in terms of reach, frequency, and duration (Flay 1987a, b).

Brinn and coll (Brinn et al. 2010) described the effectiveness of mass media campaigns compared with no intervention in influencing the young people smoking behavior, including studies that made this comparison directly (Worden et al. 1983; Bauman et al. 1991; Hafstad and Aaro 1997; Flynn et al. 2010) or used a factorial design (Flay et al. 1995). Brinn also compared the effectiveness of mass media campaigns combined with schools-based programs to schools-based programs only, to evaluate the influence in the smoking behavior of young people (two included studies made a direct comparison (Flynn et al. 1995; Longshore et al. 2006)—one study used a factorial design (Flay et al. 1995).

Brinn et al. (2010) found out a statistically and clinically significant reduction for smoking uptake in young people (three out of seven studies). These successful campaigns included common elements such as multiple channels for media delivery (e.g., television, posters, newspapers, radio), combining media and school components (school posters, school-based curriculum…) or repeating exposure to campaign messages (e.g., to the same cohort of students over a period of three years). Some successful campaigns also used provocative messages to cause effective personal reactions.

The "social influences" or "social learning theory" approach was the base of two of the three successful campaigns but it was also used in other three of four studies, which did not produce any statistically significant benefit. Characteristics of some unsuccessful studies where the short campaign durations and the less intensity than the successful campaigns but even two studies having longer durations were likely to demonstrate no benefit, probably related to the lack of a structured curriculum component to support these campaigns, such as those in the combined school-based studies.

The authors concluded that basing on the most methodologically rigorous set of studies evaluating the effectiveness of mass media campaigns directed at youth, there is some evidence that these media campaigns can be effective in preventing the uptake of smoking in young people, even if this evidence is not so strong and contains methodological flaws.

7.4.3 Characteristics of Effective Mass Media Campaigns

Latest available experience and research shows the characteristics that a public education campaign should include to be successful. First of all mass media campaigns need to stay power (advertisement must be often seen and heard to be able to influence behaviors, beliefs, or attitudes. In order to be effective, a campaign should have high frequency or long duration. According to a review of smoking cessation media campaigns from around the world conducted by WHO and CDC, media weight (reach and frequency) and campaign duration are crucial elements to insure a continued decline in smoking rates (Schar and Gutierrez 2001).

A campaign should also include various refreshed and targeted messages to motivate different people in different times.

Several elements are often incorporated in effective campaigns: special events and promotions, commissioned media reports, public relations integrated with school and community-based programs, as well as other elements of a comprehensive tobacco use reduction plan (Vartuaunen et al. 1998; Siegel 1998).

A combination of hard-hitting "why to quit" and supportive "how to quit" messages to motivate smokers and provide them with strategies to help their success are also important. Research indicated that combining these two types of messages is more successful in influencing smokers than using one message on its own (Schar and Gutierrez 2001). Campaigns should reflect internationally learned lessons about effective messages and strategies, must be based on rigorous and state-of-the art research on effectiveness, and must be planned and executed independently of any tobacco industry influence or support.

7.4.4 *Expert Conclusions on Mass Media Public Education Campaigns*

The scientific evidence on the effectiveness of public education campaigns will continue growing as soon as more countries implement campaigns and evaluate their effectiveness. Public health education is a critical component of successful comprehensive tobacco control programs. To give some example, the U.S. Guide to Community Preventive Services studied the mass media campaigns and other tobacco prevention and cessation methods impact on prevention of tobacco use. They found "strong evidence" that long-term mass media education campaigns, with high intensity counter-advertising, when combined with other interventions, are effective in reducing tobacco use initiation and consumption, and in increasing smoking cessation (The Guide to Community-Preventive Services 2003).

The US Surgeon General concluded that mass media campaigns are effective at informing youth and the public in general about the hazards of smoking, also promoting cessation actions and services (U.S. Department of Health and Human Services 2012). The U.S. Centers for Disease Control and Prevention's publication, Best Practices for Comprehensive Tobacco Control Programs, concluded that counter-marketing (i.e., public education about the negative impact of tobacco) is also an important part of efforts to both prevent initiation of tobacco use and to encourage cessation (Centers for Disease Control and Prevention 1999).

7.4.5 Identified Research Gaps

According to Brinn et al. (2010) no study directly tested the comparison between "the effectiveness of mass media campaigns combined with schools-based programs" and "no intervention" in influencing the young people smoking behavior (although one study used a factorial design in which this single comparison was made) (Flay et al. 1995).

The effectiveness of mass media campaigns combined with schools-based programs compared with media campaigns alone in influencing the smoking behavior of young people is also still untested (although one study addressed this comparison in a factorial design) (Flay et al. 1995).

The Guide to Community Preventive Services is a free resource helping to choose programs and policies to improve health and prevent disease in USA. By using systematic reviews to answer these questions, the community guide identified a research gap concerning the reduction in tobacco use initiation, particularly referred to the effectiveness of mass media campaigns when combined with other interventions.

7.5 Mass Media Campaigns: Evidence into Practice

7.5.1 Main Umbrella Organizations Involved (e.g., WHO, EU, OECD)

An overview of scientific evidences about mass media campaign effectiveness was given above. In an era increasingly dominated by technology and communications, future prosperity also relies on people making the right lifestyle choices, and the most important of them all is their health. Many international organizations are involved in putting evidences into practice about this topic.

7.5.2 The World Health Organization

The World Health Organization (WHO) Website section "Tobacco Free Initiative" provides many activities and events focused on mass media use (http://www.who.int/tobacco/en/).

The "Tobacco multimedia center" provides videos, podcasts, photos, and fact files that people can download and use as everyday life tools.

Some initiatives focused on the use of mass media campaign include the "World No Tobacco Day," the "Smoke-free movies: from evidence to action," and the "Projects on mobile health (mHealth) for tobacco control."

Concerning the "*World No Tobacco Day*" the WHO selected "The WHO Framework Convention on Tobacco Control" as the theme of World No Tobacco Day 2011 and "tobacco industry interference" as the theme of the next World No Tobacco Day (Thursday, 31 May 2012), trying to educate policy-makers and the general public about the tobacco industry's harmful tactics.

The WHO Framework Convention on Tobacco Control (WHO FCTC) is the world's foremost tobacco control instrument, the first international public health treaty developed under the auspices of WHO, provides a comprehensive approach to reduce the considerable health and economic burden caused by tobacco. It was adopted by the World Health Assembly on 21 May 2003 and entered into force less than two years later, on 27 February 2005. More than 170 of the 193 Member States of WHO are Parties to it.

An evidence-based treaty, it reaffirms the right of all people to the highest standard of health and provides new legal dimensions for cooperation in tobacco control.

The World No Tobacco Day campaign was also available on Facebook—"Make everyday World No Tobacco Day" (https://www.facebook.com/pages/WHO-Tobacco-Free-Initiative/100643340596), YouTube (http://www.youtube.com/whoeuro), and Twitter (https://twitter.com/#!/who_europe), following actual tendencies around the use of the social networks.

Concerning the "Smoke-free movies: from evidence to action," it consist in a report that calls upon all countries to enact policies to severely restrict depictions of smoking in movies (World Health Organization 2011a, b, c). In fact, in some countries many of the films targeting young people and containing tobacco imagery are the recipients of significant government production subsidies. WHO calls for enforceable policies to restrict smoking in movies, including the end of public subsidies for the production of movies with smoking. The depiction of tobacco in films is a form of tobacco promotion that can strongly influence tobacco use, particularly among young people. The report recommends specific measures to limit movie smoking such as receiving adult ratings and/or that movie studios certify they received no payoffs from tobacco companies to display tobacco products or their use, stop displaying tobacco brands onscreen, and require strong antitobacco advertisements before all movies that have tobacco imagery.

Finally, concerning the "*Projects on mobile health (mHealth) for tobacco control*" [http://www.who.int/tobacco/mhealth/en/index.html], focused on the opinion that penetration of mobile technology started to transform the way health services are delivered, the WHO plan to create applications and models using technology for social networks in order to educate and raise awareness, by using SMS messages linked to social networking sites such as Facebook and Twitter.

7.5.3 The European Community

The *European Community tobacco control*, for example, is based on two laws: the Directive 2001/37/EC (2001) on tobacco products and the Directive 2003/33/EC (2003) on tobacco advertising.

From 2005 to 2010 the Commission launched a campaign named “HELP—For a life without tobacco,” focused on smoking prevention, smoking cessation, and passive smoking, targeting young Europeans between 15 and 25 years of age. The campaign changed over time, starting as a series of television advertisements and basic institutional Website, and becoming an innovative Web-driven campaign that launched the power of text, images, video, and social media, with a collaborative Website space. To give some figures, from 2005 to 2010 121,000 TV adverts were broadcasted, 43 % of Europeans (approximately 214 million people) and 67 % of 15–24 years young Europeans (approximately 41 million) declared that they had seen one of the Help advertisements in 2010 (+14 % compared with 2005), 226,000 visits to the Smoke Screen mini-site.

By the end of the Help campaign, many national governments had adopted smoke-free legislation, and surveys indicated a decline of the number of smokers in the EU and an increase of awareness of tobacco control.

On 16 June 2011, the new campaign Help 2.0, “Ex-smokers are unstoppable,” involved ex-smokers to encourage young adults in the 25–34 age group to stop smoking. This campaign is primary targeted at young people and it promotes a tobacco-free lifestyle by delivering comprehensive information on the health and societal problems caused by tobacco consumption. It integrates television, the Internet, and new media such as mini-sites accessible via mobile phone, drawing young people to the Help Website (http://www.help-eu.com) for information on the dangers of smoking and links to organizations such as the European Network of Quitlines (ENQ), an initiative aimed at maximizing collaboration between all European Union member countries in tobacco control and smoking cessation. The aim of this campaign is also to empower young people taking control of their lifestyle and health, without remaining passive media targets.

In order to develop the campaign, help and advice were asked to the target groups, e.g., the idea for TV spots that came directly from an Internet consultation with young people (http://ec.europa.eu/health/tobacco/help/index_en.htm).

7.5.4 Main National Public Health Agencies, Including Guidance/Best Practices Delivery Agencies

7.5.4.1 The Centers for Disease Control and Prevention

The Centers for Disease Control and Prevention (CDC) is an US federal agency under the Department of Health and Human Services that works to protect public health and safety by providing information to enhance health decisions and promoting health through partnerships with state health departments and other organizations. The CDC, through its Office on Smoking and Health (OSH), a division within the National Center for Chronic Disease Prevention and Health Promotion, is the lead federal agency for comprehensive tobacco prevention and control.

In the CDC Website, the section Media Campaign Resource Center (MCRC)—Tobacco Counter-advertising Collection allows people to browse through the collection for detailed campaign information on tobacco counter-advertisements including television, radio, prints, earned media, and other collateral media material in a variety of formats (http://apps.nccd.cdc.gov/MCRC/Apps/QuickSearch.aspx).

In the section "Smoking and Tobacco Use" (http://www.cdc.gov/tobacco/index.htm) many information are also provided.

Among them, the "Surgeon General's Reports on Smoking and Tobacco Use 2012" (U.S. Department of Health and Human Services, 2012), examines in detail the epidemiology, health effects, and causes of tobacco use among youth and young adults. The report is the review of the health consequences of tobacco use by young people, examining the social, environmental, advertising, and marketing influences that not only encourage youth and young adults to initiate and sustain tobacco use (peer influences; imagery and messages that portray tobacco use; environmental cues, including those in both traditional and emerging media platforms) but also coordinated and multicomponent interventions (including mass media campaigns, community programs, statewide tobacco control programs, price increases, and school-based policies) that are effective in preventing onset and use of tobacco use among youth and young adults.

The CDC also provides several guidelines that can be used to control and prevent tobacco use such as "*Best practices for comprehensive tobacco control programs*" (Centers for Disease Control and Prevention 1999) and "*Designing and Implementing an Effective TobaccoCounter-Marketing Campaign*" (Centers for Disease Control and Prevention 2003).

The last one is designed to help state health departments, agencies, and organizations in developing and implementing tobacco counter-marketing campaigns, i.e., the use of commercial marketing tactics to reduce the prevalence of tobacco use. "Countermarketing attempts to counter protobacco influences and increase pro-health messages and influences throughout a state, region, or community" (U.S. Department of Health and Human Services 2000).

Other CDC initiatives involving media communications (http://www.cdc.gov/tobacco/data_statistics/sgr/2012/index.htm) are:

- The "eCard," that allows people to send an eCard encouraging healthy smoke-free living.
- "Button," that supports tobacco control and prevention efforts by posting buttons on people Website, blog, or social networking site.
- "Twitter": @CDCgov Official Twitter source for health and safety updates.
- "Facebook" at https://www.facebook.com/CDC.

7.5.4.2 The U.S. Preventive Services Task Force

The U.S. Preventive Services Task Force (USPSTF) is an independent panel of non-Federal experts in prevention and evidence-based medicine and is composed of primary care providers. It conducts scientific evidence reviews of a broad range of clinical preventive health care services and develops recommendations for primary care clinicians and health systems. These recommendations are published in the form of "Recommendation Statements."

Concerning tobacco use prevention, there is a recommendation released in November 2003, "Counseling to Prevent Tobacco Use and Tobacco-Caused Disease" (U.S. Preventive Services Task Force 2003), and a second one, "Counseling and Interventions to Prevent Tobacco Use and Tobacco-Caused Disease in Adults and Pregnant Women," released in April 2009 (U.S. Preventive Services Task Force 2009).

The evidence base and potential synthesis or integration of preventive strategies in mass media interventions on tobacco control in clinical and community settings have been implemented at multiple levels of influence in the social–ecological model (Ockene et al. 2007). In the tobacco control example, relevant information about effective clinical and community-level strategies and interventions have been implemented at multiple levels contributing to improvements in important behavioral and possibly health outcomes. The statewide Massachusetts Tobacco Control Program (MTCP) has been recognized by the CDC and others as a "best practice" comprehensive and coordinated tobacco treatment and control program, "incorporating clinical and community strategies, combining and connecting activities of clinical settings, the media, community agencies, academic institutions, and local and state policy makers." It included an innovative media campaign to change public opinion and community norms around tobacco use, community mobilization to change local laws and health regulations, comprehensive tobacco treatment programs based on clinics and community settings guidelines to reduce tobacco use.

7.6 Smoking Prevention: Mass Media Campaigns Worldwide

7.6.1 Worldwide Mass Media Campaigns Targeted at General Population and at Specific Demographic Groups

The World Health Organization framework Convention on Tobacco Control (WHO FCTC) is a "legally binding global treaty that provides the foundation for countries to implement and manage tobacco control programs to address the growing epidemic of tobacco use," covering 87 % of the world's population.

The success of the WHO FCTC is reported in the 2011 WHO Report on the Global Tobacco Epidemic (that refers to the period from January 2009 to August 2010), the third in a series of periodic reports about the extent and character of the epidemic and measures to stop it, identifying the countries that have applied effective tobacco control measures to save lives (World Health Organization 2011a, b, c).

The 2011 report shows the antitobacco mass media campaign is conducted worldwide, underlying that nearly 28 % of the world population is exposed to those campaigns.

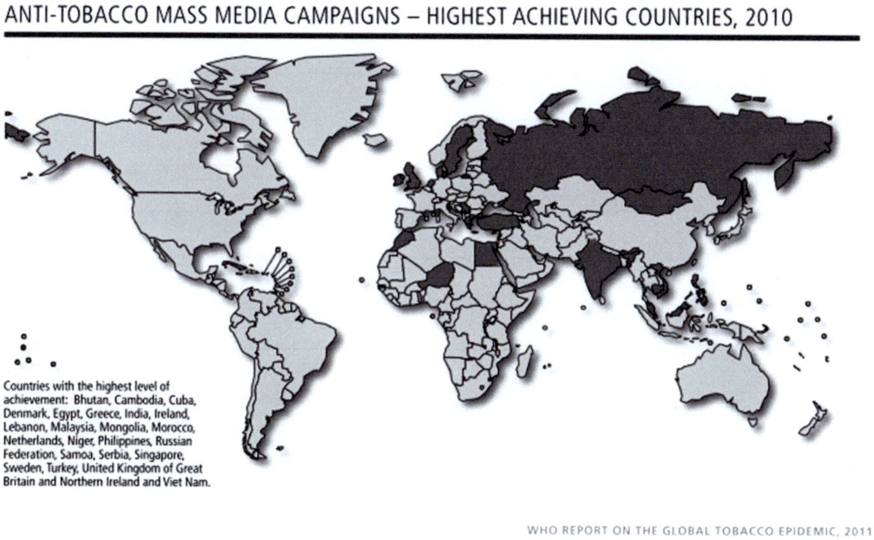

Fig. 7.4 Antitobacco mass media campaigns [from WHO Report on the Global Tobacco Epidemic (2011a, b, c)]

This year's report also provides, for the first time ever, systematically collected information about antitobacco mass media campaigns, revealing the promising work being done in this area: more than 1.9 billion people (28 % of the world's population) living in 23 countries that ran at least one strong antitobacco mass media campaign during the reporting period, were involved in them.

The mass media campaign conducted in those 23 countries were national in scope and incorporated appropriate characteristics, such as being part of a comprehensive government tobacco control program; utilizing media planning strategies; developing campaign messaging and materials; pretesting materials before use; monitoring during implementation to ensure that materials are used as planned; assessing the campaign impact; using earned media as an adjunct to the campaign. Only seven of the 23 countries that ran a strong campaign were classified as high-income—the majority reporting exemplary campaigns are low- or middle-income countries, providing evidence that all countries, regardless of income level, can run effective mass media campaigns.

Another 30 countries conducted campaigns incorporating at least five of the seven characteristics listed above. Even if high-income countries, expected to have sufficient financial resources to run media campaigns, carried out campaigns featuring most of these characteristics, lot of middle- and low-income countries also run effective campaigns incorporating most or all of them (Fig. 7.4). However, only more than a third of all countries run a national-level media campaigns during 2009–2010.

The most common implemented component was the media planning strategy utilization for the campaign, while the least frequently mentioned were evaluation

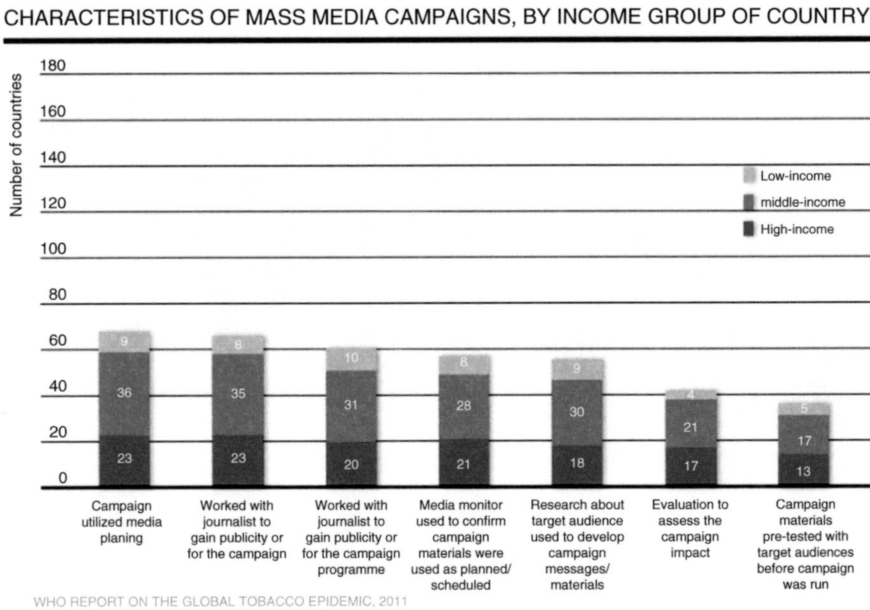

Fig. 7.5 Characteristics of mass media campaigns, by income group of Country [from WHO Report on the Global Tobacco Epidemic (2011a, b, c)]

to assess campaign impact and pretesting of materials prior to conducting campaigns (Fig. 7.5).

48 countries stated as their primary campaign objective to warn about smoking's harms, and 35 countries reported their warning about the harms of secondhand smoke exposure (over two-thirds of low-income countries). Stopping youth from using tobacco was also a common campaign objective, reported by 35 countries.

Broadcast media tend to have the widest audience reach, exposing the public to antitobacco messaging. The most commonly employed type of media in which to run antitobacco advertising campaigns was television advertising (used by 61 countries), followed by radio (42 countries). Print media were also widely used, with 42 counties using print advertising as part of their campaigns. Other media types, e.g., Internet or social media, having lower population reach, were used less frequently, but they are expected to increase in the future as their use will become more widespread (Fig. 7.6).

Concerning antitobacco mass media campaigns, 2011 WHO Report on the Global Tobacco Epidemic finally shows six examples of such a type of campaign.

Uruguay required, for example, health warning labels on cigarette packages for nearly 30 years, but labels were initially small and just displaying nonspecific message. By 2000, Uruguay's Health Ministry began to implement more effective tobacco control measures, establishing in 2005 a formal national tobacco control program, further strengthened in 2008 according to the WHO FCTC improvements.

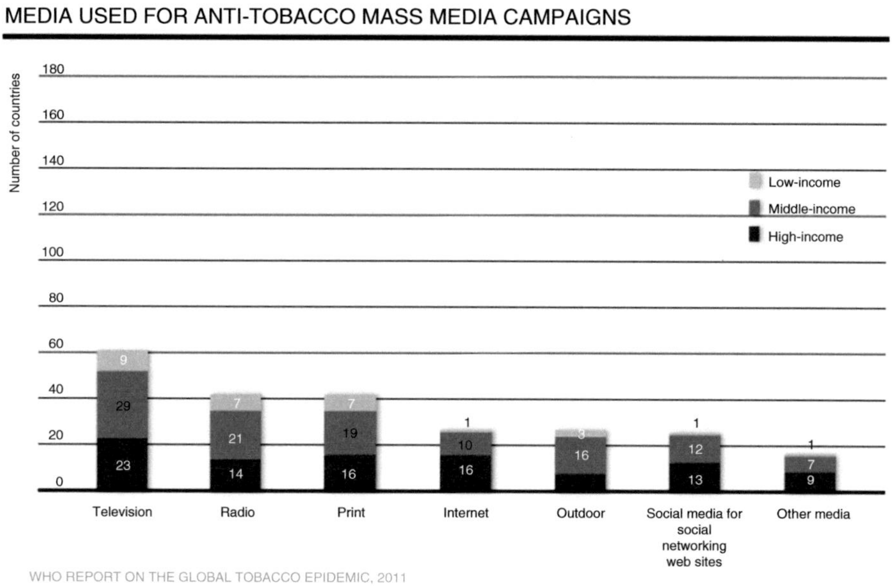

Fig. 7.6 Type of media used for antitobacco mass media campaigns [from WHO Report on the Global Tobacco Epidemic (2011a, b, c)]

Pictures were added to health warning labels, and misleading terms such as "light," "ultralight," or "mild" were prohibited, in order to avoid any false or misleading means. In 2009, the size of warning labels was increased to 80 % of primary pack surface areas.

Graphic pictorial labels covering 50 % of the front and back of packs can be found in Canada, country that recently proposed increasing their size to 75 % of primary pack surface areas, introducing new health information messages with colors and graphic elements.

Another example of a country that wants to further increase the impact of pictorial health warnings is Australia, whose Parliament was expected to adopt a bill to require generic tobacco packaging, so making Australia the first country to mandate generic packaging beginning in July 2012.

In addition, Djibouti (Africa) has implemented strong pictorial health warning labels to meet public demand for information, covering 50 % of both the front and back of packages despite tobacco industry objections: labels feature powerful images in order to raise awareness among smokers of active and secondhand tobacco smoke exposure effects, and a new series of stronger warning label images has been proposed in 2012.

Even Mauritius implemented large pictorial pack warning labels, covering on average 65 % of the total principal surface areas of the pack. Turkey increased free radio and television time for antitobacco advertising, mandating that radio and television stations provide a minimum of 90 min of free air time every month for antitobacco educational programming and advertising, during daytime and early evening hours (8:00–22:00) to reach adults and children, with a minimum of 30 min per month during 17:00–22:00.

In the Russian Federation in 2008 some advertising materials, shown to be effective in other countries, were adapted, and assistance was provided to some regional governments (e.g., Chuvashia, Krasnodarsk, Moscow, and Samara) which aired the advertising campaigns. The success of those campaigns in addition to a campaign held in Moscow, prompted several municipal and regional governments to push for smoke-free initiatives and laws, till September 2010, when the Russian Federation adopted a comprehensive national tobacco control strategy.

Furthermore, Indian government aired on television and radio between November and December 2009 first and from January to March 2011 then, in 16 local languages, an airs campaign to highlight dangers of smokeless tobacco (patients with tobacco-related disfiguring and deadly cancers, oral cancer surgeon interviews, and others).

References

Ajzen, I., & Fishbein, M. (1980). *Understanding attitudes and predicting social behavior*. Englewood Cliffs, NJ: Prentice Hall.

Atkin, C. K., & Rice, R. E. (2012). Theory and principles of media health campaigns. In R. E. Rice & C. K. Atkin (Eds.), *Public communication campaigns* (4th ed., pp. 3–16). Thousand Oaks, CA: Jossey-Bass.

Atkin, C. K., & Salmon, C. (2010). Communication campaigns. In C. Berger, M. Roloff, & D. Roskos Ewoldsen (Eds.), *Handbook of communication science* (2nd ed., pp. 419–435). Thousand Oaks, CA: Sage.

Atkin, C. K. (2001). Theory and principles of media health campaigns. In R. E. Rice & C. K. Atkin (Eds.), *Public communication campaigns* (3rd ed., pp. 49–68). Thousand Oaks, CA: Sage.

Bandura, A. (1977). *Social learning theory*. Englewood Cliffs, New Jersey: Prentice-Hall.

Bauman, K. E., LaPrelle, J., Brown, J. D., Koch, G. G., & Padgett, C. A. (1991). The influence of three mass media campaigns on variables related to adolescent cigarette smoking: Results of a field experiment. *American Journal of Public Health, 81*, 597–604.

Becker, M. H. (1974). *The health belief model and personal health behavior*. San Francisco: Society for Public Health Education.

Blackburn, S., Brownsell, S., & Hawley, M. S. (2011). A systematic review of digital interactive television systems and their applications in the health and social care fields. *Journal of Telemedicine and Telecare, 17*(4), 168–76.

Board on Health Promotion and Disease Prevention, Institute of Medicine. (2002). *The future of the public's health in the 21st century* (pp. 307–357). Washington, DC: National Academy of Sciences.

Breslow, L. (Editor-in-Chief) (2002). *The encyclopedia of public health*. New York, NY: MacMillan Publishing.

Brinn, M. P., Carson, K. V., Esterman, A. J., Chang, A. B., & Smith, B. J. (2010). Mass media interventions for preventing smoking in young people. *Cochrane Database of Systematic Reviews, 11*, CD001006.

Cappella, J., Fishbein, M., Hornik, R., Ahern, R. K., & Sayeed, S. (2001). Using theory to select messages in anti-drug media campaigns: Reasoned action and media priming. In R. E. Rice &

C. K. Atkin (Eds.), *Public communication campaigns* (3rd ed., pp. 214–230). Thousand Oaks, CA: Sage.

Centers for Disease Control and Prevention. (1999). *Best practices for comprehensive tobacco control programs*. Atlanta, GA: U.S. Department of Health and Human Services, Centers for Disease Control and Prevention, National Center for Chronic Disease Prevention and Health Promotion, Office on Smoking and Health. Available at http://www.cdc.gov/tobacco/tobacco_control_programs/stateandcommunity/best_practices/

Centers for Disease Control and Prevention. (2003). *Designing and implementing an effective tobacco counter-marketing campaign*. Atlanta, Georgia: U.S. Department of Health and Human Services, Centers for Disease Control and Prevention, National Center for Chronic Disease Prevention and Health Promotion, Office on Smoking and Health, First Edition October.

Cleary, P. D., Hitchcock, J. L., Semmer, N., Flinchbaugh, L. J., & Pinney, J. M. (1988). Adolescent smoking: Research and health policy. *The Milbank Quarterly, 66*(1), 137–71.

Davies, J. (1993) The impact of the mass media upon the health of early adolescents. *J Health Education Suppl*, S28–S35.

Derzon, J. H., & Lipsey, M. W. (2002). A meta-analysis of the effectiveness of masscommunication for changing substance-use knowledge, attitudes, and behavior. In W. D. Crano & M. Burgoon (Eds.), *Mass media and drug prevention: Classic and contemporary theories and research* (pp. 231–258). Mahwah, NJ: Erlbaum.

Directive 2001/37/EC of the European Parliament and of the Council of 5 June 2001 on the approximation of the laws, regulations and administrative provisions of the Member States concerning the manufacture, presentation and sale of tobacco products—Commission statement. Official Journal L 194, 18/07/2001 P. 0026–0035

Directive 2003/33/EC of the European Parliament and of the Council of 26 May 2003 on the approximation of the laws, regulations and administrative provisions of the Member States relating to the advertising and sponsorship of tobacco products.

Farrelly, M., Niederdeppe, J., & Yarsevich, J. (2003). Youth tobacco prevention mass media campaigns: Past, present, and future directions. *Tobacco Control, 12*, 35–47.

Fischer, P., Greitemeyer, T., Kastenmüller, A., Vogrincic, C., & Sauer, A. (2011). The effects of risk-glorifying media exposure on risk-positive cognitions, emotions, and behaviors: A meta-analytic review. *Psychological Bulletin, 137*(3), 367–90.

Flay, B. R. (1987a). *Selling the smokeless society: Fifty-six evaluated mass media programs and campaigns worldwide*. Washington, DC: American Public Health Association.

Flay, B. R. (1987b). Mass media and smoking cessation: A critical review. *American Journal of Public Health, 77*, 153–160.

Flay, B. R., Miller, T. Q., Hedeker, D., Siddiqui, O., Britton, C. F., Brannon, B. R., et al. (1995). The television, school, and family smoking prevention and cessation project. VIII Student outcomes and mediating variables. *Preventive Medicine, 24*, 29–40.

Flynn, B. S., Worden, J. K., Bunn, J. Y., Solomon, L. J., Ashikaga, T., Connolly, S. W., et al. (2010). Mass media interventions to reduce youth smoking prevalence. *American Journal of Preventive Medicine, 39*, 53–62.

Flynn, B. S., Worden, J. K., Secker-Walker, R. H., Badger, G. J., & Geller, B. M. (1995). Cigarette smoking prevention effects of mass media and school interventions targeted to gender and age groups. *Journal of Health Education, 26*(2), 45–51.

Friend, K., & Levy, D. (2002). Reductions in smoking prevalence and cigarette consumption associated with mass-media campaigns. *Health Education Research, 17*(1), 85–98.

Hafstad, A., & Aaro, L. E. (1997). Activating interpersonal influence through provocative appeals: Evaluation of a mass media based antismoking campaign targeting adolescents. *Health Communication, 9*(3), 253–72.

Kremers, S., Mudde, A., de Vries, N., Brug, J., & de Vries, H. (2004). Unplanned smoking initiation: New insights and implications for interventions. *Patient Education and Counselling, 55*, 345–52.

Kreps, G. L., & Neuhauser, L. (2010 Mar). New directions in eHealth communication: opportunities and challenges. *Patient Education and Counseling, 78*(3), 329–36.

Logan, R. A. (2004). Evaluating consumer informatics: Learning from health campaign research. *Studies in Health Technology and Informatics, 107*(Pt 2), 1147–1151.

Longshore, D., Ghosh-Dastidar, B., & Ellickson, P. L. (2006). National youth anti-drug media campaign and school-based prevention: Evidence for a synergistic effect in ALERT Plus. *Addictive Behaviors, 31*, 493–508.

Mass Media. (2010 November). *Oxford english dictionary*, online version.

McGuire, W. J. (1969). Attitudes and attitude change. In G. Lindzey & E. Aronson (Eds.), *Handbook of social psychology* (Vol. 2). Reading, Massachusetts: Addison-Wesley.

Michell, L. (1994). *Smoking prevention programs for adolescents: A literature review*. Oxford: Anglia and Oxford Regional Health Authority.

National Cancer Institute. (1991). *Strategies to control tobacco use in the United States: A blueprint for public health action in the 1990s*. Washington: National Cancer Institute.

National Cancer Institute. (2008). The role of the media in promoting and reducing tobacco use. *Tobacco Control Monograph* (No. 19. NIH Pub. No. 07-6242). Bethesda, MD: US Department of Health and Human Services, National Institutes of Health, National Cancer Institute.

Noar, S. M. (2006). A 10-year retrospective of research in health mass media campaigns: Where do we go from here? *Journal of Health Communication, 11*(1), 21–42.

Ockene, J. K., Edgerton, E. A., Teutsch, S. M., Marion, L. N., Miller, T., Genevro, J. L., et al. (2007). Integrating evidence-based clinical and community strategies to improve health. *American Journal of Preventive Medicine, 32*(3), 244–252.

Prochaska, J., & Velicer, W. (1997). The transtheoretical model of health behavior change. *American Journal of Health Promotion, 12*, 38–48.

Randolph, W., & Viswanath, K. (2004). Lessons learned from public health mass media campaigns: Marketing health in a crowded media world. *Annual Review of Public Health, 25*, 419–37.

Redman, S., Spencer, E. A., & Sanson-Fisher, R. W. (1990). The role of mass media in changing health-related behaviour: A critical appraisal of two models. *Health Promotion International, 5*, 85–101.

Reid, D. (1996). Tobacco control: Overview. *British Medical Bulletin, 52*, 108–20.

Reid, D., McNeill, A., & Glynn, T. J. (1995). Reducing the prevalence of smoking in youth: An international review. *Tobacco Control, 4*, 66–277.

Rice, R. E., & Atkin, C. K. (2009). Public communication campaigns: Theoretical principles and practical applications. In J. Bryant & M. Oliver (Eds.), *Media effects: Advances in theory and research* (3rd ed., pp. 436–468). Hillsdale, NJ: Lawrence Erlbaum.

Salmon, C., & Atkin, C. K. (2003). Media campaigns for health promotion. In T. L. Thompson, A. M. Dorsey, K. I. Miller, & R. Parrott (Eds.), *Handbook of health communication*. Mahwah, NJ: Lawrence Erlbaum.

Schar, E., & Gutierrez, K. (2001). *Smoking cessation media campaigns from around the world: Recommendations from lessons learned*. Centers for Disease Control and Prevention and World Health Organization European Tobacco-Free Initiative. Accessed May 2012, from http://www.euro.who.int/document/e74523.pdf

Schar, E., Gutierrez, K., Murphy-Hoefer, R., & Nelson, D. E. (2006). *Tobacco use prevention media campaigns: Lessons learned from youth in nine countries*. Atlanta: U.S. Department of Health and Human Services, Centers for Disease Control and Prevention, National Center for Chronic Disease Prevention and Health Promotion, Office on Smoking and Health. Available at http://www.cdc.gov/tobacco.

Siegel, M. (1998). Mass media antismoking campaigns: A powerful tool for health promotion. *Annals of Internal Medicine, 129*, 128–32.

Silver, M. Z. (2001). Efficacy of anti-tobacco mass media campaigns on adolescent tobacco use. *Pediatric Nursing May–June, 27*(3), 293–6.

Slater, M. D. (1996). Theory and method in health audience segmentation. *Journal of Health Communication, 1*(3), 267–285.

Snyder, L. B., & Hamilton, M. A. (2002). A meta-analysis of U.S. health campaign effects on behavior: Emphasize enforcement, exposure, and new information, and beware the secular trend. In R. C. Hornik (Ed.), *Public health communication: Evidence for behavior change* (pp. 357–384). Mahwah, NJ: Lawrence Erlbaum.

Stead, M., Hastings, G., & Tudor-Smith, C. (1996). Preventing adolescent smoking: A review of options. *Health Education Journal, 55*, 31–54.

Strasburger, V. C. (1995). *Adolescents and the media. Medical and psychological impact*. London: Sage Publications.

Strasburger, V. C., Jordan, A. B., & Donnerstein, E. (2010). Health effects of media on children and adolescents. *Pediatrics, 125*(4), 756–67.

The Guide to Community-Preventive Services. (2003). *The effectiveness of mass media campaigns to reduce initiation of tobacco use and to increase cessation*. Available January 3, at http://www.thecommunityguide.org/tobacco/tobac-int-mass-media.pdf

Tyas, S. L., & Pederson, L. L. (1997). *Psychosocial factors in the initiation to smoking among adolescents: A critical review and analysis of the literature*. Toronto: The Ontario Tobacco Research Unit.

U.S. Department of Health and Human Services. (2000). *Reducing tobacco use: A report of the surgeon general*. Atlanta, GA: USDHHS, Centers for Disease Control and Prevention, National Center for Chronic Disease Prevention and Health Promotion, Office on Smoking and Health.

U.S. Department of Health and Human Services. (2012). *Preventing tobacco use among youth and young adults: A report of the surgeon general*. Atlanta, GA: U.S. Department of Health and Human Services, Centers for Disease Control and Prevention, National Center for Chronic Disease Prevention and Health Promotion, Office on Smoking and Health.

U.S. Preventive Services Task Force. (2003, November). *Counseling to prevent tobacco use and tobacco-related diseases: recommendation statement*. Available at http://www.uspreventiveservicestaskforce.org/3rduspstf/tobacccoun/tobcounrs.htm

U.S. Preventive Services Task Force. (2009, April). *Counseling and interventions to prevent tobacco use and tobacco-caused disease in adults and pregnant women: reaffirmation recommendation statement* (AHRQ Publication No. 09-05131-EF-1). Available at http://www.uspreventiveservicestaskforce.org/uspstf09/tobacco/tobaccors2.htm

U.S. Department of Health, Education, and Welfare. (1964). *Smoking and health: Report of the Advisory Committee to the Surgeon General of the Public Health Service* (PHS publication no. 1103). Washington, DC: U.S. Department of Health, Education, and Welfare, Public Health Service, Center for Disease Control.

U.S. Department of Health and Human Services (DHHS). (1994). *Preventing tobacco use among young people: A report of the Surgeon General*. Atlanta, Georgia: US Department of Health and Human Services, Public Health Service, Centers for Disease Control and Prevention, National Center for Chronic Disease Prevention and Health Promotion, Office on Smoking and Health.

Valente, T. W. (2001). Evaluating communication campaigns. In R. E. Rice & C. K. Atkin (Eds.), *Public communication campaigns* (3rd ed., pp. 105–124). Thousand Oaks, CA: Sage.

Valente, T., & Schuster, D. (2002). The public health perspective for communicating environmental issue. In T. Diets & P. Stern (Eds.), *The human dimension of global change*. Washington, DC: National Academy Press.

Vartiainen, E., Paavola, M., McAlister, A., & Puska, P. (1998). Fifteen-year follow-up of smoking prevention effects in the North Karelia youth project. *American Journal of Public Health, 88*, 81–85.

Vartuaunen, E., Paavola, M., et al. (1998). Fifteen-year follow-up of smoking prevention effects in the North Karelia youth project. *American Journal of Public Health, 88*, 81–5.

Wahi, G., Parkin, P. C., Beyene, J., Uleryk, E. M., & Birken, C. S. (2011). Effectiveness of interventions aimed at reducing screen time in children: A systematic review and meta-analysis of randomized controlled trials. *Archives of Pediatrics & Adolescent Medicine, 165*(11), 979–986.

Wakefield, M. A., Loken, B., & Hornik, R. C. (2010). Use of mass media campaigns to change health behaviour. *Lancet, 376*(9748), 1261–71.

Wellings, K., & Macdowall, W. (2000). Evaluating mass media approaches to health promotion: A review of methods. *Health Education, 100*, 23–32.

Worden, J. K., Flynn, B. S., Geller, B. M., Chen, M., Shelton, L. G., & Secker-Walker, R. H. (1988). Development of a smoking prevention mass media program using diagnostic and formative research. *Preventive Medicine, 17*, 531–58.

Worden, J. K., & Flynn, B. S. (1983). *Using television messages to prevent smoking among adolescents*. American Public Health Association Annual Meeting. Dallas: Office of Health Promotion Research and Biometry Facility, College of Medicine, Department of Mathematics (Statistics Program) College of Engineering and Mathematics, University of Vermont.

World Health Organization. (2011, September). *Smoke-free movies: From evidence to action* (2nd ed.). WHO Library Cataloguing-in-Publication Data

World Health Organization. (2011b). *WHO report on the global tobacco epidemic, 2011. Warning about the dangers of tobacco. WHO Library Cataloguing-in-Publication Data*. Geneva, Switzerland: WHO Press.

World Health Organization. (2011). *WHO report on the global tobacco epidemic*. Appendix II—Table 2.3 anti-tobacco mass media campaigns (see Table 4.9). http://whqlibdoc.who.int/publications/2011/9789240687813_eng.pdf

Chapter 8
How to Tackle Smoking at the Population Level

Giuseppe La Torre, Domitilla Di Thiene, and Alice Mannocci

Objectives The concern about the tobacco pandemic raised a global public health response. The possibility to win this battle is really connected with the ability of public health to act at the population level. In order to make people able to resist at smoking pressure it is necessary to develop laws protecting individuals. Smoking or not smoking it is not only a individual choice but the result of political choice.

Another aim of this section is to summarize the health warnings on tobacco products packaging used in the different countries in the World and to report the current scientific evidence of the differences impact of these in the smokers.

Learning Outcomes

The WHO Framework Convention on Tobacco Control (WHO FCTC) (2003a, b) is the first international treaty in response to tobacco epidemic and, interestingly, the world's first public health treaty.

A central pillar of tobacco control is EU legislation on tobacco products and on tobacco advertising.

Moreover, by the end of this section the reader will be able to:

- Learn the definition of tobacco packaging warning message.
- Identify the types of warning labels.
- Learn the recommendations in the WHO Frame Work Convention on Tobacco Control Guidelines for implementation, Article11.
- Know the principal scientific evidences of effectiveness of the health pictorial warnings on tobacco products.

G. La Torre (✉) • A. Mannocci • D. Di Thiene
Department of Public Health and Infectious Diseases, "Sapienza" University of Rome, Piazzale Aldo Moro 5, Rome 00185, Italy
e-mail: giuseppe.latorre@uniroma1.it; alice.mannocci@uniroma1.it

G. La Torre, *Smoking Prevention and Cessation*, DOI 10.1007/978-1-4614-7046-5_8,

8.1 The Tobacco-Free Framework

The World Health Organization Framework Convention on Tobacco Control (WHO FCTC) is the first international treaty negotiated under the auspices of WHO. It was adopted by the World Health Assembly on 21 May 2003 and entered into force on 27 February 2005. Though data and statistics of smoking are often repeated, their impact is still shocking: tobacco kills more than five million people a year—more than tuberculosis, HIV/AIDS, and malaria combined. Without any form of control, tobacco-related deaths will increase to more than eight million per year by 2030. The Member States of the WHO joined together and unanimously committed to stopping this epidemic by taking the unprecedented step of developing a treaty on tobacco control. Utilizing and, to a certain extent, inventing and reinventing the tools of international law and global public health, they negotiated the WHO FCTC. The treaty has enjoyed global support, with more than 170 Parties (174 in march 2012), and is often called the most powerful tool in the fight against tobacco-related morbidity and mortality and it has since become one of the most rapidly and widely embraced treaties in United Nations history (Lien 2011).

The WHO FCTC was developed in response to the globalization of the tobacco epidemic and is an evidence-based treaty that reaffirms the right of all people to the highest standard of health. The convention represents a milestone for the promotion of public health and provides new legal dimensions for international health cooperation. Table 8.1 summarizes key policy provisions of the FCTC.

There are currently 21 nonparties to the treaty [11 which have not signed and 10 which have signed but not ratified (Table 8.2)].

The core demand reduction provisions in the WHO FCTC are contained in articles 6–14 which detail the price, tax, and non-price measures necessary to reduce the demand for tobacco, namely, protection from exposure to tobacco smoke; regulation of the contents of tobacco products; regulation of tobacco product disclosures; packaging and labeling of tobacco products; education, communication, training, and public awareness; tobacco advertising, promotion, and sponsorship; and demand reduction measures concerning tobacco dependence and cessation.

The core supply reduction provisions in the WHO FCTC are contained in articles 15–17, the illicit trade in tobacco products; sales to and by minors and provision of support for economically viable alternative activities.

Significant barriers to the treaty's long-term success remain in many countries, especially those in the middle and low income range. These include a lack of locally relevant evidence and data gathering/surveillance infrastructure in many countries and an inadequate expertise in relation to some areas of research, health systems development, and policy formation and implementation. Moreover a insufficient leadership and networking, a lack of national foci for tobacco control, including both governmental and nongovernmental entities and the little investment in funding for research and programs directed at the control of tobacco use and tobacco attributable disease often vanished the efforts to implement the FCTC (Wipfli et al. 2004).

Table 8.1 Key policy provisions of the framework convention on tobacco control (FCTC)

Increase tobacco taxes
Protect citizens from exposure to tobacco smoke in workplaces, public transport, and indoor public places
Enact comprehensive bans on tobacco advertising, promotion, and sponsorship
Regulate the packaging and labeling of tobacco products to prevent the use of misleading and deceptive terms such as "light" and "mild"
Regulate the packaging and labeling of tobacco products to ensure appropriate product warnings are communicated to consumers, for example, obligate the placement of rotating health warnings on tobacco packaging that cover at least 30 % (but ideally 50 % or more) of the principal display areas and can include pictures or pictograms
Regulate the testing and disclosure of the content and emissions of tobacco products
Promote public awareness of tobacco control issues by ensuring broad access to effective comprehensive educational and public awareness programs on the health risks of tobacco and exposure to tobacco smoke
Promote and implement effective programs aimed at promoting the cessation of tobacco use
Combat smuggling, including the placing of final destination markings on packs
Implement legislation and programs to prohibit the sale of tobacco products to minors
Implement policies to support economically viable alternative sources of income for tobacco workers, growers, and individual seller

Modified from Fong et al. (2006)

Table 8.2 Countries that are not party to the FCTC. Modified from Wipfli and Huang (2011)

1. Andorra	10. Indonesia	19. Switzerland
2. Argentina	11. Liechtenstein	20. Tajikistan
3. Cuba	12. Malawi	21. Turkmenistan
4. Czech Republic	13. Monaco	22. USA
5. Dominican Republic	14. Morocco	23. Uzbekistan
6. El Salvador	15. Mozambique	24. Zimbabwe
7. Eritrea	16. St. Kitts and Nevis	
8. Ethiopia	17. Saint Vincent and the Grenadines	
9. Haiti	18. Somalia	

Modified from Wipfli and Huang (2011)

8.2 EU Legislation on Tobacco

The European Union (EU) and Member States authorities work together on tobacco control.

A central pillar of tobacco control is EU legislation on tobacco products and on tobacco advertising. These laws are meant to conciliate internal market objectives with the need to ensure a high level of public health protection across the EU.

The European Commission is in charge of overseeing the implementation of these laws and of proposing necessary revisions.

The Directive on Tobacco Products (2001) requires that all tobacco products sold in the EU display two text warnings: the first compulsory warning is either "tobacco kills" or "tobacco can seriously harm you and others around you." The second warning, selected from a list of 14, includes "smoking causes fatal lung cancer." The Directive also bans misleading terms such as "light," "mild," or "low tar," and obliges manufacturers to report to Member States on the ingredients they use. It further bans oral tobacco and sets maximum limits for tar, nicotine, and carbon monoxide in cigarettes.

The Directive on Tobacco Advertising (2003) bans cross-border advertising of tobacco products in printed media, radio, and online services. It also bans sponsorship of cross-border events. In addition, tobacco advertising and sponsorship on television has already been prohibited since 1989.

For other areas of tobacco control such as prevention, cessation, and smoke-free environments, responsibility for providing the appropriate rules and structures lies with the individual Member States. In these areas, the EU's role is to support, complement, and coordinate national efforts. The EU has made the following recommendations to Member States:

1. Council recommendation on smoking prevention (2003), which encourages Member States to control all forms of tobacco promotion and sales to minors, as well as to improve awareness and health education.
2. Council recommendation on smoke-free environments (2009), the recommendation calls on Member States to act in three main fronts:

   - Adopt and implement laws to fully protect their citizens from exposure to tobacco smoke in enclosed public places, workplaces, and public transport as cited in Article 8 of the Framework Convention on Tobacco control, within 3 years of the adoption of the recommendation
   - Enhance smoke-free laws with supporting measures such as protecting children, encouraging efforts to give up tobacco use and pictorial warnings on tobacco packages.
   - Strengthen cooperation at EU level by setting up a network of national focal points for tobacco control.

Twelve EU Member States provide for comprehensive protection from exposure to tobacco smoke.

Total bans on smoking in all enclosed public places and workplaces, including bars and restaurants, are in place in Ireland, UK, and Cyprus. Italy, Malta, Sweden, Latvia, Finland, Slovenia, France, Lithuania, and the Netherlands have introduced smoke-free legislation allowing for special enclosed smoking rooms.

However, in the remaining Member States, citizens and workers are still not fully protected from exposure to tobacco smoke in indoor workplaces and public places. Bars and restaurants are a particularly difficult area of regulation.

Table 8.3 Overview of smoke-free legislation in the EU

	General workplace	Enclosed public places	Restaurants	Health care facilities	Public transport	Prisons
Austria	☺	☺	±	☺	☺	☺
Belgium	☺	☺	☺	☺	☺ ☺	☺
Bulgaria	☺	☺	±	☺	☺ ☺	☺
Cyprus	☺	☺ ☺	☺	☺ ☺	☺ ☺	±
Czech Republic	±	±	●	☺ ☺	☺	±
Denmark	☺	☺	☺	±	☺	☺
Estonia	±	±	☺	±	±	±
Finland	☺	☺	☺	☺	☺	☺
France	☺	☺	☺	☺ ☺	☺ ☺	☺
Germany	☺	☺	±	☺	☺	☺
Greece	☺ ☺	☺ ☺	☺ ☺	☺ ☺	☺ ☺	☺ ☺
Hungary	±	±	●	☺ ☺	±	±
Ireland	☺ ☺	☺ ☺	☺ ☺	☺ ☺	☺ ☺	●
Italy	☺	☺	☺	☺	☺	☺
Latvia	☺	☺ ☺	☺ ☺	☺	☺	☺
Lithuania	☺	☺ ☺	☺ ☺	☺ ☺	±	☺
Luxembourg	☺	☺ ☺	☺	☺	☺	☺
Malta	☺	☺	☺	☺ ☺	☺	☺
Netherlands	☺	☺	☺	☺	☺	☺
Poland	☺	☺ ☺	☺	☺ ☺	☺	±
Portugal	±	±	±	±	☺ ☺	±
Romania	☺	☺	±	☺ ☺	☺ ☺	☺
Slovakia	☺	☺ ☺	☺	☺ ☺	☺	☺
Slovenia	☺	☺	☺	☺ ☺	☺	☺
Spain	☺ ☺	☺ ☺	☺ ☺	☺ ☺	☺ ☺	☺
Sweden	☺	☺	☺	☺	☺	☺
UK	☺ ☺	☺ ☺	☺ ☺	☺ ☺	☺ ☺	±

Modified from http://ec.europa.eu/health/tobacco/docs/tobacco_overview2011_en.pdf
This overview is based on the analysis of the relevant legal provisions in effect in each Member State as of May 2011 but does not take into account their enforcement nor does it reflect forthcoming legislative changes in the case of Belgium, Hungary, Malta, and the Netherlands
☺ ☺ = Total ban on indoor smoking
☺ = Ban on indoor smoking, while providing for separate enclosed smoking rooms/obligation for employer to protect employees
± = Partial ban on indoor smoking, e.g., smoking zones or exemptions for certain categories of venues
● = Recommendations, suggestions, or no ban

Partial smoking bans in the hospitality sector are in place in Austria, Bulgaria, Denmark, Greece, Portugal, Romania, Belgium, Luxembourg, Slovakia, Spain, and most German Länder (Table 8.3).

The EU is a full Party to the Framework Convention on Tobacco Control (FCTC) since June 2005, as are 26 of its Member States (all but the Czech Republic) (McNeill et al. 2012).

Recently the commission is considering to put forward a proposal for the revision of the 2001 Tobacco Products Directive in 2012. Following a public consultation and the analysis of possible options for revision within an impact assessment, the directive could be strengthened, adapted to international tobacco control commitments, new developments in tobacco products and advances in science. Possible measures that are currently being examined are:

- Regulatory solutions to address novel smokeless tobacco and nicotine products.
- Better consumer information. For example, larger and double-sided picture warnings, standardized packaging, information on harmful substances.
- Regulation of ingredients in tobacco products, in particular those which make tobacco products more attractive and addictive and appeal especially to young people such as vanilla and fruit flavors.
- Revising the rules on sales of tobacco products.

8.3 Package Advertising

Tobacco packaging warning message is that message that appears on the packaging of tobacco products and that is concerning the health effects of those products.

Communicating the health effects of smoking is a primary goal of tobacco control policy and the tobacco warnings are the most common means; indeed they are appealing both for their low cost to regulators and for their unparalleled reach among smokers (Hammond et al. 2007).

The first guiding principle of WHO—FCTC states that: "Every person should be informed of the health consequences, addictive nature and mortal threat posed by tobacco consumption and exposure to tobacco smoke" (WHO 2003a).

The WHO–FCTC entered into force on 2005 and actually numbers 168 countries/Parties.

In particular the Article 11 of the guidelines produce by Convention (WHO 2011a; 2003b) requires that the Parties must implement large, rotating health warnings on all tobacco product packaging and labeling. In particular, the sections 1b and 2, cited below, are concerning the recommendations for the packaging and labeling of tobacco products:

> *1.b. Each unit packet and package of tobacco products and any outside packaging and labeling of such products also carry health warnings describing the harmful effects of tobacco use, and may include other appropriate messages. These warnings and messages:*
>
> (i) *shall be approved by the competent national authority*;
> (ii) *shall be rotating*;
> (iii) *shall be large, clear, visible and legible*;
> (iv) *should be 50 % or more of the principal display areas but shall be no less*;
> (v) *than 30 % of the principal display areas*;
> (vi) *may be in the form of or include pictures or pictograms.*
>
> *2. Each unit packet and package of tobacco products and any outside packaging and labelling of such products shall, in addition to the warnings specified in paragraph 1(b) of this Article, contain information on relevant constituents and emissions of tobacco products as defined by national authorities.*

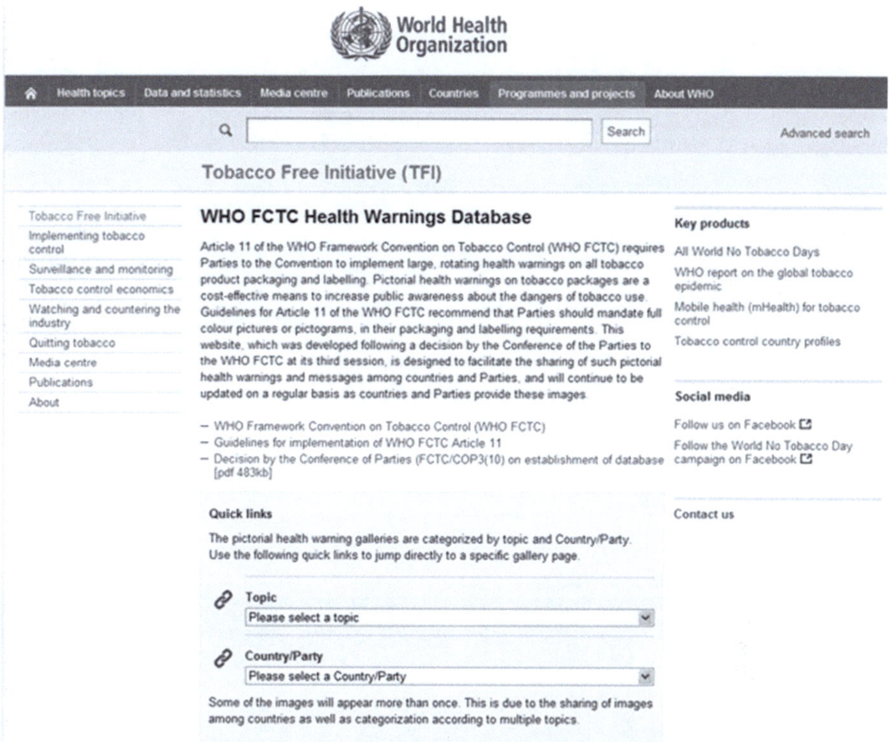

Fig. 8.1 Website of WHO for the sharing of pictorial health warnings present in the Parties. Accessed March 30, 2012, from (http://www.who.int/tobacco/healthwarningsdatabase/en/

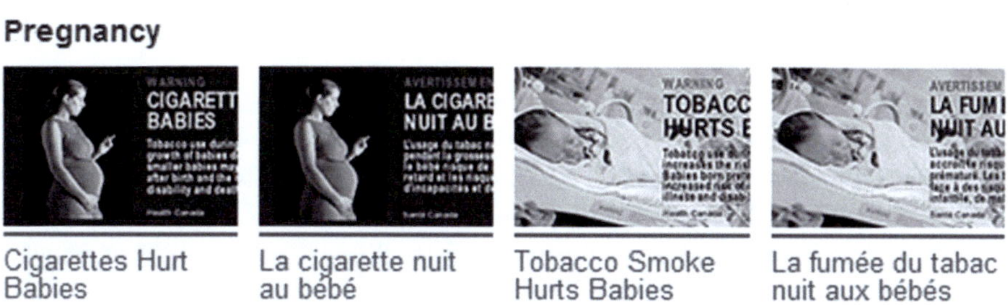
Pregnancy
Cigarettes Hurt Babies
La cigarette nuit au bébé
Tobacco Smoke Hurts Babies
La fumée du tabac nuit aux bébés

Fig. 8.2 Pictorial warnings purposed in Canada about pregnancy selecting topic "Pregnancy" and Country "Canada" on the WHO Website. Accessed March 30, 2012, from (http://www.who.int/tobacco/healthwarningsdatabase/en/)

It's possible to consult a Website that shows the sharing of such pictorial health warnings and messages among 20 countries/parties and will continue to be updated on a regular basis as countries and Parties provide these images (Figs. 8.1, 8.2, 8.3, and 8.4).

Actually it's possible to distinguish three principal methods for warnings: pictures, symbol, and texts.

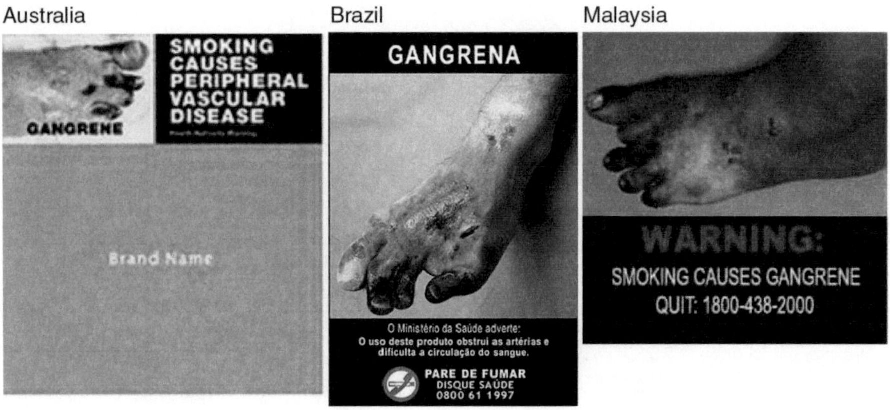

Fig. 8.3 Pictorial warnings purposed about vascular system selecting topic "vascular system/ gangrene" on the WHO Website. Accessed March 30, 2012, from http://www.who.int/tobacco/healthwarningsdatabase/en/

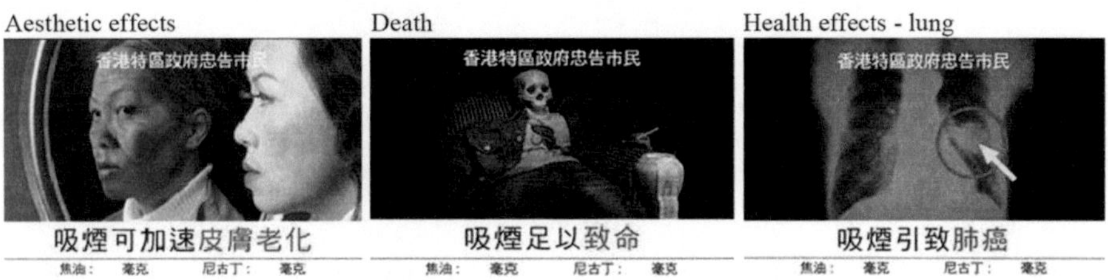

Fig. 8.4 Pictorial warnings purposed in China on the WHO Website. Accessed March 2012, from http://www.who.int/tobacco/healthwarningsdatabase/en/

In Table 8.4 some textual health warnings are reported.

In the scientific literature there is evidence that the effectiveness of the health pictorial warnings is greater in comparison with text only (Carr-Gregg and Gray 1990; Campaign for Tobacco-free Kids 2010; Wogalter et al. 2002).

The effectiveness of graphic warning can be measured in various ways, for example: the grade of the noticing of the warnings; the capacity to recall the messages or to draw the attention; change in the health knowledge; change of own smoking habits (consumption, quitting). For this reason the "look" of the tobacco products plays an important role to communicate the risks of health in the smokers (Hammond 2008a).

On the other hand the packaging represents in general a key component of marketing strategy. Indeed it underlines in the business communication the brand identity and makes a statement of the type of consumer and individual. The British American Tobacco in 1978 reported : "*One of every two smokers is not able to distinguish in blind (masked) tests between similar cigarettes … for most smokers and the decisive group of new, younger smokers, the consumer's choice is dictated more*

Table 8.4 List of health warnings from the Commission Directive 2012/9/EU of 7 March 2012

1. Smoking causes 9 out of 10 lung cancers
2. Smoking causes mouth and throat cancer
3. Smoking damages your lungs
4. Smoking causes heart attacks
5. Smoking causes strokes and disability
6. Smoking clogs your arteries
7. Smoking increases the risk of blindness
8. Smoking damages your teeth and gums
9. Smoking can kill your unborn child
10. Your smoke harms your children, family, and friends
11. Smokers' children are more likely to start smoking
12. Quit smoking—stay alive for those close to you (1)
13. Smoking reduces fertility
14. Smoking increases the risk of impotence

by psychological, image factors than by relatively minor differences in smoking characteristics" (Hammond 2008b).

Twenty-nine countries and jurisdictions have implemented policies that require pictorial health warnings on tobacco packages, and several studies were performed to evaluate the impact before and after the introduction of the new warnings. Table 8.5 reported the characteristics of health warning labels on cigarette packages in Europe. In particular in the last years many European countries are preparing a new campaign. Thanks to a directive in 2001 of the European Parliament and Council, that invited the Member States to adopt new warnings with images and texts, 13 countries had accepted to implement officially this policy (Table 8.5).

Several studies were performed to evaluate the impact of the warnings labels in smokers' knowledge or reactions. In particular after the adoption of the new pictorial warnings (the first country was Canada in 2001 followed by Brazil in 2002) many studies aimed to compare the effectiveness of these with the previous text messages (Berg et al. 2011; Borland et al. 2009; Brubaker and Mitby 1990; Chang et al. 2011; Difranza et al. 2002; Fathelrahman et al. 2009; Fischer et al. 1989; Fong et al. 2010; Goodall and Appiah 2008; Hammond et al. 2003, 2004a, b, 2006, 2012; Hitchman et al. 2011; Koval et al. 2005; Mannocci et al. 2012; Nascimento et al. 2008; O'Hegarty et al. 2006, 2007; Ozkaya et al. 2009; Portillo and Antoñanzas 2002; Qin et al. 2011; Shanahan and Elliott 2009; Sebrié et al. 2010; Sobani et al. 2010; Stockley 2001; Strahan et al. 2002; Thrasher et al. 2012, 2007a, b, 2010; Vardavas et al. 2009; Wade et al. 2011; White et al. 2008; Zaidi et al. 2011).

The work conducted by Hammond and Colleagues (2006) showed that the Canadian smokers were not fully informed about the risk of smoking. From comparing health knowledge between smokers with or without health warnings on their

Table 8.5 Table concerning the characteristics of health warning labels on cigarette packages in Europe

		Percentage of principal display area mandated to be covered by health warnings			Specific health warning labels on packages							
Country	Health warning labels mandated	Average of front and back %	Front %	Back	Does the law mandate specific health warnings on packages?	How many health warnings are approved by the law?	Do health warnings appear on each package and any outside packaging and labeling used in retail sale?	Do health warnings describe the harmful effects of tobacco us of health	Does the law mandate font style, font size and color of health warnings?	Are the health warnings rotating?	Are the health warnings written in the principal language(s) of the country?	Do the health warnings include a photograph or graphic?
Albania	Yes	50	50	50	Yes	16	Yes	Yes	Yes	Yes	Yes	No
Andorra[a]	[b]	[b]	[b]	[b]	[b]	[b]	[b]	[b]	[b]	[b]	[b]	[b]
Armenia	Yes	30	30	30	Yes	5	Yes	Yes	Yes	Yes	Yes	No
Austria	Yes	35	30	30	Yes	16	Yes	Yes	Yes	Yes	Yes	No
Azerbaijan	Yes	[c]	[c]	[c]	No	[d]	No	No	No	No	Yes	No
Belarus	Yes	30	30	30	Yes	6	Yes	Yes	No	Yes	Yes	No
Belgium	Yes	43	35	35	Yes	16	Yes	Yes	Yes	Yes	Yes	No
Bosnia and Herzegovina[e]	[b]	[b]	[b]	[b]	[b]	[b]	[b]	[b]	[b]	[b]	[b]	[b]
Bulgaria	Yes	35	30	40	Yes	16	Yes	Yes	Yes	Yes	Yes	No
Croatia	Yes	35	30	40	Yes	16	Yes	Yes	Yes	Yes	Yes	No
Cyprus	Yes	39	32	45	Yes	13	Yes	Yes	Yes	Yes	Yes	No
Czech Republic	Yes	35	30	40	Yes	16	Yes	Yes	Yes	Yes	Yes	No
Denmark	Yes	35	30	40	Yes	16	Yes	Yes	Yes	Yes	Yes	No
Estonia	Yes	35	30	40	Yes	16	Yes	Yes	Yes	Yes	Yes	No
Finland	Yes	39	32	45	Yes	16	Yes	Yes	Yes	Yes	Yes	No
France	Yes	35	30	40	Yes	16	Yes	Yes	Yes	Yes	Yes	Yes
Georgia	Yes	30	30	30	Yes	12	Yes	Yes	Yes	Yes	Yes	Yes

Germany	Yes	35	30	40	Yes	16	Yes	Yes	Yes	Yes	Yes	No
Greece	Yes	35	30	40	Yes	16	Yes	Yes	Yes	Yes	Yes	No
Hungary	Yes	35	30	40	Yes	16	Yes	Yes	Yes	Yes	Yes	No
Iceland	Yes	35	30	40	Yes	16	Yes	Yes	Yes	Yes	Yes	No
Ireland	Yes	39	32	45	Yes	16	Yes	Yes	Yes	Yes	Yes	No
Israel	Yes	30	30	30	Yes	13	Yes	Yes	Yes	Yes	Yes	No
Italy	Yes	35	30	40	Yes	10	Yes	Yes	Yes	Yes	Yes	No
Kazakhstan	Yes	40	0	40	No	[d]	No	No	No	No	No	No
Kyrgyzstan	Yes	40	40	40	Yes	9	Yes	Yes	Yes	Yes	Yes	No
Latvia	Yes	35	30	40	Yes	16	Yes	Yes	Yes	Yes	Yes	Yes
Lithuania	Yes	35	30	40	Yes	16	Yes	Yes	Yes	Yes	Yes	No
Luxembourg	Yes	39	32	45	Yes	17	Yes	Yes	No	Yes	Yes	No
Malta	Yes	39	32	45	Yes	16	Yes	Yes	Yes	Yes	Yes	Yes[f]
Monaco[g]	[b]	[b]	[b]	[b]	[b]	[b]	[b]	[b]	[b]	[b]	[b]	[b]
Montenegro	Yes	35	30	40	Yes	16	Yes	Yes	Yes	Yes	Yes	No
Netherlands	Yes	35	30	40	Yes	16	Yes	Yes	Yes	Yes	Yes	No
Norway	Yes	35	30	40	Yes	16	Yes	Yes	Yes	Yes	Yes	Yes[f]
Poland	Yes	35	30	40	Yes	16	Yes	Yes	Yes	Yes	Yes	No
Portugal	Yes	35	30	40	Yes	16	Yes	Yes	Yes	Yes	Yes	No
Republic of Moldova	Yes	35	30	40	Yes	14	Yes	Yes	Yes	Yes	Yes	No
Romania	Yes	35	30	40	Yes	16	Yes	Yes	Yes	Yes	Yes	Yes
Russian Federation	Yes	40	30	50	Yes	13	No	Yes	No	Yes	Yes	No
San Marino	No	[d]	[d]	[d]	[d]	[d]	[d]	[d]	[d]	[d]	[d]	[d]
Serbia	Yes	35	30	40	Yes	12	Yes	Yes	Yes	Yes	Yes	No
Slovakia	Yes	35	30	40	Yes	16	Yes	Yes	Yes	Yes	Yes	No
Slovenia	Yes	35	30	40	Yes	16	Yes	Yes	Yes	Yes	Yes	No
Spain	Yes	35	30	40	Yes	16	Yes	Yes	Yes	Yes	Yes	Yes
Sweden	Yes	35	30	40	Yes	14	Yes	Yes	Yes	Yes	Yes	No
Switzerland	Yes	43	35	50	Yes	16	Yes	Yes	No	Yes	Yes	Yes

(continued)

Table 8.5 (continued)

Country	Health warning labels mandated	Percentage of principal display area mandated to be covered by health warnings: Average of front and back %	Front %	Back	Specific health warning labels on packages: Does the law mandate specific health warnings on packages?	How many health warnings are approved by the law?	Do health warnings appear on each package and any outside packaging and labeling used in retail sale?	Do health warnings describe the harmful effects of tobacco us of health	Does the law mandate font style, font size and color of health warnings?	Are the health warnings rotating?	Are the health warnings written in the principal language(s) of the country?	Do the health warnings include a photograph or graphic?
Tajikistan	No	[d]	[d]	[d]	[d]	[d]	[d]	[d]	[d]	[d]	[d]	[d]
The former Yugoslav Republic of Macedonia	Yes	35	30	40	Yes	16	Yes	Yes	Yes	Yes	Yes	Yes
Turkey	Yes	48	30	65	Yes	16	Yes	Yes	Yes	Yes	Yes	Yes
Turkmeristan	No	[d]	[d]	[d]	[d]	[d]	[d]	[d]	[d]	[d]	[d]	[d]
Ukraine	Yes[f]	50[f]	50[f]	50[f]	Yes[f]	10[f]	Yes[f]	Yes[f]	No	Yes[f]	Yes[f]	Yes[f]
United Kingdom of Great Britain and Northern Ireland	Yes	35	30	40	Yes	16	Yes	Yes	Yes	Yes	Yes	Yes
Uzbekistan	Yes	30	320	30	Yes	3	No	Yes	No	Yes	Yes	No

Source: WHO (2011b)

[a]All tobacco products sold in Andorra are imported from France or Spain and therefore follow the French or Spanish laws on health warnings

[b]Data not reported/not available

[c]Not mandated

[d]Data not required/not applicable

[e]The two subnational jurisdictions of the country, Federation of Bosnia and Herzegovina and Republika Srpska, adopted separate tobacco control legislation with several differences, so no national legislation is reported

[f]Policy adopted but not implemented by 31 December 2010

[g]All tobacco products sold in Monaco are imported from France and therefore follow the French law on health warnings

packages resulted that smokers were significant more likely to say that tobacco smokers causes cancer, impotence, and stroke, when this information was printed on cigarettes packages, respectively with OR = 1.60, OR = 2.68, and OR = 1.57.

Another European study confirms these results, indicating that more than 50 % of smokers recognized the importance of health warnings in communicating health risks and that women were more impressed than men by shocking pictorial warnings OR = 2.54 (CI 95 %:1.41–4.56) (Mannocci et al. 2012).

The analysis by gender were showed in an American study published in 2006 (O'Hegarty et al. 2006). The aim of this study was investigating how US young adult smokers and former smokers respond to stronger text and graphic warnings on cigarette packages. Significantly more women than men agreed that the text-plus-graphic label with the baby would motivate them to quit (78 % and 48.6 %, respectively ($p < 0.05$)).

And what happens among adolescents? The adolescents perception was investigated in a study conducted in the high schools in Canada (Goodall and Appiah 2008). In this survey a comparison of the effects of different kind of messages loss framed and gain framed) on adolescents's smoking attitudes and behaviors was conducted. The distinction between loss and gain framed messages is essential. The first ones (loss framed) is concerning on what one may lose by engaging in the behavior (negative consequences of smoking) while the second one can be divided in gain-framed avoidance and gain-framed benefits, both emphasizing how one cam avoid a particular undesirable outcome. The gain-framed avoidance refers to the threat one can *avoid* by not smoking ("by not smoking you can avoid mouth diseases," and "if you quit smoking you reduce your risk of breathing difficulties") and the gain-framed benefits is concerning the *benefits* of not smoking ("by not smoking you improve your health and appearance," and "if you quit smoking you will breathe easier") (Goodall and Appiah 2008). The students reported favorable attitudes toward the loss-framed warnings and perceived them as more effective than other ones. It confirms a positive influence of the graphic cigarette warnings labels on adolescents' smoking-related attitudes and behavioral intentions. Similar result was found in Spanish and Pakistan studies. The first one conducted by Portillo et al. (2002), including university students, showed that youth attributed a higher health risk to smoking following the presentation of HWMs. The second one enrolled 388 high school students in 2010 (Zaidi et al. 2011) and compared the responses to questions regarding written health warnings with their associated pictures and multimedia messages. Responses were significantly greater for the pictorial/multi-media messages as deterrents from smoking, in particular about oral cavity, throat and lung cancers, and lung severe diseases, except for "Video of a person recovering from stroke" which was not significantly different from the written statement.

About the effect on cessation behavior, in a Malaysian study the impact of warnings on self-efficacy (who decided to quit) was evaluated (Fathelrahman et al. 2009). The researchers found that between factors associated there was "to quit because of the warnings labels" (OR = 2.36 CI 95 %: 1.90–2.92). Another Australian survey among former smokers suggest that health warnings promote long-term abstinence from smoking. 62 % of quitters reported that the pictorial warnings had "helped them to give up smoking" (Shanahan and Elliott 2009).

In an European study was examined the effectiveness of the text health warnings among daily cigarette smokers in four Member States (Germany, France, the Netherlands, and UK). The labels impact index was measured using a score (LII) with higher scores signifying greater impact. Effectiveness, as measured by the LII, was significant highest in France, lower in the UK, and lowest in Germany and the Netherlands, likely this difference was attributable to the least comprehensive tobacco control programs. Additionally, the impact of the health warning labels was found to be highest among low-income smokers across all countries, and among smokers with lower education in all countries except the UK, suggesting that health warnings may be more effective among low socioeconomic status groups. In this way the effectiveness of health warnings should be further investigated, particularly as some EU countries adopt pictorial warnings and the possible association with socioeconomic differences (Hitchman et al. 2011).

In a recent systematic review, conducted by Hammond (2011), about 100 studies were identified. There is evidence that health warnings can promote smoking cessation and discourage youth uptake. Indeed some smokers reported that warning labels increase their motivation to quit and help them to sustain abstinence after quitting. In addiction larger warnings on packages are significantly more effective than smaller, text-only messages.

It's clear the impact of health warnings on the awareness, but the evidences highlight the importance of contextual factors too, for example:

– Geographical regions or countries: very similar health warnings reported in different area in the World showed unequal levels of effectiveness.
– Different cultures, social norms, and health policies on tobacco consumption have a possible interaction with the effect of the labels.
– The socio-demographical characteristic: dependence, pre-existing health beliefs, personal experience with the health effects of smoking, etc., could lead to different impressions.

In this context a good regulation requires a larger number of warnings to rotate on packages in order to obtain the communication effectiveness in diverse subgroups, including among individual with low literacy/education and children.

On the other hand in some studies the messages have been found with the same appeal to different age groups, that's suggest it's not important to characterize the warnings between adult or youth.

In conclusion, health warnings on the packages, and in particular the pictorial ones, represent an important communication instrument of the risk in the current smoker, in terms of reduction of consumptions levels, increased motivation to quit. Moreover, they represent a help to the former smokers to remain abstinent and have a discouraging effect in youth to start smoking.

References

Berg, C. J., Thrasher, J. F., Westmaas, J. L., Buchanan, T., Pinsker, E. A., & Ahluwalia, J. S. (2011). College student reactions to health warning labels: Sociodemographic and psychosocial factors related to perceived effectiveness of different approaches. *Preventive Medicine, 53*(6), 427–430.

Borland, R., Wilson, N., Fong, G. T., Hammond, D., Cummings, K. M., Yong, H. H., Hosking, W., Hastings, G., Thrasher, J., & McNeill, A. (2009). Impact of graphic and text warnings on cigarette packs: Findings from four countries over five years. *Tobacco Control, 18*(5), 358–364.

Brubaker, R. G., & Mitby, S. K. (1990). Health-risk warning labels on smokeless tobacco products: Are they effective? *Addictive Behaviors, 15*(2), 115–118.

Campaign for tobacco-free kids. (2010). Pictorial warning labels by country and jurisdiction. Accessed April 30, 2012,from http://global.tobaccofreekids.org

Carr-Gregg, M. R. C., & Gray, A. J. (1990). "Generic" packaging—a possible solution to the marketing of tobacco to young people. *The Medical Journal of Australia, 153*(11–12), 685–686.

Chang, F., Chung, C., Yu, P., & Chao, K. (2011). The impact of graphic cigarette warning labels and smoke-free law on health awareness and thoughts of quitting in Taiwan. *Health Education Research, 26*(2), 179–191.

EU Council Recommendation 2003/54/EC of 2 December 2002 on the prevention of smoking and on initiatives to improve tobacco control. Available at http://eur-lex.europa.eu/LexUriServ/LexUriServ.do?uri=OJ:L:2003:022:0031:0034:EN:PDF

Difranza, J. R., Clark, D. M., & Pollay, R. W. (2002). Cigarette package design: Opportunities for disease prevention. *Tobacco Induced Diseases, 1*(2), 97–109.

EU Council Recommendation of 30 November 2009 on smoke free environments 2009/C 296/02. Available at http://eur-lex.europa.eu/LexUriServ/LexUriServ.do?uri=OJ:C:2009:296:0004:0014:EN:PDF

EU Council Recommendation on smoke-free environments. Available at http://eur-lex.europa.eu/LexUriServ/LexUriServ.do?uri=CELEX:32009H1205(01):EN:NOT

European Commission. (2001). Directive on Tobacco products 2001/37/EC http://eur-lex.europa.eu/LexUriServ/LexUriServ.do?uri=CELEX:32001L0037:EN:NOT

European Commission. (2003). Directive on Tobacco Advertising 2003/33/EC http://eur-lex.europa.eu/smartapi/cgi/sga_doc?smartapi!celexapi!prod!CELEXnumdoc&lg=EN&numdoc=32003 L0033&model=guichett

European Commission. (2012). Tobacco policy. Available at http://ec.europa.eu/health/tobacco/policy/index_en.htm

Fathelrahman, A. I., Omar, M., Awang, R., Borland, R., Fong, G. T., Hammond, D., & Zain, Z. (2009). Smokers' responses toward cigarette pack warning labels in predicting quit intention stage of change and self-efficacy. *Nicotine & Tobacco Research, 11*(3), 248–253.

Fischer, P. M., Richards, J. W., Jr., Berman, E. J., & Krugman, D. M. (1989). Recall and eye tracking study of adolescents viewing tobacco advertisements. *JAMA: The Journal of the American Medical Association, 261*(1), 84–89.

Fong, G. T., Cummings, K. M., Borland, R., Hastings, G., Hyland, A., Giovino, G. A., Hammond, D., & Thompson, M. E. (2006). The conceptual framework of the International Tobacco Control (ITC) Policy Evaluation Project. *Tobacco Control, 15*(Suppl 3), iii3–iii11.

Fong, G. T., Hammond, D., Jiang, Y., Li, Q., Quah, A. C. K., Driezen, P., Yan, M., & I. T. C China Project Team. (2010). Perceptions of tobacco health warnings in China compared with picture and text-only health warnings from other countries: an experimental study. *Tobacco Control, 19*(Suppl 2), i69–i77.

Goodall, C., & Appiah, O. (2008). Adolescents' perceptions of Canadian cigarette package warning labels: Investigating the effects of message framing. *Health Communication, 23*(2), 117–127.

Hammond, D. (2008a). Health warning on tobacco packages: Summary of evidence and legal challenges. Accessed March 30, 2012, from http://global.tobaccofreekids.org/en/

Hammond, D. (2008b). British American tobacco the vanishing media. BAT 1978. Cited in: Health warning on tobacco packages: Summary of evidence and legal challenges

Hammond, D. (2011). Health warning messages on tobacco products: a review. *Tobacco Control, 20*(5), 327–337.

Hammond, D., Fong, G. T., McDonald, P. W., Brown, K. S., & Cameron, R. (2004a). Graphic Canadian cigarette warning labels and adverse outcomes: evidence from Canadian smokers. *American Journal of Public Health, 94*(8), 1442–1445.

Hammond, D., Fong, G. T., McDonald, P. W., Cameron, R., & Brown, K. S. (2003). Impact of the graphic Canadian warning labels on adult smoking behaviour. *Tobacco Control, 12*(4), 391–395.

Hammond, D., Fong, G. T., McNeill, A., Borland, R., & Cummings, K. M. (2006). Effectiveness of cigarette warning labels in informing smokers about the risks of smoking: Findings from the International Tobacco Control (ITC) Four Country Survey. *Tobacco Control, 15*(Suppl 3), iii19–iii25.

Hammond, D., Geoffrey, T., Borland, R., Cummings, K. M., McNeill, A., & Driezen, P. (2007). Text and graphic warnings on cigarette packages: Findings from the international tobacco control four country study. *American Journal of Preventive Medicine, 32*(3), 202–209.

Hammond, D., McDonald, P. W., Fong, G. T., Brown, K. S., & Cameron, R. (2004b). The impact of cigarette warning labels and smoke-free bylaws on smoking cessation: evidence from former smokers. *Canadian Journal of Public Health, 95*(3), 201–204.

Hammond, D., Thrasher, J., Reid, J. L., Driezen, P., Boudreau, C., & Santillán, E. A. (2012). Perceived effectiveness of pictorial health warnings among Mexican youth and adults: a population-level intervention with potential to reduce tobacco-related inequities. *Cancer Causes & Control, 23*(Suppl 1), 57–67.

Hitchman, S. C., Mons, U., Nagelhout, G. E., Guignard, R., McNeill, A., Willemsen, M. C., Driezen, P., Wilquin, J. L., Beck, F., Du-Roscat, E., Ptschke-Langer, M., Hammond, D., & Fong, G. T. (2011). Effectiveness of the European Union text-only cigarette health warnings: Findings from four countries. *European Journal of Public Health, 22*(5), 693–699.

Koval, J. J., Aubut, J. L., Pederson, L. L., O'Hegarty, M., & Chan, S. S. H. (2005). The potential effectiveness of warning labels on cigarette packages: The perceptions of young adult Canadians. *Canadian Journal of Public Health, 96*(5), 353–356.

Lien, G., & DeLand, K. (2011). Translating the WHO Framework Convention on Tobacco Control (FCTC): Can we use tobacco control as a model for other non-communicable disease control? *Public Health, 125*, 847–853.

Mannocci, A., Antici, D., Boccia, A., & La Torre, G. (2012). Impact of cigarette packages warnings labels in relation to tobacco-smoking dependence and motivation to quit. *Epidemiologia e Prevenzione, 36*(2), 100–107.

McNeill, A., Craig, L., Willemsen, M. C., & Fong, G. T. (2012). Tobacco control in Europe: A deadly lack of progress. *European Journal of Public Health, 22*(Suppl 1), 1–3.

Nascimento, B. E., Oliveira, L., Vieira, A. S., Joffily, M., Gleiser, S., Pereira, M. G., Cavalcante, T., & Volchan, E. (2008). Avoidance of smoking: The impact of warning labels in Brazil. *Tobacco Control, 17*(6), 405–409.

O'Hegarty, M., Pederson, L. L., Nelson, D. E., Mowery, P., Gable, J. M., & Wortley, P. (2006). Reactions of young adult smokers to warning labels on cigarette packages. *American Journal of Preventive Medicine, 30*(6), 467–473.

O'Hegarty, M., Pederson, L. L., Yenokyan, G., Nelson, D., & Wortley, P. (2007). Young adults' perceptions of cigarette warning labels in the United States and Canada. *Preventing Chronic Disease, 4*(2), A27.

Ozkaya, S., Edinsel, S., Ozkaya, E., & Hamzaþebi, H. (2009). Effects of new warning labels on cigarette packets among high school adolescents. *Tüberküloz ve Toraks, 57*(3), 327–332.

Portillo, F., & Antoñanzas, F. (2002). Information disclosure and smoking risk perceptions. Potential short-term impact on Spanish students of the new European Union directive on tobacco products. *European Journal of Public Health, 12*(4), 295–301.

Qin, Y., Wu, M., Pan, X., Xiang, Q., Huang, J., Gu, Z., Shi, Z., & Zhou, M. (2011). Reactions of Chinese adults to warning labels on cigarette packages: A survey in Jiangsu Province. *BMC Public Health, 11*, 133.
Sebrié, E. M., Blanco, A., & Glantz, S. A. (2010). Cigarette labeling policies in Latin America and the Caribbean: Progress and obstacles. *Salud Pública de México, 52*(Suppl 2), S233–S243.
Shanahan, P., & Elliott, D. (2009). *Evaluation of the Effectiveness of the Graphic Health Warnings on Tobacco Product Packaging 2008*. Canberra: Australian Government Department of Health and Ageing.
Sobani, Z., Nizami, S., Raza, E., ul Ain baloch, N., & Bhan, J. A. (2010). Graphic tobacco health warnings: Which genre to choose? *The International Journal of Tuberculosis and Lung, 14*(3), 356–361.
Stockley, C. S. (2001). The effectiveness of strategies such as health warning labels to reduce alcohol-related harms—an Australian perspective. *The International Journal on Drug Policy, 12*(2), 153–166.
Strahan, E. J., White, K., Fong, G. T., Fabrigar, L. R., Zanna, M. P., & Cameron, R. (2002). Enhancing the effectiveness of tobacco package warning labels: A social psychological perspective. *Tobacco Control, 11*(3), 183–190.
Thrasher, J. F., Arillo-Santillán, E., Villalobos, V., Pérez-Hernández, R., Hammond, D., Carter, J., Sebrié, E., Sansores, R., & Regalado-Piñeda, J. (2012). Can pictorial warning labels on cigarette packages address smoking-related health disparities? Field experiments in Mexico to assess pictorial warning label content. *Cancer Causes & Control, 23*(Suppl 1), 69–80.
Thrasher, J. F., Hammond, D., Fong, G. T., & Arillo-Santillán, E. (2007a). Smokers' reactions to cigarette package warnings with graphic imagery and with only text: A comparison between Mexico and Canada. *Salud Pública de México, 49*(Suppl 2), S233–S240.
Thrasher, J. F., Rousu, M. C., Anaya-Ocampo, R., Reynales-Shigematsu, L. M., Arillo-Santillán, E., & Hernández-Avila, M. (2007b). Estimating the impact of different cigarette package warning label policies: The auction method. *Addictive Behaviors, 32*(12), 2916–2925.
Thrasher, J. F., Villalobos, V., Szklo, A., Fong, G. T., PÚrez, C., SebriÚ, E., Sansone, N., Figueiredo, V., Boado, M., Arillo-Santillán, E., & Bianco, E. (2010). Assessing the impact of cigarette package health warning labels: A cross-country comparison in Brazil Uruguay and Mexico. *Salud Pública de México, 52*(Suppl 2), S206–S215.
Vardavas, C. I., Connolly, G., Karamanolis, K., & Kafatos, A. (2009). Adolescents perceived effectiveness of the proposed European graphic tobacco warning labels. *European Journal of Public Health, 19*(2), 212–217.
Wade, B., Merrill, R. M., & Lindsay, G. B. (2011). Cigarette pack warning labels in Russia: How graphic should they be? *European Journal of Public Health, 21*(3), 366–372.
White, V., Webster, B., & Wakefield, M. (2008). Do graphic health warning labels have an impact on adolescents' smoking-related beliefs and behaviours? *Addiction, 103*(9), 1562–1571.
WHO. (2003a). Framework convention on tobacco control. World Health Assembly Resolution 56 h. Part II: Objective, guiding principles and general obligations. Article 4.1, 2003.
WHO. (2003b). Framework convention on tobacco control. World Health Assembly Resolution 56 h. Part III: Measures relating to the reduction of demand for tobacco. Article 11.
WHO. (2011a). Framework convention on tobacco control. Guidelines for implementation Article 11. Packaging and labeling of tobacco products, http://www.who.int/fctc/guidelines/article_11.pdf
WHO. (2011b). *Report on the global tobacco epidemic. Warning about the dangers of tobacco.* Accessed March 30, 2012, from http://www.who.int/tobacco/mpower/en
Wipfli, H., & Huang, G. (2011). Power of the process: Evaluating the impact of the framework convention on tobacco control negotiations. *Health Policy, 100*(2–3), 107–115.
Wipfli, H., Stillman, F., Tamplin, S., da Costa, L., Silva, S., Yach, D., & Samet, J. (2004). Achieving the framework convention on tobacco control's potential by investing in national capacity. *Tobacco Control, 13*, 433–437.

Wogalter, M. S., Conzola, V. C., & Smith-Jackson, T. L. (2002). Research-based guidelines for warning design and evaluation. *Applied Ergonomics, 33*(3), 219–230.

World Health Organization Framework Convention on Tobacco Control (WHO FCTC). Retrieved from, 27th March, 2011, from http://www.who.int/fctc/en/index.html; Accessed April 30, 2012, from http://www.health.gov.au/internet/main/publishing.nsf/content/F22B9115FD392DA5CA257588007DA955/$File/cover.pdf; Accessed March 30, 2012, from http://www.who.int/tobacco/healthwarningsdatabase/en/

Zaidi, S. M. A., Bikak, A. L., Shaheryar, A., Imam, S. H., & Khan, J. A. (2011). Perceptions of anti-smoking messages amongst high school students in Pakistan. *BMC Public Health, 11*, 117.

Chapter 9
Smoking Among Health Professionals

Giuseppe La Torre, Maria Rosaria Gualano, Rosella Saulle, and Claudio Bontempi

Objectives The aim of this chapter is to offer advanced data and information carried out and supported by relevant and robust scientific reports and studies on:

(a) prevalence of smokers among hospital professionals;
(b) knowledge, attitudes and behaviours towards smoking;
(c) interventions to prevent and discourage smoking in a health-care sector.

The intention is to give an overview on the prevalence of tobacco smoking among health professionals and medicals students in different countries and to show available examples of smoking prevention and cessation training. In this context, the aims of this section were to investigate and to delineate a review based on the analysis of different smoking cessation interventions aimed to health-care workers and to identify the most effective ones for health professionals and medical students and to describe the current efforts to frame policy prevention strategies smoking cessation interventions—targeted in hospital or during study course—to have a greater positive impact as an example by quitting smoking both for themselves and their patients, so for community and public health.

G. La Torre (✉) • R. Saulle • C. Bontempi
Department of Public Health and Infectious Diseases, "Sapienza" University of Rome, Piazzale Aldo Moro 5, Rome 00185, Italy
e-mail: giuseppe.latorre@uniroma1.it; rosella.saulle@uniroma1.it; claudio.bontempi@uniroma1.it

M.R. Gualano
Department of Public Health Sciences, University of Turin, via Santena 5 bis, Turin 10126, Italy
e-mail: mar.guala@gmail.com

G. La Torre, *Smoking Prevention and Cessation*, DOI 10.1007/978-1-4614-7046-5_9,

Learning Outcomes

By the end of this chapter the reader will be able to:

- Know epidemiological data about smoking in health-care workers and learn the theory underling the phenomenon "*smoking habits and attitudes toward tobacco among health-care staff and students*";
- Identify the *important role* among health-care workers staff attitudes towards smoking in determining patient education to quit smoking;
- Evaluate the most effective intervention to prevent and discourage smoking in health-care sector.

9.1 Introduction

Reducing and controlling tobacco smoking should be a primary aim for a certain population in order to reduce harms to health caused by this important risk factor, and there is a general agreement to adopt intervention tools involved in responsibility fields such as health care, education, politics, economy and media.

Tobacco smoking can be considered an old and a new challenge for public health and is both a matter of personal health and a public health concern for health-care providers (Braun et al. 2004; Slater, et al. 2006; Jenkins and Ahijevych 2003; Sarna et al. 2000a).

Health-care professionals have an important role to play both as advisers—influencing smoking cessation—and as role models. Studies have shown that patients are often responsive to counsel received from health-care professionals (Hauser, et al. 2002; Sharp and Tishelman 2005).

Health-care worker staff attitudes towards smoking have been shown to be important in determining the effectiveness of workplace smoking policies and nurses who smoke should set an example by quitting smoking both for themselves and their patients.

Health-care professionals and nurses medical doctor who smoke downplay their role in patient education and tend to show a more negative attitude towards patients (Hocking, et al. 1991). Moreover, it has been proposed that before nurses can serve as role models for positive health behaviours, they must incorporate these behaviours into their own personal lifestyles (Soeken, et al. 1989; Morra and Knobf 1983; Faulkner and Ward 1983; Spencer 1984).

Among health professionals the prevalence of tobacco smoke is extremely high, more than other professional categories, and this could be partly attributed to a low weight that tobacco smoking has in the medical curriculum of future physicians that will contribute in a determinant way to healthy choices of their patients. In order to realise that the medical students need to be adequately trained with the aim of acquire competences and skills that help patients to prevent tobacco smoking and to increase smoking cessation, through a programme oriented to specific issue related to the potential harm of tobacco products.

9.2 Smoking Among Medical Doctors

Medical doctors play a key role in the process of smoking cessation both as advisers and behavioural models for the citizens; so it is relevant to have information on their habits and attitudes towards smoking, especially concerning their role to give help to smokers who wish to quit (Hussain et al. 1993).

In fact, health professionals could better persuade patients to stop smoking if they themselves are not smokers (Smith and Leggat 2007a). Interestingly, other studies have shown that smokers who team up with their health-care providers have more chance to quit than trying on their own.

World Health Organization (WHO 1999; Working Group on Tobacco or Health 1987) has recommended that tobacco-smoking surveys be conducted among health professionals.

In spite of their important and universally accepted role of advisers and exemplars, the investigations conducted among them report that smoking rates among them are quite high. Nevertheless, international trends show physicians' smoking rates are declining in many countries (Smith and Leggat 2007b).

In the United States of America (USA) per capita tobacco consumption has increased from 1880 to 1950, in particular after the First World War (Garfinkel 1997; Giovino 2002). During this period, a lot of physicians used to smoke tobacco and even several medical journals carried out tobacco advertisements (Kawane 1993) (Fig. 9.1).

Conversely, since 1950, smoking habit in the medical profession has decreased worldwide (Smoking control among health-care workers 1993), reflecting the same phenomenon occurred in the general population, and physicians quit to take part in advertising.

In the 1950s and 1960s of last century some studies demonstrated a relationship between tobacco consumption and health risks. In the mid of the 1960s Hammond et al. (1965) showed higher death rates among cigarette smokers in comparison to non-smokers (general population). Moreover, in 1964 the Surgeon General's Advisory Committee on Smoking and Health declared that "Cigarette smoking is a health hazard of sufficient importance in the United States to warrant appropriate remedial action" (U.S. Department of Health, Education and Welfare 1964).

Since 1960, a lot of investigations about smoking habit were conducted among US medical doctors and nowadays it seems that very few physicians are current smokers in USA. In fact in 1959, 40 % of US physicians were smokers (Garfinkel 1976), while in 1975 this percentage appeared to be halved. After 1980, around 21 % of US physicians were current smokers (Garfinkel and Stellman 1986). After 1987 a drastic reduction of smokers' rates among medical doctors was registered: in 1994 prevalence of smokers' physicians was below 10 % (Lee et al. 2004) (Fig. 9.2).

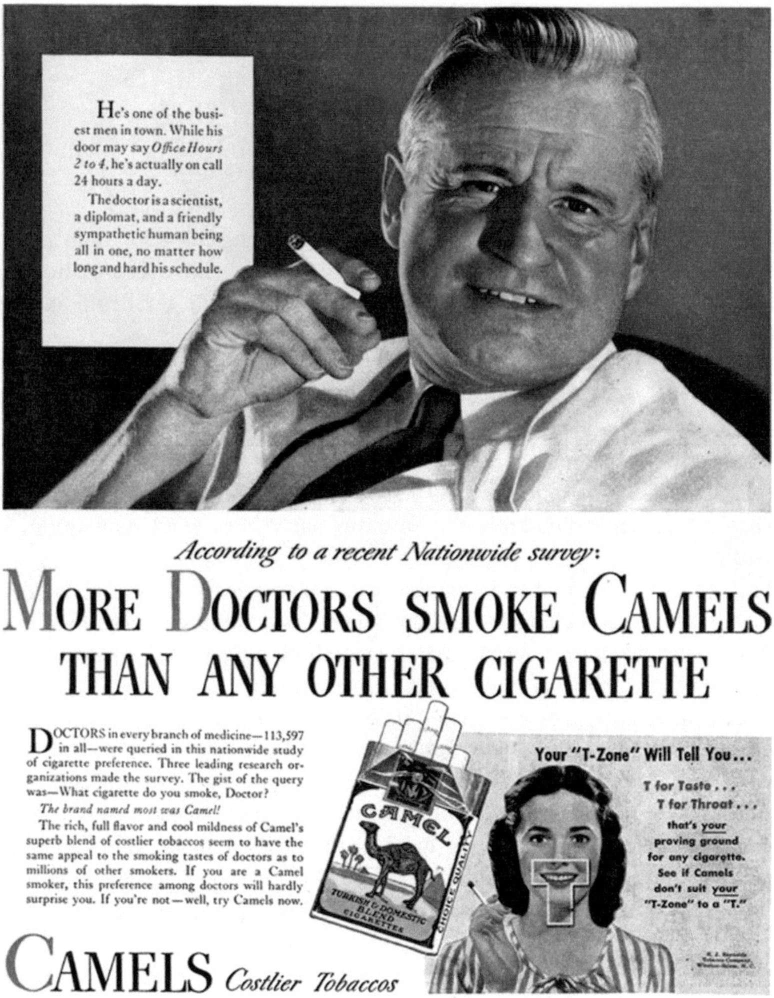
He's one of the busiest men in town. While his door may say *Office Hours 2 to 4*, he's actually on call 24 hours a day.
The doctor is a scientist, a diplomat, and a friendly sympathetic human being all in one, no matter how long and hard his schedule.
According to a recent Nationwide survey:
MORE DOCTORS SMOKE CAMELS
THAN ANY OTHER CIGARETTE
DOCTORS in every branch of medicine—113,597 in all—were queried in this nationwide study of cigarette preference. Three leading research organizations made the survey. The gist of the query was—What cigarette do you smoke, Doctor?
The brand named most was Camel!
The rich, full flavor and cool mildness of Camel's superb blend of costlier tobaccos seem to have the same appeal to the smoking tastes of doctors as to millions of other smokers. If you are a Camel smoker, this preference among doctors will hardly surprise you. If you're not—well, try Camels now.
CAMEL
TURKISH & DOMESTIC BLEND CIGARETTES
CHOICE QUALITY
Your "T-Zone" Will Tell You...
T for Taste...
T for Throat...
that's your proving ground for any cigarette. See if Camels don't suit your "T-Zone" to a "T."
CAMELS *Costlier Tobaccos*

Fig. 9.1 When "more doctors smoked Camels"

In Great Britain a long-lasting longitudinal study called the British Doctor's Study (Doll and Hill 1954, 1964; Doll and Peto 1976; Doll et al. 1980, 1994, 2004) has been conducted since the beginning of the 1950. In 1951 the British Medical Association enrolled 34,440 British doctors to investigate their smoking habits in a prospective cohort. During the first 20 years follow-up, the researchers recorded all the certified causes of deaths and subsequent changes in smoking habits. The ratio of the death rate among cigarette smokers to that among non-smokers of comparable age was, for men under 70 years, about 2:1, while for men over 70 years it was 1.5:1. This study was very important to suggest a clear association between tobacco consumption and diseases, particularly lung cancer. In fact during the period of the

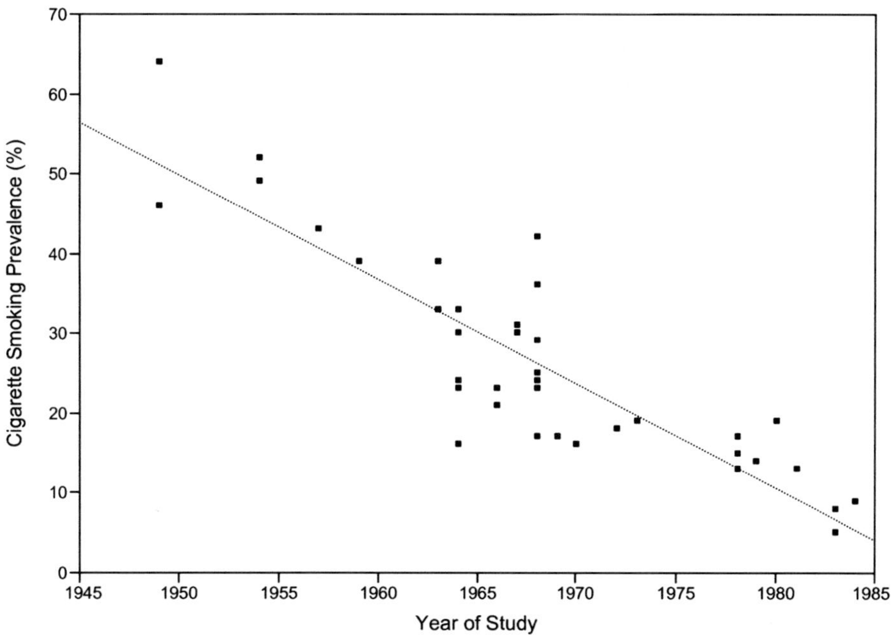

Fig. 9.2 Decreasing trend of cigarette smoking prevalence among physicians in the USA between 1949 and 1984. From: The historical decline of tobacco smoking among United States physicians: 1949–1984. Smith DR (2008) Tob Induc Dis 4:9

study all the enrolled doctors reduced its cigarette consumption and consequently lung cancer became less common as the study progressed, but other cancers did not (Doll and Peto 1976). After 40 years follow-up, Doll and colleagues found that the percentage of British physicians who smoked cigars, pipes or cigarettes declined from 62 % to 18 % between 1951 and 1990 (Doll et al. 1994).

As far concerns other countries, we can describe similar trends have also been demonstrated in other countries. In Scandinavia for example current smokers among medical doctors decreased from 74 % (1952) to 19 % (1984) in Norway, from 34 % (1969) to 19 % (1984) in Finland, and from 64 % (1970) to 28 % (1989) in Denmark and from 46 % in 1969 to 37 % in 1972 in Sweden (Faith-Ell and Wilhelmsen 1973; van Reek and Adriaanse 1991).

The research by Hay reported smoking rates of New Zealand doctors declined from 20 % in 1976 to 15 % in 1981 and to 5 % in 1996 (Hay 1998).

The prevalence of smoking among Japanese male physicians decreased from 27.1 % in 2000 to 21.5 % in 2004 and then to 15.0 % in 2008 (Kaneita et al. 2010). A systematic review conducted by Abdullah and colleagues 2011 shows that in China current smoking prevalence among physicians ranged from 14 % to 64 %, with substantial differences by gender (men: 26–61 %; women: 0–19 %).

Nevertheless, in some countries medical doctors still smoke at high rates. For example in Italy, a recent study carried out in several Italian hospital enrolling more than 1,000 health-care professionals, revealed a prevalence of current smokers accounting for 44 % and medical doctors for 33.9 %. Such smoking rate is much higher than the rate of smokers among the general Italian population (22 %) (Ficarra et al. 2011).

Only few studies focused their attention on investigating smoking habit by different medical specialties. For example in the 1960s Tate and Fulghum (1965) reported that the smoking rate among Florida physicians was 40 % in urology, 37 % in obstetrics/gynaecology, psychiatry and general practice, while Coe and Brehm (1971) registered that 31 % of internists and 29 % of general practitioners smoked. In addition in 1968 Eisinger (1972) and Tamerin and Eisinger 1972 found that 36 % of paediatricians and 42 % of psychiatrists, respectively, smoked cigarettes. Fortmann and coll (Fortmann et al. 1985) reported that primary care physicians had the highest smoking prevalence rate by speciality.

Finally we would like to underline a paradox: between 5 % and 19 % of *pulmonary* physicians were current smokers (Sachs 1984).

We can try to examine what could be the reasons of the high rates of smoking among medical doctors, especially in some countries, showing that tobacco control measures have not been uniformly successful worldwide. The main potential reason for the large smoking prevalence among health-care workers might be high occupational stress, which is considered a key factor in addition to addiction, enjoyment and peer influence.

9.3 Smoking Prevalence Among Nurses

Smoking among nurses has been recognised as a serious concern affecting the profession since the 1970s, when female registered nurses smoked at a higher rate (38.9 %) than women in the US population (32.0 %) and at a substantially higher rate than physicians (21 %) (*U.S. Department of Health and Human Services* 1980).

Smoking prevalence decreased among nurses between the early 1970s and the 1990s (Nelson et al. 1994), from 31.7 % to 18.3 % among registered nurses (RNs) and from 37.1 % to 27.2 % among licensed practical nurses (LPNs), However, the smoking rates for nurses remained higher than for physicians or dentists.

In 1999, LPNs continued to smoke at higher rates than RNs: 21.7 % versus 38 %, respectively (Collins et al. 1999). In a critical review of the literature, Rowe and Macleod-Clark (2000a) identified high smoking rates amongst nurses (39–48 %) in the 1980s, triggering an increase in the number and quality of international studies into tobacco smoking in the nursing profession.

Prevalence data from the Tobacco Use Supplement of the 1992–1993 "*Current Population Survey*" showed that among registered nurses (RNs), 18.2 % were current smokers and 21.6 % were former smokers and that among LPNs, 28.9 % were current smokers and 17.3 % were former smokers (Department of Commerce, Census Bureau, 1995).

Smith and Leggat (2007c) identified in a recent international review that the average prevalence of smoking amongst nurses was around 20 % with trends in some countries supporting greater reductions in smoking rates.

The USA, for example has been proactive with a national programme designed to help nurses quit (http://www.tobaccofreenurses.org/) and has continued to see a progressive decline in smoking prevalence amongst 237,648 women in the Nurses' Health Study, from 33.2 % in 1976 to 8.4 % in 2003 (Sarna et al. 2008). Tobacco consumption amongst nurses in Australia declined from 53 % in 1976 (Kirkby et al. 1976) to 21 % in 1999 (Hughes and Rissel 1999) and in Canada from 32 % in 1982 (Senior 1982) to 12 % in 2002. Smoking rates amongst nurses in the UK fell from 40 % in 1984 (Spencer 1984) to 20 % in 1993 (Hussain et al. 1993). Many nations remain increasingly burdened by the tobacco epidemic, for example high smoking prevalence rates can be seen amongst nurses in Italy (36 %) (Proietti et al. 2006), Greece (57 %) (Vagropoulos et al. 2006), Turkey (45 %) (Sezer et al. 2007) and Bosnia and Herzegovina (51 %) (Hodgetts et al. 2004).

Tobacco smoking in Jordan is common among both health professionals and the general population, especially among men. A recent series of surveys in Jordan estimated smoking rates of 24.9 % among youth, with a 76.3 % self-report of SHS exposure (Al Qaseer and Batarseh 2009), 22.4 % among male physicians (Merill et al. 2007) and 28.6 % among college students (Haddad and Malak 2002; Haddad and Pertro 2006) which rose to 35 % in 2008 (Khader and Alsadi 2008) Jordanian nurses had a slightly higher percentage who desired to quit smoking compared with the percentage in the Northern Ireland study (77 % vs.73 %) (McCarty et al. 2001).

The National Lifestyles, Attitudes and Nutrition Survey in Ireland (Morgan et al. 2008) found that 29 % (27 % in 2002) of respondents were smokers, 31 % men and 27 % women. The highest prevalence rates of smokers found in the age groups 20–25 years (28 %) and 26–30 years (34 %).

There has been a lag in research into the smoking prevalence amongst Australian nurses since the 1990s. In Australia in 1991, Nagle et al. (1999) conducted a survey of 388 nurses and found 22 % of them to be current smokers. Similarly in 1997 a survey of 610 nurses found 21 % of them to be current smokers (Hughes and Rissel 1999). These results were just below the smoking rates amongst women in the Australian community at the time (23.8 % in 1992; 23.2 % in 1995) (Hill and White 1995; Hill et al. 1998). Recent results, published on the New Zealand Census 2006, indicate that comparable nations have been successful in further reducing smoking rates amongst nurses, with smoking rates of 13 % amongst female nurses and 20 % amongst male nurses (Edwards et al. 2008). Nursing is a predominantly female occupation and data suggest that more than 70 % of women who smoke daily express a desire to quit regardless of age or ethnicity (Bialous et al. 2004).

Approximately half of all smokers will make a quit attempt each year and around 95 % of quitters will fail on any single attempt (Fiore and United States Tobacco Use and Dependence Guideline Panel 2000).

The majority of nurses commence smoking prior to entering nursing training and the reasons for continued smoking are similar to that of the female adolescent population (Jenkins and Ahijevych 2003; O'Connor and Harrison 1992; Rowe and

Macleod-Clark 2000a, b; Rowe and Macleod-Clark 2000a, b; Clark and McCann 2008). In a survey of 366 undergraduate nursing students, Clark and McCann (2008) found that peers and friends were an important influence on the decision to commence smoking. During their training most of the nursing students wanted to cease smoking, multiple quit attempts were common and barriers to stopping included pleasure obtained from smoking and the effects of stress.

It is important to understand the profiles and smoking behaviours of nurses, and attitudes to smoking cessation strategies, in order to improve nursing efforts towards reducing tobacco-related burden of disease.

Elements of work environment including shift work, heavy physical job strain and level of empowerment in the workplace are amongst the important factors that have an impact on smoking behaviour in nurses (Bialous et al. 2004; Sanderson et al. 2005). The prevalence of smoking has been reported as higher in certain specialty areas such as psychiatry, gerontology and emergency departments (Trinkoff and Storr 1998a). Data on smoking prevalence by nursing specialties show higher rates of smoking among psychiatric (23 %), gerontologic (18.2 %), and emergency nurses (18 %), and lower rates among paediatric critical care nurses (7.6 %) and nurses working in general paediatrics, women's health and school settings (9.6 %) (Trinkoff and Storr 1998b). Lower smoking rates have been observed in oncology nurses (4.5 %) (Lally et al. 2008) and also paediatric critical care nurses (Trinkoff and Storr 1998b).

The reasons for this are unclear, although these have been considered high stress areas for work, and the psychological level of job demands for nurses have been associated with the psychological aspects of nicotine dependence (Ota et al. 2004): for addicted tobacco users, the lack of nicotine leads to withdrawal symptoms including, but not limited to, headache, nausea, constipation or diarrhoea, fatigue, drowsiness and insomnia, irritability, difficulty concentrating, anxiety, depression and cravings.

Oncology nursing organisations have been active in research studies describing advocacy activities of nurses in the prevention of cancer (Lally et al. 2008). Whether areas of nursing which focus more on preventive health care, such as oncology and paediatrics, influence smoking behaviour of nurses remains unclear too.

Smoking among nurses, LPNs and nursing students has been described for more than 50 years but most published studies addressing smoking prevalence among nurses are limited in both sample size and setting. Moreover, research and intervention efforts focused on assisting nurses with cessation have been limited (Gorin 2001; Kitajima et al. 2002; McKenna et al. 2003).

Ironically, nurses with a smoking history have contributed to our knowledge about the impact of tobacco on women's health through their participation in the Nurses Health Study (U.S. Department of Health and Human Services 2004).

More than 70 % of the women who smoked daily expressed a desire to quit smoking regardless of ethnicity or age (U.S. Department of Health and Human Services 2004).

Women were as likely as men, or more likely, to have attempted smoking cessation in the preceding year and equally likely to have maintained abstinence (Centers for Disease Control and Prevention 1994).

9.4 Public Awareness About Smoking Habits Among Health Professionals

Smoking is very much a part of social unity, whether in the workplace or at home.

National and international statistics highlight the fact that tobacco smoke is the greatest single preventable risk factor for morbidity and mortality within the general population: each year more than five million people worldwide die from smoking-related illnesses (WHO 2003) and globally, tobacco use will kill an estimated eight million people annually by 2030 (WHO 2008).

Through both primary and secondary exposure, tobacco use affects every system in the body and every patient group to whom nurses provide care in every nation (NCI 1999; DHHS 2004; Malone 2006).

Research has found that smoking cessation interventions provided at inpatient level can improve short- and long-term morbidity and mortality rates and also reduce overall health care: tobacco use cessation gives immediate and major health benefits and is the "gold standard" in cost-effective disease prevention strategies (Eddy 1992; Maciosek et al. 2006).

The treatment of tobacco-related diseases makes up an economic burden to the health-care system as well as to society due to the fact that almost half of those who die due to smoking die before the age of 70 (Peto 1994).

A number of studies have pointed to the potential value of health professionals taking an active role in facilitating smoking cessation in general population (Padula 1992; Katz et al. 2012) and these professionals are in an ideal position for providing smoking-related counselling to their patients and could be the largest workforce providing effective smoking cessation interventions and powerful advocates for tobacco free communities; studies have shown that patients are often responsive to counsel received from health-care professionals (Hauser et al. 2002; Sharp and Tishelman 2005). As an example, there is evidence that in particular setting, i.e. the Emergency Department (ED), nurses and physicians can effectively deliver efficiently smoking cessation counselling to smokers using the 5As framework (ask–advise–assess–assist–arrange) (Katz et al. 2012). In the ED setting, Bernstein and colleagues 2011 performed a clinical trial randomising two types of treatment for smokers: (1) usual care, accompanied by giving a smoking cessation brochure or (2) enhanced care, receiving the brochure, a motivational interview, nicotine patches and a phone call at 3 days. After 3 months, differences between these two groups did not exist (quitting rates 13.2 % vs. 14.7 % in the groups, respectively), demonstrating that even low-intensity screening and referral may prompt substantial numbers of ED smokers to quit or attempt to quit.

In a systematic review conducted by Rigotti et al. 2007, the effectiveness of interventions for smoking cessation initiated for hospitalised patients was assessed. Analysing 17 randomised and quasi-randomised clinical trials, these authors found that only behavioural interventions of high intensity that begin during a hospital stay and include at least 1 month of supportive contact after discharge are effective in promoting smoking cessation among hospitalised patients (OR = 1.65; 95 % CI: 1.44–1.90) (Rigotti et al. 2007).

Another systematic review demonstrated there is evidence that medical advice increased the success of quit attempts. Offering assistance by medical doctors is more effective than opportunistic brief physician advice to stop smoking among smokers not selected by motivation to quit, both for behavioural support (RR = 1.69; 95 % CI: 1.24–2.31) and for offering medication (RR = 1.39; 95 % CI: 1.25–1.54) (Aveyard et al. 2011).

Smoking cessation guidelines, developed from best available evidence, recommend that health-care professionals should assess patients' smoking habits and give opportunistic smoking cessation advice as part of routine patient care (Fiore et al. 2000; Raw et al. 1998; Australian Department of Health and Ageing 2004; Fiore and United States Tobacco Use and Dependence Guideline Panel 2008). Nursing regulatory bodies and the community as a whole expect that nurses should counsel patients in their care on health-related issues (Saarmann et al. 2000; Shuttleworth 2004).

A meta-analysis of nurses' effectiveness in smoking cessation demonstrated a significant increase in the likelihood of people quitting (Rice and Stead 2008); however, incorporating smoking cessation care into routine practice has been difficult to achieve (Nagle et al. 1999; Gomm et al. 2002; Scanlon et al. 2008).

Acute care nurses are in a unique position to provide smoking cessation counselling as they not only comprise the largest group of health-care professionals but also administer care 24 h a day, 7 days a week.

In a survey of 415 practice nurses in Kansas found that attendance at tobacco-related continuing education was a significant predictor of respondents' implementing smoking cessation programmes with patients.

Patients in acute settings are physically vulnerable and are (on some level) contemplating or actively seeking advice on how they can improve their health, for instance by smoking cessation (Conroy et al. 2005). This "window of opportunity" has been shown to increase health motivation and has also been associated with increased abstinence from smoking while in the acute care setting.

As the largest group of health professionals, with an important role of caring for the under-served nurses play an essential role in helping patients stop smoking and in reducing disparities in access to tobacco control services and programmes. The efficacy of nurses in the delivery of tobacco cessation treatment has been supported by numerous studies (Rice and Stead 2008).

Significant progress in the reduction of cigarette smoking has been made in the past decades, but tobacco use continues to be the leading cause of preventable illness and death in the USA.

The goal of the U.S. Department of Health and Human Services, as expressed in Healthy People 2010, was to reduce overall smoking prevalence to 12 %.

Despite calls for international efforts in tobacco control, responses from nursing organisations throughout the world have been inconsistent, and nurses' involvement in tobacco control remains a promising area for growth (Percival et al. 2003). Evidence suggests that nurses are willing and able to provide health promotion activities and are regarded as highly effective in this area (Saarmann et al. 2000).

However, studies demonstrate that acute care nurses currently lack the knowledge, skills and confidence to be effective when providing smoking cessation interventions. In a qualitative study of 12 acute care nurses in Scotland, Whyte et al. (2006) identified that nurses had opportunities to advise patients about smoking but did not always recognise these or have the knowledge to respond appropriately (Gomm et al. 2002): nurses often had received no formal training in providing cessation advice. These findings are similar to those of Nagle, Schofield and Redman (1999) in New South Wales who found that 75 % of respondents believed nurses should counsel patients who wanted to stop smoking but perceived that nurses lacked the skills and knowledge necessary to provide suitable counselling. Nurses are more likely to perform smoking cessation interventions if they believe they have the necessary skills and knowledge.

Scanlon et al. (2008) showed that nurses who agreed to have a responsibility to counsel patients on health-related conditions lacked awareness that smoking contributes to a wide range of specific health conditions and lacked knowledge of smoking cessation interventions, reducing their willingness to provide cessation interventions to patients.

Also Nagle et al. (1999) found that Australian nurses had a poor knowledge of the health effects of smoking and strategies for smoking cessation. Whyte et al. (2006) found that, although nurses would participate in interactions about smoking with patients, the quality of their knowledge was poor and the nurses have many of the same misconceptions about cessation as the general public.

Indeed, although nurses have a general knowledge about the harmful health effects of tobacco use, they do not recognise the biochemical processes related to nicotine addiction and withdrawal and the benefits of scientifically based combinations of strategies to achieve cessation (Sarna et al. 2000a).

Nagle et al. (1999) found that 63 % of their sample was too busy to do this, while lack of time was not a major consideration for nurses surveyed by Gomm et al. (2002). In general, respondents were willing to implement smoking cessation interventions. Nearly one-quarter were already doing so, while over half indicated that they were ready to intervene but needed help to do so. This suggests that they would welcome additional training and support to enable them to implement effective interventions. The lack of preparation in providing smoking cessation interventions during nursing education in China (Sophia et al. 2007) could be one of the main barriers preventing nurses from such practices, although extrinsic barriers such as lack of motivation among patients, heavy workload and lack of time were also important. Lack of education about tobacco has been identified as a barrier among nurses and other health-care professionals too (Lancaster et al. 2000; Sarna et al. 2000b; Sarna et al. 2001).

There were found significant differences in perceived competence and other aspects of cessation interventions between nurses with prior training in smoking cessation counselling and others without such training. Nurses with training in smoking cessation counselling showed more positive attitudes and engaged in smoking cessation interventions more frequently, which about their roles and responsibilities towards smoking cessation interventions, intervened more frequently,and perceived greater competence. So, the positive correlation between knowledge and willingness also suggests that lack of knowledge is a factor affecting nurses' willingness to provide smoking cessation advice.

Also the literature suggests that nurses who smoke have feelings of guilt and shame about their own smoking practices and may perceive a lack of understanding by non-smoking colleagues and managers about their need of support for smoking cessation (Bialous et al. 2004).

Scanlon et al. (2008) in his study had indicated that there needs to be more emphasis on the effects of smoking in both undergraduate and post-registration nursing education, along with discussion of smoking cessation strategies, so nurses are more knowledgeable, confident and ready to provide interventions for hospitalised patients.

Numerous studies have shown that the inclusion of tobacco control in professional curricula is necessary to increase the number of nurses prepared to deliver effective smoking cessation interventions (Bakker et al. 2005; Hall et al. 2005; Hornberger and Edwards 2004; McCarty et al. 2001; Sarna et al. 2000a; Yang et al. 2006).

Recent reviews of curricula of schools of nursing in the USA (Hornberger and Edwards 2004; Sarna et al. 2001; Wewers et al. 2004) and schools of medicine (Roddy et al. 2004) showed inadequate content and time spent on smoking and smoking cessation. Gaps in nurses' education continue to persist as smoking is marginalised as a lifestyle issue and evidence-based smoking cessation interventions have not received appropriate priority in classroom teaching or clinical practice.

Previous research in western countries has shown that nurses' attitudes and self-perceived competence were significantly related to smoking cessation practice (Borrelli et al. 2001; Johnston et al. 2005). The majority of Chinese nurses in this survey reported positive attitudes towards tobacco control policies and their role and responsibility in helping patients stop smoking. Less than half (48 %) believed that only non-smokers could intervene with smoking. Sarna et al. (2000b) reported that smoking status negatively affected tobacco control attitudes. In that study, fewer smoking nurses than non-smokers supported tobacco control policies (e.g. policies that restrict tobacco use in public places, ensure smoke free environments, increase cigarette taxes, etc.). An important action will be monitoring the trends of smoking among nurses in China because this may influence their attitudes about tobacco control.

So, despite recognition of their professional responsibility as models of good health practices and known health risks associated with smoking, many nurses continue to smoke (Mackay and Eriksen 2002) and there is the evidence that nurses who smoke are not adequately fulfilling this role. Despite the emphasis on nurses serving as role models for a healthy lifestyle, entering the nursing profession did not provide an adequate incentive to quit, or the resources for cessation, as might be expected (Jenkins and Ahijevych 2003). Prepared nurses who are motivated to act can save millions of lives by helping smokers quit and by supporting more effective tobacco control measures (Sophia et al. 2007).

Smoking among nurses remains a barrier to interventions with patients because of their smoking habits (Jenkins and Ahijevych 2003; Rowe and Macleod-Clark 2000a; Sarna et al. 2000a): nurses who smoke are less likely to participate in health promotion counselling with their patients who smoke; smoking in nurses is one of the many factors acting as a deterrent to their provision of smoking cessation care (Feeney et al. 1997; Hughes and Rissel 1999; Nagle et al. 1999; Sarna et al. 2000b; McKenna et al. 2001).

Most smoking habits will have been well established prior to becoming a nurse, some of the nurses started to smoke before entering nursing school, whereas others described starting to smoke as they entered the nursing profession: there have been only isolated efforts by nursing schools to promote smoking cessation among nursing students. Thus, in addition to the identified need to increase tobacco-related content in the curricula of nursing schools (Rowe and Macleod-Clark 2000b; Sarna et al. 2000b; Wewers et al. 2004), it is important for nursing schools to provide support for students who want to quit.

Findings indicate that nurses quit smoking for many of the same reasons that other women quit (e.g. pregnancy, their children, or concern for their health) (U.S. Department of Health and Human Services 2004).

Many nurses who smoke, but desire to quit, have had multiple unsuccessful quit attempts and perceive stress, fear of weight gain and anxiety as barriers to quitting. The majority of the participants were overweight or obese, and it is consistent with the literature on women and smoking that overweight and obesity are higher among former smokers than among current smokers, lending support to the fears women express about gaining weight when they quit smoking. Thus, cessation intervention for nurses and women should address the potential for weight gain and weight management strategies.

However, research into the smoking behaviour of nurses has been inconsistent and has not kept pace uniformly with government surveys on smoking prevalence in the general population (Rowe and Macleod-Clark 2000a) and despite the evidence that nurses continue to smoke at high rates, limited support has been provided by the nursing profession to help nurses quit, and published studies have not detailed the cessation strategies used by nurses who have achieved long-term abstinence (Chalmers et al. 2001).

There is clearly a need for the nursing profession to send out strong messages to nurses about smoking, to develop a systematic approach to monitoring their smoking behaviour and to provide support for all nurses who smoke to quit.

Existing scientific findings about smoking and the best strategies to enhance cessation report that theoretical perspectives describing behavioural change have guided cessation interventions on a personal and professional level. Nurses' struggles with addiction, pattern of quit attempts and relapse were similar to what has been described in the general population (Fiore et al. 2000). To be effective in supporting nurses' quit efforts, interventions should include psychological and behavioural preparation, with reasonable expectations for withdrawal.

The development of personal factors that facilitate cessation among nurses was based on Bandura's description of self-efficacy and empowerment to quit. High perceived self-efficacy predicted individual success in taking action to quit smoking. Low self-efficacy has similarly been linked with increased risk for relapse. Thus, nurses should be convinced that their behaviour will lead to successful quitting and that social support and skills training will increase their success at cessation. However, if they are unable to access these resources, they may have low self-efficacy. The nicotine addiction model (Fiore et al. 2000) interfaces with self-efficacy and quitting behaviour because addiction could interfere with self-efficacy if not properly addressed.

Additionally, more former smokers recognised social factors as important influences on smoking behaviour, and smoke-free workplaces offered an incentive to quit. Not surprisingly, in some cases, treatment of patients suffering from tobacco-related diseases served as a motivating factor for nurses to quit.

This information was used to develop the Tobacco Free Nurses Initiative, the first ever national programme to support nurses' smoking cessation efforts (http://www.tobaccofreenurses.org).

9.5 Smoking Among Health Profession Students

Even if tobacco use is widely recognised as one of the most important preventable risk factors for the onset of several chronic diseases such as cardiovascular and respiratory disease, many types of cancer and non neoplastic pathology, health professionals are aware that tobacco smoke has a leading role as the most preventable cause of death and disability; paradoxically, they are not sufficiently conscious of their fundamental role to help their patients for quit smoking (Fiore et al. 1994; Zwar and Richmond 2006). In fact in many countries, physicians and nurses forgot their key role as behaviour model and so the prevalence of smoking is higher among health-care workers than among the general population (Ficarra et al. 2011; Ruiz-Canela et al. 2009).

In terms of public health, helping people to stop smoking is widely demonstrated to be economically opportune in term of cost-efficacy. However, only one in five patients receive advice and assistance to quit smoking, and a very low percentage receives a proper pharmacological therapy (Ferketich et al. 2006). A possible reason for such an incongruence can be recognised in the lack of complete training in smoking cessation techniques in medical curricula, while there is evidence that introducing tobacco knowledge into the curriculum is effective in reducing the prevalence of smoking among medical students (Richmond and Kehoe 1997).

In America, Europe and Asia several studies investigated knowledge, attitudes and behaviours of students towards tobacco use, especially among medical and sanitary students, which represent the future medical practitioners (Ferrante et al. 2010; Melani et al. 2000; Heras et al. 2000; Dekker et al. 1993; Waalkens et al. 1992; Clareboets et al. 2010; Tirodimos et al. 2009; Raupach et al. 2009; Borges et al. 2008).

We can recognise basic weaknesses in many of these surveys: the absence of a standardised method used for the definition of smoker status, the use of different methods in the sampling process and different questionnaires and data collection procedures (Smith and Leggat 2007c).

In order to create a standardised research method, the WHO, US Centers for Disease Control and Prevention (CDC) and the Canadian Public Health Association developed and implemented a single protocol: the Global Health Professions Student Survey (GHPSS) (Warren et al. 2009).

GHPSS is part of the Global Tobacco Surveillance System (GTSS), which collects data through three surveys: the Global Youth Tobacco Survey (GYTS), the Global School Personnel Survey (GSPS) and GHPSS.

GHPSS is a school-based survey of third-year students pursuing advances degree in dentistry, medicine, nursing or pharmacy. The GHPSS questionnaire is composed by core questions on demographics, prevalence of cigarette smoking and use of other tobacco products, exposure to second hand smoke, desire to quit smoking, and training received to provide patients counselling on cessation techniques (Warren et al. 2011a).

In this way researchers can apply this single method in many different countries around the World; this condition allows to coherently compare different geographical situations, translating and adjusting the questionnaire in the different languages.

Since 2005 the GHPSS was performed in several countries in South America, Europe, Africa and Asia, and in Table 9.1 the prevalence of current smoking in different countries is reported.

Table 9.1 Prevalence of current smokers among health professional students in GHPSS surveys

Survey year	Country	Prevalence % current smokers (95 % CI)
2005	Albania	43.3 (40.7–45.9)
2007	Algeria	9.0 (8.1–9.9)
2005	Argentina	35.5 (33.6–37.4)
2006	Armenia	20.4 (16.1–25.4)
2006	Bangladesh	27.5 (21.3–34.7)
2006	Bolivia	41.1 (35.3–47.2)
2006	Bosnia and Herzegovina	40.3 (39.2–41.5)
2006	Bangladesh	27.2 (20.8–34.8)
2006	Brazil, Rio de Janeiro	16.9 (15.6–18.2)
2005	Cambodia	6.4 (4.1–9.7)
2008	Chile	28.4 (27.1–29.6)
2006	Costa Rica	32.8 (CI missing)
2005	Croatia	36.6 (34.1–39.2)
2008	Cuba	29.5 (27.6–31.4)
2006	Czech Republic	21.7 (19.5–24.0)
2005	Egypt	7.9 (5.7–10.7)
2006	Ghana	1.3 (0.6–2.8)
2008	Guatemala	22.5 (19.8–25.4)
2005	India	11.6 (8.8–15.2)
2006	Indonesia	8.6 (5.4–13.5)
2007	Iran	5.6 (4.6–6.9)
2005	Iraq	17.5 (15.4–19.8)
2008	Jamaica	6.7 (4.3–10.3)

(continued)

Table 9.1 (continued)

Survey year	Country	Prevalence % current smokers (95 % CI)
2008	Kenya	9.8 (7.7–12.5)
2008	Kyrgyzstan	36.6 (33.9–39.4)
2006	Lebanon	28.2 (25.1–31.4)
2006	Libyan Arab Jamahiriya	10.1 (9.1–11.2)
2006	Lithuania	27.3 (23.5–31.4)
2006	Mexico	35.3 (29.8–41.3)
2006	Myanmar	12.4 (11.7–13.1)
2005	Nepal	23.5 (9.1–48.5)
2008	Niger	37.1 (33.9–41.7)
2008	Panama	11.1 (9.6–12.9)
2008	Paraguay	22.3 (20.9–23.8)
2006	Peru	32.7 (28.5–37.3)
2006	Republic of Serbia	34.7 (33.3–36.2)
2006	Russian Federation	38.8 (37.6–39.9)
2006	Saudi Arabia	11.6 (9.2–14.6)
2006	Serbia	34.7 (33.2–36.2)
2006	Slovakia	30.4 (29.0–31.9)
2006	Slovenia	20.9 (17.3–25.0)
2006	Sri Lanka	4.1 (3.4–5.0)
2006	South Korea	16.0 (12.0–21.1)
2007	Sudan	7.7 (6.3–9.4)
2006	Syrian Arab Republic	16.8 (16.2–17.5)
2006	Thailand	2.1 (1.6–2.9)
2007	Tunisia	9.9 (8.6–11.3)
2005	Uganda	2.8 (1.8–4.2)
2008	Uruguay	32.3 (31.2–33.3)
2007	Vietnam	11.2 (10.6–11.7)
2007	Gaza Strip	22.7 (19.7–26.0)
From: Tobacco use, exposure to secondhand smoke, and cessation counseling among medical students: cross-country data from the Global Health Professions Student Survey (GHPSS), 2005–2008. Warren CW, Sinha DN, Lee J, Lea V, Jones NR. BMC Public Health. 2011 Feb 1;11:72.		
2009	Greece	28.8 (24.2–33.8)
From: Tobacco Use, Exposure to Secondhand Smoke, and Cessation Counseling Among Health Professions Students: Greek Data from the Global Health Professions Student Survey (GHPSS). Barbouni A, Hadjichristodoulou C, Merakou K, Antoniadou E, Kourea K, Miloni E, Warren CW, Rahiotis G, Kremastinou J. Int J Environ Res Public Health. 2012 Jan;9(1):331–42. Epub 2012 Jan 19		
2009	Italy	31.3 (27.8–34.9)
2009	Germany	28. 0 (14.6–21.4)
2009	Spain	28.9 (24.2–33.6)
2009	Poland	28.7 (25.5–32)
From: Tobacco use among medical students in Europe: results of a multicentre study using the Global Health Professions Student Survey. La Torre G, Kirch W, Bes-Rastrollo M, Ramos RM, Czaplicki M, Gualano MR, Thümmler K, Ricciardi W, Boccia A; GHPSS Collaborative Group. Public Health. 2012 Feb;126(2):159–64. Epub 2011 Dec 15		

Warren and colleagues (2011b) applied the GHPSS from 2005 to 2009 in 44 countries, studying the behaviours of Dentistry students.

The results of his study showed a wide range of percentage of current smoker students: the highest value above 40 %, has been measured in six countries: Kyrgyzstan, Macedonia, Moldova, Russian Federation, Chile and Mexico, while in three countries has been measured rates <5 % : Libya, Thailand and Cambodia.

Regarding African countries, 10.2 % of dentistry students currently smoked cigarettes in Algeria, and 16.7 % currently smoked cigarettes in Senegal, with males significantly more likely to smoke than females in both sites. In Eastern Mediterranean regions the percentage of current smoker students ranged from 33.4 % of Gaza Strip/West Bank to 2.3 % of Libya, with two countries reporting rates over 20 %: Lebanon 31.6 % and Syria 23.6 %.

In Europe, five countries reported percentage of current smokers over 40 %: Bulgaria 52.2 %, Kyrgyzstan 44.0 %, Macedonia 52.5 %, Moldova 65.2 % and Russian Federation 43.7 %; while the lowest rates were founded in Slovenia 17.9 % and Latvia 19.6 %. In American countries current cigarette smokers was at least 20 % in all sites, except Guatemala, Guyana, Panama and Paraguay and over 40 % in Chile and Mexico.

In the South-East Asia region, current cigarette smoking ranged from over 20 % in Bangladesh and Myanmar to <5 % in Thailand.

In Western Pacific region, current cigarette smoking ranged from 33.3 % in Mongolia to 2.1 % in Cambodia.

Regarding exposure to second hand smoke in public places, over 70 % of the students reported that they had experienced such exposure in the past 7 days in 32 of the 48 sites.

In a worldwide view, in this study over 80 % of the students thought dentists have a role in giving advice about smoking cessation to patients in 37 of 46 sites, with 26 over 90 %. The lowest percentage was in Slovakia (56.8 %). Over 80 % of the students thought health professionals should get specific training on cessation techniques in 40 of the 47 sites, with 25 over 90 %. The lowest was in Myanmar (69.3 %). Less than 40 % of the students reported having ever received some kind of formal training in their professional school on cessation approaches to use with their patients in 40 of the 47 sites. This percentage was <20 % in 27 sites and <10 % in 8 sites.

Over 50 % of the students had received formal training in Fiji (100 %), India (54.8 %), Lithuania (60.0 %) and Moldova (61.3 %).

From 2005 to 2008, Warren and colleagues 2011b performed a similar survey among medical student collecting data from 47 countries.

Among medical students, in three countries the current smoking rates was above 40 % (Albania, Bosnia and Herzegovina and Bolivia) and three sites had rates <5 % (Uganda, Sri Lanka and Thailand). Males were more likely than females to smoke cigarettes in 37 of 48 sites; while females had higher rates than males in Serbia, Chile and Thailand and there were no gender differences in 8 of the 48 sites. In Africans countries, 37.7 % of medical students currently smoked cigarettes in Niger; while <10 % smoked in the other three African sites. Current cigarette smoking ranged from over 20 % in Gaza Strip/West Bank (22.7 %) and Lebanon (28.2 %) to

<10 % (Egypt, Iran, Sudan and Tunisia) in Eastern Mediterranean region. In Europe, current cigarette smoking was over 30 % in every site, except Armenia, Czech Republic, Lithuania and Slovenia. In American sites, current cigarette smoking was over 20 % in all sites, except Brazil, Jamaica and Panama. In the South-East Asia Region, current cigarette smoking was over 20 % in Bangladesh and Nepal and <5 % in Sri Lanka and Thailand. In Western Pacific region, current cigarette smoking ranged from 16.0 % in South Korea to 6.4 % in Cambodia.

Regarding health professional roles and training, over 80 % of the students thought health professionals have a role in giving advice about smoking cessation to patients in 42 of 46 sites, with 30 over 90 %. The lowest was in Slovakia (59.7 %). Over 80 % of the students thought health professionals should get specific training on cessation techniques in 41 of the 48 sites, with 33 over 90 %. The lowest was in Czech Republic (60.8 %). Less than 40 % of the students reported having ever received some kind of formal training in their professional school on cessation approaches to use with their patients in 46 of the 48 sites; <20 % in 16 sites and <10 % in 6 sites. Over 40 % of the students had received formal training in Niger (46.4 %) and Myanmar (43.7 %) (Warren et al. 2011b).

As far Europe is concerned, from March to May 2009 GHPSS was conducted in a cross-country, cross-sectional study among 12 medical schools in four European countries (Germany, Italy, Poland and Spain) (La Torre et al 2012).

The overall response rate was high: 92.0 %. The global prevalence of smoking among medical students was 29.3 % (95 % CI 28.1–34.7), with rates ranging from 28.0 % in Germany to 31.3 % in Italy. Concerning gender differences in Germany, Italy and Spain, male students were more likely to be current smokers than female students, although the difference was only significant in Germany ($P<0.0001$). The opposite was found in Polish medical students, where the prevalence of smoking was higher in females. Regarding roles and training, only 16.5 % of respondents had received smoking cessation training during their time at medical school, with significant differences between Italy (3.5 %) and the other countries ($P<0.001$). In terms of knowledge of smoking cessation methods, the vast majority (89.8 %) of medical students were aware of nicotine patches and gum (highest prevalence in Spain, 96.3 %), and 24.4 % were aware of the use of antidepressants, such as Bupropion or Varenicline (highest prevalence in Germany, 33.6 %).

Focusing on Italian condition, the 2009 survey was a multicentre cross-sectional pilot study carried out in five Italian Schools of Medicine (Sapienza University of Rome, Catholic University of the Sacred Heart of Rome and the Faculties of Medicine of Chieti, Torino and Palermo). The prevalence of current smokers was 31.4 % (95 % CI: 28.1–34.7), higher than the prevalence of 22 % in general population aged between 15 and 24 years. Regarding attitudes towards tobacco use, more than half considered health professionals as behavioural models for patients, and around 90 % thought health professionals have a role in giving advice or information about smoking cessation. Unfortunately, only 5.8 % of responders had received smoking cessation training during their medical school years. Concerning knowledge about smoking cessation methods, most students had heard about nicotine patches or gum, 45 % about counselling techniques and around 18 % about acetylcholine receptor partial agonists (such as Varenicline or Champix).

Interestingly, medical students who considered health-care professionals as behavioural models had lower likelihood of smoking (OR=0.52; 95 % CI: 0.35 to 0.77).

Finally, considering the high prevalence of smokers among health-care professionals and the their primary role as behavioural models, the results from the GHPSS Surveys in the World highlight the importance of focussing attention on the integration of smoking cessation training addressed to medical students.

References

Abdullah, A. S., Qiming, F., Pun, V., Stillman, F. A., & Samet, J. M. (2011). A review of tobacco smoking and smoking cessation practices among physicians in China: 1987–2010. *Tobacco Control*(Dec 15).

Al Qaseer, B. M., Batarseh, S. (2009). *Global school-based student health survey: Jordan global school based student health survey*. Centers for Disease Control and Prevention & World Health Organization. Accessed April, 2012 from http://www.who.int/chp/gshs/GSHS_Country_Report_Jordan_2007.pdf

Australian Department of Health and Ageing. (2004). *Smoking cessation guidelines for Australian general practice*. Canberra: Department of Health and Ageing.

Aveyard, P., Begh, R., Parsons, A., & West, R. (2011). Brief opportunistic smoking cessation interventions: A systematic review and meta-analysis to compare advice to quit and offer of assistance. *Addiction*(Dec 16).

Bakker, M. J., de Vries, H., Mullen, P. D., & Kok, G. (2005). Predictors of perceiving smoking cessation counselling as a midwife's role: A survey of Dutch midwives. *European Journal of Public Health, 15*(1), 39–42.

Bernstein, S. L., Bijur, P., Cooperman, N., Jearld, S., Arnsten, J. H., Moadel, A., et al. (2011). A randomized trial of a multicomponent cessation strategy for emergency department smokers. *Academic Emergency Medicine, 18*(6), 575–583.

Bialous, S. A., Sarna, L., Wewers, M. E., Froelicher, E. S., & Danao, L. (2004). Nurses' perspectives of smoking initiation, addiction, and cessation. *Nursing Research, 53*(6), 387–395.

Borges, A., Marques, F., Lima, J., Costa, L., Gonçalves, P., Fernandes, R., et al. (2008). Smoking habits of sixth year medical students and anti-smoking measures in Portugal. *Revista Portuguesa de Pneumologia, 14*, 379–390.

Borrelli, B., Hecht, J. P., Papandonatos, G. D., Emmons, K. M., Tatewosian, L. R., & Abrams, D. B. (2001). Smoking-cessation counseling in the home: Attitudes, beliefs, and behaviors of home healthcare nurses. *American Journal of Preventive Medicine, 21*(4), 272–277.

Braun, B. L., Fowles, J. B., Solberg, L. I., Kind, E. A., Lando, H., & Pine, D. (2004). Smoking-related attitudes and clinical practices of medical personnel in Minnesota. *American Journal of Preventive Medicine, 27*, 316–322.

Centers for Disease Control and Prevention. (1994). *Preventing tobacco use among young people—A report of the surgeon general*. Atlanta: USDHHS, CDC.

Centers for Disease Control and Prevention (CDC). (1993). Smoking control among health-care workers: World No-Tobacco Day, 1993. *MMWR. Morbidity and Mortality Weekly Report, 42*(19), 365–367.

Clareboets, S., Sivarajasingam, V., & Chestnutt, I. G. (2010). Smoking cessation advice: Knowledge, attitude and practice among clinical dental students. *British Dental Journal, 208*, 173–177.

Clark, E., & McCann, T. V. (2008). The influence of friends on smoking commencement and cessation in undergraduate nursing students: A survey. *Contemporary Nurse, 27*(2), 185–193.

Coe, R. M., & Brehm, H. P. (1971). Smoking habits of physicians and preventive care practices. *HSMHA Health Reports, 86*(3), 217–221.

Collins, R. L., Gollnisch, G., & Morsheimer, E. T. (1999). Substance use among a regional sample of female nurses. *Drug and Alcohol Dependence, 5*(1–2), 145–155.

Conroy, M. B., Majchrzak, N. E., Silverman, C. B., Chang, Y., Regan, S., Schneider, L. I., & Rigotti, N. A. (2005). Measuring provider adherence to tobacco treatment guidelines: A comparison of electronic medical record review, patient survey, and provider survey. *Nicotine & Tobacco Research, 7*(Suppl. 1), S35–S43.

Dekker, H. M., Looman, C. W., Adriaanse, H. P., & van der Maas, P. J. (1993). Prevalence of smoking in physicians and medical students, and the generation effect in the Netherlands. *Social Science & Medicine, 36*, 817–822.

DHHS. (2004). *The health consequences of smoking: A report of the surgeon general*. Atlanta, GA: Department of Health and Human Services, Centers for Disease Control and Prevention.

Doll, R., Gray, R., Hafner, B., & Peto, R. (1980). Mortality in relation to smoking: 22 years' observations on female British doctors. *BMJ, 280*(6219), 967–971.

Doll, R., & Hill, A. B. (1954). The mortality of doctors in relation to their smoking habits; a preliminary report. *BMJ, 1*(4877), 1451–1455.

Doll, R., & Hill, A. B. (1964). Mortality in relation to smoking: Ten years' observations of British doctors. *BMJ, 1*(5395), 1399–1410.

Doll, R., & Peto, R. (1976). Mortality in relation to smoking: 20 years' Observations on male British doctors. *BMJ, 2*(6051), 1525–1536.

Doll, R., Peto, R., Boreham, J., & Sutherland, I. (2004). Mortality in relation to smoking: 50 years' observations on male British doctors. *BMJ, 328*(7455), 1519.

Doll, R., Peto, R., Wheatley, K., Gray, R., & Sutherland, I. (1994). Mortality in relation to smoking: 40 years' observations on male British doctors. *BMJ, 309*(6959), 901–911.

Eddy, D. (1992). David Eddy ranks the tests. *Harvard Health Letter 17*(9) Suppl. 10, 10–11

Edwards, R., Bowler, T., Atkinson, J., & Wilson, N. (2008). Low and declining cigarette smoking rates among doctors and nurses: 2006 New Zealand Census data. *The New Zealand Medical Journal, 121*(1284), 43–51.

Eisinger, R. A. (1972). Cigarette smoking and the pediatrician. Findings based on a national survey. *Clinical Pediatrics, 11*(11), 645–647.

Faith-Ell, P., & Wilhelmsen, L. (1973). The smoking habits of Swedish doctors in 1969 and 1972. *Lakartidningen, 70*(31), 2719–2722.

Faulkner, A., & Ward, L. (1983). Nurses as health educators in relation to smoking. *Nursing Times, 79*, 47–48.

Feeney, G. F., Kelly, A., Griffin, D. K., & Young, R. M. (1997). Smoking interventions within the hospital setting: A study of demand for smoking interventions and perceived efficacy of nurses in delivery of services. *Health Promotion Journal of Australia, 7*(1), 52–56.

Ferketich, A. K., Khan, Y., & Wewers, M. E. (2006). Are physicians asking about tobacco use and assisting with cessation? Results from the 2001–2004 national ambulatory medical care survey (NAMCS). *Preventive Medicine, 43*, 472–476.

Ferrante, M., Fiore, M., Leon, L., Costantidines, F., Castaing, M., Fallico, R., et al. (2010). Age of smoking initiation, tobacco habits and risk perception among primary, middle and high school students in southern Italy. *Italian Journal of Public Health, 7*, 262–267.

Ficarra, M. G., Gualano, M. R., Capizzi, S., Siliquini, R., Liguori, G., Manzoli, L., et al. (2011). Tobacco use prevalence, knowledge and attitudes among Italian hospital healthcare professionals. *European Journal of Public Health, 21*(1), 29–34.

Fiore, M. C. (1996). US public health service clinical practice guideline: Treating tobacco use and dependence. *Respiratory Care, 45*(10), 1200–1262.

Fiore, M. C., Bailey, W. C., Cohen, S. J., Dorfman, S. F., Goldstein, M. G., Gritz, E. R., et al. (2000). *Treating tobacco use and dependence. Quick reference guide for clinicians*. Rockville, MD: U.S. Department of Health and Human Services.

Fiore, M. C., Epps, R. P., & Manley, M. W. (1994). A missed opportunity. Teaching medical students to help their patients successfully quit smoking. *Journal of the American Medical Association, 271*, 624–626.

Fiore, M., & United States Tobacco Use and Dependence Guideline Panel. (2000). *Treating tobacco Use and dependence*. Rockville, MD: U.S. Department of Health and Human Services, Public Health Service.

Fiore, M., & United States Tobacco Use and Dependence Guideline Panel. (2008). *Treating tobacco use and dependence: 2008 update*. Rockville, MD: U.S. Department of Health and Human Services, Public Health Service.

Fortmann, S. P., Sallis, J. F., Magnus, P. M., & Farquhar, J. W. (1985). Attitudes and practices of physicians regarding hypertension and smoking: The Stanford Five City Project. *Preventive Medicine, 14*(1), 70–80.

Garfinkel, L. (1976). Cigarette smoking among physicians and other health professionals, 1959–1972. *CA: A Cancer Journal for Clinicians, 26*, 373–375.

Garfinkel, L. (1997). Trends in cigarette smoking in the United States. *Preventive Medicine, 26*(4), 447–450.

Garfinkel, L., & Stellman, S. D. (1986). Cigarette smoking among physicians, dentists, and nurses. *CA: A Cancer Journal for Clinicians, 36*, 2–8.

Giovino, G. A. (2002). Epidemiology of tobacco use in the United States. *Oncogene, 21*(48), 7326–7340.

Gomm, M., Lincoln, P., Egeland, P., & Rosenberg, M. (2002). Helping hospitalised clients quit smoking: A study of rural nursing practice and barriers. *The Australian Journal of Rural Health, 10*(1), 26–32.

Gorin, S. S. (2001). Predictors of tobacco control among nursing students. *Patient Education and Counseling, 44*(3), 251–262.

Haddad, L. G., & Malak, M. Z. (2002). Smoking habits and attitudes towards smoking among university students in Jordan. *International Journal of Nursing Studies, 39*, 793–802.

Haddad, L., & Pertro, W. (2006). Predictors of intention to quit smoking among Jordanian university students. *Canadian Journal of Public Health, 97*, 9–14.

Hall, S., Vogt, F., & Marteau, T. M. (2005). A short report: Survey of practice nurses' attitudes towards giving smoking cessation advice. *Family Practice, 22*(6), 614–616.

Hammond, E. C., Van Griethuysen, T. H., Dibeler, J. B., Sneddon, A. M., & Halligan, W. (1965). Smoking habits and disease in New York State. *New York State Journal of Medicine, 65*(20), 2557–2561.

Häuser, W., Grandt, D., Schäfer, H., & Görge, G. (2002). Smoking cessation: A physician's responsibility. *MMW Fortschritte Der Medizin, 31*, 30–34.

Hay, D. R. (1998). Cigarette smoking by New Zealand doctors and nurses: Results from the 1996 population census. *New Zealand Medical Journal, 111*(1062), 102–104.

Heras, T. A., Garcıa Sanchon, C., Hernandez Lopez, M. C., Ballestın, N., & Nebot, M. (2000). Smoking among nursing students in Catalonia: Knowledge, attitudes and practice. *European Journal of Epidemiology, 16*, 607–611.

Hill, D. J., & White, V. M. (1995). Australian adult smoking prevalence in 1992. *Australian Journal of Public Health, 19*(3), 305–308.

Hill, D. J., White, V. M., & Scollo, M. M. (1998). Smoking behaviours of Australian adults in 1995: Trends and concerns. *The Medical Journal of Australia, 168*(5), 209–213.

Hocking, B., Borland, R., Owen, N., & Kemp, G. (1991). A total ban on workplace smoking is acceptable and effective. *Journal of Occupational Medicine, 33*, 163–167.

Hodgetts, G., Broers, T., & Godwin, M. (2004). Smoking behaviour, knowledge and attitudes among family medicine physicians and nurses in Bosnia and Herzegovina. *BMC Family Practice, 5*, 12.

Hornberger, C. A., & Edwards, L. C. (2004). Survey of tobacco cessation curricula in Kansas nursing programs. *Nurse Educator, 29*(5), 212–216.

Hughes, A. M., & Rissel, C. (1999). Smoking: Rates and attitudes among nursing staff in central Sydney. *International Journal of Nursing Practice, 5*(3), 147–154.

Hussain, S. F., Tjeder-Burton, S., Campbell, I. A., & Davies, P. D. (1993). Attitudes to smoking and smoking habits among hospital staff. *Thorax, 48*, 174–175.

Jenkins, K., & Ahijevych, K. (2003). Nursing students' beliefs about smoking, their own smoking behaviors, and use of professional tobacco treatment intervention. *Applied Nursing Research, 16*(3), 164–172.

Johnston, J. M., Chan, S. S., Chan, S. K., Lam, T. H., Chi, I., & Leung, G. M. (2005). Training nurses and social workers in smoking cessation counseling: A population needs assessment in Hong Kong. *Preventive Medicine, 40*, 389–406.

Kaneita, Y., Uchida, T., & Ohida, T. (2010). Epidemiological study of smoking among Japanese physicians. *Preventive Medicine, 51*(2), 164–167.

Katz, D. A., Vander Weg, M. W., Holman, J., Nugent, A., Baker, L., Johnson, S., et al. (2012). The Emergency Department Action in Smoking Cessation (EDASC) trial: Impact on delivery of smoking cessation counseling. *Academic Emergency Medicine, 19*(4), 409–420.

Kawane, H. (1993). When doctors advertised cigarettes. *Tobacco Control, 2*, 45.

Khader, Y. S., & Alsadi, A. A. (2008). Smoking habits among university students in Jordan: Prevalence and associated factors. *Eastern Mediterranean Health Journal, 14*, 897–904.

Kirkby, R. J., Bashkawi, E. B., Drew, C. A., & Foenander, G. P. (1976). Smoking in nurses. *The Medical Journal of Australia, 2*(23), 864–865.

Kitajima, T., Ohida, T., Harano, S., Kamal, A. M., Takemura, S., Nozaki, N., et al. (2002). Smoking behavior, initiating and cessation factors among Japanese nurses: A cohort study. *Public Health, 116*(6), 347–352.

La Torre, G., Kirch, W., Bes-Rastrollo, M., Ramos, R. M., Czaplicki, M., Gualano, M. R., et al. (2012). Tobacco use among medical students in Europe: Results of a multicentre study using the Global Health Professions Student Survey. *Public Health, 126*(2), 159–164.

Lally, R. M., Chalmers, K. I., Johnson, J., Kojima, M., Endo, E., Suzuki, S., et al. (2008). Smoking behavior and patient education practices of oncology nurses in six countries. *European Journal of Oncology Nursing, 12*(4), 372–379.

Lancaster, T., Silagy, C., Fowler, G. (2000). Training health professionals in smoking cessation. *Cochrane Database System Review* (3), CD000214.

Lee, D. J., LeBlanc, W., Fleming, L. E., Gomez-Marin, O., & Pitman, T. (2004). Trends in US smoking rates in occupational groups: The National Health Interview Survey 1987–1994. *Journal of Occupational and Environmental Medicine, 46*, 538–548.

Maciosek, M. V., Edwards, N. M., & Coffield, A. B. (2006). Priorities among effective clinical preventive services: Methods. *American Journal of Preventive Medicine, 31*(1), 90–96.

Mackay, J., & Eriksen, M. (2002). *The tobacco atlas*. Geneva, Switzerland: World Health Organization.

Malone, R. E. (2006). Nursing's Involvement in tobacco control: Historical perspective and vision for the future. *Nursing Research, 55*(4 Suppl.), S51–S57.

McCarty, M. C., Zander, K. M., Hennrikus, D. J., & Lando, H. A. (2001). Barriers among nurses to providing smoking cessation advice to hospitalized smokers. *American Journal of Health Promotion, 16*(2), 85–87.

McKenna, H., Slater, P., McCance, T., Bunting, B., Spiers, A., & McElwee, G. (2001). Qualified nurses' smoking prevalence: Their reasons for smoking and desire to quit. *Journal of Advanced Nursing, 35*(5), 769–775.

McKenna, H., Slater, P., McCance, T., Bunting, B., Spiers, A., & McElwee, G. (2003). The role of stress, peer influence and education levels on the smoking behaviour of nurses. *International Journal of Nursing Studies, 40*(4), 359–366.

Melani, A. S., Verponziani, W., Boccoli, E., Trianni, G. L., Federici, A., Amerini, R., et al. (2000). Tobacco smoking habits, attitudes and beliefs among nurse and medical students in Tuscany. *European Journal of Epidemiology, 16*(7), 607–611.

Merrill, R. M., Madanat, H., Layton, J. B., Hanson, C. L., & Madsen, C. C. (2007). Smoking prevalence, attitudes, and perceived smoking prevention control responsibilities and behaviors among physicians in Jordan. *International Quarterly of Community Health Education, 26*, 397–413.

Morgan, K., McGee, H., Watson, D., Perry, I., Barry, M., Shelley, E., et al. (2008). *SLAN 2007: Survey of lifestyle, attitudes and nutrition in Ireland, main report, Department of Health and Children*. Dublin: The Stationery Office.

Morra, M., & Knobf, M. (1983). Comparison of nurses' smoking habits: The 1975 DHEW survey and Connecticut nurses, 1981. *Public Health Reports, 98*, 553–557.

Nagle, A., Schofield, M., & Redman, S. (1999). Australian nurses' smoking behaviour, knowledge and attitude towards providing smoking cessation care to their patients. *Health Promotion International, 14*(2), 133–144.

NCI. (1999). *Health effects of exposure to environmental tobacco smoke: The report of the California Environmental Protection Agency*. Bethesda, MD: U.S. Department of Health and Human Services, National Institutes of Health, National cancer Institute.

Nelson, D. E., Giovino, G. A., Emont, S. L., Brackbill, R., Cameron, L. L., Peddicord, J., et al. (1994). Trends in cigarette smoking among US physicians and nurses. *Journal of the American Medical Association, 271*(16), 1273–1275.

O'Connor, A., & Harrison, M. (1992). Survey of smoking prevalence among Canadian nursing students and registered nurses. *Canadian Journal of Public Health, 83*(6), 417–421.

Ota, A., Yasuda, N., Okamoto, Y., Kobayashi, Y., Sugihara, Y., Koda, S., et al. (2004). Relationship of job stress with nicotine dependence of smokers—A cross-sectional study of female nurses in a general hospital. *Journal of Occupational Health, 46*(3), 220–224.

Padula, C. A. (1992). Nurses and smoking: Review and implications. *Journal of Professional Nursing, 8*(2), 120–132.

Peto, R. (1994). Smoking and death: The past 40 years and the next 40. *BMJ, 309*(6959), 937–939.

Percival, J., Bialous, S. A., Chan, S., & Sarna, L. (2003). International efforts in tobacco control. *Seminars in Oncology Nursing, 19*(4), 301–308.

Proietti, L., Bonanno, G., Di Maria, A., Palermo, F., Polosa, R., & Lupo, L. (2006). Smoking habits in health care workers: Experience in two general hospitals of eastern Sicily. *Clinica Terapeutica, 157*(5), 407–412.

Raupach, T., Shahab, L., Baetzing, S., Hoffmann, B., Hasenfuss, G., West, R., et al. (2009). Medical students lack basic knowledge about smoking: Findings from two European medical schools. *Nicotine & Tobacco Research, 11*, 92–98.

Rice, V. H., Stead, L. F. (2008). Nursing interventions for smoking cessation. *Cochrane Database of Systematic Reviews* (1), CD001188.

Richmond, R. L., & Kehoe, L. (1997). Smoking behavior and attitudes among Australian medical students. *Medical Education, 31*, 169–176.

Rigotti, N. A., Munafo, M. R., Stead, L. F. (2007). Interventions for smoking cessation in hospitalised patients. *Cochrane Database Systematic Reviews* (3):CD001837.

Roddy, E., Rubin, P., & Britton, J. (2004). Tobacco Advisory Group of the Royal College of Physicians. A study of smoking and smoking cessation on the curricula of UK medical schools. *Tobacco Control, 13*(1), 74–77.

Rowe, K., & Macleod-Clark, J. (2000a). The incidence of smoking amongst nurses: A review of the literature. *Journal of Advanced Nursing, 31*, 1046–1053.

Rowe, K., & Macleod-Clark, J. (2000b). Why nurses smoke: A review of the literature. *International Journal of Nursing Studies, 37*, 173–181.

Ruiz-Canela, M., Martinez-Gonzalez, M. A., Lopez-del Burgo, C., de Irala, J., Beunza, J. J., & Bes-Rastrollo, M. (2009). Are smoking habits changing among Spanish health professionals? Results from the SUN Cohort 1999–2008. *Tobacco Use Insights, 2*, 17–24.

Saarmann, L., Daugherty, J. A., & Riegel, B. (2000). Patient teaching to promote behavioral change. *Nursing Outlook, 48*, 281–287.

Sachs, D. P. (1984). Treatment of cigarette dependency. What American pulmonary physicians do. *American Review of Respiratory Disease, 129*(6), 1010–1013.

Sanderson, D. M., Ekholm, O., et al. (2005). Influence of lifestyle, health, and work environment on smoking cessation among Danish nurses followed over 6 years. *Preventive Medicine, 41*(3–4), 757–760.

Sarna, L., Bialous, S. A., Jun, H. J., et al. (2008). Smoking trends in the Nurses' Health Study (1976–2003). *Nursing Research, 57*(6), 374–382.

Sarna, L. P., Brown, J. K., Lillington, L., Rose, M., Wewers, M. E., & Brecht, M. L. (2000a). Tobacco interventions of oncology nurses: Report from a national survey. *Cancer, 89*, 881–889.

Sarna, L., Brown, J. K., Lillington, L., Wewers, M. E., & Brecht, M. L. (2000b). Tobacco-control attitudes, advocacy, and smoking behaviors of oncology nurses. *Oncology Nursing Forum, 27*, 1519–1528.

Sarna, L., Wewers, M. E., Brown, J. K., Lillington, L., & Brecht, M. L. (2001). Barriers to tobacco control interventions. *Nursing Outlook, 49*, 166–172.

Scanlon, A., Clark, E., & McGuiness, W. (2008). Acute (adult clinical inpatient) care nurses' attitudes towards and knowledge of nationally endorsed 5As smoking cessation guidelines. *Contemporary Nurse, 29*(1), 80–91.

Senior, S. L. (1982). Study of smoking habits in hospital and attitudes of medical staff towards smoking. *Canadian Medical Association Journal, 126*(2), 131–133.

Sezer, H., Guler, N., & Sezer, R. E. (2007). Smoking among nurses in Turkey: Comparison with other countries. *Journal of Health, Population, and Nutrition, 25*(1), 107–111.

Sharp, L., & Tishelman, C. (2005). Smoking cessation for patients with head and neck cancer. *Cancer Nursing, 28*, 226.

Shuttleworth, A. (2004). The role of nurses in reducing the use of tobacco. *Nursing Times, 100*(1), 26–28.

Slater, P., McElwee, G., Fleming, P., & McKenna, H. (2006). Nurses' smoking behaviour related to cessation practice. *Nursing Times, 102*, 32.

Smith, D., & Leggat, P. (2007a). An international review of tobacco smoking research in the nursing profession: 1976–2006. *Journal of Research in Nursing, 12*(165), 181.

Smith, D. R., & Leggat, P. A. (2007b). An international review of tobacco smoking in the medical profession: 1974–2004. *BMC Public Health, 7*, 115.

Smith, D. R., & Leggat, P. A. (2007c). An international review of tobacco smoking among medical students. *Journal of Postgraduate Medicine, 53*, 55–62.

Smoking and Health. (1964). *Report of the advisory committee to the surgeon general of the public health service*. Washington: U.S. Department of Health, Education and Welfare.

Soeken, K. L., Bausell, R. B., & Winklestein, M. (1989). Preventive behaviour: Attitudes and compliance of nursing students. *Journal of Advanced Nursing, 14*, 1026–1033.

Sophia, S. C., Chan, Linda Sarna, David C. N. Wong, et al. (2007). Nurses Tobacco-Related Knowledge, Attitudes, and Practice in Four Major Cities in China. *Journal of Nursing Scholarship, 39*(1), 46–53.

Spencer, J. K. (1984). Nurses' cigarette smoking in England and Wales. *International Journal of Nursing Studies, 21*(2), 69–79.

Tamerin, J. S., & Eisinger, R. A. (1972). Cigarette smoking and the psychiatrist. *The American Journal of Psychiatry, 128*(10), 1224–1229.

Tate, C. I., & Fulghum, J. E. (1965). Seventy per cent of Florida physicians Are nonsmokers. *Jounal of Florida Medical Association, 52*, 47–48.

Tirodimos, I., Georgouvia, I., Savvala, T. N., Karanika, E., & Noukari, D. (2009). Healthy lifestyle habits among Greek university students: Differences by sex and faculty of study. *Eastern Mediterranean Health Journal, 15*, 722–728.

Tobacco Free Nurses. (2006). Retrieved April, 2012 from http://www.tobaccofreenurses.org/

Trinkoff, A., & Storr, C. (1998a). Substance use among nurses: Differences between specialties. *American Journal of Public Health, 88*(4), 581–585.

Trinkoff, A., & Storr, C. (1998b). Work schedule characteristics and substance use in nurses. *American Journal of Industrial Medicine, 34*, 266–271.

U.S. Department of Health and Human Services. (1980). The health consequences of smoking for women: A Report of the Surgeon General. U.S. Department of Health and Human Services, Public Health Service, Office of the Assistant Secretary for Health, Office on Smoking and Health. Retrieved from http://profiles.nlm.nih.gov/NN/B/B/R/T/_/nnbbrt.pdf

U.S. Department of Health and Human Services. (2004). *The health consequences of smoking: A report of the surgeon general.* Atlanta, GA: U.S. Department of Health and Human Services, Centers for Disease Control and Prevention, National Center for Chronic Disease Prevention and Health Promotion, Office on Smoking and Health.

US Department of Commerce, Census Bureau. (1995). *National Cancer Institute sponsored tobacco use supplement to the current population survey.* Washington, DC: Bureau of Labor Statistics.

Vagropoulos, I., Tsilchorozidou, T., Tsinopoulos, G., Salonikidou, Z., Mouratova, M., Giavropoulou, M., et al. (2006). Smoking habits among the hospital staff of a general hospital in northern Greece: A long way for smoke-free hospitals. *Monaldi Archives for Chest Disease, 65*(3), 160–164.

van Reek, J., & Adriaanse, H. (1991). Smoking by physicians in Scandinavia: 1952–1989. *Scandinavian Journal of Social Medicine, 19*(4), 256–259.

Waalkens, H. J., Cohen Schotanus, J., Adriaanse, H., & Knol, K. (1992). Smoking habits in medical students and physicians in Groningen, the Netherlands. *European Respiratory Journal, 5*, 49–52.

Warren, C. W., Asma, S., Lee, J., Lea, V., & Mackay, J. (2009). *Global tobacco surveillance system. The GTSS Atlas*. Atlanta: CDC Foundation.

Warren, C. W., Sinha, D. N., Lee, J., Lea, V., & Jones, N. R. (2011a). Tobacco use, exposure to secondhand smoke, and cessation counseling among medical students: Cross-country data from the Global Health Professions Student Survey (GHPSS), 2005–2008. *BMC Public Health, 11*, 72.

Warren, C. W., Sinha, D. N., Lee, J., Lea, V., Jones, N., & Asma, S. (2011b). Tobacco use, exposure to secondhand smoke, and cessation counseling training of dental students around the world. *Journal of Dental Education, 75*(3), 385–405.

Wewers, M. E., Kidd, K., Armbruster, D., & Sarna, L. (2004). Tobacco dependence curricula in U.S. baccalaureate and graduate nursing education. *Nursing Outlook, 52*(2), 95–101.

Whyte, R. E., Watson, H. E., & McIntosh, J. (2006). Nurses' opportunistic interventions with patients in relation to smoking. *Journal of Advanced Nursing, 55*(5), 568–577.

Working Group on Tobacco or Health. (1987). *Guidelines for the conduct of tobacco-smoking surveys among health professionals* (pp. 3–19). Tokyo, Japan: World Health Organization Regional Office for Western Pacific.

World Health Organization. (1999). *Leave the pack behind* (pp. 33–39). Geneva, Switzerland: World Health Organization.

World Health Organization. (2003). *The World Health Report 2003*. Geneva: WHO.

World Health Organization. (2008). *World Health Organization report on the global tobacco epidemic, 2008: The MPOWER package 2008*. Geneva: World Health Organization.

Yang, Y., Jiang, Y., Wu, Y. H., Nan, Y., Wang, J., Yu, S., et al. (2006). Evaluation on quitting intervention in health professionals of six cities. *Wei Sheng Yan Jiu, 35*(1), 89–91.

Zwar, N. A., & Richmond, R. L. (2006). Role of the general practitioner in smoking cessation. *Drug and Alcohol Review, 25*, 21–26.

Chapter 10
Basic Principles of Smoking Cessation Techniques

Giuseppe La Torre and Maria Caterina Grassi

Objectives The aim of this chapter is to give an overview on the basic smoking cessation techniques, including counseling and use of medications

Learning Outcomes

Through this section the reader will be provided:
Some general approach to counseling for people who wants to quit smoking.
An overview of the drugs actually available for treating smokers who wants to stop smoking.

10.1 Introduction

Cigarette Smoking remains the most important health hazard (Jha et al. 2013; Thun et al. 2013), and quitting smoking is beneficial to health at any age (CDC 2011). The motivation to quit is the first essential step in stopping smoking, but not all the smokers want to quit. Then, how to understand if the smoker is ready to quit? How can we help him/her in trying the right way in implementing an effective cessation intervention?

In order to be ready for change, the smoker need to perceive the importance of the problem as well as to increase his/her confidence in the ability to change.

G. La Torre (✉) • M.C.Grassi
Department of Public Health and Infectious Diseases, "Sapienza" University of Rome, Piazzale Aldo Moro 5, Rome 00185, Italy
e-mail: giuseppe.latorre@uniroma1.it; caterina.grassi@uniroma1.it

G. La Torre, *Smoking Prevention and Cessation*, DOI 10.1007/978-1-4614-7046-5_10,

Moreover, we want to underline the relevant importance of a direct interaction with the medical schools aimed to provide adequate information to students on nicotine dependence and treatment and smoking-associated risks (Grassi et al. 2012; La Torre et al. 2012).

This chapter addresses three basic principles of smoking cessation, giving first of all an overview on the Transtheoretical approach Model (TTM) of behavior change developed by Prochaska and DiClemente (1983) and then a broader view on cessation techniques including counseling and drug therapies.

10.2 Transtheoretical Approach Model

This approach was developed at the beginning of the1980s of last century by two researchers that identify five stages an individual passes through with the aim of changing an established behavior.

According to Prochaska and DiClemente, the model can be easily applied to a wide range of problem behaviors, including smoking cessation, physical exercise and weight control, low cholesterol diet, abuse of alcohol, drug abuse.

In the field of smoking cessation, following the TTM, the smoker can progress through five stages (Fig. 10.1):

1. Precontemplation
2. Contemplation
3. Preparation
4. Action
5. Maintenance

Moreover, considering tobacco dependence as a chronic medical illness (McLellan et al. 2000) in which smokers experience periods of relapse and remission, two additional stages need to be considered in order to give a full picture of the smoking cessation process, i.e.,

- Relapse
- Termination

In this approach, the TTM consider change as a process in which different progresses are reached through a series of five stages.

Following the theory of Prochaska and DiClemente (1992), the stage of change is a key variable for the design of individual and public health interventions for smoking cessation (Velicer et al. 1998).

In other words, the stage of change is a variable that involves past behavior and behavioral intention to characterize an individual's readiness to change.

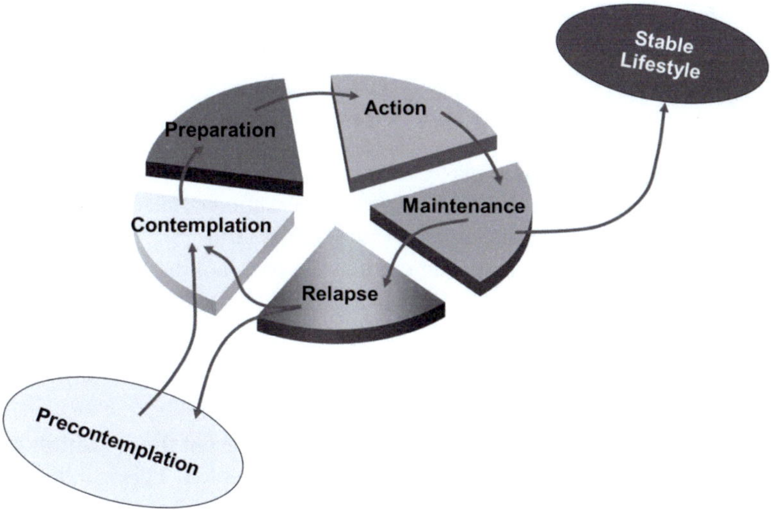

Fig. 10.1 The transtheoretical model in smoking cessation (from: AFMC Primer on Population Health. A virtual textbook on public health concepts for clinicians. Chapter 8 illness prevention and health promotion)

10.2.1 Precontemplation

This is the stage during which smokers do not want to take action in quitting smoking in the next future (i.e., 6 months). This typology of smoker can be applied to different kind of people:

(a) Uninformed or under-informed on the consequences of their behavior.
(b) Who tried to change several times and actually consider themselves as unable to change.

Smokers belonging to these groups tend to avoid reading, talking, or thinking about their high smoking habits, and according to other theories they can be classified as resistant or unmotivated or as not ready for a smoking cessation program.

10.2.2 Contemplation

This is the stage during which smokers declare their intention to change in the next future (i.e., six months). They are ambivalent toward smoking, and this could last a long period, since there is the awareness of the pros of changing, but there is also the awareness of the cons.

10.2.3 Preparation

In this stage smokers are willing to quit in the next future (i.e., next month). They have a plan of action. Examples of this plan could be:

- Attending a health education class.
- Consulting a health professional for smoking cessation counseling.
- Talking to the family doctor (General Practitioner, GP).
- Reading a self-help book or surfing the Internet for smoking cessation help.

10.2.4 Action

At this stage smokers have changed their behaviors in recent times (within the past 6 months). In this case, action means becoming a no-smoker. This is a very critical stage, and a great attention must be paid to possible relapse.

10.2.5 Maintenance

Finally, maintenance is the stage in which people are trying to prevent relapse. Usually, if the smoking cessation works, former smokers are less tempted to relapse, so becoming more confident in their ability to maintain their change.

This is the theoretical framework, but health professionals need to be aware of possible actions to implement in each of these stages. In Fig. 10.2, a suggested approach to smoking cessation is described. This approach is based on the TTM.

10.3 What Is Counseling?

Counseling in the health sector can be described as a wisdom and advice offered by a counselor to the patient as a regular part of the healthcare process.

Different types of counseling can be described:

(a) Individual counseling
(b) Group counseling
(c) Telephone counseling (telephone quitlines)

In tobacco cessation, individual, group, and telephone counseling are effective and their effectiveness increases with increasing intensity of treatment.

We have to recognize that three types of counseling are particularly effective:

- Practical counseling, in which problem-solving and/or skills training is provided to the smoker.

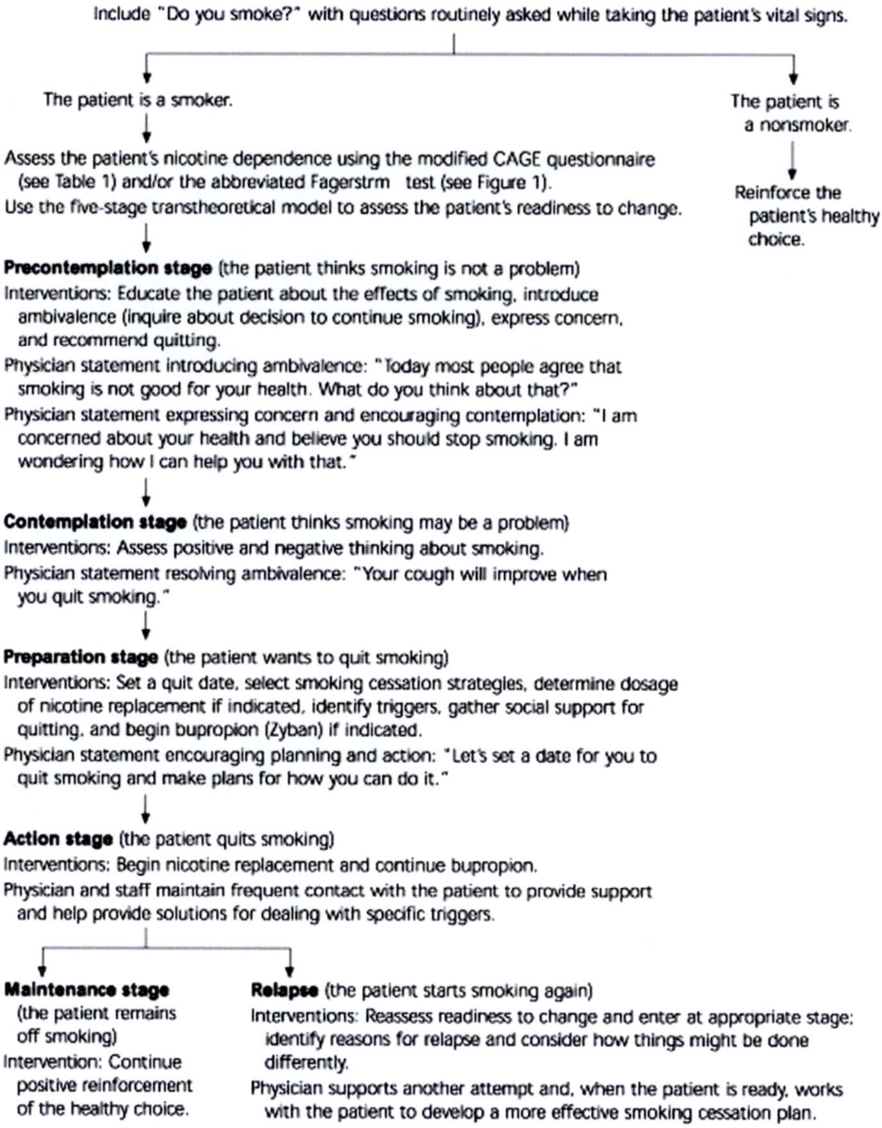

Fig. 10.2 A smoking cessation approach based on TTM. (from Mallin, R. (2002) Smoking cessation: Integration of behavioral and drug therapies. *American Family Physician, 65*(6), 1107–1115)

- Social support delivered to the patient as being part of the treatment approach.
- Motivational interviewing or motivational enhancement that is focused on approaches which are effective in increasing future quit attempts in smokers currently unwilling to quit (precontemplation stage).

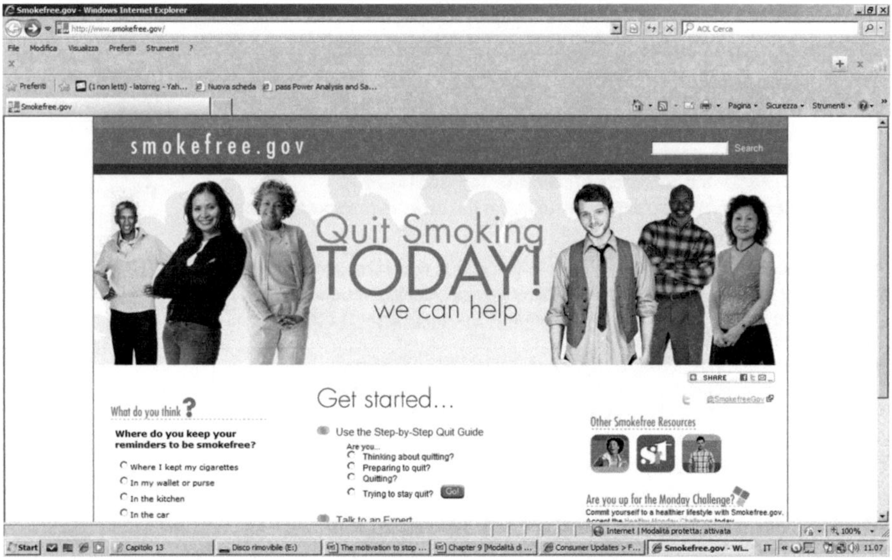
Smokefree.gov - Windows Internet Explorer
smokefree.gov
Search
Quit Smoking
TODAY!
we can help
What do you think?
Where do you keep your reminders to be smokefree?
Where I kept my cigarettes
In my wallet or purse
In the kitchen
In the car
Get started...
Use the Step-by-Step Quit Guide
Are you...
Thinking about quitting?
Preparing to quit?
Quitting?
Trying to stay quit?
Go!
Other Smokefree Resources
Are you up for the Monday Challenge?
Commit yourself to a healthier lifestyle with Smokefree.gov.

Fig. 10.3 An example of quitline

10.3.1 Counseling for Smoking Cessation

Counseling in the field of tobacco smoking cessation plays an important role. According to the National Health Interview Survey in the USA (Schiller et al. 2012), 48.3 % of smokers received a health professional's advice to quit smoking, 5.9 % received counseling, 31.7 % counseling and/or medication.

According to Jorenby, both individual counseling and group counseling are useful to increase the success rates for tobacco smoking cessation, while self-help materials, the most common type of counseling, is not particularly effective (Jorenby 2001).

Moreover, proactive telephone calls are also an effective way of delivering counseling. Several countries are providing quitlines (see an example in Fig. 10.3 concerning USA) that can give concrete help in quitting smoking at no charge.

It is well recognized that some information can substantially increase the chance of success, regardless of the type of counseling offered to the smoker. In this field, a problem-solving approach is effective for a lot of patients. Jorenby (2001) reports as useful the following example:

- The smoker has to think about times of the day he/she is likely to smoke.
  - When: first thing in the morning or after meals.
- And after that he/she needs to plan something that can be useful for distracting him/herself when the urge strikes.
  - What to do: leaving the situation or deep breathing.

Table 10.1 Who can give counseling in the healthcare sector

Healthcare professionals	References
Medical doctors	McIvor et al. (2009)
Dentistry	Needleman et al. (2010)
Nurses	Rice and Stead (2008)
Pharmacists	Sinclair et al. (2004)
Physical therapists	Bodner and Dean (2009)
Dental hygienists	Ramseier and Fundak (2009)

The social support in quitting smoking has been found very effective. It can be delivered in the form of caring, concern, and encouragement and is strictly related to the increasing of the success rate of tobacco smoking cessation. This kind of support can be classified as:

- Intratreatment social support, i.e., delivered by healthcare providers after a hospital discharge for a smoking-related illness or in the general practitioner environment (see Table 10.1 for finding which type of healthcare professional can give this counseling).
- Extratreatment social support, given by non healthcare subjects, such as family, friends, and other members of the community to whom the smoker belongs.

10.3.2 Administrative Aspects of Counseling

In the USA, the program Medicare (Part B) covers different levels of counseling, intermediate and intensive, for quitting smoking and tobacco use. In Box 10.1 Counseling codes for individuals and groups are reported.

Box 10.1 Counseling Codes for Individuals and Groups

Counseling codes for	
Individuals	Groups
CPT 99406 intermediate: Smoking and tobacco-use cessation counseling visit (more than 3 min, up to 10 min) for symptomatic patients	*CPT S9453 Smoking cessation classes:* Nonphysician provider, per session
CPT 99407 intensive: Smoking and tobacco-use cessation counseling visit (more than 10 min) for symptomatic patients	*CPT 99078 Physician educational services:* In a group setting
ICD-9 305.1 Nondependent tobacco-use disorder	
ICD-9 V15.82 History of tobacco use	*ICD-9 305.1 Nondependent tobacco-use disorder*

Medicare covers tobacco cessation counseling for asymptomatic outpatient and hospitalized beneficiaries that, alternatively use tobacco, whether or not they have signs or symptoms of tobacco-related disease are competent and alert during counseling or receive counseling from a Medicare-recognized practitioner.

It is important to underline that this coverage is limited only to patients who:

- Use tobacco and have a disease or adverse health effect linked to tobacco use.
- Are taking drugs whose metabolism is influenced by tobacco use.

Concerning the number of attempts covered each year by Medicare Part B, the maximum is 2, and for every attempt a maximum of 4 intermediate or intensive sessions can be included, reaching a maximum of 8 sessions in one year. For billing purposes, Medicare produced two new G Codes covering intermediate smoking and tobacco cessation counseling visit (more than 3 min, up to 10 min) for asymptomatic patients (G0436) and intensive smoking and tobacco cessation counseling visit (more than 10 min) for asymptomatic patients (G0437).

10.4 The 5A's and 3A's Approaches

Smoking cessation advice and assistance by physicians play an important role in helping smokers quit (Fiore et al. 2008). Brief interventions provided by healthcare professionals for helping the patient quitting smoking can be structured or unstructured.

The first ones are widely use in different healthcare setting, such as the family medicine (GP) or in a clinical ward in the hospital.

10.4.1 5A's

This is a common use brief intervention by healthcare professionals suggested by many guidelines (Glynn et al. 1990; American Psychiatric Association 1996; American Medical Association 1994; Mecklenburg et al. 1991). The 5A's is structured in the following steps (Fig. 10.4):

1. Ask the patient about tobacco use.
2. Advice the smoker to quit.
3. Assess the readiness to quit.
4. Assist the patient willing to stop smoking in quitting.
5. Arrange a follow up to check his/her status.

However, it has been recognized that this kind of brief intervention can be useful and successful mostly for smokers who are highly motivated to stop smoking. If the health professional is facing with a smoker that is not ready to quit, an effective intervention is only giving advice to quit (precontemplation stage).

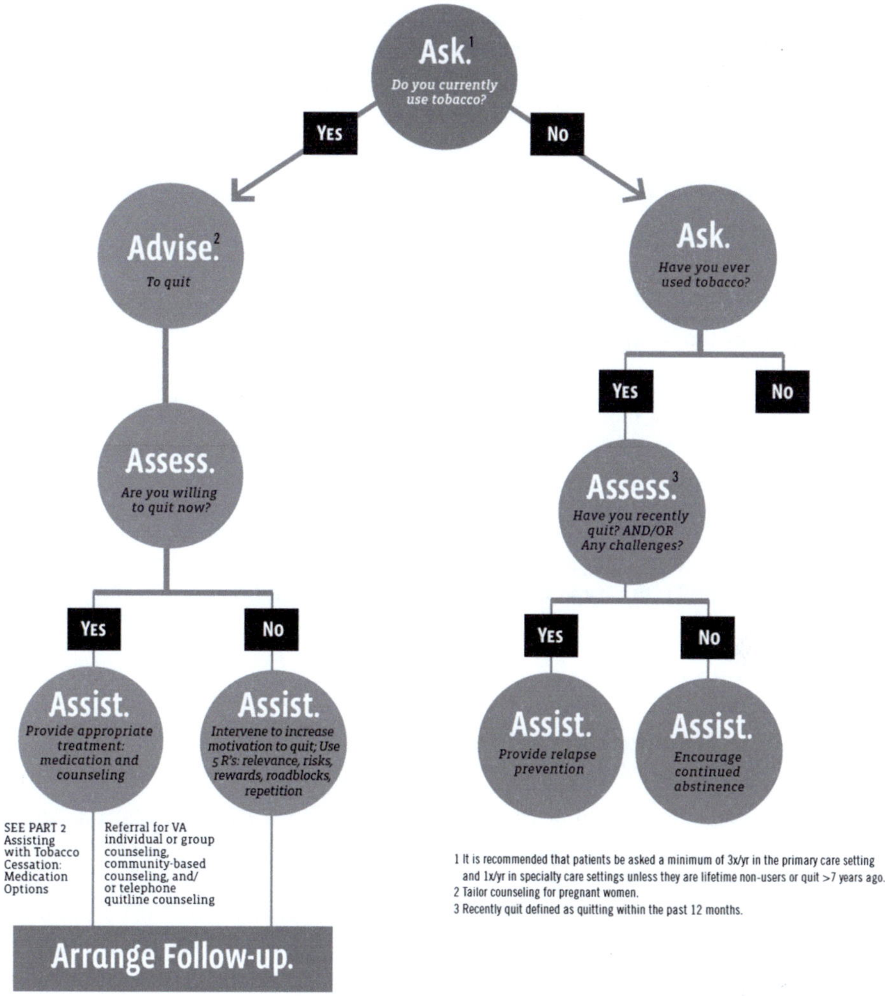

Fig. 10.4 The structure of 5A's brief intervention (from U.S. Department of Veterans Affairs Office of Public Health and Environmental Hazards (13B) at http://vaww.publichealth.va.gov/smoking/index.asp

It is important to underline that a key factor for the success of brief intervention is motivation. Many clinical practice guidelines (Fiore et al. 2008) stress the importance of motivation when it comes to quitting smoking. The TTUD clinical practice guideline (2008) suggests the use of the "5R's" strategy in order to help the smoker quitting:

- Relevance: Why is quitting personally relevant?
- Risk: What are the potential negative consequences that for the smoker are particularly relevant?

- Rewards: What are the benefits of stopping smoking for the patient?
- Roadblocks: What are possible barriers to quitting?
- Repetition: Repeat at every treatment session.

10.4.2 3A's

The 3A's protocol is another brief intervention for smoking cessation, that is a modification of the 5A's clinical guideline (Ask, Advise, Assess, Assist, Arrange).

It consists of the following steps:

1. Ask and record a patient's smoking status.
2. Advise to quit smoking.
3. Assess, sending the patient to Stop Smoking Service (SSS), giving information to smokers on type, and effectiveness of drug use.

This abbreviated version of the 5A's can be used by healthcare providers who have not much time to interact with their patients. However, as demonstrated by Gordon et al. (2007), this type of intervention is not significantly different by the 5A's approach.

10.5 The Evidence of Counseling

Individually delivered smoking cessation counseling can assist smokers to quit. This is the conclusion of a Cochrane systematic review that included 30 clinical trials and more than 7,000 patients (Rice and Stead 2008). In this review 22 trials compared two different interventions (a) individual counseling and (b) a minimal behavioral intervention. Counseling delivered to individuals (a) was more effective than the control intervention (b). The "risk" for quitting smoking in the long run for the individual counseling was higher than 39 % (RR = 1.39; 95 % CI: 1.24–1.57).

Considering in this review only a subgroup of 4 RCT in which participants received nicotine replacement therapy the probability of stopping was higher than 27 % (RR = 1.27; 95 % CI: 1.02–1.59).

Moreover, another Cochrane review (Stead, L. F., Perera, R., Lancaster, T. (2007). A systematic review of interventions for smokers who contact Quitlines. *Tobacco Control 16* Suppl 1:i3–i8.) including 65 trial, led to identify quitlines effectiveness for smoking cessation effective, and this happens particularly for patients who are interested in quitting.

This review highlighted there is evidence of a dose response: three or more calls increase the probability of quitting if compared to a minimal intervention (standard self-help materials, brief advice) or to pharmacotherapy alone.

An effect of motivation can be seen. In fact, among smokers who actively contacted helplines for telephone counseling, the cessation rates were higher for groups randomized to receive multiple sessions of proactive counseling (RR for cessation at longest follow up equal to 1.37, 95 % CI: 1.26–1.50). On the other hand, telephone counseling not initiated by calls to helplines had a smaller effect, even if significant (RR = 1.29; 95 %CI: 1.20–1.38).

10.6 Medication for Drug Cessation

According to Fiore et al. (US Public Health Service Guideline 2008), the combination of counseling and medication is more effective than either alone, while other methods were found to be ineffective (see Box 10.2).

Box 10.2 Evidence from Other Methods

Hypnotherapy

A Cochrane systematic review (Barnes et al. 2010) was conducted in 2010 with the aim of assessing the efficacy of hypnotherapy for smoking cessation, since the results of the impact of this method were controversial. Only RCTs of hypnotherapy were considered, in which smoking cessation rates at least six months after the beginning of treatment were reported. Barnes and coll. found 11 studies in which one harm was hypnotherapy compared with 18 different control interventions. The authors found significant heterogeneity between studies, confirming the results were conflicting for the efficacy of this method if compared to no treatment, or to advice, or psychological treatment.

Mobile Phone-Based Interventions

Whittaker et al. (2009) conducted a Cochrane systematic review with the aim of assessing the efficacy of mobile phone-based interventions in helping smokers to quit. The authors considered randomized or quasi-randomized trials involving any type of mobile phone-based intervention. They included in the analysis 4 trials concerning the use of:

- A text message program (New Zealand)
- A text message program (UK)
- An Internet and mobile phone program (Norway)

Whittaket and coll. found no evidence of effect of mobile phone-based smoking cessation interventions on long-term outcome. On the other hand short-term results are positive. The text message program RCT showed a significant increase in the probability of self-reported quitting in the short term (RR=2.18; 95 %CI: 1.80–2.65). Combining data from the Internet and mobile phone programs trials there is evidence of an increase in self-reported quitting both in the short and long term (RR=2.03; 95 % CI: 1.40–2.94).

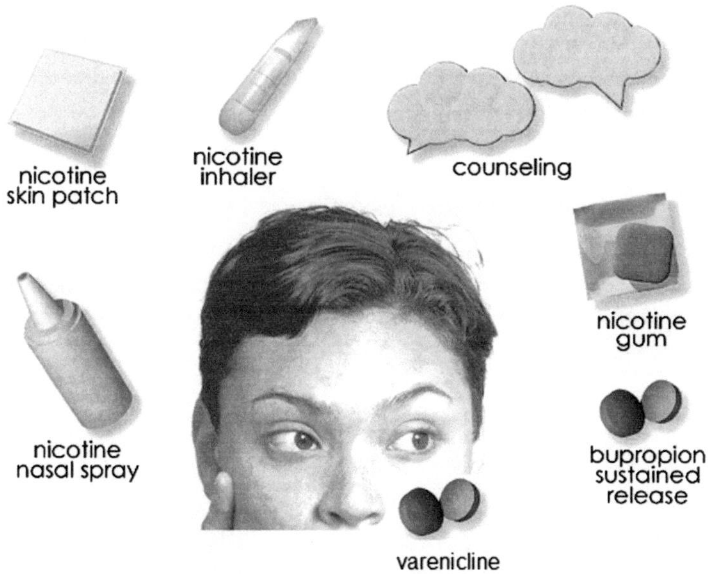

Fig. 10.5 What are the available medication to quit smoking (Modified by Jorenby, D. E. (2001). Smoking cessation strategies for the twenty-first century. *Circulation,* 104, e51–e52)

So, it is important to give some information on type, efficacy, and safety of medications that are currently used in this context (Fig. 10.5).

Two regulatory agencies at the international level (Medscape education), the US Food and Drug Administration (FDA) and the European Medicines Agency (EMEA), include the use of:

(a) Nicotine replacement therapy (NRT).
(b) Bupropion sustained release (BUP) (in the USA from 1997; in Europe from 1999).
(c) Varenicline (VAR) (in the USA from May 2006; in Europe from September 2006).

These medications (NRT, BUP, VAR) can be used as first-line therapies as suggested by US (Fiore et al. 2008) and European guidelines (NICE 2002; Tønnesen et al. 2007). Moreover, some guidelines recommend the use of nortriptyline or clonidine as a second-line therapy for smokers for whom first-line drugs are contraindicated, not effective or intolerable (Tønnesen et al. 2007; Fiore et al. 2008). Counseling and pharmacotherapy in combination have been found to achieve the highest rate of smoking cessation (Nides et al. 2008; Rigotti 2002; Grassi et al.

Box 10.3 Cost Effectiveness of Varenicline and Treatments for Major Smoking-Related Morbidities

A recent review published in 2011 examined economic evaluations of varenicline, from 2006 to 2009 to compare the reported cost effectiveness of varenicline with that of treatments for major smoking-related diseases (Zimovetz et al. 2011).

The results of this study showed that varenicline cost-effectiveness ratios were substantially lower than those reported for interventions used for treatment of smoking-related diseases, with an incremental cost-effectiveness ratios (ICER) for varenicline ranging from dominance (more effective and cost saving) to €18 582 per quality-adjusted life-year-QALY* (including indirect costs).

These estimates appeared substantially lower when compared with ICERs reported for secondary prevention of smoking-related diseases, which in some cases were as high as €66,218 per QALY.

In another study published in 2011 too, Javitz et al. aimed to compare the cost effectiveness of three behavioral smoking cessation modalities based on varenicline treatment: web-based counseling, proactive telephone counseling (PTC), and combination of the two modalities.

Costs per additional 6-month nonsmoker and per additional lifetime quitter were $1,278 and $2,601 for web, $1,472 and $2,995 for PTC, and $1,617 and $3,291 for PTC–web. Cost per life-year (LY) and QALY saved were $1,148 and $1,136 for web, $1,320 and $1,308 for PTC, and $1,450 and $1,437 for PTC–web.

The web intervention was the least expensive followed by the PTC and PTC–web groups. Moreover, smoking cessation treatment consisting of varenicline combined with a telephone-based or web-based counseling program were as cost effective as many other smoking cessation interventions discussed in the literature, quite likely including generic bupropion SR combined with a PTC program. The cost per LY and QALY saved were sufficiently low for all modalities to rate any of these smoking cessation interventions as among the most cost effective of lifesaving medical treatment (Javitz et al. 2011).

*The acceptable thresholds of cost effectiveness are approximately €22,000—€33,000 per QALY in the UK

2006, 2011), and clinical practice guidelines recommends the use of both for all quit attempts (Fiore et al. 2008).

In Box 10.3 the economic evaluation of varenicline is reported.

10.6.1 First-Line Medications

10.6.1.1 Nicotine Replacement Medications

The rationale for the use of nicotine replacement medications is to supply the smoker who wants to quit with nicotine in controlled amounts, avoiding other chemicals present in the smoke, derived from the tobacco plant or the combustion. This kind of medication is particularly useful for taking under control some symptoms of nicotine craving and withdrawal (i.e., urge to smoke, depression, trouble sleeping, irritability, anxiety, and increased appetite) and can be used through different type of deliver.

Nicotine replacement products include transdermal patches, chewing gum, lozenges, nasal spray, and vapor inhaler. The first three types are the most used, since they can be delivered without prescription (Over The Counter, OTC), while nasal spray and vapor inhaler are prescription-only products.

Skin patches, also known as transdermal nicotine patches, are affixed to the skin, similar to how one would apply an adhesive bandage; the nicotine gum and the lozenges are products in which the nicotine is delivered directly to the bloodstream via absorption by oral mucosa.

It is important to consider some aspects before starting a NRT. First of all, this kind of therapy must be stopped if some symptoms appear, such as persistent redness or swelling of the skin around the patch, nausea, vomiting, dizziness, weakness, fast or irregular heartbeat.

Moreover, the patient must not use other product containing nicotine while using NRT. Furthermore, pregnant or breast-feeding women should use NRT only under medical control. Finally, NRT must be considered with caution if the patients suffer from some chronic diseases, such as diabetes, hypertension, heart disease, asthma, or stomach ulcers.

10.6.1.2 Products Not Containing Nicotine

Two drugs that do not contain nicotine have been approved for smoking cessation, i.e., VAR (2006) and BUP. Both are available in tablet form on a prescription-only basis.

VAR (trade name Chantix in the USA and Champix in other countries) acts as a selective partial agonist at alpha 4 beta 2 nicotine acetylcholine receptor, VAR inhibits nicotine-induced dopaminergic activation in a dose-dependent manner, a mechanism that may account for the observation that VAR devalues the rewarding effects of smoking (Coe et al. 2005; Rollema et al. 2007). In other words, VAR has the capacity to stimulate nicotine receptors, even if more weakly than nicotine. It reduces symptoms of nicotine craving and decreases the pleasurable effects of tobacco smoking.

Concerning side effects, patients using VAR experience mostly nausea and less commonly headache, difficulty sleeping, and abnormal dreams.

It is important to report that VAR in some patients is associated with changes in behavior, agitation, depressed mood, suicidal thoughts or actions, as now reported as safety information in the black box warning.

BUP (trade name Aplenzin, Budeprion, Voxra, Wellbutrin, or Zyban) is an antidepressant that inhibits the catecholamine (dopamine and norepinephrine) reuptake, then decreases cravings and withdrawal symptoms. It acts as a nicotinic acetylcholine receptor antagonist, resulting as a mild psychostimulant.

Concerning side effects, patients using BUP experience mostly insomnia and dry mouth and less frequently allergic reactions, hypertension, and seizures. Rare side effects of BUP are psychotic symptoms, mania and suicidal ideation.

The use of BUP should be avoided in individuals who are also taking monoamine oxidase inhibitors and patients with epilepsy, anorexia nervosa, and bulimia; in Table 10.2 first-line medication guidelines for smoking cessation are reported, including dosage, duration of use, administration instructions, cautions for patients, and side effects.

10.6.1.3 The Evidence of Efficacy of First-Line Medications

Cahill et al. (Cochrane 2012) in a recent systematic review demonstrated VAR and BUP are highly effective in quitting smoking, with more participants that quit successfully with VAR than with BUP.

Considering a follow-up period of 6 months or longer and including 14 trials (6,166 patients), the pooled "risk" for continuous or sustained abstinence for VAR (standard dose) versus placebo is more than double (RR = 2.27; 95 %CI: 2.02–2.55) and double at lower or variable doses including 4 RCT and 1,272 smokers (RR = 2.09; 95 %CI: 1.56–2.78).

Comparing the effect of VAR versus BUP at 1 year the probability of quitting is higher for VAR (RR = 1.52; 95 %CI: 1.22–1.88).

No statistically significant difference was found between VAR and NRT for point prevalence abstinence at 24 weeks including 2 RCT and 778 smokers (RR = 1.13; 95 %CI: 0.94–1.35).

Another drug actually used for tobacco dependence is cytisine. Cytisine has been used to treat tobacco dependence for 40 years in Eastern Europe and is a drug extracted from *Cytisus laborinum* plant that acts as its derivative VAR: it is a partial agonist of alpha 4 beta 2 nicotinic receptors. Actually two recent trials (Cahill et al. 2012) (937 people) found that more subjects taking cytisine stopped smoking compared with placebo at longest follow up, with a pooled RR of 3.98 (95 % CI: 2.01–7.87).

Table 10.2 First-line medication guidelines for smoking cessation

Medications (brand examples)	Dosage	Duration	*OR* (95 % CI)
Nicotine gum (i) [Nicorette®] 2 mg, 4 mg OTC	2 mg: *<25 cigarettes/day* 4 mg: ≥25 cigarettes/day Weeks 1–6: 1 piece q 1–2 h – Minimum: 9 pieces/day – Maximum: 24 pieces/day Weeks 7–9: 1 piece q 2–4 h Weeks 10–12: 1 piece q 4–8 h	Up to 12 weeks	*1.5 (1.2–1.7)*
Nicotine lozenge (i) [Nicorette®] 2 mg, 4 mg OTC	2 mg: *first cigarette >30 min after waking* 4 mg: *first cigarette ≤30 min after waking* Weeks 1–6: 1 lozenge q 1–2 h – Minimum: 9 lozenges/day – Maximum: 20 lozenges/day Weeks 7–9: 1 lozenges q 2–4 h Weeks 10–12: 1 lozenges q 4–8 h	Up to 12 weeks	2 mg: *2.0 (1.4–2.8)* (iii) 4 mg: *2.8 (1.9–4.0)* (iii)
Nicotine patch, 24 h (i) [Nicoderm CQ®] 7 mg, 14 mg, 21 mg OTC	*If >10 cigarettes/day: (ii)* 21 mg/day × 4–6 weeks; 14 mg × 2 weeks; 7 mg × 2 weeks *If ≤10 cigarettes/day (ii)* 14 mg/day × 6 weeks; 7 mg/day × 2 weeks	8–10 weeks *PATCH plus:* + bupropion HCI SR + ad lib gum or spray + lozenge + inhaler	*1.9 (1.7–2.2)* 2.5 (1.9–3.4) (iii) 3.6 (2.5–5.2) (iii, iv) 2.3 (1.5–3.6) (iii, iv) 2.2 (1.3–3.6) (iii, iv)
Nicotine nasal spray (i) [Nicotrol NS®] (4 bottles/package) 200 sprays/10 ml bottle 0.5 mg/metered spray Rx	1 dose = 2 sprays (one spray in each nostril) Start with 1–2 doses/h (Maximum: 5 doses/h) – Minimum: 8 doses/day – Maximum: 40 doses/day Taper at end suggested	12 weeks; up to 6 months in selected patients	*2.3 (1.7–3.0)*

Nicotine inhaler (i) [Nicotrol®] (168 cartridges/package) 10 mg/cartridge Rx	10 mg cartridge (delivers 4 mg) ~ 20 min of active puffing – Minimum: 6 cartridges/day – Maximum: 16 cartridges/day Taper at end suggested	12 weeks; up to 6 months In selected patients	*2.1 (1.5–2.9)*
Bupropion HCI SR [Zyban®] 150 mg SR tablet Rx	Start 1–2 weeks before quit date Days 1–3: 150 mg q AM Day 4 until end: 150 mg BID (v) – Maximum: 300 mg/day	7–12 weeks; up to 6 months in selected patients	*2.0 (1.8–2.2)*
Varenicline [Chantix®] 0.5 mg, 1 mg tablet Rx	Start 1 week before quit date Days 1–3: 0.5 mg q AM Days 4–7: 0.5 mg BID Days 8 until end: 1 mg BID (vi)	12 weeks; up to 6 months in selected patients	*3.1 (2.5–3.8)* (vi)

	Administration Instructions	Cautions *(Pregnancy)*	Side effects/comments
Nicotine gum	• Chew gum slowly until tingles (~ 15–30 chews), then park between cheek and gum	• Caution in patients with recent myocardial infarction (within 2 weeks), serious arrhythmias, unstable angina	• Mouth soreness; jaw ache
	• Resume chewing when tingle fades	• Caution with dentures, dental caps, partial bridges, temporomandibular joint disease	• Hiccups
	• Repeat "chew-park" process until tingle is gone/does not return (~ 30 min)	• *FDA: C; Briggs: Compatible—maternal benefit >> embryo/fetal risk*	• Dyspepasia
	• No food or beverages except water 15 min before or during use		• Gastrointestinal disturbances: – Associated with improper use and swallowing large amounts of nicotine
Nicotine lozenge	• Dissolve slowly in mouth (~ 20–30 min); may notice warm tingling sensation	• Caution in patients with recent myocardial infraction (within 2 weeks), serious arrhythmias, unstable angina	• Nausea; hiccups heartburn; indigestion
	• Occasionally move to other side of mouth • Do not chew or swallow • No food or beverages except water 15 min before or during use	• *FDA: C; Briggs: Not available*	• 4 mg: cough (<10 %) and headaches (<10 %)

(continued)

Table 10.2 (continued)

	Administration Instructions	Cautions (*Pregnancy*)	Side effects/comments
Nicotine Patch, 24 h	• Apply patch to clean, hairless, dry skin on trunk or upper limbs	• Caution in patients with recent myocardial infarction (with 2 weeks), serious arrhythmias, unstable angina	• Insomnia
	• Rotate application sites	• Avoid in patients with severe eczema or psoriasis	• Local skin reaction (50 %): – Usually mild
	• If sleep disturbances, remove patch at bedtime	• Remove metal containing patches (e.g., tancolored) prior to MRI	– Rarely leads to discontinuation
	• Do not cut patch	• *FDA: D; Briggs: Compatible—maternal benefit >> embryo/fetal risk*	– Rotate application site to minimize
Nicotine nasal spray	• Prime pump before first use or if not used for >24 h	• Caution in patients with recent myocardial infarction (within 2 weeks), serious arrhythmias, unstable angina	• Nasal irritation (94 %), nasal congestion
	• Shake nasal spray before using	• Avoid in patients with severe reactive airway disease and chronic nasal disorders	• Smell and taste alterations
	• Deliver with head tilted slightly back	• Wait 5 min before driving	
	• Avoid sniffing, inhaling, or swallowing	• Highest dependence potential	
		• *FDA: D; Briggs: Compatible—maternal benefit >> embryo/fetal risk*	
Nicotine inhaler	• Inhale into back of throat or puff in short breaths; do not inhale into lungs	• Caution in patients with recent myocardial infarction (within 2 weeks), serious arrhythmias, unstable angina	• Mouth and throat irritation (40 %)
	• Open cartridge retains potency for 24 h	• Caution in patients with severe bronchospastic disease	• Cough (32 %)
	• Use inhaler at room temperature	• *FDA: D; Briggs: Compatible—maternal benefit >> embryo/fetal risk*	• Rhinitis (23 %)
	• No food or beverages except water 15 min before or during use		

Bupropion HCl SR	• Take second dose in afternoon to reduce insomnia • Allow at least 8 h between doses	• Contraindicated in patients with history of seizure or eating disorders • Monitor blood pressure when combined with nicotine replacement therapy • Monitor for changes in mood, behavior, psychiatric symptoms, and suicidal ideation • *FDA: C; Briggs: Human data suggest low risk*	• Insomnia (30–40 %) • Dry mouth (10 %) • Seizures (rare) reported in smoking cessation trials
Varenicline	• Take after eating (with a full glass of water) to reduce nausea • Take second dose at supper to reduce insomnia	• Caution in patients with significant renal impairment, serious psychiatric illness • Caution driving/operating machinery • Monitor for changes in mood, behavior, psychiatric symptoms, and suicidal ideation • *FDA: C; Briggs: No human data—animal data suggest low risk*	• Nausea (up to 30 %) – Dose related – May diminish over time – Reduced with initial titration • Insomnia; abnormal, vivid, strange dreams • Rare serious skin/allergic reactions

Modified from SCORxE. Evidence-based best practices for promoting smoking cessation in South Carolina (http://www.sccp.sc.edu/SCORxE)

References

American Medical Association. (1994). *American Medical Association guidelines for the diagnosis and treatment of nicotine dependence: How to help patients stop smoking*. Washington DC: American Medical Association.

American Psychiatric Association. (1996). Practice guideline for the treatment of patients with nicotine dependence. *The American Journal of Psychiatry, 153*(10 Suppl), S1–S31.

Barnes, J., Dong, C. Y., McRobbie, H., Walker, N., Mehta, M., & Stead, L. F. (2010). Hypnotherapy for smoking cessation. *Cochrane Database Systematic Reviews* (10): CD001008.

Bodner, M. E., & Dean, E. (2009). Advice as a smoking cessation strategy: A systematic review and implications for physical therapists. *Physiotherapy Theory and Practice, 25*(5–6), 369–407.

Cahill, K., Stead, L. F., & Lancaster, T. (2012). Nicotine receptor partial agonists for smoking cessation. *Cochrane Database Systematic Reviews* (44): CD006103.

CDC. (2011). Quitting smoking among adults—United States, 2001–2010. *Morbidity and Mortality Weekly Report, 60*, 1513–1519.

Coe, J. W., Brooks, P. R., Wirtz, M. C., Bashore, C. G., Bianco, K. E., Vetelino, M. G., et al. (2005). 3,5-Bicyclic aryl piperidines: A novel class of alpha4beta2 neuronal nicotinic receptor partial agonists for smoking cessation. *Bioorganic and Medicinal Chemical Letters, 15*, 4889–4897.

Fiore, M. C., Jaén, C. R., Baker, T. B., et al. (2008). *Clinical practice guideline: Treating tobacco use and dependence—2008 update*. Rockville, MD: US Dept of Health and Human Services, Public Health Service.

Glynn, T. J., Manley, M. W., & Pechacek, T. F. (1990). Physician-initiated smoking cessation program: The National Cancer Institute trials. *Progress in Clinical and Biological Research, 339*, 11–25.

Gordon, J. S., Andrews, J. A., Crews, K. M., Payne, T. J., & Severson, H. H. (2007). The 5A's vs 3A's plus proactive quitline referral in private practice dental offices: Preliminary results. *Tobacco Control, 16*(4), 285–8.

Grassi, M. C., Chiamulera, C., Baraldo, M., Culasso, F., Ferketich, A. K., Raupach, T., et al. (2012). Cigarette smoking knowledge and perceptions among students in Four Italian medical schools. *Nicotine & Tobacco Research, 14*(9), 1065–1072.

Grassi, M. C., Enea, D., Ferketich, A. K., Pasquariello, S., & Nencini, P. (2011). Effectiveness of varenicline for smoking cessation: A 1-year follow-up study. *Journal of Substance Abuse Treatment, 41*(1), 64–70.

Grassi, M. C., Enea, D., Marchetti, R., Caricati, A. M., & Nencini, P. (2006). Combined counseling and bupropion therapy for smoking cessation: Identification of outcome predictors. *Drug Development Research, 67*, 271–279.

Javitz, H. S., Zbikowski, S. M., Deprey, M., McAfee, T. A., McClure, J. B., Richards, J., et al. (2011). Cost-effectiveness of varenicline and three different behavioral treatment formats for smoking cessation. *Translational Behavioral Medicine, 1*(1), 182–190.

Jha, P., Ramasundarahettige, C., Landsman, V., Rostron, B., Thun, M., Anderson, R. N., et al. (2013). 21st-century hazards of smoking and benefits of cessation in the United States. *The New England Journal of Medicine, 368*, 341–350s.

Jorenby, D. E. (2001). Smoking cessation strategies for the 21st century. *Circulation, 104*, e51–e52.

La Torre, G., Kirch, W., Bes-Rastrollo, M., Mateos Ramos, R., Czaplicki, M., Gualano, M. R., et al. (2012). Epidemics of tobacco use among medical students in Europe: Results of a multicentre study global health professions students survey. *Public Health, 126*(2), 159–164.

Mallin, R. (2002). Smoking cessation: Integration of behavioral and drug therapies. *American Family Physician, 65*(6), 1107–1115.

McIvor, A., Kayser, J., Assaad, J. M., Brosky, G., Demarest, P., Desmarais, P., et al. (2009). Best practices for smoking cessation interventions in primary care. *Canadian Respiratory Journal, 16*(4), 129–34.

McLellan, A. T., Lewis, D. C., O'Brien, C. P., & Kleber, H. D. (2000). Drug dependence, a chronic medical illness: Implications for treatment, insurance, and outcomes evaluation. *JAMA: The Journal of the American Medical Association, 284*(13), 1689–1695.

Mecklenburg, R. E., Christen, A. G., Gerbert, B., & Gift, M. C. (1991). *How to help your patients stop using tobacco: A National Cancer Institute manual for the oral health team 1990* (NIH Publication No. 91–3191). Bethesda, MD: US DHHS Public Health Service, National Institutes of Health, National Cancer Institute.

Medscape education (smoking cessation—multimodal techniques: Efficacy, utilisation, guidelines. Accessed from http://www.medscape.org/viewarticle/585737_3)

NICE. (2002). *Guidance on the use of nicotine replacement therapy (NRT) and bupropion for smoking cessation.* NICE technology appraisal 39. Available from: www.nice.org.uk/TA039.

Needleman, I. G., Binnie, V. I., Ainamo, A., Carr, A. B., Fundak, A., Koerber, A., et al. (2010). Improving the effectiveness of tobacco use cessation (TUC). *International Dental Journal, 60*(1), 50–59.

Nides, M., Glover, E. D., Reus, V. I., Christen, A. G., Maker, B. J., BillingC, B., et al. (2008). Varenicline versus bupropion SR or placebo for smoking cessation: A pooled analysis. *American Journal of Health Behavior, 32*, 664–675.

Prochaska, J. O., & DiClemente, C. C. (1983). Stages and processes of self-change of smoking: Toward an integrative model of change. *Journal of Consulting and Clinical Psychology, 51*, 390–395.

Prochaska, J. O., & DiClemente, C. C. (1992). Stages of change in the modification of problem behaviors. *Progress in Behavior Modification, 28*, 183–218.

Ramseier, C. A., & Fundak, A. (2009). Tobacco use cessation provided by dental hygienists. *International Journal of Dental Hygiene, 7*(1), 39–48.

Rice, V. H., & Stead, L. F. (2008). Nursing interventions for smoking cessation. *Cochrane Database Systematic Reviews* (1): CD001188.

Rigotti, N. A. (2002). Treatment of tobacco use and dependence. *The New England Journal of Medicine, 346*, 506–512.

Rollema, H., Chambers, L. K., Coe, J. W., Glowa, J., Hurst, R. S., Lebel, L. A., et al. (2007). Pharmacological profile of the alpha4beta2 nicotinic acetylcholine receptor partial agonist varenicline, an effective smoking cessation aid. *Neuropharmacology, 52*, 985–994.

Schiller, J. S., Lucas, J. W., & Peregoy, J. A. (2012). Summary health statistics for U.S. adults: National Health Interview Survey, 2011. National Center for Health Statistics. *Vital and health statistics, 10*(256). pp 218.

Sinclair, H. K., Bond, C. M., & Stead, L. F. (2004). Community pharmacy personnel interventions for smoking cessation. *Cochrane Database Systematic Reviews* (1):CD003698.

Tønnesen, P., Carrozzi, L., Fagerström, K., et al. (2007). Smoking cessation in patients with respiratory diseases: A high priority, integral component of therapy. *The European Respiratory Journal, 29*, 390–417.

Thun, M. J., Carter, B. D., Feskanich, D., Freedman, N. D., Prentice, R., Lopez, A. D., et al. (2013). 50-year trends in smoking-related mortality in the United States. *The New England Journal of Medicine, 368*, 351–364.

Velicer, W. F., Prochaska, J. O., Fava, J. L., Norman, G. J., & Redding, C. A. (1998). Smoking cessation and stress management: Applications of the transtheoretical model of behavior change. *Homeostasis, 38*, 216–233.

Whittaker, R., Borland, R., Bullen, C., Lin, R. B., McRobbie, H., & Rodgers, A. (2009) Mobile phone-based interventions for smoking cessation. *Cochrane Database Systematic Reviews* (4): CD006611.

Zimovetz, E. A., Wilson, K., Samuel, M., & Beard, S. M. (2011). A review of cost-effectiveness of varenicline and comparison of cost-effectiveness of treatments for major smoking-related morbidities. *Journal of Evaluation in Clinical Practice, 17*(2), 288–297.

Chapter 11
Smoking Cessation Among Different Settings

Giuseppe La Torre and Luca Calzoni

Objectives This section aims to address the role and the efficacy of smoking cessation interventions among different settings and concerning health professionals as well as workplace.

Learning Outcomes

By the end of this section the reader will be able to:

- Understand how smoking cessation interventions work in different settings.
- Understand how smoking cessation interventions among healthcare personnel can play a fundamental role in supporting similar policies addressed to the general public.
- Learn what strategies have been adopted in real healthcare settings to promote smoking cessation.

11.1 Smoking Cessation in the General Population

In order to reverse the tobacco epidemic, concerted efforts are needed from a wide range of sectors. National health systems and health workers are called to play a fundamental role in the process, implementing measures to prevent and treat tobacco dependence (WHO 2011a, b).

G. La Torre (✉)
Department of Public Health and Infectious Diseases, "Sapienza" University of Rome, Piazzale Aldo Moro 5, Rome 00185, Italy
e-mail: giuseppe.latorre@uniroma1.it

L. Calzoni
Department of Public Health and Infectious Diseases, "Sapienza" University of Rome, Via Lazio 69, Latina, LT 04100, Italy
e-mail: luca.calzoni.1@gmail.com

G. La Torre, *Smoking Prevention and Cessation*, DOI 10.1007/978-1-4614-7046-5_11,

However, many health systems do not integrate tobacco prevention and treatment into routine patient care. Medical professional training includes only a minimum of time devoted to treatment of tobacco dependence, and many health professionals do not even consider tobacco control as part of their job (Martinez et al. 2008). In some countries, a considerable number of health workers are users of tobacco themselves (WHO 2011a, b).

This last aspect is particularly striking, since medical professionals have been recognized to possess the greatest potential of any group in society to promote a reduction in tobacco use (WHO 2011a, b). Their participation to tobacco control efforts is of vital importance: this is why one of the strategies to reduce the number of smoking-related deaths in the general population is to encourage the involvement of health professionals in tobacco-use prevention and cessation programs.

Smoking cessation in the general population has beneficial effects on several outcomes, economic, clinical, and humanistic ones. According to Sherman (2005) the economic gains are concerning not only money saved through having fewer overall healthcare costs, but also through not perpetuating the addiction.

At the clinical level, smoking cessation has clinical relevant effects, going from attenuation of depression and decreased blood pressure and triglyceride levels, to enhanced glycemic control. Moreover, considering the possible effect on these pathologies, quitting smoking has a great impact also on the reduction of morbidity and mortality in this patient population.

Finally, the humanistic impact of smoking cessation deals with the development of a greater sense of control over one's own health (Sherman 2005).

In Fig. 11.1 a simplified model of the cessation process is presented. There is evidence that the main population-based cessation effect of physician advice and media campaigns concerns the promotion of cessation attempts.

On the other hand there is less evidence supporting an effect of these interventions on longer term cessation success.

It is important to underline that the predominant effects of restrictions where tobacco smoking is permitted, the increase of cost of cigarettes, as well as pharmacological interventions and comprehensive tobacco-control campaigns are in promoting longer term cessation success (Burns 2012).

According to WHO (2011a, b), in the field of smoking cessation the public health approaches at the general population level must involve mass media campaigns, Quit and Win competitions and telephone helplines, as tools for changing societal norms and promoting better health.

Health promotion campaigns delivered through mass media can increase knowledge about the health effects of smoking tobacco products and the benefits of quitting. This kind of campaign has the potential of changing and reinforcing attitudes toward quitting smoking, giving examples of simple action that can influence smoking behavior.

Quit and Win campaigns have been using innovative communication methods and partnerships, including the involvement of community organizations and health services, to achieve cessation rates of around 20 %. Usually a special Website is available together with a special call center, guaranteeing a complete information service

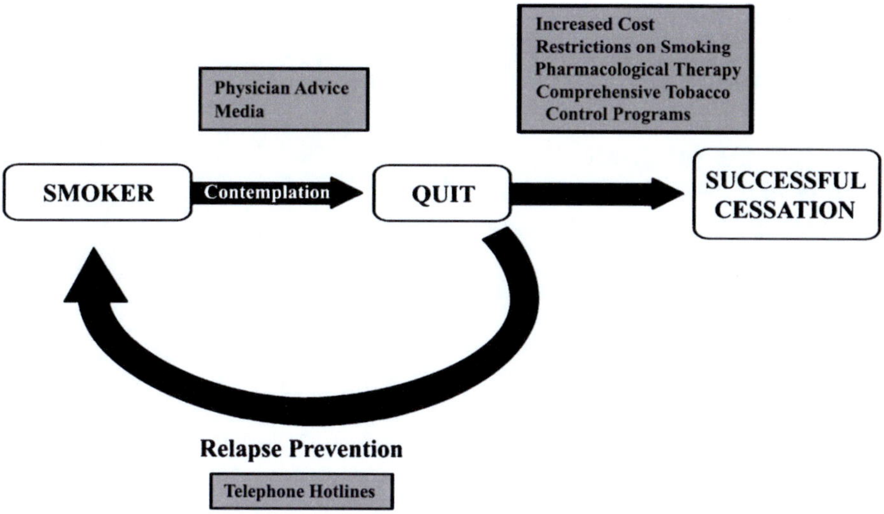

Fig. 11.1 Smoking cessation at the population level (from Burns 2012)

(Gianti et al. 2007). The smoker who wants to participate with the aim of quitting must agree to remain nonsmokers for a given period. This agreement must be witnessed by a relative, a friend who can enforce and validate the smoker's statement. At the end of the period, the winners are chosen and their abstinence is then measured by biological tests, such as urinary cotinine and respiratory carbon monoxide.

Quitlines (proactive and reactive) also play an important role in a comprehensive smoking cessation program. This kind of tool is intended to provide a service with peculiar characteristics, i.e., reasonable cost and good accessibility. Proactive quitlines can provide immediate "reactive" assistance when a smoker first calls. Moreover, they also provide more comprehensive services through outbound ("proactive") calls. On the other hand reactive quitlines respond to callers' immediate requests for assistance, even though they do not provide outbound counseling calls. This strategy has not been recommended by the various guidelines, since the evidence is still limited (CDC 2005). Many quitlines are provided by public entities (Figs. 11.2 and 11.3) and the service is for free.

11.2 Smoking Cessation in the Clinical Setting

Tobacco smoking can contribute to several health problems that are the causes of hospitalization, including cardiovascular diseases, respiratory diseases, and cancer. Moreover, tobacco smoking is associated with increased risk during hospitalizations for surgical procedures. Considering these facts, it is important to foresee and provide tobacco dependence treatments in hospitals, even if at an early stage (Rigotti et al. 2012).

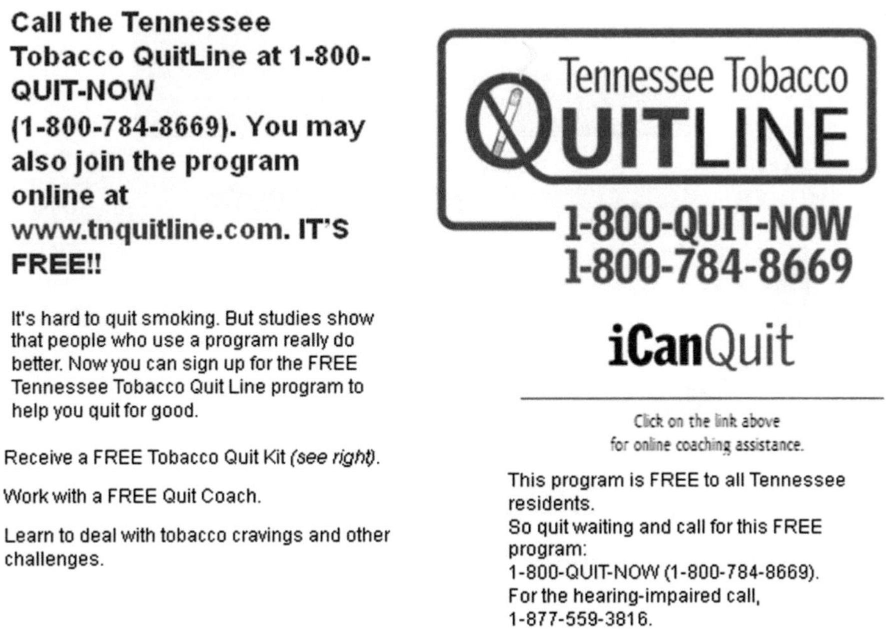
Call the Tennessee Tobacco QuitLine at 1-800-QUIT-NOW (1-800-784-8669). You may also join the program online at www.tnquitline.com. IT'S FREE!!
It's hard to quit smoking. But studies show that people who use a program really do better. Now you can sign up for the FREE Tennessee Tobacco Quit Line program to help you quit for good.
Receive a FREE Tobacco Quit Kit (see right).
Work with a FREE Quit Coach.
Learn to deal with tobacco cravings and other challenges.
Tennessee Tobacco QUITLINE
1-800-QUIT-NOW
1-800-784-8669
iCanQuit
Click on the link above for online coaching assistance.
This program is FREE to all Tennessee residents.
So quit waiting and call for this FREE program:
1-800-QUIT-NOW (1-800-784-8669).
For the hearing-impaired call,
1-877-559-3816.

Fig. 11.2 Example of public quitline (Accessed from, http://health.state.tn.us/tobaccoquitline.htm)

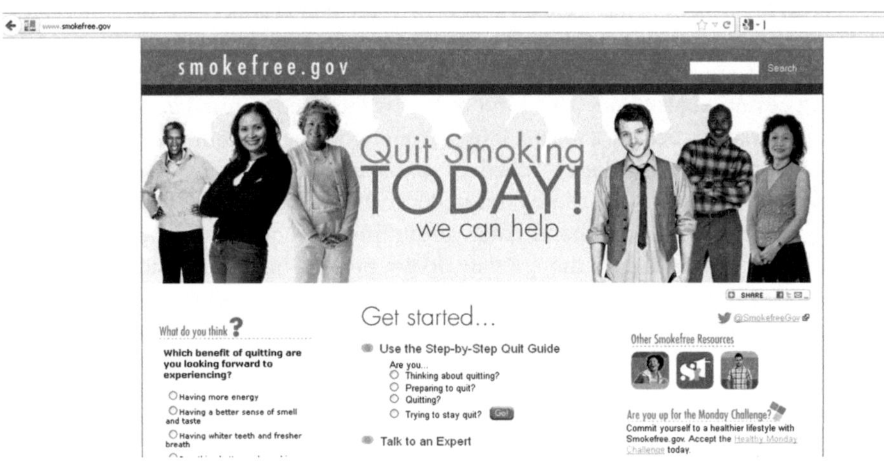
smokefree.gov
Search
Quit Smoking TODAY! we can help
What do you think?
Which benefit of quitting are you looking forward to experiencing?
Having more energy
Having a better sense of smell and taste
Having whiter teeth and fresher breath
Get started...
Use the Step-by-Step Quit Guide
Are you...
Thinking about quitting?
Preparing to quit?
Quitting?
Trying to stay quit?
Talk to an Expert
Other Smokefree Resources
Are you up for the Monday Challenge?
Commit yourself to a healthier lifestyle with Smokefree.gov. Accept the Healthy Monday Challenge today.

Fig. 11.3 National quitline created by the U.S. Department of Health and Human Services

11.2.1 Hospitalized Patients

A Cochrane systematic review of the literature in 2012 had the aim of summarizing tobacco cessation interventions for hospitalized patients, including 50 trials (Rigotti et al. 2012). The authors found that intensive counseling interventions starting during the hospital stay and continuing with supportive contacts for at least 1 month after hospital discharge (25 trials) can increase smoking cessation rates after discharge by almost 40 % (RR = 1.37; 95 % CI: 1.27–1.48) Adding nicotine replacement therapy to an intensive counseling intervention (6 trials) revealed an increase of smoking cessation rates compared with intensive counseling alone (RR = 1.54; 95 % CI: 1.34–1.79).

11.2.2 Cardiovascular Diseases

The systematic review conducted by Rigotti et al. (2012) shows that for patients admitted to hospital due to cardiovascular disease, intensive intervention with follow-up support has a positive impact on smoking cessation rates (RR = 1.42; 95 % CI: 1.29–1.56). Moreover, in the same review, the authors found in one trial efficacy of intensive intervention including both counseling and pharmacotherapy for smokers who were admitted to hospital with a cardiovascular disease. In these patients a reduction in all-cause mortality and hospital readmission rates over a 2-year follow-up period was found.

11.2.3 Cancer

A systematic review of the literature in 2011 had the aim of summarizing tobacco cessation interventions for cancer patients (Nayan et al. 2011). Eight randomized clinical trials were used for the review, accounting for 1304 patients.

Considering the studies with longer follow-ups, the authors found that the risk of quitting smoking was almost 20 % higher in the intervention group compared with the control group (RR = 1.19; 95 % CI: 0.78–1.78). In a sensitivity analysis, excluding the oldest research (conducted in 1993), the authors found a significant increase in the probability of quitting (pooled RR = 1.42; 95 % CI: 1.05–1.94).

Anyway, it is fundamental to assess smoking habits among cancer patients. It is well known that cancer survivors are not likely to receive any question about their smoking status by their medical doctors. In a survey conducted in the USA more than half of these patients who are smokers use smoking cessation treatments (Coups et al. 2009) (Table 11.1).

The assessment must be provided by medical doctors in order to adequately set the stage for discussing smoking, giving quit advice, and delivering cessation interventions. One must not forget that smoking relapse is common among patients who recently have quit smoking.

11.2.4 Respiratory Diseases

Tønnesen et al. (2007) demonstrated that smoking cessation is a priority for patients with respiratory diseases in order to improve the prognosis in this kind of patients.

Table 11.1 Use of smoking cessation treatments among cancer survivors who are current smokers and tried to quit in the last year (*N* = 130), 2005 National Health Interview Survey (from Coups et al. 2009)

	Sample (%)
Pharmacotherapy	
Nicotine gum	9.3
Nicotine patch	26.1
Another nicotine replacement product[a]	6.5
Prescription pill[b]	7.9
Any nicotine replacement product and prescription pill[b]	4.6
Any type of pharmacotherapy	33.5
Evidence-based behavioral treatment	
Telephone help line	2.0
Stop smoking clinic, class, or support group	2.4
One-on-one counseling	1.9
Any behavioral treatment	3.8
Any pharmacotherapy or evidence-based behavioral treatment	33.8
Both pharmacotherapy and evidence-based behavioral treatment	3.5
Other treatment/assistance	
Help or support from family or friends	25.6
Internet	3.5
Books, pamphlets, videos, or other materials	9.0
Acupuncture or hypnosis	5.3
None of the treatments listed above	51.4

[a] Nasal spray, inhaler, lozenge, or tablet.
[b] For example, Zyban, buproprion, or Wellbutrin.

Table 11.2 Evidence-based recommendations on smoking cessation interventions in respiratory patients (from Tønnesen et al. 2007)

1. Patients with respiratory disease have a greater and more urgent need to stop smoking than the average smoker, so respiratory physicians must take a proactive and continuing role with all smokers in motivating them to stop and in providing treatment to aid smoking cessation
2. Smoking cessation treatment should be integrated into the management of the patient's respiratory condition
3. Therapies should include pharmacological treatment (i.e., nicotine replacement therapy, bupropion, or varenicline) combined with behavioral support
4. Respiratory physicians should receive training to ensure that they have the knowledge, attitudes, and skills necessary to deliver these interventions or to refer to an appropriate specialist
5. Although the cost of implementing these recommendations will partly be offset by a reduction in attendance for exacerbations, etc., a budget should be established to enable implementation

A special task force elaborated guidelines for smoking cessation in patients with respiratory diseases, based on the available evidence, as well as the results of the consensus of an expert panel. The main recommendations are summarized in Table 11.2.

Table 11.3 Strategies for smokers with diabetes (from Sherman 2005)

Behavioral techniques
• Cigarettes signal the end of a meal, so some former smokers tend to continue to eat after they are full. Patients should set an ending time to the meal before sitting down to eat and should push away from the table at that time regardless of whether they are though eating
• An activity should be planned in advance for immediately after each meal, preferably one that incorporates exercise. Good suggestions are going for a walk, working in the garden, or continuing some large project, such as painting the rooms of the house most damaged from smoking
• Because patients are no longer buying cigarettes at the store, why stop there? Encourage them to now begin a healthy lifestyle that includes a stockpile of fruits and vegetables. They should be trained to not allow themselves access to cigarettes for when the cravings occur, so this principle could be extended to include diet as well
Cognitive techniques
• Patients should control cravings by refocusing their thoughts before a craving leads to a slip. For example, when a recent quitter begins actively thinking about tobacco products or unhealthy snacks, he or she could be trained to think of the word "STOP" or snap a rubber band around the wrist. As the craving subsides, the patient could verbalize a reinforcing message, such as "I am in control of my actions"
• Recent quitters should remind themselves when they wake up every day with a phrase such as "I made it through another day without smoking or eating unhealthily"
• Through visualization, prepare for situations in which the temptation to smoke exists

11.2.5 Diabetes

According to Sherman (2005) patients who have diabetes and are smokers are more likely to develop microvascular complications that localize at kidney and nervous system. Both micro- and macroalbuminuria can have a progression of the disease more rapidly in smokers in comparison with former or never smokers (Ikeda et al. 1997). In this case, it is important to use the right strategy to the diabetic patient, including behavioral and cognitive techniques (Table 11.3).

11.3 Smoking Cessation in the Workplace

Bans on smoking in the workplace are one of the most effective measures to reduce the prevalence of smoking among the general population (see Chap. 5). This is one of the starting points of a Cochrane systematic review published in 2008 by Cahill et al. (2008). This review includes 51 studies concerning 53 interventions, and the results are similar to those obtained in other settings. In fact, the vast majority of workplace interventions was directed toward individual workers and includes:

(a) Group therapy
(b) Individual counseling

(c) Production and distribution of self-help materials
(d) Nicotine replacement therapy
(e) Social support

In this setting, group programs, as well as individual counseling and NRT increase quitting smoking rates in comparison to no treatment or minimal intervention controls, while self-help materials have a lower effect. Considering the studies testing interventions applied to the workplace as a whole (16 trials), there is no evidence that comprehensive programs have the capability of reducing the prevalence of tobacco smoking among workers. On the other hand, there is an increasing rate of attempts to stop smoking using incentive schemes.

According to Burns (2012), smoking cessation success is facilitated by referral to cessation assistance and by other factors that include restrictions on smoking in the workplace. It is important to underline that linking local cessation assistance activities with workplaces, in which voluntary changes in smoking restrictions are made, would have the impact to increase the efficiency of the efforts to recruit smokers into these programs. Moreover, this could also increase the effectiveness of the workplace change in performing a successful smoking cessation (Burns 2012).

However, the real situation in smoking cessation in the workplace is far from being acceptable. In a cross-sectional study carried out in the USA in 2008 (Healthy Worksite Survey) Hughes et al. found that among the involved employers, 38.6 % promoted quitting tobacco, 33.8 % provided insurance coverage for cessation medications and counseling, and 5.7 % included the state-sponsored quitline in health promotion messages. There is a lack of tobacco cessation promoting practices at small businesses, restaurants, and bars.

The use of the workplace, as a space where giving prevention efforts in the field of smoking cessation, could be a very effective tool, with reduced costs. As an example, employers can help employees quit smoking with the promotion of the state-sponsored tobacco cessation quitline (Hughes et al. 2011), and doing so, assist in improving employee health and lower medical costs.

Moreover, we need to consider that the work environment influences aspects of smoking behavior. Albertsen et al. (2006) demonstrated that high job demands are associated with higher amount of tobacco smoke and with increased likelihood of cessation. In this context, resources available at the workplace, as well as social support, are associated positively with cessation and negatively with relapse and the amount of tobacco smoked.

Finally, we have to underline that social capital at work is associated with an increased likelihood of smoking cessation in baseline smokers. Kouvonen et al. (2008) carried out a prospective cohort study involving 4853 employees who reported to be smokers at baseline, in which they demonstrated that there exists a significant association between individual-level social capital and smoking cessation in the high socioeconomic group (OR = 1.63; 95 % CI: 1.01–2.63). The same effect was not found in intermediate (OR = 1.10; 95 % CI; 0.83–1.47) or low socioeconomic groups (OR = 1.28; 95 % CI: 0.86–1.91).

11.4 Smoking Cessation Among Healthcare Professionals

11.4.1 Introduction

In this section we intend to discuss the role and the efficacy of smoking cessation interventions addressed to health professionals.

To start with, we are going to describe the key role potentially played by this category of workers in smoking cessation strategies, both as advisers and as role models for the general population.

We will then see how the high prevalence of tobacco consumption among nurses in particular, and health professionals in general, actually ends up impairing their role in setting an example for their patients. We will also underline how more effective preventive policies are needed, and how, if implemented, these would carry social and economical benefits for the entire community.

We will then display the results of a recent scientific literature search we performed, with the aim of identifying what smoking cessation strategies have been actually implemented among healthcare workers, and illustrate their outcomes.

Finally, a comparison of the efficacy of these interventions will be carried out, and suggestions made about identified research gaps in the field.

11.4.2 The Key Role of Healthcare Providers in Smoking Cessation

Comprehensive tobacco programs usually consider not only a mix of interventions, including legislation and pricing measures, but also prevention and other demand reduction attempts. Health professionals, including doctors, dentists, nurses, pharmacists, and others, can intervene in all of these ambits, thus giving a fundamental contribution to tobacco control goals (WHO 2004).

Multiple reasons concur to explain the importance of their role.

To start with, health professionals are seen as trusted sources of advice and information in matters related to health. Many of them are respected, influential community leaders and are considered role models for others (WHO 2004). This means that they have a unique potential to contribute to tobacco control in several complementary ways: for example, by speaking out publicly and lobbying for comprehensive health policies or by influencing health and educational institutions to include tobacco control in curricula (Chapman et al. 2007).

Besides, healthcare workers come into contact with a high percentage of the population in their professional lives, thus having the opportunity to concretely help people change their behavior, particularly in quitting tobacco use. In fact, they can increase awareness on hazards that tobacco consumption imposes on health through public education, informational campaigns, and other demand reduction measures.

They are also able to give guidance, advice, and answers to questions concerning the consequences of tobacco use (WHO 2004).

Smoking cessation advice from health professionals, in particular, has a fundamental role: it is considered by WHO as one of the three types of treatment that should be included in any tobacco prevention effort—the other two being quitlines and pharmacological therapy (WHO 2009). Moreover, studies have shown that even simple, brief counseling by health professionals on the dangers of smoking and the importance of quitting can increase smoking cessation rates by up to 30 % (USDHHS 2000; Lancaster et al. 2000). Similarly, interventions for smoking cessation led by nurses have shown to increase the chance of successfully quitting smoking by up to 50 % (Lancaster et al. 2000).

Finally, health professionals can also play an important role in preventive strategies, especially when considering the youth. In fact, they have the opportunity to promote social norm change and forewarn children and adolescents of the dangers of tobacco (WHO 2004).

11.4.3 Prevalence of Tobacco Consumption Among Healthcare Professionals

Despite their professional responsibility as models of good health practices and their being aware of the risks associated with smoking, health professionals have not always set a good example for patients (Davis 1993). In the twentieth century for instance, some physicians even advertised cigarettes (Gardner and Brandt 2006) (Fig. 11.4).

Still nowadays, many health workers are users of tobacco themselves (WHO 2011a, b).

For instance, while smoking in the medical profession has substantially declined worldwide since the 1950s (Brackbill et al. 1988; CDC 1993; Smith 2008), tobacco control measures have not been uniformly successful, and physicians in some countries still consume tobacco at relatively high rates (Smith and Leggat 2007).

The majority of developed countries have shown a steady decline in physicians' smoking rates during the last 50 years. The lowest smoking prevalence rates have been consistently documented in Australia, the UK, and the USA (Smith 2008). The national smoking rate for physicians in the USA, in particular, has fallen dramatically between 1987 and 1994, and is now below 10 % (Nelson et al. 1994; Lee et al. 2004; WHO 2011a, b).

Similar descending trends were also seen in Scandinavia (Van Reek and Adriaanse 1991) and the Netherlands (Adriaanse et al. 1985, 1986) during the latter half of last century.

On the other hand, physicians in some developed and newly developing countries still appear to be smoking at high rates.

As documented by Smith and Leggat in their international review of tobacco smoking in the medical profession (2007), multiple investigations from Italy

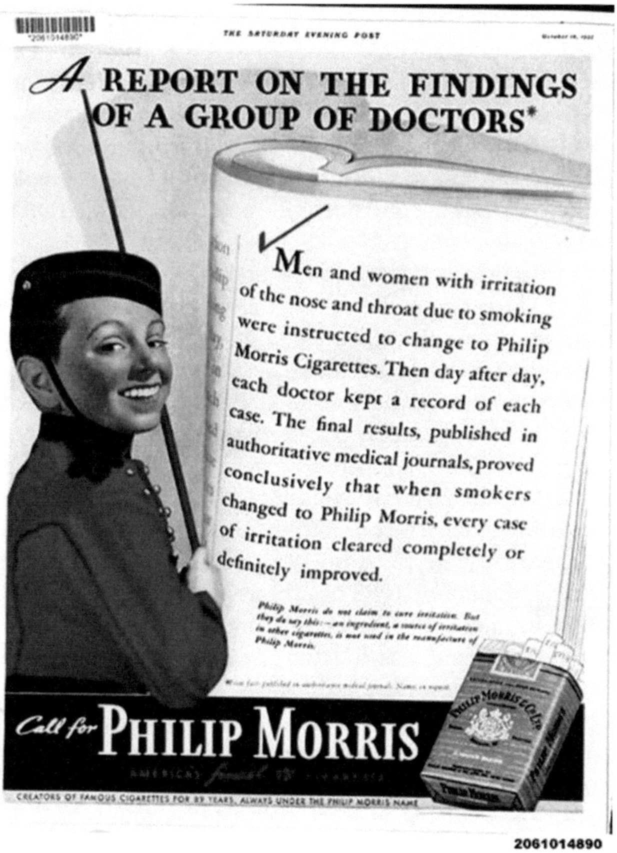
THE SATURDAY EVENING POST
A REPORT ON THE FINDINGS OF A GROUP OF DOCTORS*
Men and women with irritation of the nose and throat due to smoking were instructed to change to Philip Morris Cigarettes. Then day after day, each doctor kept a record of each case. The final results, published in authoritative medical journals, proved conclusively that when smokers changed to Philip Morris, every case of irritation cleared completely or definitely improved.
Philip Morris do not claim to cure irritation. But they do say this:—an ingredient, a source of irritation in other cigarettes, is not used in the manufacture of Philip Morris.
Call for PHILIP MORRIS
2061014890

Fig. 11.4 Advertisement: "A report on the findings of a group of doctors." From: "Saturday Evening Post"—October 16, 1937. In the mid twentieth century a large percentage of American physicians, like the general population, were smokers. This led to various advertising campaigns referring directly to physicians, with the aim of assuring consumers that tobacco products were safe. Various American medical journals also published tobacco advertisements during this period

(Pizzo et al. 2003; Nardini et al. 1998; Zanetti et al. 1998), Japan (Ohida et al. 2001; Kawahara et al. 2000; Kawane and Soejima 1996; Kaetsu et al. 2002; Kawane 2001), and France (Josseran et al. 2000, 2005), for example, have consistently reported smoking prevalence rates over 25 %.

A similar trend is also evident in some newly developing countries: physicians appear to be smoking at high rates in China (Li et al. 1999), Estonia (Parna et al. 2005), Bosnia/Herzegovina (Hodgetts et al. 2004), and Turkey (Gunes et al. 2005). In China for example, Li et al. (1999) reported that tobacco consumption rates among physicians have been increasing in recent years.

Almost half of all Chinese (45 %) (Li et al. 1999) and Japanese physicians (43 %) (Kaetsu et al. 2002) were revealed to be current smokers in two separate studies.

Similar results were also documented in Kuwait (38 %) and the United Arab Emirates (36 %) (Bener et al. 1993). Almost half (48 %) of all male Indian physicians from one study (Sarkar et al. 1990) were smoking, too. The highest smoking prevalence rate was recorded in Greece, where roughly half of all physicians (49 %) reported themselves to be current smokers (Polyzos et al. 1995).

Such figures demonstrate that, while health professionals' smoking habits vary from region to region, they are still not uniformly low, viewed from an international perspective.

Another important aspect deserves to be underlined. Interestingly, prevalence of tobacco consumption varies among the different categories of healthcare professionals, with nurses generally smoking at a much higher rate than physicians and other health workers (USDHHS 2000).

Smoking among nurses has been recognized as a serious concern affecting the profession since the 1970s, when studies showed that female registered nurses smoked at a higher rate (38.9 %) than women in the US population (32.0 %) and at a substantially higher rate than physicians (21 %) (USDHHS 1980).

Further supporting evidence comes from a multicenter cross-sectional study we personally conducted in Italy (Ficarra et al. 2011). We investigated the prevalence of smoking in a population of 1082 healthcare workers, demonstrating that nurses represent the profession with the largest prevalence of tobacco consumption. The probability of smoking was found to be more than double for nurses when compared to medical doctors (OR = 2.48, 95 % CI: 1.51–4.08). Interestingly, a higher prevalence (above 60 %) was shown among women, with a statistically significant difference compared to men. Overall, the prevalence of smoking in the sample was 44 %, more than double the corresponding rate estimated in the Italian general population older than 15 years (22 % in 2008) (ISS-DOXA 2008).

The figures and data reported should raise deep concerns, as they show a substantial failure to adhere to a healthy lifestyle by the same professionals who are in charge to support patients in improving their behavior (Ficarra et al. 2011).

This does not come without risks and negative effects. As we have considered before, health workers should lead the way as public health role models (Smith 2008). Since they are generally viewed as exemplars by the community, it has been suggested that their smoking behavior may potentially impair their role in altering patterns of smoking in the general public (Kottke et al. 1985; Dawley et al. 1981).

Smoking undermines the message to smokers that quitting is important (CDC 1993): in 1983, Sachs stated that 80 % of US citizens expected their physicians to be nonsmokers (Sachs 1983), and as early as 1976 it was suggested that physicians could best persuade patients to quit if they themselves did not smoke (Garfinkel 1976). In fact, campaigns to inform the public of the damage to health caused by smoking will not be convincing if doctors as individuals and as a profession are seen as smokers (Chapman 1995).

Moreover, healthcare workers who smoke are less likely to recognize their role as health educators (USDHHS 1979). As a proof, several studies have shown that healthcare providers who smoke are less likely to initiate cessation interventions and to counsel smokers about quitting (Pipe et al. 2009; Gómez-García and Grimaldi-Carpio 1998).

Beside its significant impact on patients' health, tobacco usage also represents an important occupational health issue in the health professions.

In fact, the main potential reason for the large smoking prevalence among healthcare providers might be occupational stress, which is considered by many authors a key factor in addition to addiction, enjoyment, and peer influence (McKenna et al. 2003; Pelkonen and Kankkunen 2000; Charlton et al. 1997).

Besides, according to the International Labour Office (ILO), the promotion of smoke-free environments represents a key part of any healthy and safe workplace (Håkansta 2004).

For all these reasons, it is particularly important that smoking in the health professions declines in future years. How can this goal be achieved?

Research has shown that smoking cessation measures among healthcare workers can be effective (Fowler 1993). A detailed description about a series of interventions that were actually implemented in real workplace settings, and about their efficacy, will be presented in the next section.

Generally speaking, however, measures should be initiated well before "the stage of becoming a smoker" in order to obtain valid and durable results (Dalsgareth et al. 2004; Zellweger et al. 2005). Effective, specifically adapted methods for accurately communicating health risks to young people (and especially medical students) are particularly needed (Dawley et al. 1981). In fact, it is now clear that smoking prevalence tends to increase during academic studies in the healthcare sector (Boccoli et al. 1997). A recent study we conducted (La Torre et al. 2012), whose aim was to examine smoking prevalence and tobacco cessation training among university students attending 12 medical schools in four European countries (Germany, Italy, Poland, and Spain), found an overall prevalence of smoking among medical students of 29.3 % (95 % confidence interval 28.1–34.7), with percentages ranging from 28 % in Germany to 31.3 % in Italy.

Nevertheless, information on tobacco use and training to provide cessation counseling among medical students are still scarce (being only reported by 16.5 % of students in the same study). Marked deficits are present in the amount and type of training they receive in smoking cessation, with little attention paid to determination of effective training methods (Roche et al. 1996). It would undoubtedly be important to introduce specific information and education programs in a formal way during regular courses (Ficarra et al. 2011): in fact, health professional students who are trained on tobacco control during their educational years have proved to become more efficient at treating patients in tobacco-related issues and are able to act as informers who can prevent tobacco use and can support their patients' cessation efforts (WHO 2004).

Furthermore, it would be necessary to implement training programs among healthcare personnel in general in order to develop ability in smoking cessation techniques (Ficarra et al. 2011; Roche et al. 1996).

It is essential to undertake effective interventions aimed to the implementation of an adequate culture of smoking cessation among health professionals, who represent role models and points of reference for patients and society (Ficarra et al. 2011). These measures can result, ultimately, in a drastic reduction of smoking prevalence, not only among health workers, but in the general population as well, proving socially and economically beneficial to the whole community (La Torre et al. 2011).

11.4.4 Implementation of Smoking Cessation Strategies: A Review of Current Scientific Literature

In order to identify what are to be considered the most effective smoking cessation interventions addressed to healthcare workers, a systematic review of current scientific literature on the subject was recently performed (La Torre et al. 2011). The findings from this review are presented here.

Study selection process—Electronic journal databases MEDLINE and Scopus were searched for studies on smoking cessation interventions among healthcare workers, according to PRISMA criteria (Liberati et al. 2009). The keywords used are shown in Fig. 11.5.

This set of inclusion criteria was adopted: prospective studies, observational studies, and clinical trials evaluating smoking cessation interventions among nurses and other healthcare workers, published in English. Reviews and studies not pertaining to smoking cessation interventions were excluded.

After removing all duplicates and excluding non-relevant and non-adequate records (a study selection flow diagram is shown in Fig. 11.5), only eight studies (out of the 1,671 records initially found) were selected for inclusion in our quantitative synthesis.

The eight articles reviewed are shown in Table 11.4.

Considering the study design, we found a total of three randomized clinical trials (Dalsgareth et al. 2004; Zellweger et al. 2005; Glavas et al. 2003), one nonrandomized clinical trial (Rowe et al. 1999), three observational studies (Bloor et al. 2006; Etter et al. 2008; Kannegaard et al. 2005), and one prospective study (Sarna et al. 2009).

Considering the type of smoking cessation intervention described, three studies discussed the efficacy of smoking restriction policies at the workplace (Bloor et al. 2006; Etter et al. 2008; Kannegaard et al. 2005), two studies considered bupropion SR (Dalsgareth et al. 2004; Zellweger et al. 2005), one study considered an Internet assistance program (Sarna et al. 2009), one study considered the efficacy of supportive interviews (Rowe et al. 1999) and one study considered transdermal nicotine patches (Glavas et al. 2003).

Quality assessment of the studies–Quality assessment of the clinical trials included in this review was performed according to Jadad scale (Jadad et al. 1996), ranging from 0 (poor) to 5 (rigorous).

Prospective and observational studies were evaluated for response rate, study design, and data analysis according to 11 scoring items (shown in Table 11.4) modified from the Angelillo-Villari criteria (Angelillo and Villari 1999). Studies were given a score from 0 (poor) to 11 (rigorous) based on the number of satisfied criteria.

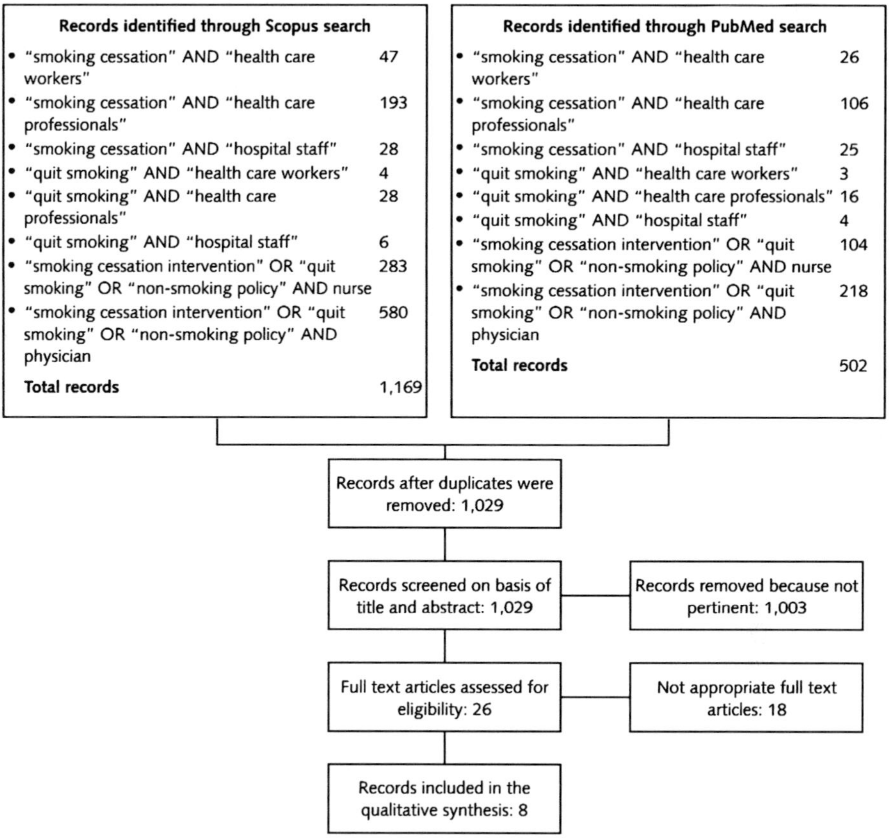

Fig. 11.5 Study selection flow diagram

Table 11.4 shows the results of the quality scoring procedures.

Each of the three clinical trials (Dalsgareth et al. 2004; Zellweger et al. 2005; Glavas et al. 2003) scored 5/5 on the Jadad scale, being randomization described and appropriate, blinding described and appropriate, and withdrawals and dropouts described in each of the studies.

As for prospective and observational studies, three studies (Rowe et al. 1999; Sarna et al. 2009) scored 9/11 on the modified Angelillo–Villari score system, three studies (Etter et al. 2008; Kannegaard et al. 2005) scored 7/11 and one study (Bloor et al. 2006) scored 3/11. Response rate was excellent in every study, but only one article properly described the subjects lost during follow up, while no study described nonparticipant population characteristics. Study design was poor or very poor in most cases, only two studies describing properly the criteria for being included in the "smoker" population and only one study assessing smoking cessation with a proper method. Data analysis was appropriate in four out of five studies.

Table 11.4 Details and quality assessment of the studies included in the review

Author, year	Study design	Workers involved (subjects included)	Methods	Main results	Quality assessment
Bloor (2006)	Observational study with anonymous questionnaire	Nurses (92)	All the nurses of a psychiatric hospital were administered a questionnaire after the introduction of a smoking restriction policy. The questionnaire consisted of questions on smoking habits (number of cigarettes per day, previous attempts of smoking cessation, etc.), 21 questions investigating nurses opinion on the smoking restriction policy in public places (evaluated with a five level Likert scale) and items addressed only to smoking nurses about their competence with smoking cessation educational interventions	71.8 % of the nurses believed that the restriction policy was not effective in motivating to quit smoking. 82.5 % believed that staff should have the right to smoke at work. 82.6 % believed that nonsmokers should not be in contact with smoke. 75 % declared that being a smoker didn't affect the ability to give advice on smoking. Only 11 (34.3 %) of the 32 nurses who smoke planned to quit smoking	Modified Angelillo-Villari score: 3/11 Response rate: 2 Study design: 0 Data analysis: 1
Etter (2008)	Observational study with anonymous questionnaire	Nurses and physicians (57)	To assess the impact of a partial smoking ban followed by a total smoking ban in a psychiatric hospital, anonymous questionnaires were administered. The target sample included all patients and staff present at the time of data collection. The questionnaires covered age, sex, and smoking status, opinions about the no-smoking policy, perceived exposure to environmental tobacco smoke, smoking behavior and smoking cessation interventions received from hospital staff	Exposure to environmental tobacco smoke decreased after the partial ban and further decreased after the total ban. Among nurses and physicians many participants (59.6 %) commented that the total ban was too strict, and most preferred the partial ban. The total ban was not followed by any change in smoking prevalence or cigarette consumption	Modified Angelillo-Villari score: 7/11 response rate: 2 study design: 1 data analysis: 4

Kannegaard (2005)	Observational study with anonymous questionnaire and comparison with a similar study	Hospital staff (729)	Results of two surveys about smoking among hospital staff. Results are compared in order to provide changes in smoking habits in a hospital which was about to start a smoking restriction policy 2 years after the first survey and a few months after the second survey. Both surveys utilized an anonymous questionnaire sent via ordinary mail to every member of the staff (both fulltime and part-time workers). Questions investigated smoking habits, passive smoking, discomfort caused by smoking in the hospital, age, gender, occupation	Number of smokers among hospital staff diminished from 33 to 26 % after 2 years. According to the survey those who kept on smoking were less willing to quit smoking at the end of the study and were also reluctant to accept any smoking cessation intervention	Modified Angelillo-Villari score: 7/11 response rate: 2 study design: 1 data analysis: 4
Dalsgareth, (2004)	Randomized clinical trial	Hospital staff (336)	Randomized double-blind clinical trial. The study lasted 26 weeks. 222 patients in the experimental group were administered bupropion SR for 7 weeks, 114 patients in the control group were administered a placebo. Follow-up visits were set at 3, 7 and 19 weeks after the end of the treatment protocol. Diary cards and measurement of the carbon monoxide concentration in the exhaled air were used to assess the abstinence	After 7 weeks 43 % of the patients in the experimental group and 18 % of the patients in the control group were abstinent ($p<0.001$). The number of continuous abstinents declined during the observation period to 23 % in the experimental group and 11 % in the control group at the end of the study ($p=0.007$)	Jadad scale: 5/5 Randomization: described, appropriate (+2) Blinding: double blind, appropriate (+2) Withdrawals and dropouts: described (+1)

(continued)

Table 11.4 (continued)

Author, year	Study design	Workers involved (subjects included)	Methods	Main results	Quality assessment
Zellweger (2005)	Prospective clinical trial	Psychiatrists and nurses (687)	Prospective double-blind randomized clinical trial. Bupropion SR was administered to the control group (170 subjects). The treatment lasted 7 weeks. They were also administered two questionnaires to measure anxiety, smoking addiction, anger, and withdrawal. Participants were followed for 52 weeks with phone calls and medical visits	Treatment with bupropion SR was well tolerated by participants and adverse events were comparable to those of previous studies. Bupropion SR was superior to placebo in reducing smokers prevalence (50 % vs. 40 % at week 4; $p = 0.013$). Statistical differences were not maintained after withdrawal of the treatment due to high placebo response	Jadas scale: 5/5 Randomization: described, appropriate (+2) Blinding: double blind, appropriate (+2) Withdrawals and dropouts: described (+1)
Glavas (2003)	Prospective clinical trial	Physicians and nurses (112)	Prospective randomized double-blind clinical trial. Each patient in the experimental group (56 subjects) was administered daily transdermal nicotine system patches. The control group patients (56 subjects) were administered identical placebo patches. Follow-up visits were set at 7, 14, and 21 days and after 5 years. Abstinence was assessed through a questionnaire and measuring carbon monoxide concentration in the exhaled breath	After 3 weeks the amount of cigarettes consumed decreased by 74.7 % in the experimental group (CO in exhaled air = −61.3 %) and by 50.7 % in the control group (CO in exhaled air = −37.4 %). Abstinence rate was 39 % in the experimental group and 20 % in the control group ($p = 0.038$). After 5 years abstinence rate was 17.8 % in the experimental group and 14.3 % in the control group ($p = 0.797$)	Jadad scale: 5/5 Randomization: described, appropriate (+2) Blinding: double blind, appropriate (+2) Withdrawals and dropouts: described (+1)

Rowe (1999)	Quasi-experimental non randomized study	Nurses and student nurses (110)	Quasi-experimental study to evaluate the effectiveness of individual interventions for smoking cessation. The individual intervention consisted of a weekly supportive interview and measurement of alveolar carbon monoxide and assessment of salivary nicotine to objectively verify abstinence at 6 and 12 months. Experimental group included 22 nurses and 32 student nurses; control group included 23 nurses and 33 student nurses. There is no randomization	24 % of the subjects in the intervention group stopped smoking vs. 7 % of the subjects in the control group. In detail, 22.7 % of the nurses in the intervention group ceased smoking vs. 8.6 % in the control group ($p<0.05$) and 25 % of the student nurses in the intervention group ceased smoking vs. 6 % in the control group ($p<0.05$)	Modified Angelillo-villari score: 9/11 Response rate: 2 Study design: 3 Data analysis: 4
Sarna (2009)	Quasi-experimental prospective study without a control group	Nurses and student nurses (246)	Prospective study assessing the efficacy of a smoking cessation Internet assistance program with a 3, 6, and 12 months follow up. The study analyzed the correlations with demographic data (age, sex, ethnicity, education) and the types of departments in which the patients worked. The demographic and professional characteristics of the sample according to smoking status were reported to each follow up	Nurses who quit smoking were 43 % after 3 months, 45 % after 6 months, and 53 % after 12 months	Modified Angelillo-Villari score: 9/11 response rate: 3 study design: 2 data analysis: 4

From La Torre et al. (2011)

11.4.5 Compared Efficacy of Various Smoking Cessation Interventions

We analyzed the results of the various types of interventions described in the eight studies (smoking restriction policies at workplace, bupropion SR, transdermal nicotine patches, supportive interviews, Internet assistance programs), with the aim of understanding how they compare, in terms of efficacy in reducing the prevalence of smokers among healthcare professionals.

Efficacy of smoking restriction policies at workplace—The observational study by Bloor et al. (2006) showed that even if smoking restriction policies might prove effective in reducing environmental tobacco smoke exposure, these interventions are unpopular and ineffective in reducing prevalence of smokers among healthcare workers. In fact, only 11 (34.3 %) out of the 32 nurses who smoked, planned to quit smoking, while 71.8 % of the nurses believed that the restriction policy was not effective in motivating to quit smoking. Even though 82.5 % of the sample believed that staff should have the right to smoke at work, 82.6 % affirmed that nonsmokers should not be in contact with smoke.

Etter et al. (2008) came to similar conclusions in their observational study on a partial smoking ban followed by a total ban. From their work is clear that exposure to environmental tobacco smoke decreased after the partial ban and further decreased after the total ban. However, among nurses and physicians many participants (59.6 %) commented that the total ban was too strict, and most preferred the partial ban. Moreover, the total ban was not followed by any change in smoking prevalence or cigarette consumption.

Better results were obtained by Kannegaard et al. (2005), who noticed in their observational study that the number of smokers among hospital personnel decreased (from 33 % at baseline to 26 % after 2 years), when workers were informed that the hospital was going to enact a restriction policy at the end of the study. However, according to the survey, those who kept on smoking were less willing to quit smoking at the end of the study and were also reluctant to accept any smoking cessation intervention.

Efficacy of bupropion SR—Bupropion SR is an atypical antidepressant, and the first non-nicotine treatment to have been specifically licensed for smoking cessation (McRobbie et al. 2007). Its action in helping people to stop smoking is independent of its antidepressant effects. The exact mechanism of action for aiding smoking cessation is still unknown, but it is thought to act via its ability to inhibit the neuronal reuptake of dopamine and noradrenaline. It may also have some action as a noncompetitive inhibitor of the nicotinic acetylcholine receptor (McRobbie et al. 2007).

The randomized, double blind clinical trial by Dalsgareth et al. (2004) proved that buproprion SR is more effective than placebo in reducing smoking prevalence in healthcare workers, at 26 weeks from the beginning of treatment. After 7 weeks, 43 % of the patients in the experimental group versus 18 % of the patients in the control group were abstinent ($p<0.001$). During the observation period, lasting 19 weeks, the number of continuous abstainers decreased to 23 % in the experimental group and to 11 % in the control group at the end of the study ($p=0.007$).

Efficacy of bupropion SR didn't seem to last longer in the prospective double blind clinical trial carried out by Zellweger et al. (2005). In their study bupropion SR proved to be superior to placebo in reducing smokers' prevalence at week 4 (50 % vs. 40 %; $p=0.013$), but statistical differences were not maintained after discontinuation of treatment (week 52), confirming that measures to prevent recurrence are necessary to continue the long-term abstention.

Efficacy of transdermal nicotine patches—Nicotine replacement therapy has been used to help smokers stop for over 20 years. Its primary mechanism of action is to diminish the severity of withdrawal symptoms associated with smoking cessation (McRobbie et al. 2007), making quitting more tolerable and the attempt more likely to succeed (Silagy et al. 2004).

The prospective randomized clinical trial by Glavas et al. (2003) proved that transdermal nicotine patches are more effective than placebo in reducing smoking prevalence in healthcare workers in the short term. However, statistical differences are not maintained years after treatment. In fact, after 3 weeks the amount of consumed cigarettes decreased by 74.7 % in the experimental group (CO in exhaled air = −61.3 %) and by 50.7 % in the control group (CO in exhaled air = −37.4 %), while abstinence rate was 39 % in the experimental group and 20 % in the control group ($p=0.038$). However, after 5 years abstinence rate was 17.8 % in the experimental group and 14.3 % in the control group ($p=0.797$).

Efficacy of supportive interviews—Rowe et al. (1999) studied the efficacy of individualized supportive interviews among nurses and student nurses. The study lasted 1 year, at the end of which 24 % of the subjects in the intervention group versus 7 % of the subjects in the control group quit smoking. In detail, 22.7 % of the nurses in the intervention group ceased smoking versus 8.6 % in the control group ($p<0.05$), and 25 % of the student nurses in the intervention group ceased smoking vs. 6 % in the control group ($p<0.05$).

Efficacy of Internet assistance programs—Sarna et al. (2009) used an Internet assistance program to help nurses and student nurses quit smoking. Patients had full-time access to a Website which provided skills to enhance smoking cessation success, no-cost smoking cessation services, evidence-based medication information and options for one-to-one counseling. Nurses who quit smoking were 43 % after 3 months, 45 % after 6 months, and 53 % after 12 months.

Considerations and comparison—The following conclusions can be drawn from the reported results for the various smoking cessation interventions.

Smoking restriction policies at workplace, while effectively reducing environmental tobacco smoke exposure, can't be considered as smoking cessation interventions (La Torre et al. 2011). According to the results of this review, healthcare workers barely tolerate smoking bans at the workplace, despite being in favor of smoking restrictions in public areas such as hospitals (Bloor et al. 2006; Kannegaard et al. 2005; Martinez et al. 2008). Such interventions also turned out to reduce willingness to quit smoking in subjects who kept on smoking (Kannegaard et al. 2005). Beside seeming to be unpopular, they also proved ineffective in reducing prevalence of smokers among healthcare workers (Bloor et al. 2006; Etter et al. 2008). Only Kannegaard et al. noticed a decreasing trend in smoking prevalence in their 2 year-long observational study. However, it is to be remarked that no restriction policy at all was actually applied during these 2 years: workers were only informed that the hospital "was about" to start a restriction policy at the end of the study.

Bupropion SR and transdermal nicotine patches have proven more effective than placebo in reducing smoking prevalence, but statistical differences were not maintained after discontinuation of treatment: therefore, they both require measures to prevent recurrence. In fact, their effects are superior to other methods only in the first months after the treatment (Dalsgareth et al. 2004; Glavas et al. 2003).

On the contrary, individualized supportive interviews and Internet assistance programs seem to grant the best long-term effects, although further studies are needed to assess their effectiveness in periods longer than 1 year (Rowe et al. 1999; Sarna et al. 2009).

11.4.6 Conclusions

As we have seen, smoking among healthcare workers is undoubtedly a serious concern affecting the profession (La Torre et al. 2011). The high prevalence of smokers in the category might be viewed as particularly striking, if we consider that medical professionals are thought to possess the greatest potential of any group in society to promote a decrease in tobacco consumption (WHO 2011a, b). In fact, beside personally providing their patients with effective smoking cessation interventions, healthcare providers should set an example for the general population by not smoking and becoming powerful advocates for tobacco-free communities (USDHHS 1979). Their participation to tobacco control efforts is of fundamental importance, their involvement in tobacco-use prevention and cessation programs being one of the main strategies to reduce the number of smoking-related deaths in the general population.

However, smoking cessation among health professionals has some barriers specific to healthcare workers, such as the high prevalence of smokers and their low awareness of being a role model in tobacco consumption control (Martinez et al. 2008).

Targeted policies and smoking cessation services are therefore needed (Chiatti et al. 2010; Eriksen et al. 2005), including improvements to the education system that trains professionals, since it has been demonstrated that smoking prevalence tends to increase during academic studies in the healthcare sector (Boccoli et al. 1997).

The most effective smoking cessation interventions in the long term seem to be individualized supportive interviews and Internet assistance programs, while smoking restriction policies have proven unpopular and ineffective, and pharmacological therapies (bupropion SR and transdermal nicotine patches) seem to have high smoking recurrence rates (La Torre et al. 2011).

However, further studies are needed on the effectiveness of the various interventions in the long term (La Torre et al. 2011).

In conclusion, if in future years health professionals and researchers will focus as much on prompting attempts at tobacco cessation as on creating new approaches to treatment, many additional tobacco users will certainly be motivated to quit, and much more lives will be saved (WHO 2004).

References

Adriaanse, H., Halfens, R., Drop, M. J., & van Reek, J. (1985). Physicians, smoking, and health in the Netherlands. *New York State Journal of Medicine, 85*, 394–395.

Adriaanse, H., Van Reek, J., & Metsemakers, J. (1986). Smoking behaviour of Dutch general practitioners in the period 1977–1983. *Scandinavian Journal of Primary Health Care, 4*(3), 151–156.

Albertsen, K., Borg, V., & Oldenburg, B. (2006). A systematic review of the impact of work environment on smoking cessation, relapse and amount smoked. *Preventive Medicine, 43*(4), 291–305.

Angelillo, I. F., & Villari, P. (1999). Residential exposure to electromagnetic fields and childhood leukaemia: A meta-analysis. *Bulletin of the World Health Organization, 77*, 906–915.

Bener, A., Gomes, J., & Anderson, J. A. D. (1993). Smoking habits among physicians in two gulf countries. *Journal of the Royal Society of Health, 113*, 298–301.

Bloor, R. N., Meeson, L., & Crome, I. B. (2006). The effects of a non-smoking policy on nursing staff smoking behaviour and attitudes in a psychiatric hospital. *Journal of Psychiatric and Mental Health Nursing, 13*, 188–196.

Boccoli, E., Federici, A., Trianni, G. L., & Melani, A. S. (1997). Changes of smoking habits and beliefs during nurse training: A longitudinal study. *European Journal of Epidemiology, 13*, 899–902.

Brackbill, R., Frazier, T., & Shilling, S. (1988). Smoking characteristics of U.S. workers, 1978–1980. *American Journal of Industrial Medicine, 13*, 5–41.

Burns, D. M. (2012). *Smoking cessation: Recent indicators of what's working at a population level*. In Population based smoking cessation proceedings of a conference on what works to influence cessation in the general population (Monograph 12). National Cancer Institute 2012.

Cahill, K., Moher, M., & Lancaster, T. (2008). *Workplace interventions for smoking cessation (Review)*. Cochrane Database of Systematic Reviews Issue 4. Art. No. CD003440.

CDC—Centers for Disease Control and Prevention. (1993). Smoking control among health care workers—World No-Tobacco Day. *MMWR Morbidity and Mortality Weekly Report, 42*(19), 365–367.

CDC—Centers for Disease Control and Prevention. (2005). *Telephone quitlines. A resource for development, implementation, and evaluation*. Accessed from, http://www.cdc.gov/tobacco/quit_smoking/cessation/quitlines/index.htm

Chapman, S. (1995). Doctors who smoke. *British Medical Journal, 311*, 142–143.

Chapman, S., & Hans-Werner, S. (2007). *Public health advocacy and tobacco control: Making smoking history*. London: Blackwell.

Charlton, A., While, D., & Mochizuki, Y. (1997). A survey into the smoking habits of nursing students. *Nursing Times, 93*, 58–60.

Chiatti, C., Chiadò Piat, S., Federico, B., Capelli, C., Di Stanislao, F., Di Giovanni, P., et al. (2010). Cigarette smoking in young-adult workers: A cross-sectional analysis from Abruzzo, Italy. *Italian Journal of Public Health, 3*, 243–248.

Coups, E. J., Dhingra, L. K., Heckman, C. J., & Manne, S. L. (2009). Receipt of provider advice for smoking cessation and use of smoking cessation treatments among cancer survivors. *Journal of General Internal Medicine, 24*(Suppl 2), 480–486.

Dalsgareth, O. J., Gerner Hansen, N. C., Søes-Petersen, U., Evald, T., Høegholm, A., Barber, J., et al. (2004). A multicenter, randomized, double-blind placebo-controlled, 6-month trial of bupropion hydrochloride sustained-release tablets as an aid to smoking cessation in hospital employees. *Nicotine and Tobacco Research, 6*, 55–61.

Davis, R. M. (1993). When doctors smoke. *Tobacco Control, 2*, 187–188.

Dawley, H. H., Cartel, S., & Morrison, J. (1981). The discouragement of smoking in a hospital setting: The importance of modelled behaviour. *International Journal Addiction, 16*, 901–910.

Eriksen, W. (2005). Work factors and smoking cessation in nurses' aides: A prospective cohort study. *BMC Public Health, 5*, 142.

Etter, M., Khan, A. N., & Etter, J. (2008). Acceptability and impact of a partial smoking ban followed by a total smoking ban in a psychiatric hospital. *Preventive Medicine, 46*, 572–578.

Ficarra, M. G., Gualano, M. R., Capizzi, S., et al. (2011). Tobacco use prevalence, knowledge and attitudes among Italian hospital healthcare professionals. *European Journal of Public Health, 21*, 29–34.

Fowler, G. (1993). Educating doctors in smoking cessation. *Tobacco Control, 2*, 5–6.

Gardner, M. N., & Brandt, A. M. (2006). The doctors' choice is America's choice: The physician in US cigarette advertisements, 1930–1953. *American Journal of Public Health, 96*, 222–232.

Garfinkel, L. (1976). Cigarette smoking among physicians and other health professionals, 1959–1972. *CA: A Cancer Journal for Clinicians, 26*, 373–375.

Gianti, A., Vianello, S., Casinghini, C., Roncarolo, F., Ramella, F., Maccagni, M., et al. (2007). The "Quit and Win" campaign to promote smoking cessation in Italy: Results and one year follow-up across three Italian editions (2000–2004). *Italian Journal of Public Health, 4*, 59–64.

Glavas, D., Rumboldt, M., & Rumboldt, Z. (2003). Smoking cessation with nicotine replacement therapy among health care workers: Randomized double-blind study. *Croatian Medical Journal, 44*, 219–224.

Gómez-García, R., & Grimaldi-Carpio, A. (1998). Smoking in health personnel: Study in a hospital unit. *Salud Pública de México, 40*(1), 53–57.

Gunes, G., Karaoglu, L., Genc, M. F., Pehlivan, E., & Egri, M. (2005). University hospital physicians' attitudes and practices for smoking cessation counseling in Malatya, Turkey. *Patient Education and Counseling, 56*, 147–153.

Håkansta, C. (2004). *Workplace smoking working paper: A review of national and local practical and regulatory measures* (pp. 1–89). Geneva: International Labor Office (ILO).

Hodgetts, G., Broers, T., & Godwin, M. (2004). Smoking behaviour, knowledge and attitudes among family medicine physicians and nurses in Bosnia and Herzegovina. *BMC Family Practice, 5*, 12.

Hughes, M. C., Yette, E. M., Hannon, P. A., Harris, J. R., Tran, N. M., & Reid, T. R. (2011). Promoting tobacco cessation via the workplace: Opportunities for improvement. *Tobacco Control, 20*(4), 305–308.

Ikeda, Y., Suehiro, T., Takamatsu, K., Yamashita, H., Tamura, T., & Hashimoto, K. (1997). Effect of smoking on the prevalence of albuminuria in Japanese men with non-insulin-dependent diabetes mellitus. *Diabetes Research and Clinical Practice, 36*, 57–61.

Istituto Superiore di Sanità-DOXA. (2008). *Il fumo in Italia 2008*. Accessed from, http://www.iss.it/fumo/doxa/cont.php?id=175&lang=1&tipo=18

Jadad, A. R., Moore, R. A., Carroll, D., Jenkinson, C., Reynolds, D. J., Gavaghan, D. J., et al. (1996). Assessing the quality of reports of randomized clinical trials: Is blinding necessary? *Controlled Clinical Trials, 17*, 1–12.

Josseran, L., King, G., Guilbert, P., Davis, J., & Brucker, G. (2005). Smoking by French general practitioners: Behaviour, attitudes and practice. *European Journal of Public Health, 15*, 33–38.

Josseran, L., King, G., Velter, A., Dressen, C., & Grizeau, D. (2000). Smoking behavior and opinions of French general practitioners. *Journal of the National Medical Association, 92*, 382–390.

Kaetsu, A., Fukushima, T., Moriyama, M., & Shigematsu, T. (2002). Change of the smoking behavior and related lifestyle variables among physicians in Fukuoka, Japan: A longitudinal study. *Journal of Epidemiology, 12*, 208–216.

Kannegaard, P. N., Kreiner, S., Gregersen, P., & Goldstein, H. (2005). Smoking habits and attitudes to smoking 2001 among hospital staff at a danish hospital—Comparison with a similar study in 1999. *Preventive Medicine, 41*, 321–327.

Kawahara, K., Ohida, T., Osaki, Y., Mochizuki, Y., Minowa, M., Yamaguchi, N., et al. (2000). Study of the smoking behavior of medical doctors in Fukui, Japan and their antismoking measures. *Journal of Epidemiology, 10*, 157–162.

Kawane, H. (2001). Smoking among Japanese physicians. *JAMA: The Journal of the American Medical Association, 286*, 917.

Kawane, H., & Soejima, R. (1996). Smoking among doctors in a medical school hospital. *Kawasaki Medical Journal, 22*, 211–216.

Kottke, T. E., Hill, V., Heitig, C., Brekke, M., Blake, S., Arneson, S., et al. (1985). Smoke-free hospitals, attitudes of patients, employees and faculty. *Minnesota Medicine, 68*, 53–55.

Kouvonen, A., Oksanen, T., Vahtera, J., Väänänen, A., De Vogli, R., Elovainio, M., et al. (2008). Work-place social capital and smoking cessation: The Finnish public sector study. *Addiction, 103*(11), 1857–1865.

La Torre, G., Kirch, W., Bes-Rastrollo, M., Ramos, R. M., Czaplicki, M., Gualano, M. R., et al. (2012). Tobacco use among medical students in Europe: Results of a multicentre study using the Global health professions student survey. *Public Health, 126*(2), 159–164.

La Torre, G., Saulle, R., Di Nardo, F., & Germani, T. (2011). Smoking cessation interventions in nurses and other health care workers. *Reviews in Health Care, 2*(1), 97–107.

Lancaster, T., Stead, L., Silagy, C., et al. (2000). Effectiveness of interventions to help people stop smoking: Findings from the Cochrane Library. *British Medical Journal, 321*, 355–358.

Lee, D. J., LeBlanc, W., Fleming, L. E., Gómez-Marín, O., & Pitman, T. (2004). Trends in US smoking rates in occupational groups: The National Health Interview Survey 1987–1994. *Journal of Occupational and Environmental Medicine, 46*(6), 538–548.

Li, H. Z., Fish, D., & Zhou, X. (1999). Increase in cigarette smoking and decline of anti-smoking counselling among Chinese physicians: 1987–1996. *Health Promotion International, 14*, 123–131.

Liberati, A., Altman, D. G., Tetzlaff, J., Mulrow, C., Gøtzsche, P. C., Ioannidis, J. P. A., et al. (2009). The PRISMA statement for reporting systematic reviews and meta-analyses of studies that evaluate health care interventions: explanation and elaboration. *Italian Journal of Public Health, 4*, 94–131.

Martinez, C., Garcia, M., Mendez, E., Peris, M., & Fernandez, E. (2008). Barriers and challenges for tobacco control in a smoke-free hospital. *Cancer Nursing, 31*, 88–94.

McKenna, H., Slater, P., McCance, T., et al. (2003). The role of stress, peer influence and education levels on the smoking behaviour of nurses. *International Journal of Nursing Studies, 40*, 359–366.

McRobbie, H., Bullen, C., Whittaker, R., Wallace-Bell, M., & Fraser, T. (2007). *Best practice for smoking cessation: Background report for the Tasmanian department of health and human services*. Tasmania: Department of Health and Human Services.

Nardini, S., Bertoletti, R., Rastelli, V., Ravelli, L., & Donner, C. F. (1998). Personal smoking habit and attitude toward smoking among the health staff of a general hospital. *Monaldi Archives for Chest Disease, 53*, 74–78.

Nayan, S., Gupta M. K., & Sommer, D. D. (2011). Evaluating smoking cessation interventions and cessation rates in cancer patients: A systematic review and meta-analysis. *ISRN Oncology, 7*, Article ID 849023.

Nelson, D. E., Giovino, G. A., Emont, S. L., Brackbill, R., Cameron, L. L., Peddicord, J., et al. (1994). Trends in cigarette smoking among US physicians and nurses. *JAMA: The Journal of the American Medical Association, 271*(16), 1273–1275.

Ohida, T., Sakurai, H., Mochizuki, Y., Kamal, A. M., Takemura, S., Minowa, M., et al. (2001). Smoking prevalence and attitudes toward smoking among Japanese physicians. *JAMA: The Journal of the American Medical Association, 285*, 2643–2648.

Parna, K., Rahu, K., & Rahu, M. (2005). Smoking habits and attitudes towards smoking among Estonian physicians. *Public Health, 119*, 390–399.

Pelkonen, M., & Kankkunen, P. (2000). Work stress, smoking habits and competence in supporting clients to cease smoking—A survey among Finnish nurses. *Public Health, 114*, 464–467.

Pipe, A., Sorensen, M., & Reid, R. (2009). Physician smoking status, attitudes toward smoking, and cessation advice to patients: An international survey. *Patient Education and Counseling, 74*(1), 118–123.

Pizzo, A. M., Chellini, E., Grazzini, G., Cardone, A., & Badellino, F. (2003). Italian general practitioners and smoking cessation strategies. *Tumori, 89*, 250–254.

Polyzos, A., Gennatas, C., Veslemes, M., Daskalopoulou, E., Stamatiadis, D., & Katsilambros, N. (1995). The smoking-cessation promotion practices of physician smokers in Greece. *Journal of Cancer Education, 10*, 78–81.

Rigotti, N. A., Clair, C., Munafò, M. R., & Stead, L. F. (2012). Interventions for smoking cessation in hospitalised patients. *Cochrane Database Systematic Reviews* (5), CD001837.

Roche, A. M., Eccleston, P., & Sanson-Fisher, R. (1996). Teaching smoking cessation skills to senior medical students: A block-randomized controlled trial of four different approaches. *Preventive Medicine, 25*(3), 251–258.

Rowe, K., & Macleod Clark, J. (1999). Evaluating the effectiveness of a smoking cessation intervention designed for nurses. *International Journal of Nursing Studies, 36*, 301–311.

Sachs, D. P. (1983). Smoking habits of pulmonary physicians. *The New England Journal of Medicine, 309*, 799.

Sarkar, D., Dhand, R., Malhotra, A., Malhotra, S., & Sharma, B. K. (1990). Perceptions and attitude towards tobacco smoking among doctors in Chandigarh. *The Indian Journal of Chest Diseases and Allied Sciences, 32*, 1–9.

Sarna, L., Bialous, S., Wewers, M. E., Froelicher, E. S., Wells, M. J., Kotlerman, J., et al. (2009). Nurses trying to quit smoking using the internet. *Nursing Outlook, 57*, 246–256.

Sherman, J. J. (2005). The impact of smoking and quitting smoking on patients with diabetes. *Diabetes Spectrum, 18*(4), 202–208.

Silagy, C., Lancaster, T., Stead, L., Mant, D., & Fowler, G. (2004). Nicotine replacement therapy for smoking cessation. *Cochrane Database Systematic Reviews* (3), CD000146.

Smith, D. R. (2008). The historical decline of tobacco smoking among United States physicians: 1949–1984. *Tobacco Induced Diseases, 4*(1), 9.

Smith, D. R., & Leggat, P. A. (2007). An international review of tobacco smoking in the medical profession: 1974–2004. *BMC Public Health, 7*, 115.

Tønnesen, P., Carrozzi, L., Fagerstrom, K. O., Gratziou, C., Jimenez-Ruiz, C., Nardinie, S., et al. (2007). Smoking cessation in patients with respiratory diseases: A high priority, integral component of therapy. *The European Respiratory Journal, 29*, 390–417.

USDHHS - United States Department of Health and Human Services. (1979). *Smoking and health: A report of the surgeon general*. Rockville, MD: US Department of Health, Education, and Welfare.

USDHHS - United States Department of Health and Human Services. (2000). *Reducing tobacco use: A report of the surgeon general*. Atlanta, GA: US Department of Health and Human Services, CDC.

USDHHS—United States Department of Health and Human Services (1980). *The health consequences of smoking for women: A report of the surgeon general*. U.S. Department of Health and Human Services, Public Health Service, Office of the Assistant Secretary for Health, Office on Smoking and Health.

Van Reek, J., & Adriaanse, H. (1991). Smoking by physicians in Scandinavia: 1952–1989. *Scandinavian Journal of Social Medicine, 19*(4), 256–259.

WHO - World Health Organization. (2009). *WHO report on the global tobacco epidemic, 2009: Implementing smoke-free environments*. Geneva, Switzerland: World Health Organization.

WHO - World Health Organization. (2011). *The world health report 2011*. Geneva, Switzerland: World Health Organization.

WHO—World Health Organization. (2011). Building capacity for smoking cessation and treatment of tobacco dependence. In: Policy recommendations for smoking cessation and treatment of tobacco dependence. Accessed from http://www.who.int/tobacco/resources/publications/en/chapter5_to_annex2.pdf

WHO—World Health Organization. (2004). *Health professionals and tobacco control: WNTD 2005*. Geneva, Switzerland; WHO Informal Meeting on Health Professionals and Tobacco Control, 28–30 January 2004.

Zanetti, F., Gambi, A., Bergamaschi, A., Gentilini, F., De Luca, G., Monti, C., et al. (1998). Smoking habits, exposure to passive smoking and attitudes to a non-smoking policy among hospital staff. *Public Health, 112*, 57–62.

Zellweger, J., Boelcskei, P. L., Carrozzi, L., Sepper, R., Sweet, R., & Hider, A. Z. (2005). Bupropion SR vs placebo for smoking cessation in health care professionals. *American Journal of Health Behavior, 29*, 240–249.

Chapter 12
Media and Smoking Cessation

Giuseppe La Torre and Silvia Miccoli

Objectives This section intends to describe the impact of the media on smoking cessation. In particular, this section will discuss the impact on reducing smoking prevalence using books and the Web.

Learning Outcomes

At the end of this chapter the reader will be able to:

- Know what is the impact of information present in books on smoker behavior.
- Know what is the impact of information on the Web about smoker behavior.
- Know the main Websites search engines and the Internet impact on decision to stop smoking.

12.1 Introduction

Tobacco dependence shows many characteristics of a chronic disease. Although a minority of tobacco users reaches permanent abstinence in a preliminary quit attempt, the majority persists in tobacco use for many years and typically cycle through multiple periods of relapse and remission. A failure to appreciate the chronic nature of tobacco dependence may reduce clinicians' motivation to treat tobacco use resolutely.

Much smoking cessation research and clinical practice over the last three decades has focused on identifying the ideal intervention that would turn all smokers into permanent nonsmokers. This effort may have inadvertently communicated two messages of dubious validity: first, that there is one treatment that will be effective

G. La Torre (✉) • S. Miccoli
Department of Public Health and Infectious Diseases, "Sapienza" University of Rome, Piazzale Aldo Moro 5, Rome 00185, Italy
e-mail: giuseppe.latorre@uniroma1.it; silvia.miccoli@uniroma1.it

G. La Torre, *Smoking Prevention and Cessation*, DOI 10.1007/978-1-4614-7046-5_12,

for virtually all smokers; and second, that success should be defined only on the basis of permanent abstinence. These messages may have masked the true nature of tobacco addiction; it is typically a chronic disorder that carries with it a vulnerability to relapse that persists for weeks, months, and perhaps years (Fiore et al. 2000).

Quitting tobacco is not easy as tobacco dependence is a cluster of behavioral, cognitive, and physiological phenomena. Very few tobacco users successfully quit the habit in their first attempt.

Social norms do not support tobacco users to quit in many countries. The Global Adult Tobacco Survey (GATS) shows that in China only 23.2 % of Chinese adults believe smoking causes serious illnesses. Only 24.6 % believe exposure to tobacco smoke causes heart disease and lung cancer in adults and lung illnesses in children. Only 16.1 % of current adult smokers plan to or are thinking about quitting in the next 12 months. In India, about 26 % of current adult smokers plan to or are thinking about quitting in the next 12 months.

Evidence-based support to quit tobacco use (tobacco dependence treatment) includes methods from simple medical advice to pharmacotherapy, along with quit-lines and counseling. However, tobacco users have low levels of awareness of the evidence about these tobacco dependence treatment interventions (WHO 2012).

The benefits of quitting are often well known, but outweigh by the downsides for most. Again, smokers tend to focus on short-term gain, including saving money and not smelling. Several are unconvinced of substantial health gain if they stop smoking (and believe fatalistically that any damage to health was already done and irreversible).

The perceived downsides of quitting included weight gain, cravings, increased stress, boredom and anxiety, social exclusion and loss of a luxury and reward, with no suitable replacement (Jackson et al. 2002).

Good prevention and health promotion should be based on other aspects, not only on the simple information or coercion, but it should also work on cognitive variables on the individual and his emotions.

Some researchers conducted studies to establish the links that may exist between smoking and personality. For example, they have asked whether it was possible to identify certain personality traits that share smoking or whether certain personality traits can predict the success of arrest or the intensity of withdrawal symptoms experienced in the stop (Fig. 12.1).

In 2003 and in 2010, the Website manager Stop-tabac.ch led two studies on the association between personality traits depending on the model of Cloninger and smoking (Etter et al. 2003; Etter 2010). In the first study in 2003, the results indicated that the trait of novelty seeking (novelty seeking, NS) and especially the extravagance that is a personality trait subject to novelty seeking were associated with the smoking. The second 2010 study also showed that smokers had a higher score than former smokers or nonsmokers in issues related to novelty seeking, but also those related to the tendency to avoid the danger (harm avoidance, HA): smokers, more anxious, would seek in the anxiolytic effects of smoking and antidepressants. Conversely, smokers have a lower score on self-determination. In summary, smokers have a higher score in novelty seeking and harm avoidance, so they are described

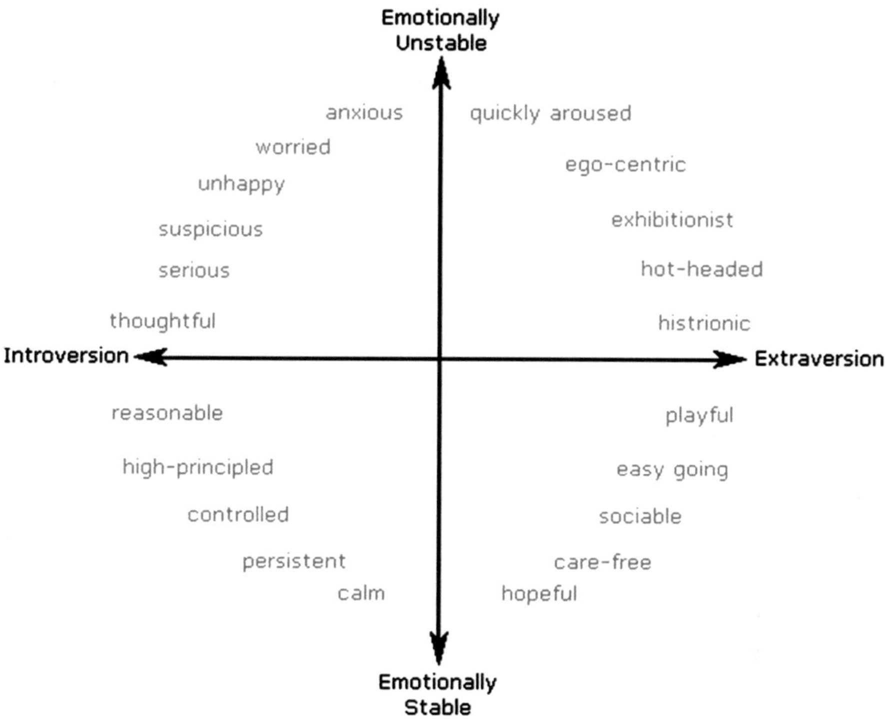

Fig. 12.1 Links between smoking and personality

as people sometimes impulsive, exploratory, excitable, extravagant, disorderly, cautious, fearful, tense, anxious, and inhibited (Stop tabach 2012).

12.2 The Allen Carr Book "How to Quit Smoking"

Allen Carr enjoyed the status of being the world's foremost antismoking guru, claiming he had helped millions to kick their deadly habit. Despite this reputation—or perhaps because of it—he remained at odds with the medical profession to the day he died. In the minds of the public and much of the media, however, his unconventional approach to quitting smoking was accepted as something of a revelation. Allen Carr was a strong smoker for 33 years, coming to smoke 100 cigarettes daily.

He also noted that even heavy smokers such as himself were able to go without cigarettes quite easily in situations where lighting up would be unthinkable. This demonstrated that nicotine addiction was not a powerful one in the sense that it led to serious withdrawal symptoms. Instead, he speculated that nicotine provoked a light but rapidly acquired addiction that gave rise to a devious psychological dependence, which he called "the little voice" in the head of addicts, coaxing them to light up whenever the opportunity arose.

He borrowed money from a friend and published "The Easy Way to Stop Smoking" 2 years later. Famously, the book deconstructs, one by one, the myths—and many of the accepted truths—about smoking and dismisses the lies that smokers tell themselves. Memorably, one chapter of the book entitled "The benefits of smoking" contains a single, blank page. Cleverly, readers are encouraged to continue smoking until they reach the very end of the book, by which stage most are relishing the prospect of quitting (Obituaries Allen Carr 2006).

Nevertheless, he died of lung cancer. According his statement, the method based on "positive thinking," applies to any addiction, provided you follow the instructions correctly.

Instead of other methods, based on the awareness development that smoking is a health damage and an antisocial behavior, Easyway method, that provides for the persistence in smoking until the end of therapy without the use of medicaments or NRT (nicotine replacement therapies) as nicotine patches, chewing gums, is based on the contrast to psychological mechanisms of smoking desire and also uses techniques borrowed from cognitive psychology. What is the approach of this book? Festinger talks about *cognitive dissonance* (Festinger 1978). The cognitions are the knowledge, opinions, believes concerning the environment, themselves, and their behaviors. Everyone aims for consistency within himself. When there is a dissonance between two cognitions, if one of these causes emotional stress, people restore the consistent state by changing the fewer resistant element of the system.

In the smokers case, we can consider the following points:

- Cognitions: They smoke. They know that smoking harms health.
- Cognitive behavioral element: I smoke.

There are many strategies for restoring the balance. The first step consists of changing inconsistent behavior, quitting to smoke. This is really difficult: a behavior may not be under total control of the will, it can have strong emotional components in itself that once changed new discomfort (the idea that the cigarette gives security and helps to focus). As an alternative, people can change environmental cognition and external informations: you can't change that smoking causes damage to health, but you tend to pay attention, for example, in those cases where a smoker has lived up to 100 years.

Fotuhi and colleagues (2012) conducted a study to assess whether smokers adjust their beliefs in a pattern that is consistent with cognitive dissonance theory. This is accomplished by examining the longitudinal pattern of belief change among smokers as their smoking behaviors change. Smokers with no history of quitting across the three waves exhibited the highest levels of rationalizations for smoking. When smokers quit smoking, they reported having fewer rationalizations for smoking compared with when they had previously been smoking. However, among those who attempted to quit but then relapsed, there was once again a renewed tendency to rationalize their smoking. This rebound in the use of rationalizations was higher for functional beliefs than for risk-minimizing beliefs, as predicted by social psychological theory. Smokers are motivated to rationalize their behavior through the endorsement of more positive beliefs about smoking, and these beliefs change systematically with changes in smoking status. More work is needed to determine if this cognitive dissonance-reducing function has an inhibiting effect on any subsequent intentions to quit (Fotuhi et al. 2012).

The free choice feeling is Allen Carr key. Allen Carr doesn't appeal to fear.

When people feel tensions and threats to the self, they react with an unpleasant emotional reaction leading to search responses can reduce the voltage.

The appeal to fear is effective if it is followed a recommendation reassuring that reduces the tension created and can thereby strengthen the adaptive response.

If the appeal to fear is too intense, the subject will activate defensive inferences (Attili 2000).

Many smokers motivated to quit are still caught in a vicious circle driven by fear (to stay addicted, to get sick, etc.) and every time they think of quitting they associate the craving and the fear of losing something they are used (Hutter et al. 2006).

Furthermore, the method described in the books "The Easy Way to Stop Smoking" and "The Only Way to Stop Smoking Permanently" written by the former heavy smoker and author Allen Carr (1934–2006) was never tested in controlled trials. Although individual reports attest to the success of these methods, they cannot be generally recommended without the necessary scientific evidence (Ramseier and Fundak 2009).

University may be a good place and time for smoking cessation, because younger, lighter smokers are more successful for stopping (Willcox 1997).

More traditional booklets (Raw 1992) seem less popular—one respondent who did not request the book said, "they don't normally tell you anything new." Many students may not be interested in conventional "stop smoking" advice.

In search of less time-consuming methods of smoking cessation, Allen Carr' seminars (17 seminars lasting 6 h each) performed at workplaces in Austria were evaluated; these seminars offered in many countries have not been evaluated before. Hutter et al. decided to analyze the 1-year success rate of all courses performed by this method in Austrian enterprises during a 4-month period. The results of this study show that in subjects that participated in the cessation seminar but did not consent to take part in the study (overall 49, 31 of which could be contacted by telephone 18 months after the seminar) the 1-year quit rate was 48 %.

Frequently high smoking cessation rates are due to the selection of highly motivated persons for intervention, e.g., from the first symptoms of smoking-related disease. Also for young people and certain occupational groups working as multipliers (e.g., journalists, teachers, health professionals) special courses should be developed. Another possible strategy to further increase success rates could be a quitline on which the trainer should be able to give further advice at least for 1 week after the seminar, as most relapses occurred shortly afterwards (25 % within 3 days, 46 % within a week).

There is consensus that group therapy of tobacco dependence is cost effective, but Allen Carr' seminars have not been evaluated independently before.

Work seminars seem to be capable of helping every second smoker who is motivated to participate (Hutter et al. 2006).

Cummings et al. (1988) propose that self-help interventions need to contain the following information: (1) information about the health and social consequences of smoking; (2) specific strategies and exercises for successful quitting; and (3) specific strategies and exercises for the maintenance of nonsmoking and the prevention of and coping with relapse.

12.3 Information on the Web

Through an examination of the conceptual bases of persuasion, it is posited that the World Wide Web and other Internet-based resources have many of the characteristics necessary for persuasive communication and may, in fact, constitute a hybrid channel that combines the positive attributes of interpersonal and mass communication. The notion that the Internet features many of the persuasive qualities of interpersonal communication makes it a prime candidate for the application of key behavioral science theories and principles to promote healthier behaviors. The broad reach that the Internet shares with many mass communication channels indicates an economy to Internet-based efforts to communicate with large audiences. It is concluded that if the Internet can be used for persuasive health communication and its reach continues to expand, it is time for public health professionals to explore the design and evaluation of Internet-based interventions directed at health behavior change (Cassell et al. 1998).

The global impact of the Internet continues to grow each year, with recent reports showing that global *usage* is much higher than individual *access* (Internet World Stats 2011) (Fig. 12.2).

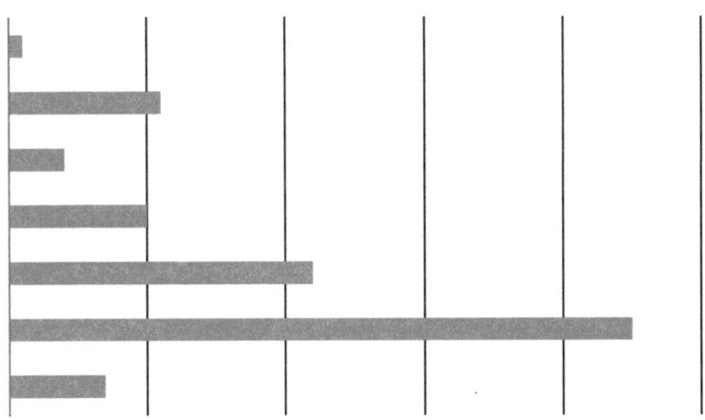

Fig. 12.2 Internet users in the World. Distribution by world regions 2011

There are an estimated 1.3 billion smokers worldwide, of whom 650 million are expected to die prematurely of a tobacco-related disease (World Health Organization 2006). Most smokers attempt to quit on their own even though cessation aids can substantially increase their chances of success. Millions of smokers seek cessation advice on the Internet, so using it to promote cessation products and services is one strategy for increasing demand for treatments. Little is known, however, about what cessation aids these smokers would find most appealing or what predicts their preferences (e.g., age, level of dependence, or timing of quit date) (Westmaas et al. 2011). The National Tobacco Cessation Collaborative, an American and Canadian consortium of leading nonprofit and government agencies dedicated to reducing the burden of tobacco use, delineated several core strategies to increase demand for available treatments. One of these strategies includes the recommendation to understand what smokers need and want, instead of viewing them as "passive treatment beneficiaries rather than treatment consumers" (Backinger et al. 2010).

"Health seekers"—Internet users search online for information on health topics, whether they are acting as consumers, caregivers, or e-patients. Millions of smokers seek cessation information on the Internet (Fox 2006).

In a random-digit dial survey conducted in 2004, 7 % of Internet users in the USA reported using the Web to search for information on "how to quit smoking" (Fox 2005); more women reported to have looked than men (10 % vs. 7 %), and unlike other health-related information seekers, they tended to be younger. At the time, this represented approximately 10.2 million people who had ever turned to the Internet for smoking cessation–related information or services. Little is known about these individuals, including their basic demographic characteristics, smoking status (e.g., current smokers seeking cessation treatment, recent quitters seeking support to maintain abstinence), readiness to quit, quitting history, and treatment preferences. With the proliferation of antismoking sentiments and restrictive smoking policies, a diverse group of individuals may be turning to the Internet for assistance. In order to provide individually tailored and effective cessation treatment services via the Internet, it is necessary to better understand the characteristics and needs of this population (Cobb and Graham 2006).

Online social networks for smoking cessation have become ubiquitous and, thus, may represent a promising modality for smokers to both receive and provide the kind of support necessary for cessation and relapse prevention (Fig. 12.3). Through Internet-based social networks, smokers have round-the-clock access to thousands of other individuals who are actively quitting smoking, struggling to maintain abstinence, or celebrating various milestones of abstinence. Access in real time to a diverse mix of individuals in all stages of the cessation journey is a unique aspect of online social networks. No other cessation treatment modality provides an ongoing opportunity for current and former smokers to interact and influence each other. In addition, smokers benefit not only from active interactions with other network members but also from various passive sources of social influence and social support. Smokers can establish personal connections with other network members or can browse ("lurk") the messages and profiles of others. These kinds of active and passive interactions may influence an individual's motivation to quit, reinforce

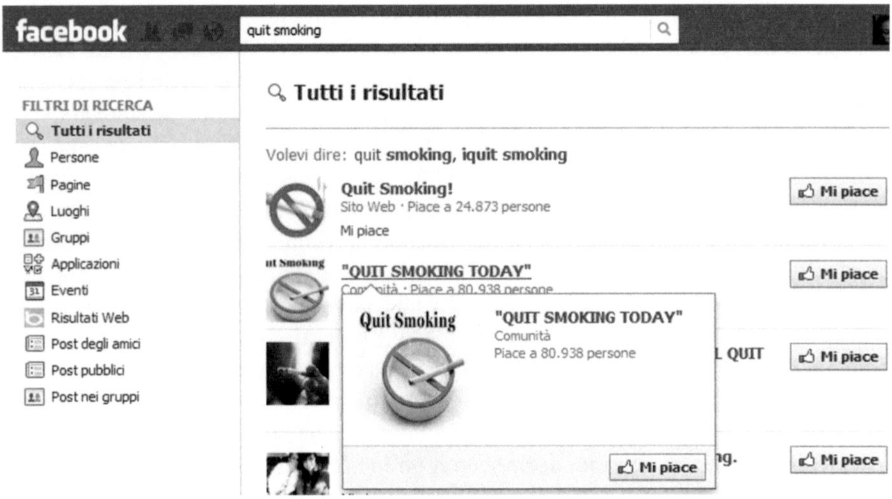

Fig. 12.3 Smokers and social networks (http://www.facebook.com/nycquits?sk=wall)

the undesirability of smoking, assist in buffering cessation-related stressors, enhance coping skills, and provide suggestions for eliminating smoking cues (Graham et al. 2011).

These associations appear to be relatively robust, with higher levels of social exchanges (e.g., messages, forum posts, and blog posts) and social connectedness (e.g., number of buddies and number of people sending messages to and receiving messages from) associated with higher likelihood of abstinence. While these associations are compelling, we know of no studies that have examined whether interactions in an online social network for cessation do, in fact, lead to changes in perceived social support. If observational findings are to be harnessed in interventions that attempt to manipulate social support to improve cessation outcomes, a measure of perceived social support from online social networks is needed, both as a manipulation check and also as a measure of a potentially important mediating mechanism. Smoking cessation Websites can therefore reach an audience that otherwise would not have access to any kind of smoking cessation support. These Websites can reach large audiences at a low cost per visitor, are operational at all times (24 h per day), available ubiquitously, and if they are developed by qualified professionals, they can provide information and advice of high quality (Etter 2006).

To date there have been few published studies of online social networks for cessation. Several studies have described the frequency, intensity, and nature of interactions among online social network members (Burri et al. 2006; Etter 2006; Cobb et al. 2010; 2005; Vallone et al. 2011).

Other studies have examined the association of participation in online communities with cessation outcomes (Cobb et al. 2005; An et al. 2008; Zbikowski et al. 2008).

For the enhanced Internet condition, participants were provided free access to QuitNet.com (http://www.QuitNet.com), an interactive, commercial cessation

Website that provides evidence-based cessation treatment in accordance with national guidelines (Clinical Practice Guideline Treating Tobacco Use and Dependence 2008 Update Panel, Liaisons, and Staff 2008).

QuitNet provides:

1. Advice to quit.
2. Assistance in setting a quit date.
3. Assessment of motivation, smoking history, demographics, and nicotine dependence.
4. Individually tailored information.
5. Problem solving/skills training content.
6. Tailored assistance in using pharmacotherapies approved by the US Food and Drug Administration.
7. Social support within its large online social network (Cobb et al. 2010).

For over 10 years, QuitNet has enrolled individuals into a network of current and former smokers seeking to quit or stay quit and provided multiple mechanisms of social support and social influence. QuitNet's community features allow for multiple forms of social support and social influence. Communication can occur through asynchronous channels, such as private internal email ("Q-Mail") or one-to-many messaging in the threaded forums, as well as synchronous channels such as chat rooms.

Social influence regarding cessation is conveyed through profile pages, journals (similar to a blog), anniversary lists, and testimonials. Users are encouraged to publically share their quit dates, which are set through a "wizard" tool, and users are prompted for updates at each login. QuitNet maintains a complete transactional history of all events, including communications that occur throughout the site. Active events (e.g., sending internal email or posting a public message) and passive actions (e.g., reading messages or viewing another individual's profile) are logged into a relational database (Graham et al. 2011). Despite their huge audience, Websites will have no impact if the interventions they provide are not effective. But there is no simple answer to the question of efficacy. Strong claims for efficacy can be found on the major smoking cessation Websites, but these claims do not rely on published scientific evidence. Overall, the evidence for the efficacy of smoking cessation Websites is at best mixed, it covers only a few Websites (and none of the major ones), and data cover the short-term only. There is therefore an urgent need to conduct more research in this field (Etter 2006).

Stop-tabac.ch (Stop-Tabac, Institute of Social and Preventive Medicine, University of Geneva, Switzerland 1998), (http://www.stop-tabac.ch) is a smoking cessation Website, established in 1996 and constantly updated and expanded since then (Wang and Etter 2004). It contains coach individualized smoking cessation, discussion forums, chat, FAQ, and testimonials.

This Website was initially developed in French and was later partly translated in English, German, Italian, Danish, Chinese, Spanish, Serbo-Croat, and Georgian. The site is listed first in *Google.fr* when typing "tabac", "fumer", or "arrêter de fumer" (tobacco, smoking or quit smoking) (Etter 2006).

By late 2010 Help institutional Website (http://www.help-eu.com) was an innovative, Web-driven campaign that unleashed the power of text, images, video, and social media. The Website had become a vibrant, collaborative online space in which young people could not only learn about tobacco control but could also find inspiration. The number of visits to the Help Website between 2005 and 2010 was 15.6 million.

A separate online campaign was also put into action during May and June 2010, targeting a young female audience through the network of media Websites owned by Elle magazine. A special advertising campaign for Help was developed for the 12 separate Elle sites in Europe to promote the tobacco control message with a link to the Help campaign home page, yielding over 6.7 million page impressions for the 2-week duration of the campaign. The click-through rate (CTR) from the Elle sites to Help-eu.com reached as high as 5.07 %, whereas the CTR for the health sector is normally 0.1 %.

The Help site had an "infotainment" aspect in that it provided a home for the pictures/videos produced by young people themselves in support of the campaign and offered a launchpad for viral marketing across the Web. It also included the participative Tips section, a range of computer games (which could also be downloaded as apps onto mobile phones), and an online animation series launched in 2009 called "Helpers."

Helpers aside, other campaign material was permanently hosted on a Facebook group page and on YouTube. External Websites were also used in campaigns on national sites and pan-European portals like Yahoo! and MSN. Equally important, though, was an online partnership with MTV, which particularly flourished with the development of the MTV Smoke Screen campaign.

This changing face of the online campaign was reflected in a viral video series during 2007–2008 called "Nicomarket," which caught the unique approach taken by Help in combining humor with a deadly serious message. The viral promoted a series of imaginary products that actually provided the effects of smoking, such as a face cream that made women look 10 years older, an air "freshener" that gave off cigarette smoke, and a toothpaste that made teeth turn brown, mimicking the look of smokers' teeth. Another product gave men the "opportunity" to diminish their sexual capacities. Available from a fictitious company called Nicomarket, the spoof adverts could be forwarded to friends or posted on blogs/Websites. At the end of the Nicomarket advertisement, users were redirected to the official Help Website for more information and advice (Siquier 2010) (Fig. 12.4).

12.4 Web-Based Courses

Currently, there exist multiple ways to help individual smokers quit, but limited resources often impede access to these cessation aids, especially in some regions of the world (Barrera et al. 2009).

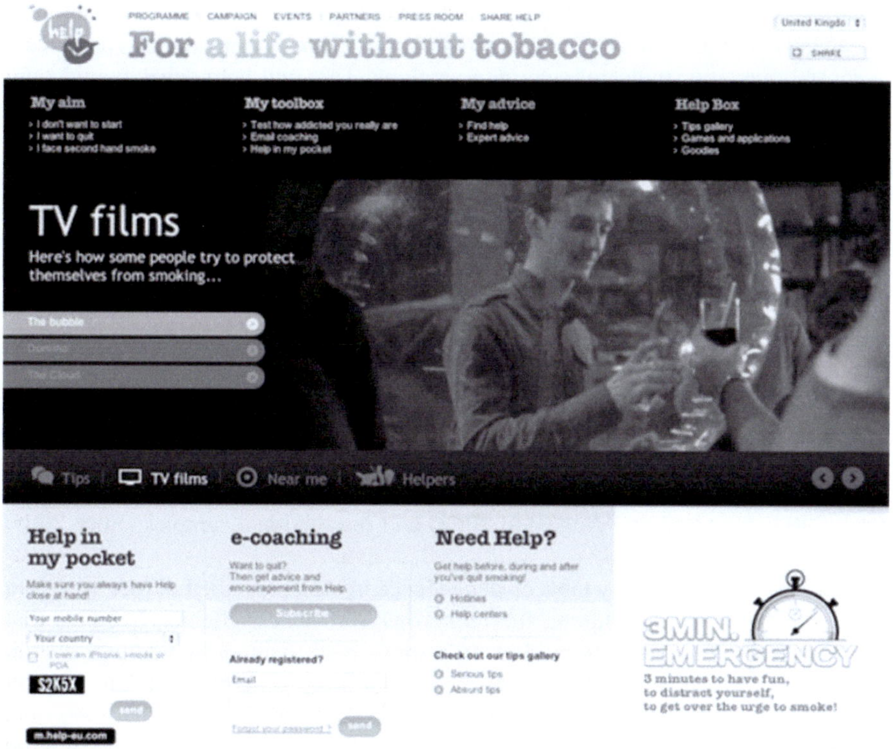

Fig. 12.4 The Help Website

Substantial numbers of smokers from numerous countries seek Web-based smoking cessation resources and add to the growing support for Web-assisted tobacco interventions as an additional tool to address the need for global smoking cessation efforts.

The Internet is a viable means through which evidence-based smoking cessation interventions can be delivered (Walters et al. 2006).

The Internet has opened up new possibilities in public health (Sorensen 2001) and it is increasingly being recognized as a powerful tool for intervention and prevention program delivery (Levy and Strombeck 2002). The Web is a promising channel to reach a large number of smokers (Bock et al. 2004).

There are several ways in which an individual who is considering stopping tobacco use might find assistance on the Internet. Website visitors may find useful information on how to quit smoking. A recent meta-analysis suggests that simply providing general self-help materials results in a modest increase in quit rates (OR = 1.24; 95 % CI: 1.07–1.45) (Lancaster and Stead 2005).

A series of randomized studies have demonstrated a modest benefit in providing individually tailored self-help information via the Internet (Etter 2005; Strecher et al. 2005; Swartz et al. 2006; Muñoz et al. 2006).

Given the increasing number of Internet smoking cessation interventions, researchers need to examine the characteristics of individuals who decide to participate in formal outcome studies of such interventions. This will help develop evidence-based interventions for international samples of smokers using the Web to quit, as well as focus attention on those not reached, to develop campaigns that increase their participation (Barrera et al. 2009).

In a typical format, smokers are surveyed via a computerized or paper assessment, and the results are tailored to some characteristic of the individual, such as gender, dependence level, perceived barriers to quitting, or stage of change. Based on a theoretical model of motivation and change, e.g. Transtheoretical Model, (Prochaska et al. 1994) the algorithm library generates instructions for each possible survey response. The resultant feedback, information, or advice is then presented on a computer screen or through printed materials.

A consistent pattern in the demographics of Web-based smoking cessation participants indicates that a majority of participants are White women and are highly educated. This pattern is evident in both US (Graham et al. 2006; Lemmonds et al. 2004; Stoddard and Auguston 2006) and international samples (Etter 2005; West et al. 2006).

Smokers seeking quality tobacco dependence treatment on the Internet may have difficulty distinguishing among the numerous Websites available. Websites that provide direct treatment often fail to fully implement treatment guidelines and do not take full advantage of the interactive and tailoring capabilities of the Internet (Bock et al. 2004).

Backinger et al., in a survey about Youtube as a source of quitting smoking information, show that almost 60 % of videos contained a message about quitting smoking. Differences were found across search terms for videos about quitting smoking, with "stop smoking" yielding the highest percentage (80.8 %) of videos about quitting smoking. Almost half of the videos (48.9 %) contained EBPs (evidence-based practices) for cessation strategies; however, a significant portion contained either non-EBPs (28.4 %) or both EBPs and non-EBPs (22.7 %). The number of views per an individual video across the six categories ranged from a low of 8 in the "relevance" strategy and "smoking cessation" search term to a high of 1,247,540 in the "view count" strategy and "stop smoking" search term. Of the top three most viewed videos by strategy and search term, 66.7 % included a specific mention of quitting smoking and, of these, the majority included EBPs.

Results highlight the need to develop and upload videos containing EBPs both to increase the overall proportion of EBP videos in all categories, particularly in "quit smoking" and "stop smoking." Research is needed to study whether YouTube videos influence knowledge, attitudes, and behaviors regarding quitting smoking (Backinger et al. 2011).

The Internet is a powerful delivery channel that has the potential to deliver behavior change interventions on a population-wide basis to help people modify risk factors such as smoking. There are limited, but encouraging, data to indicate that Web-based cessation interventions are effective in controlled trials. However, it is not known if these approaches are appealing to or appropriate for the broader population of Internet users seeking cessation assistance. For example, approximately 30 % of visitors to a widely utilized smoking cessation Website indicated that they had quit smoking within the past week (Graham and Abrams 2005; Strecher et al. 2005; Etter 2005; Swartz et al. 2006; Cobb et al. 2005).

Self-help materials may reach more eligible persons, but they typically result in lower cessation rates (Lancaster and Stead 2005; Silagy and Stead 2001). In recent years, a few intervention trials have begun to test more sophisticated methods. Studies now describe multiple iterations of feedback, specific advice, or a tailored plan for quitting, computer generated e-mail reminders, or other multimedia experiences. Such aspects are particularly apparent in computer programs targeted at youth, some of which incorporate Flash technology, interactive responses, chat rooms, or video streaming (Walters et al. 2006).

These newer interventions are noteworthy both because of their sophisticated presentation (i.e., they look and feel different), as well as their ability to customize the intervention ipsitively based on the user's responses to the program (i.e., they ask questions and respond to the user). By soliciting information and allowing the program to respond with visual or audible responses, a computer can better mimic the transactional qualities of human communication (Cassell et al. 1998).

Such interventions are also thought to be more persuasive than static text. That is, if the receiver feels there is a "give and take" in the transaction, they will be more likely to attend to the message, comprehend the argument, and consider the position (O'Keefe 1990).

While the number of smoking cessation programs is growing (high dissemination), there is little understanding of how, why, and under what conditions, such interventions might work (low evaluation). To estimate and improve the effectiveness of computer- and Internet-based interventions, it will be important for future research efforts to emphasize the importance of theoretical foundations to design and develop computer-based programs and rigorous evaluation methods to determine their effectiveness (Walters et al. 2006).

The possibilities for tailoring smoking interventions using interactive computer programs are vast, but the development costs can be high (Science Panel on Interactive Communication and Health 1999).

These costs may be justified if the program impacts populations as effectively as other programs or reaches populations which have typically been resistant to other kinds of interventions.

Because the number of computer-based health education programs has increased significantly over the past 10 years, there is a need for smoking prevention and cessation programs that are theoretically and empirically based (Revere and Dunbar 2001; Rhodes et al. 1997; Skinner and Kreuter 1997). Explanatory models of behavior change propose various factors that are thought to underlie adoption or rejection of a given behavior. Such a theory should be the basis for specifying program objectives, health behaviors, cognitive determinants of behavior (e.g., knowledge, attitudes, social perceptions, self-efficacy), change methods, and evaluation and measurement protocols (Lieberman 1997; Revere and Dunbar 2001; Rhodes et al. 1997; Skinner and Kreuter 1997). Program design must further impact the array of behavioral determinants by offering an engaging experience and thereby optimize the chance for translation of computer messages to real-world application (Shegog et al. 2001).

To tailor interventions, programs use a variety of variables, such as gender, level of problem severity, and motivational readiness (e.g., Stage of Change) for change. However, because many of these studies did not find a differential effect of the intervention across gender, ethnicity, or problem severity, future studies will need to determine which types of tailoring are most effective, and for whom.

Increased rigor in the design of evaluation studies is also necessary to determine which computer-based smoking programs best affect behavioral outcomes. Adler and Johnson (2000) have noted some of the shortfalls of existing computer-based research, including demonstration articles over comparison studies, inexperience of investigators studying computer applications, and studies that compare interventions that vary in both content and media formats. Future research directions include investigations of user–media–message interactions to understand effective educational strategies rather than comparisons of different media approaches, economic analyses regarding the cost and time benefits of computer-based applications, and diffusion studies that examine how technology might be best integrated into educational and healthcare settings (Adler and Johnson 2000; Street and Rimal 1997).

In the scope of public health interventions, computer-based applications have been available for a relatively brief time. During this time, however, generations of applications have evolved that have demonstrated some effectiveness in changing smoking behavior. Increased rigor in design, development, and evaluation of future programs will provide better insight into how to affect this persistent public health problem (Walters et al. 2006).

Through an examination of the conceptual bases of persuasion, it is posited that the World Wide Web and other Internet-based resources have many of the characteristics necessary for persuasive communication and may, in fact, constitute a hybrid channel that combines the positive attributes of interpersonal and mass communication. The notion that the Internet features many of the persuasive qualities of interpersonal communication makes it a prime candidate for the application of key behavioral science theories and principles to promote healthier behaviors.

In the Boxes 12.1 and 12.2 advices to stop smoking on the Web, and some Website and quitline are reported.

Box 12.1 Advices to Stop Smoking on the Web

Insomnia is also one of the problems arising from the smoking cessation and on the Web there are some tips may be useful to overcome these problems (http://www.stoptabac.ch/fr/Insomnies/Brochure-Insomnies_finale 20090114.pdf) (Fig. 12.5).

Booklet for women who smoke, about how to quit, and the health consequences of smoking on women (http://www.stoptabac.ch/fr/order_suisse_poste.html) (Fig. 12.6).

(continued)

Box 12.1 (continued)

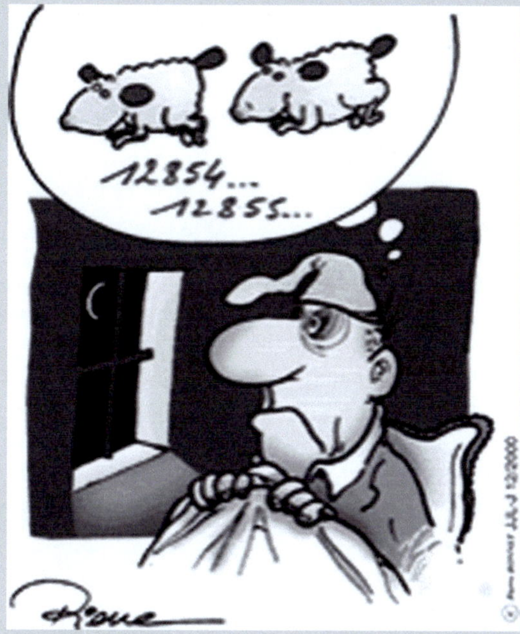
12854...
12855...

Fig. 12.5 About insomnia

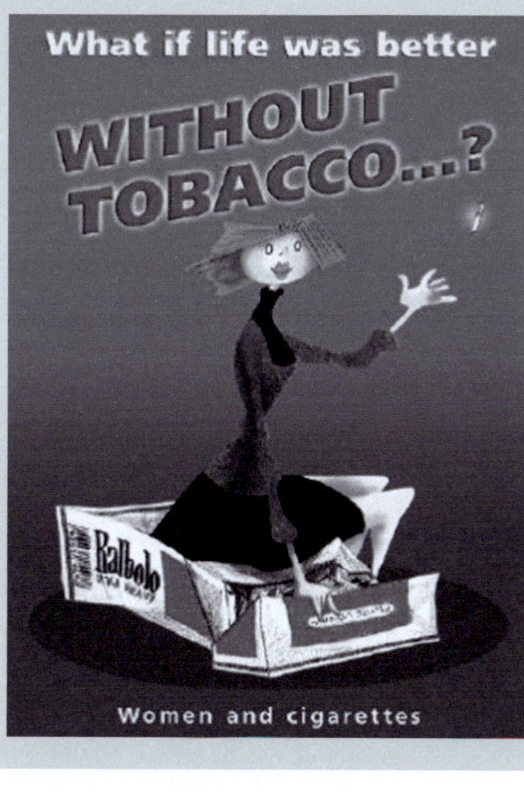
What if life was better
WITHOUT TOBACCO...?
Women and cigarettes

Fig. 12.6 Women and tobacco

Box 12.2 Some Website and Quitline

- American Cancer Society: http://www.cancer.org
- The American Lung Association: http://www.lungusa.org/stop-smoking/about-smoking/
- Ministero della Salute: http://www.salute.gov.it/stiliVita/paginaInterna-MenuStiliVita.jsp?id=465&menu=fumo
- Rauchen—Intervention in der zahnmedizinischen Praxis: http://www.dental-education.ch/smoking
- Campagne de l'Office fédéral de la santé publique: http://www.bravo.ch
- National Cancer Institute (NCI): http://www.cancer.gov/pinkbook
- Campaign for Tobacco-free Kids: http://www.tobaccofreekids.org
- CDC Office on Smoking and Health: http://www.cdc.gov/tobacco/
- CDC Division of Adolescent and School Health: http://www.cdc.gov/healthyyouth/tobacco/index.htm
- Centers for Disease Control and Prevention's Media Campaign Resource Center: http://www.cdc.gov/tobacco/mcrc
- World Health Organization Tobacco-Free Initiative: http://www.who.int/tobacco
- Health Education Council: http://www.healthedcouncil.org
- Children Opposed to Smoking Tobacco: http://www.costkids.org
- National SAFE KIDS Campaign: http://www.Safekids.org
- United Nations International Children's Fund: http://www.unicef.org/lifeskills/index_7197.html
- Tobacco-Free Coalition of Oregon's site: http://www.tobaccofreeoregon.org
- Osservatorio Fumo, Alcol e Droga dell'Istituto Superiore di Sanità: http://www.iss.it/ofad/
- Lega Italiana per la Lotta contro i Tumori (LILT): http://www.legatumori.it/page.php?id=1053&area=955

Quitline

- http://www.stopsmokingcoach.eu/home.ashx?lang=it#registertab-tab
- http://www.quitnow.gov.au/internet/quitnow/publishing.nsf
- http://www.quit.org.au/ways-to-quit/call-the-quitline.aspx
- http://doh.wa.gov/tobacco/quit/quitline.htm
- http://www.quit.org.nz/
- http://www.ctri.wisc.edu/quitline.html
- http://www.cancer.org/Healthy/StayAwayfromTobacco/GuidetoQuittingSmoking/index

References

Adler, M. D., & Johnson, K. B. (2000). Quantifying the literature of computer-aided instruction in medical education. *Academic Medicine, 75*(10), 1025–1028.

An, L. C., Schillo, B. A., Saul, J. E., Wendling, A. H., Klatt, C. M., Berg, C. J., et al. (2008). Utilization of smoking cessation informational, interactive, and online community resources as predictors of abstinence: Cohort study. *Journal of Medical Internet Research, 10*(5), e55.

Attili, G. (2000). *Introduzione alla psicologia sociale*. Roma: Edizioni SEAM.

Backinger, C. L., Pilsner, A. M., Augustson, E. M., Frydl, A., Phillips, T., & Rowden, J. (2011). YouTube as a source of quitting smoking information. *Tobacco Control, 20*(2), 119–122.

Backinger, C. L., Thornton-Bullock, A., Miner, C., Orleans, C. T., Siener, K., DiClemente, C. C., et al. (2010). Building consumer demand for tobacco-cessation products and services: The national tobacco cessation collaborative's consumer demand roundtable. *American Journal of Preventive Medicine, 38*(3), S307–S311.

Barrera, A. Z., Pérez-Stable, E. J., Delucchi, K. L., & Muñoz, R. F. (2009). Global reach of an internet smoking cessation intervention among Spanish- and English-speaking smokers from 157 countries. *International Journal of Environmental Research and Public Health, 6*(3), 927–940.

Bock, C., Graham, A., Sciamanna, C., Krishnamoorthy, J., Whiteley, J., Carmona-Barros, R., et al. (2004). Smoking cessation treatment on the internet: Content, quality, and usability. *Nicotine & Tobacco Research, 6*(2), 207–219.

Burri, M., Baujard, V., & Etter, J. F. (2006). A qualitative analysis of an internet discussion forum for recent ex-smokers. *Nicotine & Tobacco Research, 8*(1), S13–S19.

Cassell, M. M., Jackson, C., & Cheuvront, B. (1998). Health communication on the Internet: An effective channel for health behavior change? *Journal of Health Communication, 3*(1), 71–79.

Clinical Practice Guideline Treating Tobacco Use and Dependence 2008 Update Panel, Liaisons, and Staff. (2008). A clinical practice guideline for treating tobacco use and dependence: 2008 update. A U.S. Public Health Service report. *American Journal of Preventive Medicine, 35*(2), 158–176.

Cobb, N. K., & Graham, A. L. (2006). Characterizing internet searchers of smoking cessation information. *Journal of Medical Internet Research, 8*(3), e17.

Cobb, N. K., Graham, A. L., & Abrams, D. B. (2010). Social network structure of a large online community for smoking cessation. *American Journal of Public Health, 100*(7), 1282–1289.

Cobb, N. K., Graham, A. L., Bock, B. C., Papandonatos, G., & Abrams, D. B. (2005). Initial evaluation of a real-world Internet smoking cessation system. *Nicotine & Tobacco Research, 7*(2), 207–216.

Cummings, K. M., Emont, S. L., Jaen, C., & Sciandra, R. (1988). Format and quitting instructions as factors influencing the impact of a self-administered quit smoking program. *Health Education Quarterly, 15*(2), 199–216.

Etter, J. F. (2005). Comparing the efficacy of two internet-based, computer-tailored smoking cessation programs: A randomized trial. *Journal of Medical Internet Research, 7*(1), e2.

Etter, J. F. (2006). Internet-based smoking cessation programs. *International Journal of Medical Informatics, 75*(1), 110–116.

Etter, J. F. (2010). Smoking and Cloninger's temperament and character inventory. *Nicotine & Tobacco Research, 12*(9), 919–926.

Etter, J. F., Pélissolo, A., Pomerleau, C., & De Saint-Hilaire, Z. (2003). Associations between smoking and heritable temperament traits. *Nicotine & Tobacco Research, 5*(3), 401–409.

Festinger, L. (1978). *Teoria della dissonanza cognitiva*. Milano: FrancoAngeli.

Fiore, M. C., Bailey, W. C., Cohen, S. J., Dorfman, S. F., Goldstein, M. G., Gritz, E. R., et al. (2000). *Smoking cessation: Clinical practice guideline no. 18*. Rockville, MD: US Dept of Health and Human Services, Public Health Service.

Fotuhi, O., Fong, G. T., Zanna, M. P., Borland, R., Yong, H. H., & Cummings, K. M. (2012). Patterns of cognitive dissonance-reducing beliefs among smokers: A longitudinal analysis from the International Tobacco Control (Itc) Four Country Survey. *Tobacco Control, 22*(1), 52–58. doi:10.1136/tobaccocontrol-2011-050139.

Fox, S. (2005). *Health information online*. Washington, DC: Pew Internet & American Life Project. Cited April 29, 2012, from http://www.pewinternet.org/~/media/Files/Reports/2005/PIP_Healthtopics_May05.pdf.pdf

Fox, S. (2006). *Pew internet*. Washington, DC: Pew Internet & American Life Project. Cited April 29, 2012, from http://www.pewinternet.org/~/media/Files/Reports/2006/PIP_Online_Health_2006.pdf.pdf

Graham, A. L., & Abrams, D. B. (2005). Reducing the cancer burden of lifestyle factors: Opportunities and challenges of the internet. *Journal of Medical Internet Research, 7*(3), e26.

Graham, A. L., Bock, B. C., Cobb, N. K., Niaura, R., & Abrams, D. B. (2006). Characteristics of smokers reached and recruited to an internet smoking cessation trial: A case of denominators. *Nicotine & Tobacco Research, 8*(1), S43–S48.

Graham, A. L., Papandonatos, G. D., Kang, H., Moreno, J. L., & Abrams, D. B. (2011). Development and validation of the online social support for smokers scale. *Journal of Medical Internet Research, 13*(3), e69.

Hutter, H. P., Moshammer, H., & Neuberger, M. (2006). Smoking cessation at the workplace: 1 year success of short seminars. *International Archives of Occupational and Environmental Health, 79*(1), 42–48.

Internet World Stats. (2011). *Internet usage statistics—The Internet big picture world Internet users and population stats*. Cited April 29, 2012, from http://www.internetworldstats.com/stats.htm

Jackson, N., Prebble, A., & Rose, C. S. (2002). *Perceptions of smoking cessation products and services among low income smokers*. Health Development Agency.

Lancaster, T., & Stead, L. F. (2005). Self-help interventions for smoking cessation. *Cochrane Database Systematic Review* (3), CD001118.

Lemmonds, C. A., Mooney, M., Reich, B., & Hatsukami, D. (2004). Characteristics of cigarette smokers seeking treatment for cessation versus reduction. *Addictive Behaviors, 29*(2), 357–364.

Levy, J. A., & Strombeck, R. (2002). Health benefits and risks of the Internet. *Journal of Medical Systems, 26*(6), 495–510.

Lieberman, D. A. (1997). Interactive video games for health promotion: Effects on knowledge, self-efficacy, social support, and health. In R. Street, W. Gold, & T. Manning (Eds.), *Health promotion and interactive technology: Theoretical applications and future directions*. Mahwah, NJ: Lawrence Erlbaum Associates.

Muñoz, R. F., Lenert, L. L., Delucchi, K., Stoddard, J., Perez, J. E., Penilla, C., et al. (2006). Toward evidence-based internet interventions: A Spanish/English Web site for international smoking cessation trials. *Nicotine & Tobacco Research, 8*(1), 77–87.

Obituaries Allen Carr. (2006). *BMJ bmj.com, 333*, 1273–1274.

O'Keefe, D. J. (1990). *Persuasion*. Newbury Park, CA: Sage.

Prochaska, J. O., Norcross, J. C., & DiClemente, C. C. (1994). *Changing for good: The revolutionary program that explains the six stages of change and teaches you how to free yourself from bad habits*. New York: W. Morrow.

Ramseier, C. A., & Fundak, A. (2009). Tobacco use cessation provided by dental hygienists. *International Journal of Dental Hygiene, 7*(1), 39–48.

Raw, M. (1992). *Stopping smoking made easier*. London: HEA.

Revere, D., & Dunbar, P. J. (2001). Review of computer-generated outpatient health behavior interventions. *Journal of the American Medical Informatics Association, 8*(1), 62–79.

Rhodes, F., Fishbein, M., & Reis, J. (1997). Using behavioral theory in computer-based health promotion and appraisal. *Health Education & Behavior, 24*(1), 20–34.

Science Panel on Interactive Communication and Health Eng TR, & Gustafson, D. H. (1999). *Wired for health and well-being: The emergence of interactive health communication*. Washington DC: HHS.

Shegog, R., Sockrider, M., Bartholomew, L. K., Masse, L., Parcel, G., & Abramson, S. (2001). Impact of a computer-assisted self-management education program on factors related to asthma self-management behaviour. *Journal of the American Medical Informatics Association, 8*(1), 49–61.

Silagy, C, Stead L. F. (2001). Physician advice for smoking cessation. *Cochrane Database Syst Rev. (2)*:CD000165.

Siquier, P. (2010). *Help-For a life without tobacco-A legacy*. Cited April 29, 2012, from http://ec.europa.eu/health/tobacco/docs/help_legacy.pdf

Skinner, C. S., & Kreuter, M. (1997). Using theories in planning interactive computer programs. In R. Street, W. Gold, & T. Manning (Eds.), *Health promotion and interactive technology: Theoretical applications and future directions*. Mahwah, NJ: Lawrence Erlbaum Associates.

Sorensen, A. A. (2001). Promoting public health through electronic media: A challenge for schools of public health. *American Journal of Public Health, 91*(8), 1183–1185.

Stoddard, J. L., & Auguston, E. M. (2006). Smokers who use internet and smokers who don't: Data from the Health Information and National Trends Survey (HINTS). *Nicotine & Tobacco Research, 8*(1), S77–S85.

Stop tabach. (2012). *Tabagisme et traits de personnalité*. Cited April 26, 2012, from http://www.stop-tabac.ch/fra/autour-du-tabac/personnalite-et-tabagisme.html

Strecher, V. J., Shiffman, S., & West, R. (2005). Randomized controlled trial of a web-based computer-tailored smoking cessation program as a supplement to nicotine patch therapy. *Addiction, 100*(5), 682–688.

Street, R. L., & Rimal, R. N. (1997). Health promotion and interactive technology: A conceptual foundation. In R. Street, W. Gold, & T. Manning (Eds.), *Health promotion and interactive technology: Theoretical applications and future directions*. Mahwah, NJ: Lawrence Erlbaum Associates.

Swartz, L. H. G., Noell, J. W., Schroeder, S. W., & Ary, D. V. (2006). A randomised control study of a fully automated internet based smoking cessation programme. *Tobacco Control, 15*(1), 7–12.

Vallone, D. M., Duke, J. C., Cullen, J., McCausland, K. L., & Allen, J. A. (2011). Evaluation of EX: A national mass media smoking cessation campaign. *American Journal of Public Health, 101*(2), 302–309.

Walters, S. T., Wright, J. A., & Shegog, R. (2006). A review of computer and Internet-based interventions for smoking behavior. *Addictive Behaviors, 31*(2), 264–277.

Wang, J., & Etter, J. F. (2004). Administering an effective health intervention for smoking cessation online: The international users of Stop-Tabac. *Preventive Medicine, 39*(5), 962–968.

West, R., Gilsenan, A., Coste, F., Zhou, X., Brouard, R., Nonnemaker, J., et al. (2006). The ATTEMPT cohort: A multi-national longitudinal study of predictors, patterns and consequences of smoking cessation; introduction and evaluation of internet recruitment and data collection methods. *Addiction, 101*(9), 1352–1361.

Westmaas, J. L., Abroms, L., Bontemps-Jones, J., Bauer, J. E., & Bade, J. (2011). Using the internet to understand smokers' treatment preferences: Informing strategies to increase demand. *Journal of Medical Internet Research, 13*(3), e58.

Willcox, M. L. (1997). Tobacco control programmes for universities: A feasibility study. *Journal of Public Health Medicine, 19*(1), 37–44.

World Health Organization. (2006). *Facts and figures about tobacco*. First Conference of Parties to the WHO Framework Convention on Tobacco Control Geneva. Cited April 29, 2012, from http://www.who.int/tobacco/fctc/tobacco%20factsheet%20for%20COP4.pdf

World Health Organization. (2012). *Quitting tobacco*. Cited April 26, 2012, from http://www.who.int/tobacco/quitting/background/en/index.html

Zbikowski, S. M., Hapgood, J., Smucker Barnwell, S., & McAfee, T. (2008). Phone and web-based tobacco cessation treatment: Real-world utilization patterns and outcomes for 11,000 tobacco users. *Journal of Medical Internet Research, 10*(5), e41.

Chapter 13
Ethical Aspects of Tobacco Smoking

Giuseppe La Torre and Rosella Saulle

Aim of the Chapter This chapter discusses the bioethical basis for cooperative approaches to the global tobacco epidemic. It discusses the use of legal instruments to address global public health threats and the ethical basis for implementation of acts for smoking cessation. In addition, the aims are to describe the major ethical issues surrounding tobacco taxation and to identify policy responses to minimize any ethical dilemmas.

Learning Objectives

After completing this section, the reader will be able to:

1. Make a review on the ethical aspect related to tobacco smoking.
2. Examine the main ethical parameters of the arguments pertaining to the alleged "right" to advertise tobacco products and those maintaining that it should be banned. In particular, will explore the ethics of the adoption of "partial" bans on tobacco advertising.
3. Know the action to behave as a role model to promote patient and community health by abstaining from or quitting smoking and encouraging and assisting patients and colleagues to quit smoking.
4. Assume more responsibility for advocating for smoke-free environments and policies that combat smoking-related health threats in the community.
5. Actively support international policies and interventions that expand tobacco cessation and smoke-free environments.

G. La Torre (✉) • R. Saulle
Department of Public Health and Infectious Diseases, "Sapienza" University of Rome, Piazzale Aldo Moro 5, Rome 00185, Italy
e-mail: giuseppe.latorre@uniroma1.it; rosella.saulle@uniroma1.it

G. La Torre, *Smoking Prevention and Cessation*, DOI 10.1007/978-1-4614-7046-5_13,

13.1 Tobacco Smoking and Public Awareness: What Are the Risks?

Philosophically, smoking has long been regarded as a paradigmatically private-regarding vice, best treated as such.

Folk wisdom has long held tobacco smoking to be unhealthy and it actually is axiomatic that tobacco smoking is hazardous to health.

The statistics are well documented and often very grim. In the 2008 World Health Organization Report on the global tobacco epidemic presented the following statistics: a 100 million people died of tobacco-related diseases globally in the twentieth century; there are approximately over five million tobacco-related deaths every year and without intervention an estimated one billion could die of tobacco-related diseases in this twenty-first century. By any standard, tobacco is no ordinary product. A recent US Surgeon General stated in the preface to the 1990 Surgeon General's report on smoking: "it is safe to say that smoking represents the most extensively documented cause of disease ever investigated in the history of biomedical research."

The 1964 surgeon general's report addresses this question of causation at length, arguing, inter-alia, that just as cause precedes consequence, smoking precedes cancer. "*About a quarter of the young men who smoke a pack a day or so of cigarettes are killed before their time by smoking*"*; and* "*on average … [they] have lost ten to fifteen years of life*" *(*Peto 1980).

Strictly speaking, all that that proves is that smoking correlates with many diseases: as any first course in statistics teaches, correlation is not causation.

13.1.1 Tobacco Is Not Just Killing Smokers

That it is a merely private-regarding vice, harming only smokers themselves (Ackerman 1977) is challenged by evidence of the harmful effects of "passive smoking" (i.e., nonsmokers' inhalation of smoke given off by others smoking around them).

Inhaling secondhand smoke (SHS) increases the risk for lung cancer in nonsmokers by 30 % American Thoracic Society. Asia Pacific Society of Respirology (1995). Canadian Thoracic Society. European Respiratory Society, and International Union Against Tuberculosis and Lung Disease 1995.

Most significantly, environmental tobacco smoke (ETS) harbors over 4,000 mostly unsavory chemicals, ranging from arsenic, benzene, cadmium, chromium, beryllium, carbon monoxide, ammonia, hydrogen, cyanide, to formaldehyde. Of these chemicals, 50 are known to cause cancer, while at least 250 are generally harmful to health. The great irony, however, is that sidestream smoke, to which nonsmokers are exposed, is reputedly "richer in known carcinogens than is the smoke that smokers themselves inhale." Individuals exposed to ETS would inevitably inhale nicotine, which would be absorbed directly into their bloodstream, where it would degrade relatively quickly, and through ensuing metabolism, morph into cotinine (Oriola 2009).

Study has shown that passive smokers would typically have cotinine levels of about 1 % of those found in active smokers (Le Souëf 2000).

Nearly half the world's children—700 million—breathe tobacco smoke, often in their own homes. Furthermore, adolescents who grow up in smoking homes are more likely to smoke themselves (Muilenburg Legge et al. 2009; Schlein 2008).

Infants and nonsmoking children who are chronically exposed to in utero and ETS have an increased risk of respiratory diseases, malignancy, and other health problems that result in increased hospitalizations and days lost from school (White et al. 1991).

More troublingly, an average nonsmoking person at work who is constantly exposed to multiple cigarette smokers would receive close to four times the dose of ETS than the nonsmoking spouse would receive at home (Goodin 1989). This would resonate well with workers who operate in work environments where cigarette smoking is the norm. These would include restaurant workers, bar attendants, and waitresses, for example, and is arguably one of the reasons that cities across the world now prohibit smoking at such venues.

Half of the countries in the world, representing two-thirds of the world's population, allow smoking in the workplace (Food and Agriculture Organization of the United Nations 2009) and about 200,000 workers die each year because of smoke-filled workplaces.

Nonsmoking adults who are exposed also have more respiratory symptoms that are likely to contribute to work absenteeism due to illness.

The question is simply whether, in the case of smoking, the active cooperation of the smoker really is such as to constitute voluntary acceptance of the consequent risks of illness and death.

Given that passive smoking is characterized as involuntary smoking, it is literally nothing short of assault on nonsmokers, and a fatal one at that, in light of the well-documented health hazards posed to nonsmokers by high levels of nicotine and cotinine in their bloodstream (Smith 2007).

A 1990 Dutch Health Council Advisory Report found inter-alia that inhaled ETS or passive smoking could increase the risk of lung cancer by 20 %; significantly increase the risk of other forms of cancer; or the risk of cardiovascular disease by 20–30 %; increase the risk of underweight children by pregnant women by 20–40 %; and double (by 100 %) the risk of sudden infant death syndrome (Health Council of the Netherlands 2003).

Furthermore, in the USA, secondhand tobacco smoke is held accountable for an estimated 3,400 annual lung cancer deaths and approximately between 22,700 and 69,600 annual heart disease deaths among adult nonsmokers (Bosky 2008; Goodin 1989; Smith 2007; Oriola 2009).

Tobacco-related deaths kill more people than AIDS, tuberculosis, and malaria together (*World Health Organization* 2009a, b). Smoking cessation has immediate and substantial health benefits, both symptomatically and pathophysiologically, and dramatically reduces the risk of most smoking-related diseases (*US Dept of Health and Human Services* 1989).

13.1.2 Do Smokers Voluntarily Accept the Risks?

It is sacrosanct that ETS causes harm to nonsmokers and impairs public health. Human rights and public health are powerful and modern approaches with intrinsic connections, which share the common objective of protecting the health and the well being of all individuals. The Calcutta Declaration adopted at the Regional Public Health Conference in 1999 had, in its agenda for action, recommended using a rights approach to health. Upholding human rights and the dignity of all human beings and adoption of an intergenerational approach are important prerequisites for improving public health and ensuring sustainable development.

Given what we know of the health risks from smoking, we may well be tempted to "ban cigarette manufacturers from continuing to manufacture their product on the grounds that we are preventing them from causing illness to others in the same way that we prevent other manufacturers from releasing pollutants into the atmosphere, thereby causing danger to members of the community." As Dworkin (1972) continues, "*The incurring of the harm requires the active cooperation of the victim.*"

Certainly there is, morally speaking, a world of difference between the harms that others inflict upon you and the harms that you inflict upon yourself.

The question is simply whether, in the case of smoking, the active cooperation of the smoker really is such as to constitute voluntary acceptance of the consequent risks of illness and death.

This question is decomposable into two further ones. The first concerns the question of whether smokers knew the risks. That is essentially a question of "informed consent."

People can be held to have consented only if they knew to what they were supposedly consenting. The second concerns the question of whether, even if smoking in full knowledge of the risks, they could be said to have "accepted" the risks in a sense that was fully voluntary (Goodin 1989).

Courts have been as sensitive to this distinction as moral philosophers, appealing to the venerable legal maxim, *volenti non fat injuria*, to hold that through their voluntary assumption of the risk smokers have waived any claims against cigarette manufacturers.

13.2 Individual Rights

13.2.1 Types and Importance of Individual Rights: Public Health and Other Perspectives

Individual rights are actions that society judges to be moral entitlements of each of its members. These entitlements revolve around life, liberty, and use of property.

A public health perspective generally looks at these rights in descending order of priority, namely that rights to life trump those of liberty, which trump use of property. While agreeing that other perspectives and the rights priority they endorse are important and widely held, the perspective here largely assigns precedence to the public health viewpoint. Yet it also recognizes, and wherever possible seeks to foster, liberty and use of property as individuals see fit.

Three subtypes of individual rights can be distinguished: *the right to life, liberty, and use of private property*.

All three aspects of individual rights are central to efforts to *control ETS* but in different ways. It is clear that ETS interferes with an individual's physical and mental health and thus can be construed as violating one's right to life. This interference occurs whether or not ETS is sanctioned by governmental or corporate policies. Another interference caused by those who smoke is that their activity (i.e., creating ETS) violates the rights of others to be let alone to pursue their own interests and activities—that is, it harms their liberty. The third individual rights subtype is to use one's own property as one wishes. This may include producing, marketing, and using a commercial product, such as tobacco. Here ETS restrictions limit the individual rights of property, but also do so, at least in part, to safeguard other individual rights.

No rights are unlimited, and the polity and courts must at times give priority to some rights over others. For instance, as important as liberty is, it usually is considered secondary to the right of life. Although commercial activity in some form is vital to modern society, it still can exist only at society's sufferance. As such it may be and usually is regulated. Common commercial activities are regulated through positive regulatory steps and through torts; in contrast to political rights (life and liberty), property rights are generally much more narrowly construed by regulators, legislators, and the courts. It should be noted from a normative perspective that tobacco is one of the least regulated dangerous substances. The impression promoted by the tobacco industry is to the contrary (Katz 2005).

13.2.2 Human Rights

Smokers and nonsmokers all have right. Nonsmokers and employers are becoming less tolerant of smokers. Non smokers are speaking up their rights and demanding protection from smoke hazard. As the Surgeon General stated in the 1986 report: "*the right of smokers to smoke ends where their behaviour affects the health and well-being of others.*"

The accumulation of evidence on the risks and health consequences of involuntary exposure to ETS emphasizes the need for stronger regulation to protect nonsmokers, particularly children. An example of this regulation is presented in Box 13.1.

Box 13.1 The European Strategy for Tobacco Control (ESTC) Recommended That Strategic National Action Should Include

- Introducing or strengthening legislation to make all public places smoke-free, including public transport and workplaces.
- Banning smoking indoors and outdoors in all educational institutions and their premises for children up to the age of 18 years and indoors in all other educational institutions.
- Banning smoking in all places of healthcare delivery and their indoor and outdoor premises.
- Banning smoking at all public events arranged indoors and outdoors.
- Banning or severely restricting smoking in restaurants and bars to protect owners, employees, and clients from serious damage to their health.
- Classifying ETS as a carcinogen to protect the rights of workers (nonsmokers and smokers), particularly those working in smoking environments, and to speed up the banning of smoking in all workplaces.
- It was also suggested that Member States review and strengthen the mechanisms for enforcing their legislation and increase compliance through comprehensive information campaigns and litigation.

There is also evidence that smoke-free legislation will help current smokers to stop smoking and reduce the average consumption of tobacco by those that continue to smoke (Katz 2005).

13.2.3 Assumption: The Concept of "Public Health"

The Framework Convention on Tobacco Control (FCTC) emphasizes that contracting states have the right to protect their populations' health, that individual rights should be respected, and that the "widest possible international cooperation is necessary to control tobacco-caused illnesses" (Tobacco Advisory Group of the Royal College of Physicians. 2005).

However, there is no specific mention of the bioethical basis for this global approach to tobacco control.

Understanding the jurisprudential, ethical, and conceptual parameters of "public health" is vital to grasping public health justificatory grounds for tobacco smoking discouragement policy in general, and tobacco smoking proscription in enclosed public spaces in particular.

The term "public health" tends to be characterized by a myriad of "public health problems," ranging from infectious diseases, cigarette smoking, pollution, inadequate sanitation, societal inequalities, domestic violence, teenage pregnancy, gambling, to suicide.

Thus, the term "public health" seems to cover every conceivable social and economic problematic that put the society or public at risk (Goodin 1989).

Definition proffered by James F. Childress et al. was:

> *Public health is primarily concerned with the health of the entire population, rather than the health of individuals. Its features include an emphasis on the promotion of health and the prevention of disease and disability; the collection and use of epidemiological data, population surveillance, and other forms of empirical quantitative assessment; a recognition of the multidimensional nature of the determinants of health; and a focus on the complex interactions of many factors—biological, behavioral, social and environmental—in developing effective interventions.* (Childress et al. 2002)

Thus, without doubt, public health protection is the critical mass of the general governmental tobacco smoking discouragement policy (Wilson and Thompson 2005) or the bourgeoning global wave of tobacco smoking proscription in enclosed public spaces (Bosky 2008), which is arguably buoyed by the 2005 World Health Organizations' FCTC (The WHO Framework Convention on Tobacco Control 2009).

Consequently, if public health issues were mainly about concerns for, and the protection of the health of the general public rather than that of individuals, then the best entity most suited to safeguard public health is the government, due to its inherent legal and moral authority to do so. Indeed, government's legitimacy to regulate public health issues is directly anchored on its authority to govern and protect public interest (Bayles 1978; Locke 1999).

13.3 Bioethical Basis for Global Tobacco Control

13.3.1 Principles of Bioethics

There are four main principles of bioethics that apply to tobacco control:

(a) Autonomy
(b) Beneficence
(c) Non-maleficence
(d) Justice

Persons are deemed to have autonomy on the basis of their nature as rational and moral beings. Preservation of individual autonomy requires both information about a health risk behavior and voluntary choice (i.e. without nicotine addiction).

Beneficence is the obligation for national governments to promote public well being, and non-maleficence refers to the obligation of governments to avoid harm (embodied, for example, in the "Precautionary principle," by which a government may preclude population exposure to a likely hazard even without absolute proof of the hazard). The principle of justice requires the fair and equitable distribution of social goods and, accordingly, the fair and equitable distribution of social and biological burdens.

13.3.2 Political Outcomes

There is no doubt that tobacco use or cigarette smoking is an autonomous and indeed, very private act (Smith 2007).

Therefore, the central question is: should political intervention in a private affair as basic as tobacco smoking in enclosed public spaces be justified in the name of public health protection?

The role of government includes protecting its population. The ASPECT Consortium, established by the European Commission, states that:

> *Parties recognize that scientific evidence has unequivocally established that exposure to tobacco smoke causes death, disease and disability... Each Party shall adopt and implement in areas of existing national jurisdiction as determined by national law and actively promote at other jurisdictional levels the adoption and implementation of effective legislative, executive, administrative and/or other measures, providing for protection from exposure to tobacco smoke in indoor workplaces, public transport, indoor public places and, as appropriate, other public places* (European Commission 2004).

Because of the massive harm caused by active and passive exposure, laws and regulations for tobacco control can be considered a requirement of good governance. The banning of all forms of tobacco advertising and promotion has long been regarded as a central platform of comprehensive tobacco control policy.

The goals of these policies are:

1. *To prevent the initiation of smoking and the development of nicotine addiction.*
2. *To encourage the cessation of tobacco use among those who already smoke cigarettes or use other tobacco products.*
3. *To protect nonsmokers.*

Such policy includes (1) *taxes on cigarettes*; (2) *restrictions on advertising*; (3) *restriction on cigarette sales to children and teenagers*; (4) *prohibition of smoking in specified public places*; (5) *assurances that smoke-free environments will be available in workplaces*; (6) *regulation of content and packaging of tobacco products*; (7) *public education*; (8) *promotion of smoking cessation services*; (9) *assistance for tobacco farmers;* (10) *restriction of international trade in tobacco*; (11) *health warnings on cigarette packages*; *and* (12) *abolition of "kiddie" packages of cigarettes.*

This range of government intervention illustrates that restrictions on advertising represent only one strategy in the attempt to control the use of products that have known potential to affect adversely either those who use them or the general public. There is no more a "right" to advertise than there is a "right" to sell. Both activities are frequently subsumed by broader considerations of public benefit, welfare, and safety. These considerations can be paternalistic (Dworkin 1972) (justified by concern to protect individuals from the consequences of their own behavior, particularly when it can be demonstrated that individuals have inadequate or erroneous knowledge about the range, probability, and severity of these consequences), or Millean (Mill 1975) (based on concerns to restrain individual liberty if its expression has adverse consequences for others). Some libertarians argue that paternalism is ethically unjustified—people should be free to risk harm to themselves provided that they can demonstrate that they are fully informed about the probability of, and the nature of, the harm they risk. While many people living in nations which have histories of health education about the risks of tobacco use are informed in general terms about smoking, their knowledge is often inadequate to any usual test of informed consent.

Legal paternalism has its roots in the Latin word pater, which means to act like a father or treat someone like a child (Hospers 1980).

The term has been adapted by modern legal and political philosophers to describe situations where authority figures make decisions or act for another person or persons, ostensibly in their best interests or for their general good or welfare, and usually without their consent (Suber and Gray 1999).

13.3.3 Legal Paternalism, Nanny-Statism, and the Defense of Public Health Against ETS

Legal and ethical subquestions: Is there a right to tobacco use or to freely smoke as such? If there were such a right, wouldn't political intervention in the free use of tobacco products smack of paternalism or undermine smokers' privacy or their right to freely smoke?

According to Peter Suber (Suber and Gray 1999), paternalism advances societal interests such as life, health, and safety, at the expense of their liberty, but it is controversial because it is necessarily coercive, albeit with benevolent objectives. Gerald Dworkin's (Dworkin 1983) definition echoes similarly liberty-restraining feature of paternalism, while it purportedly serves societal general welfare and good: [the] interference with a person's liberty of action justified by reasons referring exclusively to the welfare, good, happiness, needs, interests, or values of the person being coerced (Dworkin 1983).

In the context of the general tobacco-smoking discouragement policy, the flip side of soft paternalism is "hard" paternalism, and in the context of restrictive tobacco use policy, it would necessarily override or undermine the autonomy or privacy of tobacco users, who have no intention of quitting, but who are being frustrated by spiraling tobacco prices and the ever-shrinking public space to smoke at will and in comfort.

Therefore, in the context of public health policies such as tobacco smoking proscription in enclosed public places, "hard" paternalism, which has been described as the "real paternalism," (Pope. 2000) would still impinge on autonomy, liberty, or personal freedoms of smokers, even if the policy was designed to save them from harming themselves, as well as for the protection of the public from harmful ETS (Hayry et al. 1989). Significantly, not all paternalistic actions aimed at curbing tobacco use stem from political authorities, and such curbs could be driven more by economics than by public health imperatives or the agenda to save the smoker from harming himself.

More crucially, legal paternalistic strictures such as tobacco smoking proscription in enclosed public places do carry sanctions with punitive undertones. According to Peter Suber, the inherent punitive or criminalizing nature of paternalistic legislations make paternalistic policies as instruments of behavioral change even more divisive. In the context of tobacco smoking prohibition in enclosed public spaces, for example, smokers would not only suffer the concomitant inconvenience of not being able to smoke in enclosed public spaces but also could be fined or imprisoned if they flouted the law. However, it is arguable that since the prohibited act is not victimless or harmless as exemplified by the ills of ETS cataloged above, any restrictions placed on the act would appear morally justifiable.

13.3.4 Social Action: Is There a "Right" to Advertise?

Many communities have recognized the social implications of smoking and have, therefore, enacted public policy and legislation. Such legislative issues are complex and involve balancing the rights and privileges of various heterogeneous groups.

According to the evidence, a fully comprehensive ban, covering all media and all forms of advertising (direct or indirect), promotion, sponsorship, and use of product brand names or characteristics contributes to the reduction of tobacco consumption and lessens the social desirability of smoking, particularly among young people.

Defenders of tobacco advertising tend to assume a free marketing philosophy where any restrictions on advertising are seen as ethically offensive to the sovereignty of business interests.

At one extreme of regulation, governments frequently exercise their rights to ban products outright, typically citing consumer protection from unsafe goods as their rationale.

The cornerstone of arguments used by proponents of the continuation of tobacco advertising is that the only factor relevant to whether a product should be advertised is its current legal status. By this argument, the industry would agree that illicit drugs should not be advertised, but would presumably (along with most in public health) support the lifting of any restrictions on the advertising of condoms. This insistence on the current legal status of tobacco is indifferent to the history of research into tobacco whereby its consequences to health only became established long after its use and manufacturing infrastructure became widespread. As many have argued, if tobacco had been recently "invented" and subject to the tests of safety required of food and drugs, no nation would release it onto the market in the way it is sold today.

The rejoinder to this by defenders of tobacco advertising is to make hollow calls for governments to declare tobacco illegal if they are sincere in their concerns. When governments ignore such taunts, supporters of tobacco advertising allege hypocrisy on the part of governments, pointing to their appetite for tobacco excise tax.

As argued above, concern to control use of any product can be addressed through a variety of policies, of which outright banning is the furthest extreme. Considerations of proportionality—making sure that restrictions and controls imposed are no broader than necessary to achieve the desired ends—can make a decision to ban advertising while not banning the product entirely reasonable (WHO. The European tobacco control report 2007).

At the European level, the ESTC recommended that strategic national action should include:

- Prohibiting all forms of direct and indirect advertising for tobacco products and smoking, including promotion, "brand-stretching," and sponsorship.
- Adopting national measures and imposing appropriate regulatory restrictions to ensure that tobacco advertising, promotion, and sponsorship do not promote a tobacco product by any means that are false, misleading or deceptive or that are likely to create an erroneous impression about its characteristics, health effects, hazards, or emissions.

It was also suggested that Member States ban indirect advertising and cooperate effectively at the integrational and intergovernmental levels to phase out cross-border advertising.

13.3.5 Tobacco Taxation and Public Health: Ethical Problems, Policy Responses

The WHO treaty stresses the imperatives of protecting all persons from exposure to tobacco smoke.

The taxing of tobacco has been recently described as the most cost effective tobacco control option in all regions of the world (Shibuya et al. 2003). Tobacco taxation contributes substantial benefits at the population level by protecting health (i.e., by deterring the uptake of smoking by youth, by promoting quitting, and by reducing harm from exposure to SHS). However, tobacco taxation may contribute to an unjust tax burden, may increase financial hardship for low-income populations, and may impair the autonomy of smokers.

Such taxes can contribute to autonomy, by reducing SHS exposure to nonsmokers, and by allowing freedom from nicotine dependency for those who quit smoking or do not start regular smoking as a result of high tobacco prices. Furthermore, *increases* in tobacco taxation may reduce health inequalities and so contribute to justice. Nevertheless, the additional tax burden imposed on smokers who wish to continue to smoke, or are unable to quit, can be considered unjust. The autonomy of such smokers may be partly impaired.

Although tobacco tax can be regarded as ethically justifiable because of its substantial overall benefit to society, there is substantial scope for policy changes to further reduce any harms and injustices for those populations who continue to smoke.

13.3.6 Restrictions on Smoking in Public Places

Smoking is increasingly being regulated in public places in the WHO European Region. This trend has moved from restrictions on smoking in specific institutions, such as schools and hospitals, to separating smokers and nonsmokers in a larger number of places and finally to legislation banning or restricting smoking in public places, including workplaces. The main reasons for these developments are the increasing evidence about the risks of ETS and growing public support among both smokers and nonsmokers for regulation (WHO. The European tobacco control report 2007).

Since 2002, major developments have also occurred in the area of smoke-free policies. Several countries have introduced bans on smoking in public places which for the first time extended to bars and restaurants. The regulation of smoking in public places has become more restrictive in the WHO European Region. On 29 March 2004 these restrictions were led by the example of Ireland and Norway in Ireland when smoking bans in public places were extended for the first time in the Region to pubs, bars, and restaurants as well as all workplaces. Since then, legislation banning smoking in all indoor premises, including bars and restaurants, has been passed in Italy, Malta, Norway, Spain, Sweden, and the UK.

Nearly 20 countries have passed stricter laws covering smoking in bars and restaurants, and currently, nearly two-thirds of countries have bans or restrictions on smoking in most indoor public places—a substantial improvement since 2001. By October 2006, seven countries: Ireland, Italy, Malta, Norway, Spain, Sweden, and the UK (Scotland) had introduced smoke-free bars and restaurants and more countries were planning to do so. The legislation varies in its comprehensiveness.

Recent years have also been characterized by significant and increasing public support for strong tobacco control policies and action at both national and international levels. Smokers as well as nonsmokers are now in favor of tougher controls (Table 13.1)

Since 2002, 24 Member States have reinforced legislation on direct advertising by either passing new laws or implementing existing provisions. EU Directive 2003/33/EC totally banned advertising in the press, on the radio, and in the sponsorship of sporting or cultural events with cross-border effect from 31 July 2005. Advertising remains less regulated in the Commonwealth of Independent States (CIS), although there has been notable progress in most countries since 2002.

There have also been significant developments in the regulation of tobacco products. Since December 2002, EU Directive 2001/37/EC (Directive 2001/37/EC of the European Parliament and of the Council) has required EU tobacco manufacturers to disclose the nature and quantities of all the ingredients used in tobacco products. In 2006, 32 countries and, in particular, the EU are regulating the levels of tar at 10 mg per cigarette, nicotine at 1 mg, and carbon monoxide at 10 mg in cigarettes, a decrease compared with the 2001–2002 levels of 12 mg of tar and carbon monoxide per cigarette and 1.2 mg of nicotine per cigarette.

The CIS countries and those in south-eastern Europe (SEE) in the main still set higher levels: 1.2–1.4 mg for nicotine and 12–16 mg for tar per cigarette.

Table 13.1 Regulation of smoking in public places, October 2006

County	Health care facilities	Educational facilities	Government facilities	Restaurants	Pubs and bars	Indoor workplaces and offices	Theaters and cinemas
Albania	Voluntary agreement	Voluntary agreement	Voluntary agreement	No restriction	No restriction	Voluntary agreement	Voluntary agreement
Andorra	Ban	Ban	Ban	No restriction	No restriction	No restriction	Ban
Armenia	Ban	Ban	Restriction	Restriction	Restriction	Restriction	Restriction
Austria	Ban	Ban	Ban	Voluntary agreement	Voluntary agreement	Ban	Ban
Azerbajan	Ban	Ban	Restriction	Restriction	Restriction	Restriction	Ban
Belarus	Ban	Ban	Ban	Restriction	Restriction	No Restriction	Restriction
Belgium	Ban	Ban	Ban	Restriction	Restriction	Ban	Ban
Bosnie and Herzegovina	Ban	Ban	Ban	Ban	Restriction	Ban	Ban
Bulgaria	Ban	Ban	Ban	Restriction	Restriction	Ban	Ban
Croatia	Ban	Ban	Ban	Restriction	Restriction	Restriction	Ban
Cyprus	Ban	Ban	Ban	Restriction	Restriction	Restriction	Ban
Czech Republic	Ban	Ban	Ban	Restriction	Restriction	Ban	Ban
Denmark	Restriction	Restriction	Restriction	No restriction	No restriction	Restriction	Restriction
Estonia	Ban	Ban	Ban	Restriction	Restriction	Ban	Ban
Finland	Ban	Ban	Ban	Restriction	Restriction	Ban	Ban
France	Ban	Ban	Ban	Restriction	Restriction	Restriction	Ban
Georgia	Restriction	Restriction	Restriction	Restriction	Restriction	Restriction	Restriction
Germany	Voluntary agreement	Restriction	No restriction	Voluntary agreement	Voluntary agreement	Ban	No restriction
Greece	Ban	Ban	Ban	Restriction	Restriction	Ban	Ban
Hungary	Ban	Ban	Ban	Restriction	Restriction	Ban	Ban[a]
Iceland	Ban	Ban	Ban	Restriction	Restriction	Ban	Ban
Ireland	Ban[b]	Ban	Ban	Ban	Ban	Ban	Ban
Israel	Ban	Ban	Ban	Restriction	Restriction	Ban	Restriction

(continued)

Table 13.1 (continued)

County	Health care facilities	Educational facilities	Government facilities	Restaurants	Pubs and bars	Indoor workplaces and offices	Theaters and cinemas
Italy[c]	Ban	Ban	Ban	Ban	Ban	Ban	Ban
Kazakhstan	Ban	Ban	Ban	Restriction	Restriction	Restriction	Ban
Kyrgyzstan	Ban	Restriction	Restriction	No restriction	No restriction	No restriction	No restriction
Labvia	Restriction	Ban[d]	Restriction	Restriction	Restriction	Restriction	Restriction
Lithuania	Ban	Ban	Ban	Restriction	Restriction	Restriction	Ban
Luxembourg	Ban	Ban	No restriction	Restriction	Restriction	Restriction	Ban
Malta[e]	Ban	Ban	Ban	Ban	Ban	Ban	Ban
Montenegro	Ban	Ban	Ban	Restriction	Restriction	Restriction	Restriction
Netherlands	Ban	Ban	Ban	Voluntary agreement	Voluntary agreement	Ban	Ban
Norway	Ban	Ban	Ban	Ban[f]	Ban	Ban	Ban
Poland	Restriction	Restriction	Restriction	Restriction	Restriction	Restriction	Restriction
Portugal	Ban	Ban	Voluntary agreement	Voluntary agreement	Voluntary agreement	Voluntary agreement	Ban
Republic of Moldova	Ban	Ban	Restriction	No restriction	No restriction	Restriction	Restriction
Romania[g]	Ban	Ban	Ban	Restriction	Restriction	Ban	Ban

Note. Shading indicates that the legislation entered into force during 2002–2006

[a]Except for the bar

[b]Except for prisons, psychiatric hospitals and homes for the elderly

[c]Smoking is banned in all enclosed public spaces. It is allowed in areas specially arranged for smoking which comply with the terms specified in the legislation

[d]Except for universities and colleges which have only a partial restriction

[e]Separate smoking rooms are allowed, but not in bars and restaurants, any other place food is served, or in most educational facilities

[f]Only a partial ban since bars and restaurants under 100 m^2 are exempted

[g]The complete ban entered into force in March 2006 in Scotland, will enter into force in Northern Ireland in April 2007 and in England in August 2007. In Wales the law is still being drafted

13.3.7 Education, Information, and Physician's Responsibility in Promoting the patient's Health in the Community, Strongly Supported by Ethical Arguments Grounded in Medical Professionalism

Smoking cessation is an important component of tobacco control policy. Evidence shows that brief advice and behavioral support are effective in motivating smokers to quit and that the use of nicotine replacement therapy increases the rate of success.

There is no sign that tobacco consumption is declining in the under-resourced world; the under-resourced world will consume 71 % of all tobacco products. Numerous reaffirmations of medical professionalism expand this responsibility from improving the healthcare system to promoting health in the physician's own community.

This commonsense view about an oncologist's responsibility to his or her community is strongly supported by ethical arguments grounded in medical professionalism.

As the Medical Professionalism Physician Charter states, "To maintain the fidelity of medicine's social contract during this turbulent time, we believe that physicians must reaffirm their active dedication to the principles of professionalism, which entails not only their personal commitment to the welfare of their patients but also collective efforts to improve the healthcare system for the welfare of society."

Physicians have the duty to inform and advise the public and policymakers about the dangers of smoking, especially Oncologists with their expertise because they know the consequences of tobacco use and the role of tobacco in increasing cancer risk.

Each physician is expected by the public, the medical profession, and by each of his or her patients to prevent disease when possible (Patients who are nonsmokers should receive positive reinforcement for decreasing their risk of smoking-related disease) and to give the best available treatment once disease is present, so they have often played an important role in combating major public health problems. Pediatricians, obstetricians, and family practitioners have a special opportunity to influence the health of both young parents and children. Education of pregnant women regarding harmful effects of smoking on themselves and their fetuses, and the risk of lower respiratory tract illness and symptoms in children growing up with smoking parents may help motivate women to stop smoking before becoming severely addicted.

Physicians have a contract with society (Gruen et al. 2004); the physician's primary responsibility to his or her patient requires participation in promoting the patient's health in his or her own community (US Dept of Health and Human Services 1989).

Multiple studies have shown that physicians who smoke are less likely to counsel their patients against smoking and to assist their patients in smoking cessation. It is not surprising that a physician smoker may be conflicted and is less likely to offer the advice and assistance to his or her patients for smoking cessation. This is critical, because providing cessation assistance is considered standard of care.

The Hippocratic view arguably requires that physicians be role models of healthy living. The practice of medicine is one of the three classic professions, along with law and religion. Lawyers and religious leaders are required to uphold the values of their profession in their personal lives—lawyers the value of law and religious leaders the values of their faith. Lawyers and religious leaders risk being removed from their profession if they personally act contrary to these values. So what is required of physicians who profess the value of health? It may be hard to identify exactly which health risks are so egregious that a physician must avoid them in order to profess and live in accord with health values. Advising patients about the health risks of smoking is the standard of care. A great deal of research and policy has been devoted to increasing clinical interactions aimed at tobacco control (Penz and Berg 2010).

The ESTC recommended that strategic national action should include:

- Implementing age- and gender-based promotional and educational programs aimed at encouraging the cessation of tobacco use.
- Developing and integrating best practices in the treatment of tobacco dependence and prevention of relapse (i.e., behavioral support, counseling services, "quitlines," and routine advice on cessation of tobacco use) into national health programs, plans, and strategies, including those for primary health care, alcohol and drugs control, reproductive health, tuberculosis control, etc.
- Establishing and strengthening programs of training in smoking cessation techniques for health professionals, including physicians, nurses, dentists, and pharmacists as well as teachers and community and social workers.
- Establishing in healthcare facilities programs for diagnosis, medical advice, and treatment of tobacco dependence, with a priority focus on primary health care.

13.3.7.1 National Campaigns

Evidence suggests that continuous and intensive information and education programs increase the social acceptance of tobacco control policy measures.

The ESTC recommended that strategic national action should include:

Developing and implementing effective and appropriate basic curricula and training programs on tobacco control for policy-makers, health professionals, students, educators, and other relevant persons; facilitating and strengthening education, training and public awareness campaigns, including counter-advertising.

13.3.7.2 EU Information and Communication Campaigns

In 2002, in the framework of a strengthened comprehensive and multisectorial tobacco control policy, the EU embarked on an important antismoking publicity campaign targeting teenagers in the EU. Between 2002 and 2004 the EU spent 18€ million on the "Feel Free to Say No" campaign. Evaluation has shown that through this campaign more than a billion contacts with its target audience were made.

Box 13.2 The ESTC Recommended That Strategic National Action Should Include

- Adopting standards for the regulation of tobacco products, including standards for the testing and measuring, design, manufacture and processing of such products, and cooperating in the development and harmonization of such standards.
- Introducing and enforcing measures for the disclosure of tobacco products by all manufacturers, including details of major ingredients and additives and the major constituents of tobacco smoke, as well as of their toxicity, carcinogenicity and addictiveness, and promoting the availability of clear and meaningful information to the public.
- Banning the terms "low tar," "light," "ultra light," "mild" or any other similar confusing term that has the aim or the direct or indirect effect of conveying the impression that a particular tobacco product is less harmful than others; steps should also be taken to ensure that tobacco packaging and labeling does not otherwise promote a tobacco product by any means that are false, misleading or deceptive.
- Ensuring that each unit, packet, or package of tobacco products carries a strong health warning in accordance with international and integrational agreements.
- Ensuring that these warnings provide clear information about the toxic contents of the tobacco product, specifically tar, nicotine, and carbon monoxide, including actual measurements of smoke yields; appear in the principal language or languages of the country in whose territory the product is on sale; and progressively occupy not less than 40 % of the front and 40 % of the back of tobacco packages.

More accurate assessment is required of the content of tobacco products and stronger regulation of the substances being delivered to smokers. Through visible, specific, and unequivocal health warnings, consumers should be adequately informed so that they understand the risks.

In Box 13.2 the strategic national actions recommended by the ESTC are presented.

13.4 Burden of Disease Attributable to Tobacco Use and Tobacco-Related Costs

Even though consideration of quality of life and health status of the population should be essential to the determination of health policy in relation to prevention, usually the determining factor is evidence that future savings in health and other social costs will offset the investments (McGinnis et al. 2002). For tobacco control, that evidence is available. A growing body of health economists calculates that societies would experience net benefits if tobacco use decreased in line with increased taxation (Jha and Chaloupka 2000).

In addition, economists point out that money not spent on tobacco does not disappear from the economy but is spent or invested in other products or services (Lightwood et al. 2000). There would be few economic incentives to grow tobacco in the European Union if it was not subsidized. Tobacco manufacturing is capital intensive, that is, it does not need a large work force or create jobs. Tobacco distributors and retailers are often counted as working in a tobacco economy, but they distribute and sell other items as well, so their jobs are not entirely dependent on tobacco products. Costs to society of decreased tobacco use would be transferred from tobacco-related healthcare costs to costs related to a population living longer.

Significantly, tobacco smoking foists concomitant economic burdens on individuals, corporate bodies, and the society as a whole (Winokur 2007).

Between 2002 and 2006, most European Union Member States made significant progress in relation to banning advertising, increasing the size of health warnings, strengthening product regulation, and, to a certain extent, raising taxes on tobacco. The price of tobacco products rose by an average annual rate of 6.8 % above inflation between 2001 and 2005 in the European Union (EU) countries—good progress when compared to the previous annual rate of increase of 2.7 %. The data are less encouraging in the countries in the eastern part of the Region where, in some cases, tobacco became cheaper over this period. Most countries still do not earmark tobacco taxes for tobacco control. Real price increases do not necessarily mean that tobacco products are becoming less affordable. Variations in per capita income also have to be taken into account.

In 2002, tobacco was the leading contributor to the burden of disease in 31 Member States of the European Region (particularly in the western part of the Region), the second in 8, and the third in 6 (Table 13.2).

The most recent available data indicate that tobacco use accounts for 57,227.000 DALYs for both sexes, representing 3.7 % of the global burden (5.4 % for males and 1.9 for females). This vast amount of DALYs is differently distributed in the world (Table 13.3) (WHO 2009a, b).

The estimates of healthcare costs related to smoking cited in World Bank publications range from 0.1 % to 1.1 % of the gross domestic product (GDP) (Prahbat and Chaloupka 2000). Studies recently conducted in the WHO European Region suggest that these costs could be even higher. The direct and indirect costs of smoking in the EU were estimated to range from 97.7€ to 130.3€ billion in 2000, corresponding between 1.04 % and 1.39 % of the EU GDP (European Commission 2004). Available data show that the costs are more substantial in the new EU member states, where the burden of disease and the death rates related to smoking are higher.

As far as concerns prices and taxes, in the Box 13.3 the strategic national actions recommended by the ESTC are presented.

Table 13.2 Rank and proportion of the burden of DALYs attributable to tobacco by country, 2002

Country	Rank	DALYs (%)	Country	Rank	DALYs (%)
Albania	1	9.2	Latvia	3	12.0
Andorra	1	11.2	Lithuania	3	11.5
Armenia	1	12.3	Luxembourg	1	11.3
Austria	1	11.0	Malta	3	9.7
Azerbaijan	2	6.9	Monaco	1	10.4
Belarus	4	11.6	Netherlands	1	16.7
Belgium	1	15.8	Norway	1	11.8
Bosnia and Herzegovina	1	14.7	Poland	1	11.8
Bulgaria	2	12.4	Portugal	2	10.4
Croatia	1	15.8	Republic of Moldova	4	9.7
Cyprus	2	5.6	Romania	2	13.1
Czech Republic	1	15.5	Russian Federation	3	13.4
Denmark	1	17.7	San Marino	1	11.0
Estonia	3	11.9	Serbia and Montenegro	2	15.3
Finland	3	7.7	Slovakia	2	12.2
France	1	12.4	Slovenia	1	13.7
Georgia	4	9.2	Spain	1	12.3
Germany	1	13.7	Sweden	2	8.0
Greece	1	12.9	Switzerland	1	10.7
Hungary	1	20.9	Tajikistan	8	2.3
Iceland	1	12.6	The former Yugoslav Republic of Macedonia	1	11.1
Ireland	1	11.8	Turkey	1	7.0
Israel	1	6.1	Turkmenistan	5	5.1
Italy	1	12.0	Ukraine	3	12.8
Kazakhstan	1	13.4	UK	1	14.2
Kyrgyzstan	1	6.6	Uzbekistan	7	3.1

Table 13.3 Attributable DALYs for tobacco smoking in WHO regions, estimates for 2004

WHO region	DALYs attributable to tobacco use
Africa	1,930
South-East Asia	12,764
The Americas total	8,837
High income	5,681
Low and middle income	3,157
Eastern Mediterranean total	2,793
High income	31
Low and middle income	2,762
Europe total	17,725
High income	5,526
Low and middle income	12,199
Western Pacific total	12,848
High income	1,871
Low and middle income	10,976

Box 13.3 The ESTC Recommended That, as Far as Concerns Prices and Taxes, Strategic National Action Should Include

- Maintaining high prices and taxes for tobacco products.
- Raising taxes in order to bring the price of tobacco products above the average rates of inflation and income growth, to ensure their constantly decreasing affordability.
- Prohibiting all tax-free and duty-free sales of tobacco products.
- Allocating and sustaining a significant part of government revenues, including those from tobacco taxes, to funding national tobacco control programs.
- Harmonizing taxation and prices of all tobacco products to discourage the substitution of one tobacco product by another.

References

American Thoracic Society, Asia Pacific Society of Respirology. (1995). Canadian Thoracic Society. European Respiratory Society, and International Union Against Tuberculosis And Lung Disease. Smoking and health: Physician responsibility. A statement of the Joint Committee on Smoking and Health. American College of Chest Physicians. *Chest 108*, 1118–1121.

Ackerman, B. A. (1977). *Private property and the constitution*. New Haven, CT: Yale University Press.

Bayles, M. D. (1978). *Principles of legislation: The uses of political authority* (pp. 95–118). Detroit, MI: Wayne State University Press.

Bosky, A. (2008). Ashes to ashes: Secondhand smoke meets a timely death in Illinois. *Loyola University Chicago Law Journal, 39*(4), 847–907.

Childress, J. F., Faden, R. R., Gaare, R. D., Gostin, L. O., Kahn, J., Bonnie, R. J., et al. (2002). Public health: Mapping the terrain. *The Journal of Law, Medicine & Ethics, 30*(2), 170–178.

Commission, E. (2004). *Tobacco or health in the European Union. Past, present and future. The ASPECT consortium*. Luxembourg: Office for Official Publications of the European Communities.

Directive 2001/37/EC of the European Parliament and of the Council on the approximation of the laws, regulations and administrative provisions of the Member States concerning the manufacture, presentation and sale of tobacco products. *Official Journal of the European Communities*, 2001, L 194, 26–34.

Dworkin, G. (1972). Paternalism. *The Monist, 56*(1), 64–84 (Reprinted in Sartorius, ed., 1983, pp. 19–34).

Food and Agriculture Organization of the United Nations. (2009). *Higher world tobacco use expected by 2010—Growth rate slowing down: Number of smokers growing—production shifting to developing countries*.

Goodin, R. E. (1989). *No smoking: The ethical issues*. Chicago: The University of Chicago Press. 1989.

Gruen, R. L., Pearson, S. D., & Brennan, T. A. (2004). Physician-citizens—Public roles and professional obligations. *Journal of the American Medical Association, 291*, 94–98.

Hayry, H., Hayry, M., & Karjalainen, S. (1989). Paternalism and Finnish anti-smoking policy. *Social Science and Medicine, 28*(3), 293–297.

Health Council of the Netherlands. (2003). The impact of passive smoking on public health (Publication No. 2003/21).

Hospers, J. (1980). Libertarianism and legal paternalism. *Journal of Libertarian Studies, IV*(3), 255–265.

Jha, P., & Chaloupka, F. (2000). The economics of global tobacco control. *BMJ, 321*, 358–361.
Katz, J. E. (2005). Individual rights advocacy in tobacco control policies: An assessment and recommendation. *Tobacco Control, 14*(Suppl II), 31–37.
Le Souëf, P. N. (2000). Review series paediatric origins of adult lung diseases-tobacco related lung diseases begin in childhood. *Thorax, 55*, 1063–1067.
Lightwood, J., Collins, D., Lapsley, H., & Novotny, T. E. (2000). Estimating the costs of tobacco use. In P. Jha & F. J. Chaloupka (Eds.), *Tobacco control in developing countries*. Oxford: Oxford University Press.
Locke, J. (1999). Political Power. In M. Rosen & J. Wolff (Eds.), *Political Thought*. Oxford: Oxford University Press.
McGinnis, J. M., Williams-Russo, P., & Knickman, J. R. (2002). The case for more active policy attention to health promotion. *Health Affairs, 21*, 78–93.
Mill, J. S. (1975). On liberty. In R. Wollheim (Ed.), *Three essays* (pp. 1–141). Oxford: Oxford University Press.
Muilenburg Legge, J., Latham, T., Annang, L., Johnson, W. D., Burdell, A. C., West, S. J., et al. (2009). The home smoking environment: Influence on behaviors and attitudes in a racially diverse adolescent population. *Health Education & Behavior, 36*, 777–793.
Oriola, T. A. (2009). Ethical and legal analyses of policy prohibiting tobacco smoking in enclosed public spaces. *The Journal of Law, Medicine & Ethics, 37*(4), 828–840.
Penz, R., & Berg, C. J. (2010). Smoking and ethics: What are the duties of oncologists? *Oncologists, 15*(9), 987–993.
Peto, R. (1980). Possible ways of explaining to ordinary people the quantitative dangers of smoking. *Health Education Journal, 39*, 45–46.
Pope, T. M. (2000). Balancing public health against individual liberty: The ethics of smoking regulations. *University of Pittsburgh Law Review, 61*(2), 419–498.
Prahbat, J., & Chaloupka, F. J. (2000). *Tobacco control in developing countries*. Oxford: Oxford University Press.
Schlein, L. (2008, February 4). World said to be on the brink of cancer epidemic. *Voice of America*.
Shibuya, K., Ciecierski, C., Guindon, E., Bettcher, D. W., Evans, D. B., Murray, C. J., et al. (2003). WHO framework convention on tobacco control: Development of an evidence based global public health treaty. *BMJ, 327*(7407), 154–157.
Smith, G. P. (2007). Cigarette smoking as a public health hazard: Crafting common law and legislative strategies. *Michigan State University Journal of Medicine and Law, 11*(2), 251–335.
Suber, P., & Gray, C. B. (1999). *The philosophy of law: An encyclopedia* (pp. 632–635). New York, NY: Garland.
The WHO Framework Convention on Tobacco Control. *The European tobacco control report 2007*. Accessed April, 2012, from http://www.euro.who.int/__data/assets/pdf_file/0005/68117/E89842.pdf
Tobacco Advisory Group of the Royal College of Physicians. (2005). *The medical case for clean air in the home, at work, and in public places*. London: Royal College of Physicians.
US Dept of Health and Human Services. (1989). *Reducing the health consequences of smoking: 25 years of progress. A Report of the Surgeon General* (DHHS Publication (CDC) 89–8411). Washington, DC: Office of Smoking and Health, US Government Printing Office.
White, J. R., Froeb, H. F., & Kulik, J. A. (1991). Respiratory illness in nonsmokers chronically exposed to tobacco smoke in the work place. *Chest, 100*, 39–43.
Wilson, N., & Thompson, G. (2005). Tobacco taxation and public health: Ethical problems, public responses. *Social Science and Medicine, 61*, 3649–3659.
Winokur, S. J. (2007). Seeing through the smoke: The need for national legislation banning smoking in bars and restaurants. *George Washington Law Review, 754*, 662–693.
World Health Organization. (2009a). *WHO report on the global tobacco epidemic—The mPower package*. Accessed January, 2012, from http://www.who.int/
World Health Organization. (2009b). *Global health risks—Mortality and burden of disease attributable to selected major risks*. Geneva: World Health Organization.

Chapter 14
Economic Issues Related to Tobacco Smoking

Guido Citoni, Maria Lucia Specchia, Alice Mannocci, Silvio Capizzi, and Giuseppe La Torre

Objectives The aim of this chapter is to give an overview on the economic aspects related to tobacco smoking, including production and supply of tobacco products.

Learning Outcomes

Through this section the reader will be provided:

- Some general data concerning, production and supply of tobacco products, as well as healthcare costs—both direct and indirect—attributable to smoking.
- An overview of scientific literature available about smoking-related illnesses economic costs.

G. Citoni
Department of Molecular Medicine, "Sapienza" University of Rome,
Viale Regina Elena 324, Rome 00161, Italy
e-mail: guido.citoni@uniroma1.it

M.L. Specchia
Istituto di Igiene, Università Cattolica del Sacro Cuore,
Largo Francesco Vito, n. 1, Rome 00168, Italy
e-mail: marialucia.specchia@rm.unicatt.it

A. Mannocci • G. La Torre (✉)
Department of Public Health and Infectious Diseases, "Sapienza" University of Rome,
Piazzale Aldo Moro 5, Rome 00185, Italy
e-mail: alice.mannocci@uniroma1.it; giuseppe.latorre@uniroma1.it

S. Capizzi
Institute of Hygiene, Catholic University of the Sacred Heart,
L.go F. Vito 1, Rome 00168, Italy
e-mail: silvio.capizzi@rm.unicatt.it

G. La Torre, *Smoking Prevention and Cessation*, DOI 10.1007/978-1-4614-7046-5_14,

14.1 Production and Supply of Tobacco Products

14.1.1 Growing and Manufacturing Tobacco

Tobacco is grown mainly in warm climates: farming can yield satisfactory results in different areas, so that its diffusion is widespread among countries.[1] The soil needed, though, should be sufficiently rich and well drained: about 1 % of global world agricultural land is devoted to it and farms tend to be concentrated inside countries. Moreover there has been a considerable shift in land cultivation, with advanced countries, such as the USA, that reduce their importance as producers either in relative or in absolute term: instead, emerging markets, have increased their share of production, becoming as is the case for China, the biggest world producer.[2] The specific behavior of different countries that decreased land use is nonetheless very scattered: sometimes a strong reduction in land used was coupled with increased yields, such as in Albania, so that production decreased less, sometimes the mild reduction in land use coupled with increased yields led to increased production such as in China, sometimes a decreased land use coupled with a nearly stationary yield brought about a mild reduction in production (USA), and sometimes both land use and yields decreased strongly as in Turkey. More homogeneous, instead, was the behavior of countries that increased land use, such as Argentina and Brazil, that faced nonetheless nearly stationary yields, and of those countries, mainly Africans, that increased both land use and yields (Uganda more than doubled yields in 20 years). The most astonishing case of exceptionally high yields' increase is Peru in the last decade: its land use, though, is becoming negligible.

We report in two graphs (Figs. 14.1 and 14.2) the top increases and decreases in land used during last decade.

The increases are mainly concentrated in African countries, while the decreases are scattered around the world. This raises the question, which will be dealt later on, if such a shift is advantageous for the countries, for the companies, and for the environment.

The pattern of production is reflected in that of the value of production of tobacco leaves: in Appendix are reported the statistics of the value of production at constant prices, reflecting strictly the volume and quality of production, and the corresponding rates of increase. We observe that many countries experienced a decrease in the real value of production, though the monetary value may have increased because of a corresponding increase in prices.[3] A global picture of big producers is given in Fig. 14.3.

[1] According to WHO Tobacco Atlas, in 2000, tobacco farming was present in more than 125 countries and cultivated land measured over four million hectares.

[2] To have a global outlook, we propose in Appendix the data for 2010, 2000, and 1990 of FAO concerning hectares of land use, yield and tons produced, together with the rates of increase/decrease in the decades. Pay attention, because the rates of growth and decline, being calculated on specific years and not as averages, may reflect unusual high/low yields due to peculiar climate conditions.

[3] See Appendix.

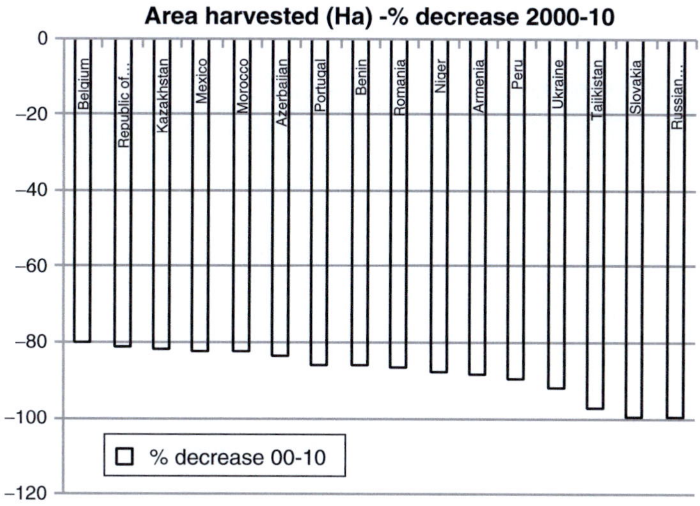

Fig. 14.1 The top increases in land used during last decade

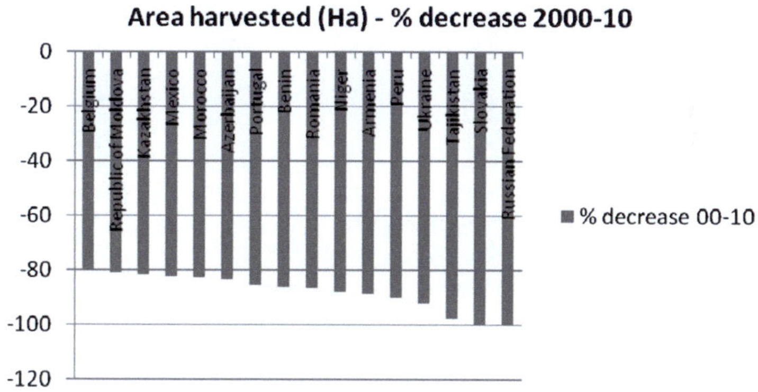

Fig. 14.2 The top decreases in land used during last decade

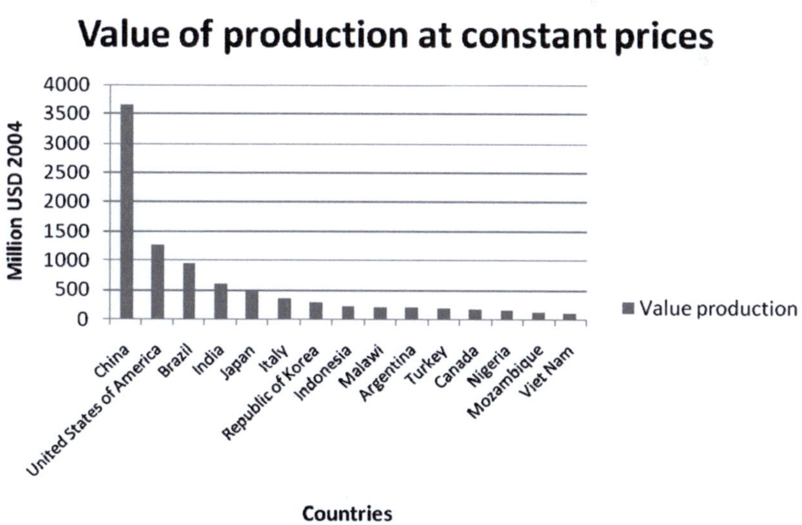

Fig. 14.3 Value of production at constant prices

Table 14.1 Global tobacco market Share: %share, by value, 2010

Company	% Share
China National Tobacco Corporation	36.1 %
Philip Morris International Inc.	14.2 %
Japan Tobacco Inc.	9.4 %
Others	40.3 %

Source: Datamonitor

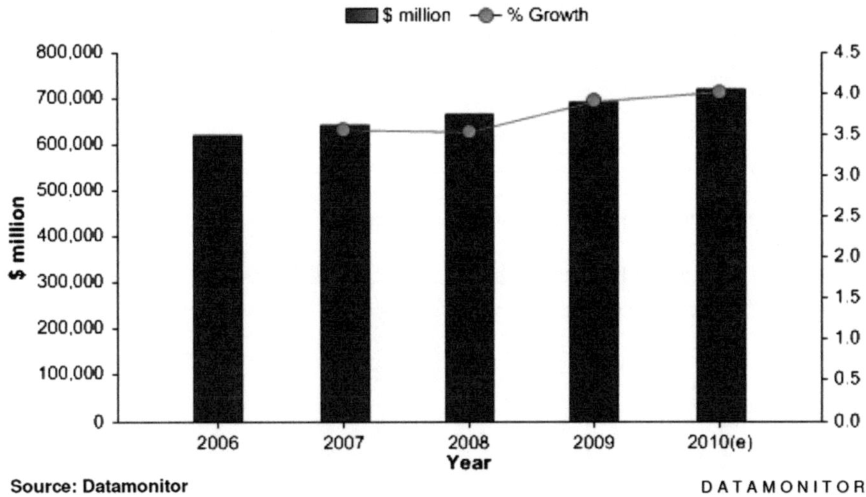

Fig. 14.4 Global tobacco market value ($ million, 2006–2010)

Production prices, where available, permit to analyze fully the side of production of leaves. We saw, for example, that Albania reduced steadily land use, production, and the real value of production: this decline was coupled with a corresponding increase in the price recognized to producers, so that their global revenue did not change dramatically. There are, nonetheless, specific countries in which the price conditions of producers deteriorated, such as in Spain. In any case, the rise of the new century brought about a nearly general price increase for producers, while at the end of the last century the evidence was more mixed. Among the big producers the farmers most advantaged by price increases can be found in Brazil and China.

We shall explore later on the pattern of trade. While the production of raw tobacco leaves is widespread, the manufacturing of tobacco is more concentrated among countries. China is the biggest player, followed by the USA and Japan (Table 14.1).

The tobacco market is made mainly of cigarettes, whose share was in 2010 about 94.5 %, followed by loose tobacco (2.5 %), chewing tobacco (1.7 %), and cigars/ cigarillos (1.3 %), and has faced no crisis at all in recent years. In fact, according to Datamonitor (2011), its global worth was in 2010 542,813.7 Millions of Euros and its annual compound growth rate during the period 2006–2010 has reached 3.8 %, with an increasing trend in latest years (Fig. 14.4).

14.1.2 The Costs of Production

The breakdown of costs of production of tobacco is a difficult job: it is heavily dependent on countries, methods of production and of curing leaves, tobacco qualities, manpower costs, and property of land. One of the tools that can be used is surveyed later on, namely the input–output approach, while other approaches are specific surveys: to give just an example of the latter, look at the study (CSO-Acop 2008) of a small producer the Republic of Mauritius. In 2005 the Tobacco-Amarello cost components were: intermediate costs 40.1 % (of which fertilizers 32.8 %, pesticides 19.5 %, fuel–lubricants 8.9 %, machines' rental 25 %, others 13.8 %), value added (wages, profits, and rents) 59.9 %. The Tobacco-Virginia quality had instead a different breakdown: intermediate costs 45.6 % (fuel–lubricants 53.9 %, fertilizers 15.8 %, rental of machines 13 %, pesticides 8.6 %, others 8.7 %), value added 54.4 %. The big difference in Fuel–lubricants usage is justified because, for the quality Virginia, diesel oil is used to cure tobacco leaves in the barn, while, for Amarello quality, curing of leaves is done in the open air.

Tobacco crops may or may not be a convenient business for farmers, due to a host of different factors such as price support, production quotas, monopoly and monopsony powers of manufacturers, and taxation. According to a study (Hu et al. 2006) looking at Chinese farmers, by far the biggest tobacco producers, in the counties of Sichouan and Guizhou, the 2002 revenues/cost ratio for Tobacco was, in the total sample made of about 1,003 farms, equal to 2.6, higher than that for Grain (2.5) but lower than that for beans (4.3), vegetable oil (3.7), and fruits (3.7).[4] In fact, tobacco farming is generally labor intensive while requiring suitable equipment to cure the leaves. The central question is then: why do farmers still go on in planting tobacco? Ruling out explanations such as custom and ignorance, soil characteristics that can explain only a minor portion of the choices, the two biggest possible explanations are: (1) price stability and (2) stability of demand (quantity). We detailed before that price increases for farmers were common feature since the beginning of the Century (China experienced such an increase) and that price decreases were rare: the reason can be found in the widespread monopolistic and monopsonistic power of big companies that prefer to buy at given prices rather than facing the risk of decreased farmers' production. The second point is interlinked with the first: the demand for cigarettes though attacked by tobacco control policies hardly faces big falls for prevalent smokers, and the increasing world population, assuming a decreased incidence, is still able to replace smokers lost for deaths or choices. The expected revenue for farmers growing tobacco is then not influenced by fluctuating prices and quantities: it is the low revenue–low risk asset in their portfolio.

[4] In the same study, it is reported that for Yunnan county of China (Jiang et al. 2004) the ratio was lower among all the crops, scoring only 0.99, compared to 4 for mulberry and silkworm, 2 for fruits, 1.99 for rice and wheat, and 1.7 for vegetable oil. For India (Chari 1992) the same may be true: the revenue-to-cost ratio was 4.01 for sunflower, 1.33 for mustard, and only 1.2 for flue-cured tobacco leaf. Finally, the already cited Acop study shows that, according to which cost definition is chosen, the price can cover costs or not (not fully covered are the imputed costs of family workers).

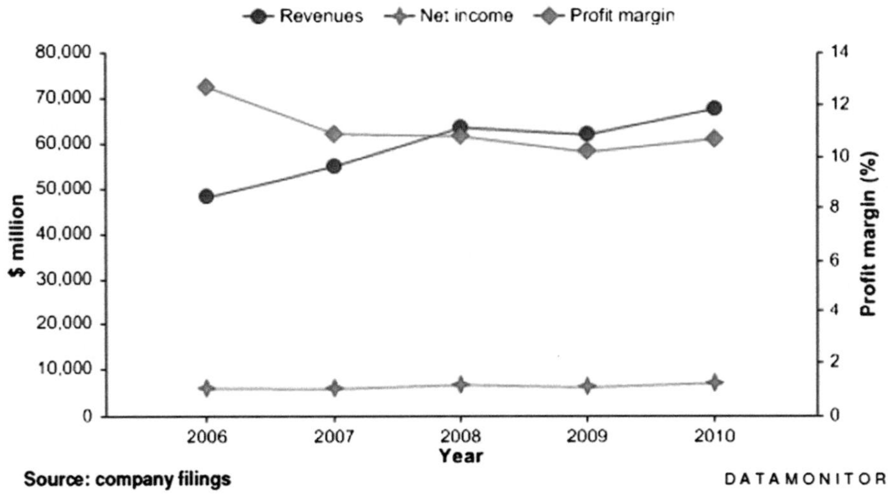

Fig. 14.5 Philis Morris International Inc: revenues and profitability

The manufacturing costs, revenue, and profits are sometimes difficult to assess, as is the case for the leading brand, that is a nationalized company from China and for other companies that do not disclose easily data. We know that the cost of cigarettes production (cost of goods sold COGS), according to Philips Morris International inc. 2012, can be split in the following components: (1) Tobacco Leaf (35 %), (2) Direct Materials (27 %), (3) Others (Conversion, fixed manufacturing expenses and other costs) (30 %), Shipping and Distribution (8 %). Revenues and the profit margin are remarkably stable during business cycles, as shown by Datamonitor graph (Fig. 14.5).

Moreover looking at shares' value of PM int.,[5] that significantly outperformed global S&P index, we can notice a fall in 2009, but by 2010 the pre-crisis value was regained and since then the price is continously rising. It is confirmed that Tobacco business is not sensitive to the cycle.

14.1.3 Tobacco Growing and Manufacturing External Effects

14.1.3.1 Negative: Deforestation, Chemical Pollution, Fires

One of the first effects that have been reported is the increasing deforestation, taking place mainly in developing countries because of tobacco growing and curing of leaves. In particular the flue-cured variety of tobacco Virginia, requires lot of wood

[5] The values, taken at the beginning of May are: 2008, 50.83; 2009, 36.28; 2010, 49.32; 2011, 69.81; 2012, 89.31.

Table 14.2 Proportion of deforestation (1999)

Country	Proportion (%)
Republic of Korea	45
Uruguay	41
Bangladesh	31
Malawi	26
Jordan	25
Pakistan	19
China, Syrian Arab Republic	18
Zimbabwe	16

for drying and curing leaves. Moreover barns construction requires poles and sticks from wood. In tropical countries, tobacco used as consumption good requires high nicotine content, obtained by practices (topping, desuckering) that heavily deplete soils and constrain to clear continously new land. Finally, paper for cigarettes involves use of wood.

Geist (1999) studies worldwide deforestation, by means of country-specific estimates of woodlands depleted because of needed woody biomass and wood consumption of tobacco and of secondary statistics on forest cover, deforestation, and population development, and concludes that about 200,000 ha of woodlands are removed by tobacco farming each year, that deforestation mainly occurs in the developing world (1.7 % of global net losses of forest cover) and that environmental criticality exists or is emerging in 35 countries (mainly in southern Africa, middle east, south and east Asia, South America, and the Caribbean).

According to Tobacco Atlas (2002), in 1999 the proportion of deforestation that in given countries was attributable to tobacco is illustrated in Table 14.2.

Land use shift from developed to low-income countries raises a question: which are the links between production efficiency, biodiversity, and resources management?

By studying a small-scale tobacco production in Tanzania, Sauer and Abdallah (2007) suggest that there could be a vicious circle between poor technology of production, often found in developing countries, deforestation, and loss of biodiversity. In fact, most power-driven equipments, fertilizers, and sustainable crop processing are beyond the reach of most small-scale growers, who need, in order to expand their production, to increase their use of wood, clearing an increasing amount of woodlands: the results of their study confirm that there is a positive association between efficiency, mainly in curing of leaves technology and in designing the barns and the source of firewood. Given the evident increasing returns to scale in production there is room to believe that an increase in agricultural production efficiency is conducive to environmental sustainability and maintenance of biodiversity. A similar link, between efficiency and sustainability of agriculture, is found for Turkey by Abay et al. (2004) that use the Data Envelopment Analysis (DEA) approach to study farms.

A related but different point of view looks at increased yields obtained in production, guessing that this can be done by increasing the use of fertilizers, pesticides, and increased technologies: according to this view increased production efficiency is bad for environment. In fact, many of the fertilizers and pesticides are highly toxic,[6] either for animals or for men, and the channels of transmission can be various (air, water).[7] The shift in production from advanced countries to low-income countries, where the efficacy of control on production is often low, may seriuosly damage such countries creating environmental problems.

Deforestation, of course, has a relevance also for climate change, in that depletion of forests reduces the power of land to absorb carbon dioxide and the burning of fires for curing leaves and for clearing lands adds carbon dioxide.

A quite different environmental issue is the disposal of butts. Filters are made of a plastic material, cellulose acetate, that is not biodegradable but is photodegradable: it takes up to 10 years to decompose and is toxic for aquatic organisms, pets, wildlife, and humans.

- Environmental problem derives from the huge number of butts and from their spatial concentration (Novotny and Zhao 1999). If the yearly number estimated of cigarettes smoked summing up to more than five trillion makes the butts disposal a serious pollution problem, their concentration makes the problem an emergency. On beaches and waterways they are the most important littering agent (Ocean Conservancy 2009). In cities there is usually a high concentration and a recent study of Marah and Novotny (2011) found that, inside the cities there is an important variability, with high-risk sites where cigarettes are sold or consumed showing a mean number of butts of 38.1, while low-risk sites have a concentration much lower (4.8) and that a model can be used to predict concentration, in order to estimate costs of clean up and strategies of removal. Costs of clean up are substantial: the city of San Francisco has estimated an annual cost of $7.4 million (Health Economics Consulting Group 2009). Companies have long feared of being deemed responsible for such littering and charged for the costs and have enacted strategies to mitigate their involvement (Harris 2011), such as developing biodegradable filters, distributing portable ash-trays to smokers, proposing antilittering campaigns: all attempts have failed because smokers do not like other filters and want to feel free to throw away butts (littering may even increase with biodegradable filters, Smith and Novotny 2011).

A final negative environmental effect is due to fires generated by lighted cigarettes, either outdoor or indoor. There is scattered evidence about both of them (ASH Fact Sheets 2009; Non-smokers Rights Association 2010):

- Vancouver Sun reports that 10 % of forest fires are due to unproperly extinguished cigarettes.
- A forest fire in China in 1987, caused by cigarettes, killed 300 people, caused 5,000 homeless, and destroyed 1.3 million hectares of land.

[6] Among them imidacloprid, chlorpyrifos, 1,3-dichloropropene, aldicarb, dithane DF, and methyl bromide.

[7] A review of adverse environmental effects of tobacco farming is found in Lecours et al. 2010.

- Estimates report that 17,000 people worldwide are killed annually by fires caused by cigarettes or cigarette lights: associated property damage is more than $27 billion.
- In Alberta, fires caused by smokers caused for 5 months in 2010 damages equal to $4.1 million.
- Health Canada, reporting data from 1995 to 1999 collected by the Canadian Association of Fire Chiefs, says that 14,030 fires were started by smokers' materials, that 356 people were killed and 1,615 injured, and that property damages amount to more than $200 million.
- Smokers' materials killed, in 2005 in UK, 110 people in homes (one-third of all deaths in domestic fires in the UK), and the average cost per fire in 2004 was £24,900.

14.1.3.2 Positive: Economy and Trade Activation

As we have shown, tobacco farming is an income stabilizing device for farmers, and cigarettes production is a business not affected by downturns. Given their remarkable stability, it is contended that they could be a structural source of support for other business: discouraging tobacco production and consumption could lead to serious crisis either for farms and countries/states living on that production or for business activated by tobacco production and sale.

The point is tricky: of course big companies' interest is in commissioning studies showing their contribution to the overall economy at either country/state or city level (employment, incomes, tax revenues), and in convincing general public that an attack to them is conducive to a loss for the whole society. The analytical problem is twofold.

First, the counterfactual has to be defined: it is in fact not correct to compare the "without" tobacco, with the "with" option; instead it has to be understood what could happen if the money withdrawn from tobacco industry is diverted to alternative productions. Some independent studies, analyzing the impact of policy-driven decline in tobacco consumption, are available for the USA. One of them, the Michigan REMI model (Warner and Fulton 1994; Warner et al. 1996), showed a mixed picture: (1) in a nontobacco producer (importer) State, such as the Michigan, accelerated decline in tobacco consumption may actually *increase* employment, by substituting consumption activating employment elsewhere with consumption activating employment inside the State; (2) in heavily tobacco-producing States, such as in the south-east, the decline in consumption would obviously lead to a decline in employment, but the amount of losses are often exaggerated (only 0.2 % employment loss). Also in other countries (Allen 1993; Buck et al. 1995) there is evidence that tobacco does not generate greater employment than alternative spending patterns.

Second, the methodology of defining the counterfactual can be either statistical, using also dynamic simulation models, or based on national accounts. The latter is mainly based on input–output tables, showing the pattern of activation of the economy. In the Appendix we report the US benchmark table for 2002 issued by the Bureau of Economic Analysis of the U.S. Department of Commerce: the industry/commodity

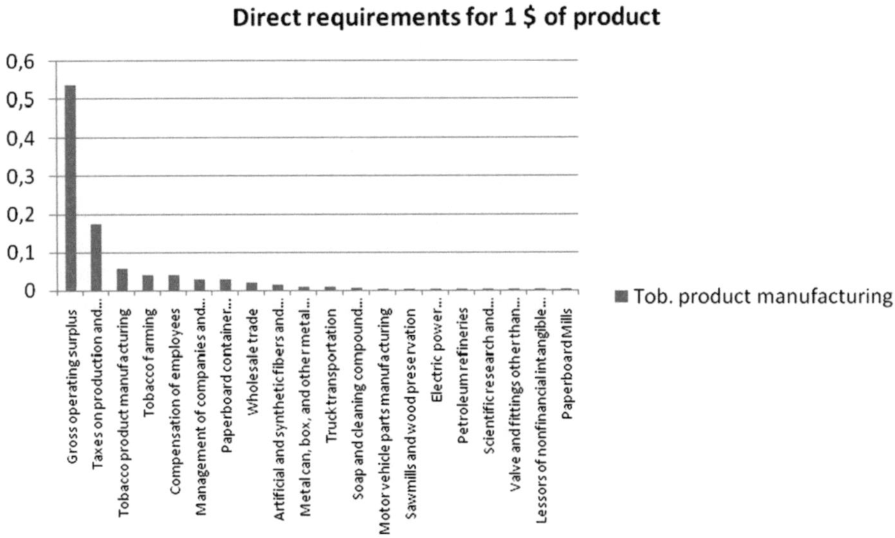

Fig. 14.6 Direct requirements for $1 of product for tobacco manufacturing

table contains the inputs that are used by the industries Tobacco Farming and Tobacco Products Manufacturing (reported in the columns); these inputs are coming from the commodities reported in the rows. The numbers represent the direct coefficients, namely the value at production prices of inputs coming from commodities and needed to produce $1 of product of each industry (all the coefficients sum to 1 by column). The final rows represent the labor compensation, taxation, and operating margin contents of tobacco farming and manufacturing: it can be seen that the operating margin is impressive in tobacco manufacturing (53 %) but is hardly noticeable in farming (0.2 %), while for labor income activation the inverse is true (farming 16 %, manufacturing about 4 %). Remarkable is also the high tax content of manufacturing (17 %).

The latter figure becomes of great interest, because it is a further line of defense used by tobacco companies: tax revenues coming from excises and ad valorem taxes on tobacco are a huge source of revenue for public sector and their reduction and/or replacement may seriously increase public deficit. We shall deal with it in the following paragraph.

We report in two graphs (Figs. 14.6 and 14.7) the main unit requirements for tobacco manufacturing and tobacco farming.

We see, for example, that for farming about 18 cents per dollar of product were spent for payments of land use, about 6 cents were spent for petrol, and 5 cents went in pesticides and other 2 in fertilizers.

For cigarettes production, instead, internal production costs accounted for more than 5 %, tobacco leaves costed <4 cents per dollar of production and that paperboard containers made <3 % of costs.

A more detailed analysis of the ability of production to activate the economy should derive multipliers based on direct and indirect requirements: it is beyond the

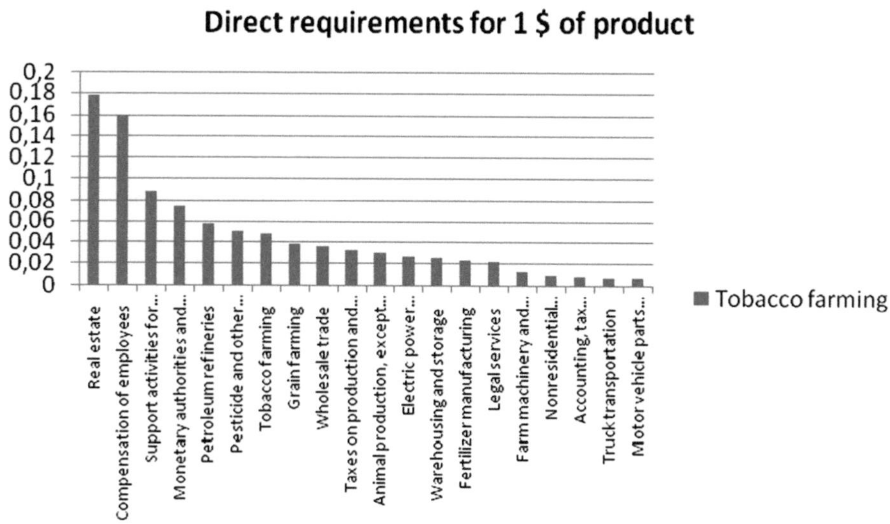

Fig. 14.7 Direct requirements for $1 of product for tobacco farming

scope of this chapter. What is evident is that cigarettes' production generates a huge profit margin, net of taxes, and that profits can heavily concentrate power in the hands of producers.

Two other issues deserve attention. The first is the companies' claim that an attack on tobacco farming can disrupt local communities dependent on tobacco. The answer is dependent on the Country/State: in advanced countries such as USA, local communities in high production States (North Carolina, Kentuky) have today a much more diversified pattern of production and can better face declines in production. According to Chaloupka and Warner (2000), for US tobacco belt: (1) From 1964 to 1993 the number of tobacco farms declined from 330,000 to 124,000, but their average acreage devoted to tobacco increased; (2) The value of domestically grown tobacco, adjusted for inflation declined; (3) For most farmers, tobacco growing is only a seasonal activity (two-third of them work outside the farm); (4) Most tobacco farms are small and the share of income from farming is declining; (5) Only 27 out of 424 tobacco counties are classified as "farm dependent," i.e., having at least 1/5 of counties earnings from farm earnings, and only one derived the majority of farm income from tobacco (4 had a share 25–35 % and 22 less than 5 %); (6) Calculated ratio of tobacco gross receipts to total proprietor and labor income within a county is in almost half of tobacco counties (199) <0.01 and only 33 counties have a ratio exceeding 0.1 (Gale 1998); (7) Finally, the index of capacity of substitution of tobacco income with income deriving from growth in other sectors is >1 in half of tobacco counties, meaning that growth in other sectors can fully compensate the decline in tobacco earnings. The conclusion is that tobacco farms in the USA are less dependent on tobacco today than before: realistic tobacco control policies would affect mildly local communities.

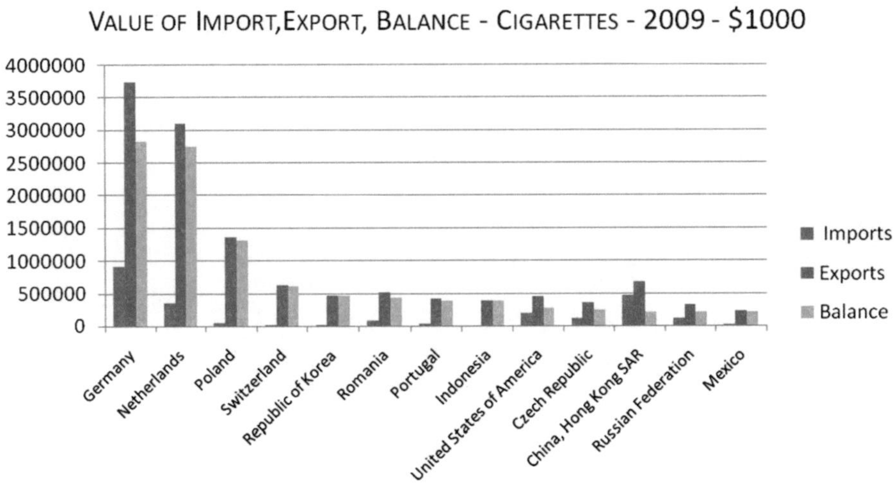

Fig. 14.8 The positive trade balance of the biggest net exporters of cigarettes in 2009

The second issue is the trade activation of tobacco business. In principle, tobacco trade is beneficial to the country only if the value of exports outweighs that of imports: this is true in just a few countries, such as Zimbabwe. Assume that tobacco leaves, as an input in cigarettes production, are, as reported by Philips Morris International inc., 35 % of the value: a developing Country producing leaves but not cigarettes would need to export 3 ton of leaves in order to be able to afford to import 1 ton of cigarettes, keeping its balance of trade in equilibrium. Data about trade flows both in quantity and in value are given by FAO, and value data, together with overall balance for 2009, are reported in the Appendix.

By looking at data some facts emerge, such as the nature of net importers of tobacco leaves and net exporters of cigarettes of three European countries: Germany, Netherland, and Poland. Vice versa a big trade deficit for cigarettes is experienced by Italy, Japan, France, and Spain: among these countries Italy is a net exporter of tobacco leaves, while Japan is also net importer of tobacco. Big tobacco producers not necessarily have big trade flows: this is the case of China that used to protect internal monopolistic cigarettes' company, while the reverse is true for Brazil that is by far the biggest net exporter of tobacco unmanufactured. Developed countries are often involved in big flows of trade, while developing countries more often are net importers with reduced flows: some exceptions are Malawi and Zimbabwe that get from net export of tobacco (and cigarettes for Zimbabwe) enough to finance other imports.

In Figs. 14.8 and 14.9 the trade balance of the biggest net exporters and net importerters of cigarettes in 2009 are reported.

The same can be done for the trade of unmanufactured tobacco (Figs. 14.10 and 14.11).

We see, for example, that Germany, which has the biggest positive value of the Balance of trade for cigarettes, has the second biggest deficit in the trade of unmanufactured tobacco.

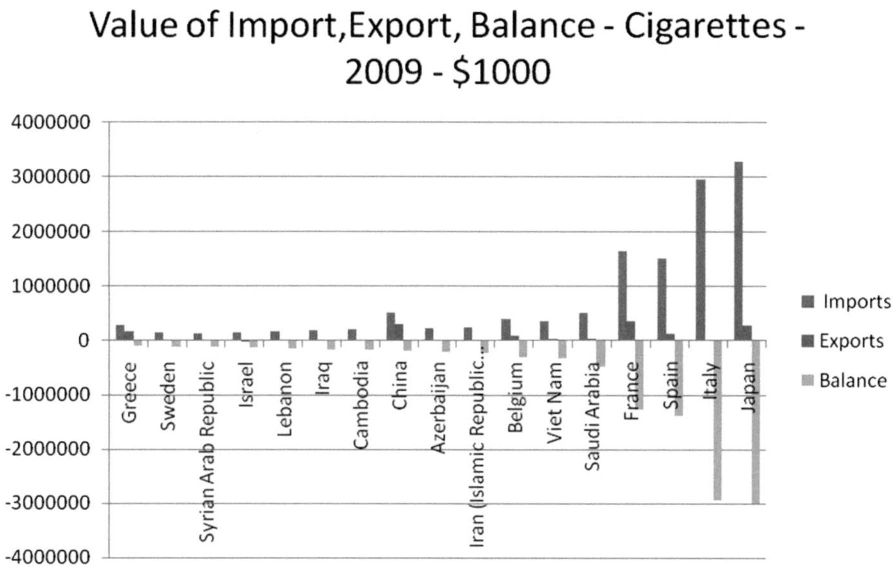

Fig. 14.9 The negative trade balance of the biggest net importers of cigarettes in 2009

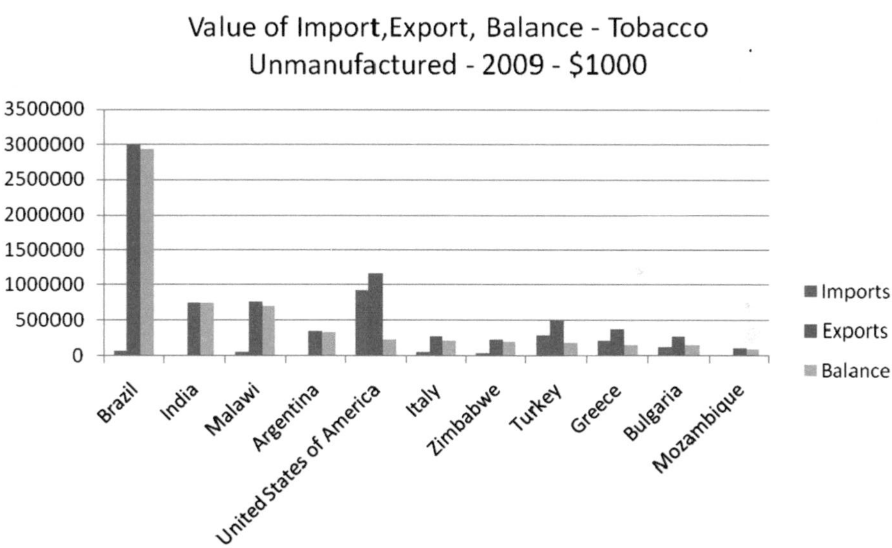

Fig. 14.10 The positive trade balance of the biggest net exporters of tobacco unmanufactured in 2009

A quite related point is that trade can be beneficial to a country, even if the balance is negative, because competition due to trade may induce changes in the quality of products. An example comes from China, which having the biggest internal market had, up to recently, protected her monopoly company and never struggled

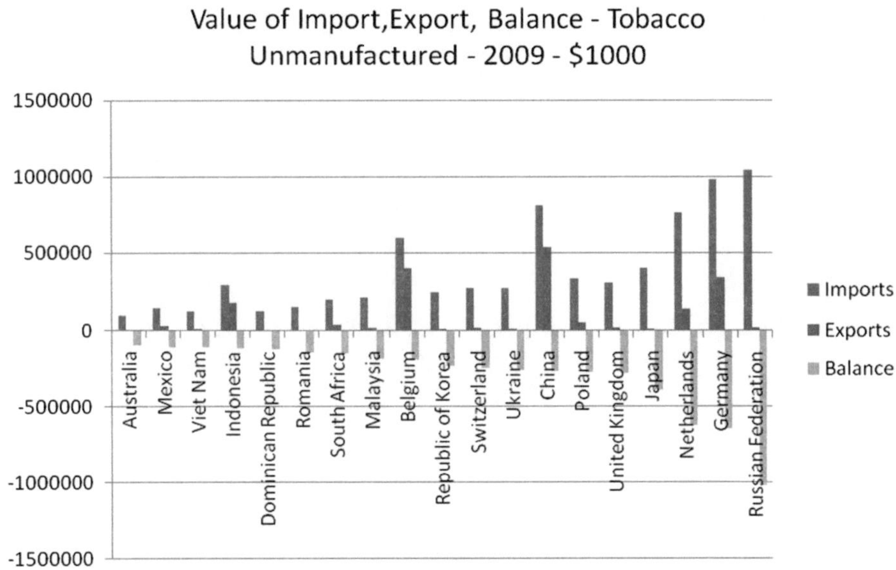

Fig. 14.11 The negative trade balance of the biggest net importers of tobacco unmanufactured in 2009

for gaining big shares of international trade, at the cost of low-quality cigarettes produced by the Chinese monopoly. Since the opening to trade, mainly induced by agreements forced by China entrance in WTO in 2001, the number of domestic brands has been reduced and the production process has been concentrated. More important for consumers, innovation in packaging and paper quality, imports of leaves of better quality from Zimbabwe, and the very same process of production, turning to low tar–low nicotine cigarettes, have taken place (Hu et al. 2006).[8]

14.1.4 Production Policies

Policies whose aim is to affect the extent of land used for tobacco growing and the amount of production may also affect prices of raw tobacco. In many countries agricultural production of tobacco is highly regulated: among the policies we find:

- Production quotas/Allotments: consisting in licenses to grow, which can or cannot be marketable. They are intended to protect farmers from overproduction and fall of prices.
- Price support: consisting in subsidizing prices of tobacco, in order to keep revenues for farmers adequate and stable.

[8] Though, as we see later, production may release nicotine in the environment, being polluting.

As an example, the US Price Support Program, abolished after 2004, fixed marketing quotas that were linked to the land, so that tobacco could be grown only by buying or renting lands which had a quota. The global amount of marketing quotas was estimated taking account of expected sales, of anticipated exports and imports (restricted by means of law on domestic content of tobacco in cigarettes sold in USA), of inventories of tobacco to be kept. Price support was guaranteed if at auctions for quantities not pre-sold (usually about 80 % was sold under contract) the price was below a minimum: a farmer's cooperative was mandated to buy tobacco at minimum price with money loaned by USDA—Commodity Credit Corporation (CCC), to store it, to resell later on (it could take years), and to repay with interests the loan received. Any loss of the program was initially refunded by taxpayer and after 1982, under the No Net Cost Tobacco Program Act, farmers and buyers had to make an assessment per pound of tobacco (in 2004 it was 10 cents for flue-cured tobacco) to cover any loss.

The net effects of the program were: (1) income stability for farmers, (2) restriction of tobacco supply, (3) restriction of farm size and more labor-intensive farming, (4) increase in the price of tobacco and of cigarettes, (5) reduction of export flows of leaves, and (6) creation of a political lobby of allotment holders.

The main results of Price Support Program were two:

- Keeping tobacco prices sufficiently high led to increases in prices of cigarettes and had a favorable effect of *reducing* consumption. The effect was nonetheless modest, because a 20–30 % increase in tobacco price, given the small (<10 %) cost component of tobacco in cigarettes, raised prices of cigarettes of 1–3 % according to estimates, and given a reduced elasticity of demand, had a final impact of reduction of cigarettes use of <0.5–1 %.
- Allocating rights to grow tobacco created highly concentrated interests, which had a negative effect on smoking, because lobby opposed laws against smoke.

Such interventions, altering the functioning of the market, are very debated: some contend that allowing production to increase and prices to decrease can lead to more use of domestic tobacco by cigarettes' producers and to more export, improving farmers' incomes.

14.2 Selling Strategies and Demand of Tobacco Products

14.2.1 Models of Demand for Tobacco Products

The economic theory has long debated the issue of the nature of demand for tobacco products: is addiction a rational choice or rather addiction stems from a partial or full myopic/irrational choice? The three leading dimensions in this field are: tolerance, reinforcement, and withdrawal. The first implies gradual rather than immediate adaptation of addictive consumption to changes of relevant variables such as prices, the second the positive effect on utility of habits that have been acquired in the past, and the third the irreversibility of choices because to abandon consumption is often too costly. We shall debate the issues in a very synthetic way.[9]

14.2.2 Imperfectly Rational Addiction Models

This group of models postulates that there is a chronic incoherence between short-term and long-term preferences of individuals: this inconsistency is nonetheless stable in time. Long-term preferences are assumed to be rational, implying a desire of individuals of quitting smoking, because of the adverse health consequences. Short-term preferences, instead, look at the pleasure that can be gained instantly by smoking, implying irrationality: individuals throw away, for a bit of enjoyment and underscoring of the risk of addiction, the long-term happiness they have planned and are willing to construct. These models, very difficult to put to empirical validation, anticipate the creation of (anti)-markets, either individually or institutionally operated, aimed to help individuals to quit smoking.

14.2.3 Myopic Rational Addiction Models

Individuals, according to this kind of models, look at current consumption as fully determined by past consumption habits but fail to understand that current consumption is determining, setting new habits, future consumption. This theory, initially used to explain the downward rigidity of consumption in years of economic crisis, has been successfully applied to cigarettes consumption, though addiction is a bit downgraded, becoming a simple "habit." Preferences are then endogenous in these models, allowing tastes to change over time and can be seen as influenced by the stock of past consumption, or by other adjustment mechanisms. The empirical validation of this group of models is more easy, because it requires either that the data confirm the dependence of current cigarette consumption on past consumption, that is setting the "habits," or that there is an asymmetric response of demand to price increases and decreases.

14.2.4 Rational Addiction

The models of rational addiction are based on a rational choice with interdependence between past, present, and future: they postulate that future consequences of today's behavior are not discounted at an infinite rate, so that they have no value today

[9] For a good synthesis look at Chaloupka and Warner 2000.

(as in a myopic choice), but at a positive, though high, rate. Individuals maximize a life-cycle utility, taking account of today and tomorrow's prices and tomorrow's consequences of their choices. In the basic model of Becker and Murphy (1988) current utility depends on current addictive consumption, current nonaddictive consumption, and the stock of past addictive consumption. Tolerance is represented by the negative marginal utility of addictive stock; reinforcement by the fact that increases in addictive stock raises the utility of current addictive consumption while withdrawal postulates that the cessation of addictive consumption is associated with a fall in total utility. Adding to the basic model the assumption of "adjacent complementarity," i.e., the fact that, due to reinforcement, the quantities of goods with addiction consumed in different periods are linked by a complementarity relationship, the model predicts that the long-run effect on consumption of any price change is greater than the short-run effect, and that this difference is greater for more addicted individuals. Moreover price responsiveness is greater for: anticipated price changes, permanent price changes, and higher time preference, implying that younger, less educated, lower income individuals are more responsive to price changes. The model predicts also unstable long-run equilibrium, explaining binge behavior of addicted, and predicts that temporary events such as price reductions, peer pressure, or stressful events may generate addiction.

Empirical evidence seems to confirm, by and large, the validity of the model (younger and less educated people behave more myopically and are more responsive to price changes); nonetheless the model is unable, implying rational choice and perfect foresight, to deal with a common trait of addicted individuals, the "regret" for their choices perceived as wrong. This could be due to the imperfect knowledge of the individuals about their specific reaction to addictive consumption (this could only be guessed looking at others): once addicted, they regret to have started believing to be able to resist to addiction. Moreover as "adjacent complementarity" implies a cost of effort for quitting smoking, individuals say they want to quit but continue to smoke or use nicotine patch that reduces quitting effort. If the model is corrected, assuming only bounded rationality, with choice limited to current consumption, the model predicts that age is often sufficient for quitting and that for heavily addicted individuals sudden quit is required but for lightly addicted individuals, a gradual consumption decrease and quit is more likely.

14.2.5 Behavioral Models

These models, sprung from economic psychology, and are mainly experimental, studying the reactions of already addicted individuals to constructed prices, where prices are intended as the physical effort necessary to gain a dose of the needed drug. For example, price could be represented by the number of complete pulls and reset of a plunger needed to receive a puff of cigarette or two, or by money gained from pulls, etc. These models confirm that smoking is inversely related to prices, and that price elasticity rises with prices.

14.2.6 Policy Issues: Prices, Taxation, and Incentives

The empirical assessment of price elasticity of demand for cigarettes has been at the core of research: results are extremely variable, and can be so summarized:

- Own price elasticity is low but different from zero, so that increases in price can reduce demand. According to Chaloupka and Warner (2000) and Chaloupka et al. (2012) the range of variation is from –0.14 to –1.23, but in most studies the average value is comprised in the –0.25/–0.5 range with a cluster around –0.4.
- Elasticity diminishes with age,[10] is bigger for men, for poor, for black, and for hispanic, and is lower for rich and educated.[11]
- Elasticity may be higher in low-income and middle-income countries than in developed. For China the estimate by Hu et al. (2006) is in the range –0.35/–0.66.
- Elasticities are usually higher if estimated on individuals, taken from cross-sectional data, than on longitudinal/aggregate data.
- Elasticity is usually greater in the long run than in the short run, because of the addictive nature of consumption.
- The money price is just one component of the full price that includes time costs, cost to face restrictions (smoking outside), law bans infraction costs, etc.
- Other factors, such as incomes (cigarettes seem to have changed in nature in recent years, being no longer a normal good and becoming an inferior good, whose consumption declines with rising incomes), advertising, and tastes, may affect consumption.
- Cross-price elasticities with other tobacco products are usually positive, pointing to a substitutability among tobacco products (substitution of hand-rolled cigarettes with bought cigarettes).

Taxation of tobacco products, by raising prices to consumers, is seen by economists as the most suitable way of discouraging consumption and has been for this reason extensively studied. The main issues regarding taxation are:

- Types of taxation
- Full or partial transfer of taxes on prices
- Taxation across countries and smuggling
- Tax revenues
- The effectiveness to public health purposes and the support of citizens
- The fairness of taxation.

Three types of taxes are used for tobacco and cigarettes: excise taxes, ad valorem taxes, and import/export duties. Excises, being taxes of a fixed amount and levied

---

[10] According to Kostova et al. 2011, the elasticity for young estimated with a two part model is very high: *the estimated price elasticity of smoking participation is −0.74, and the estimated price elasticity of conditional cigarette demand is approximately −1.37. The total price elasticity of cigarette demand is −2.11 implying that an increase in price of 10% would reduce youth cigarette consumption by 21.1% at the mean.*

[11] For a different view, see Tenn et al. 2010.

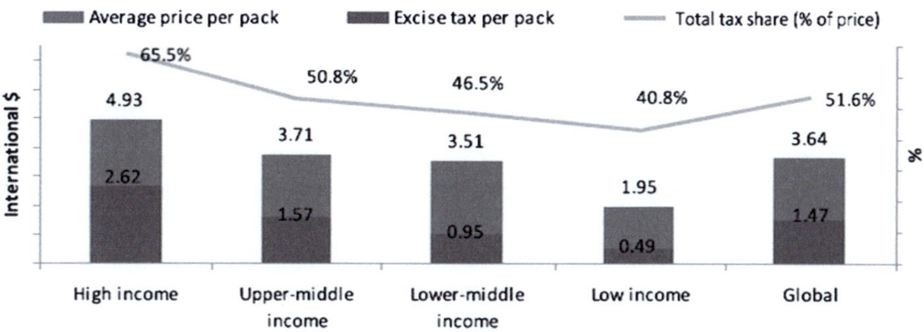

Fig. 14.12 Simple average price, excise tax per pack and total tax share of the most sold brand, by income group (International Dollars)

either on quantity (specific excises) or on values (ad valorem excises), can be structured in different ways: given amount per number of cigarettes, such as per pack of 20; amount levied on the weight of tobacco content of cigarette/pack; different amounts of taxes according to the tar/nicotine content of cigarettes, filtered or nonfiltered, price, scale of production, and cigarettes' length; and amounts given as a percentage of factory/retail price of cigarettes. Ad valorem taxes are in general a percentage of the value of the pack, and include Value added taxes and Sales taxes. Finally Import/Export duties are levied in different ways: over imported cigarettes, in order to protect internal producers and/or to raise public revenues and over exports, mainly to obtain revenues. Tobacco leaves are also taxed, with taxes on the value of tobacco crops and import/export duties. Tax revenues obtained by cigarettes can be targeted: this was the case in Norway, Finland, and other countries, where taxes were used for tobacco-related education, for counter-advertising, and for other health-related activities, and in Australia and New Zealand that created public institutions to promote health and to sponsor events instead of big tobacco companies. At present, about 90 % of Countries adopt excise taxes for cigarettes, almost so ad valorem taxes, and nearly 100 % use import duties.

Excise taxes are nearly completely transferred on prices: there is moreover a direct relationship between the amount of excises levied and the level of prices and the average income of the Country. The amount of excise and other taxes in the final price of cigarettes ranges from 65.5 % for advanced countries to 40.8 % in low-income countries and average price ranges from about $5 in PPP for high-income countries to about $2 in PPP in low-income countries (Chaloupka et al. 2012). We report a graph (Fig. 14.12) of the above authors that summarizes the tax content of cigarettes' price.

The most effective tax form, if our goal is to raise prices, in order to discourage consumption, is a specific, uniform excise tax of a relevant amount (about 70 % of final price). Care should be given to anchor the amount of tax to inflation, otherwise its value declines in real terms and as a share of final price, permitting to the companies to keep prices relatively stable with respect to other competing goods, increasing the competitiveness of cigarettes and leading to increases in consumption. If instead excises are raised, there is not certainty that prices will raise accordingly:

in fact companies that act in an oligopolistic environment, may decide either to collude, and increase prices more than taxes, if demand is sufficiently anelastic or to share tax increases with consumers, increasing prices less than taxes if demand is scarce or quite elastic. The behavior of companies is crucial in another respect: though price increases have shown their efficacy in reducing smoking initiation, in favoring smoke cessation by smokers and in reducing the amount smoked by addicted, companies by keeping prices below profit-maximizing levels, may hook new customers and once they are addicted they can raise prices, or they can prefer to exploit now already addicted smokers with inelastic demand by rising strongly prices and loosing, according to the rational addiction model, potential new smokers.

Things are more difficult if excises are ad valorem, or different for different types of product. In principle, from a harm-reducing point of view, a reduced taxation of products that reduce risks for smokers is deserving, but it may be difficult to implement because of the reduced scientific evidence on qualities necessary to be selected as a harm-reducing product. What is certain is that, with differential tax rates vast substitution effects may appear. A quite common effect is evident when excises are higher for high-price cigarettes and lower for low-price products: a shift from the former to the latter, mainly for poor appears when excises are increased.[12] Other examples are decisions to levy less taxes on small producers, in order to protect them from big tobacco companies (Indonesia), or to do the same for specific tobacco products such as Bidis in India, or to reduce excises according to oriental tabacco content of cigarettes, in order to protect domestic growers of oriental tabacco in Turkey.

As a further example of tax differentiation, leading or not to consumption effects according to the behavior of companies, can be cited the excises at State level in the USA. Such taxes, dishomogeneous (unlike federal taxes) in the amounts, are often compensated by companies, by means of cross-subsidization among States, in order to keep prices equal across States, avoiding cross-border shopping by consumers.

This leads to third issue regarding taxes, taxation across Countries and smuggling. Due to combined effects of excises, ad valorem taxes and import duties, in some Countries taxation is up to 80 % of final price, while in others is far lower. This incentivate smuggling and tax evasion, favored by globalization and ease of transport and circulation of goods and by lack of strong contrast because it is considered a minor risk with respect to drug traffic.[13] Smuggling has a long tradition in low-income countries and in geographically strategic countries such as Italy and is encouraged by tobacco companies, aiming to show that taxes are not effective in reducing consumption. Because of illicit nature of smuggling, few studies are available: they point to the direction of flows from low to high price countries and confirm that in high tax Countries a significant share of sales comes from smuggling.

[12] This reflects, as we shall see later on, a concern for other goals, sometimes pushed by specific groups of interest, different from public health or public revenue raising, equity being the official motivation for such differentiation.

[13] Following Joossens and Raw (2012) smuggling is changing in nature: the issue is shifting from pure smuggling to: "*illegal manufacturing, including counterfeiting and the emergence of new cigarette brands, produced in a rather open manner at well known locations, which are only or mainly intended for the illegal market of another country.*"

A natural experiment is available for Canada, that in the years 80–90 increased taxes, shifting from ad valorem to excises, and from 1994 on experienced smuggling, before nearly absent, in a specific way: as Canadians like the taste of their cigarettes, they were first exported tax free to the USA and then smuggled back to Canada (Chaloupka and Warner 2000).

A huge and stable tax revenue is coming from tobacco products taxation. Nonetheless companies oppose increases in taxation claiming that they would be mostly ineffective because elasticities are bigger than measured and that tax evasion and smuggling can subtract public revenues. The evidence is contrary, pointing to a nominal increase in revenues, even if other tobacco control policies are effective in furtherly curbing demand: as an example, in California, before 1989, excises were 10 cents and overall revenues about $250 millions; after three increases in excise taxes (1989 up to 35 cents, 1994 up to 37 cents and 1999 up to 87 cents) in 2000 revenues become $845 million, tripling with respect to 1988 and this coupled with a decrease in sales of more than 60 % (Chaloupka et al. 2012). A related issue is the extent and effectiveness of the targeting of revenues from tobacco products to tobacco control policies and education campaigns. The extent is up to now reduced: though 38 Countries earmark at least some resources to specific health programs few of them devote to tobacco control policies more than negligible resources (among them California and Thailand). The effectiveness is instead proven (Chaloupka et al. 2012): moreover targeting, though in a paternalistic way, resources subtracted to smokers to campaign that reduce their addiction improving their health is in line with the benefit principle of taxation.

The effectiveness of taxation to public health purposes is discussed in studies that try to project the short and long-run effects of increased taxation on reduced illnesses and related costs of care and of reduced mortality on income production, consumption and costs of care.[14] Such studies show that quite substantial increases in taxation are needed both to face all the direct and indirect individual and societal costs of smoking—such as direct costs of health care, indirect costs due to loss of current production and less future production due to premature deaths,[15] external costs imposed on others (environmental smoke), intangible costs of pain and sufferance for victims and their families—and to discourage youth from starting smoking. Quite delicate measurement issues are at stake such as the use of the prevalence (current burden of smoke) or the incidence (intervention that interrupt smoking illnesses and future tobacco related costs) approach, the elasticities of demand considered, the range of costs included.[16] As examples, Chaloupka (1998) study estimate that an increase of $1.5 in US taxes and prices of cigarettes would reduce consumption of 30 %, drop the

---

[14] All the issues about the costs of smoking are dealt with in the paragraph about costs of smoking and caring for smoking related illnesses.

[15] Though other researchers add to these costs the advantages of less healthcare consumption and less social security benefits paid due to earlier death.

[16] Often overlooked are the issues of costs on child of mother's smoke (low-birth weight children), of intangible costs, of costs of cigarettes' ignited fires, of environmental smoke, of smoke as a complicance for other illnesses, of industry costs for smoking-related maintenance, of increased laundering and hygiene consumption of individuals, and of the costs of butts disposal.

prevalence of young smokers of a half and prevent 2.5 million deaths, while an econometric study by Moore (1996) postulates that an increase of 10 % of excise taxes in the USA would save about 5,200 lives each year. A related point is the construction, on pure efficiency grounds, of an optimal tax on smoke that equates, at the margin, revenues generated to external costs produced by smoking: the main methodological point here is if and when Environmental tobacco smoke (ETS) can be considered as an external effect,[17] and about the rationality of the choice of smoking, with the inclusion of youth ignorance as a justification for choices that are regretted in adulthood.[18]

The final point does not look at efficiency of taxation but at fairness of taxation itself. Taxation hardly involves horizontal equity issues (unequal treatment of identical individuals) but has straightforward vertical equity implications: being the consumption of cigarettes more important among lower income people, they are also more damaged by taxation, implying regressivity of taxes on tobacco. Regressivity is partially mitigated because (1) rich usually buy more expensive products: if excises are ad valorem or if other ad valorem taxation is important the amount paid by rich could be similar to that paid by poor; (2) poor have higher elasticity of demand (closer to 1) than rich (closer to 0), and taxes reduce more the consumption of poor so that tax burden falling on poor is reduced; (3) if the above point is true and if reduced consumption is good in itself, taxation improves poor situation more than that of rich; (4) if taxes are earmarked to tobacco control policies or feeded back to poor because of health services are targeted to them a further positive effect is added; (5) if price increases generated by taxation affect income tax brackets, poor may receive more benefits and pay less income taxes, reversing regressivity. Nonetheless, if, according to the benefit principle, we believe that excise taxes have the nature of "user fees" that individuals have to pay for their future healthcare costs, the counterargument is that such future costs are not certain, individuals can give up smoking before any adverse health consequence is experienced, and future costs have to be heavily discounted.[19]

14.2.7 Advertising

Cigarettes are one of the most heavily advertised product in the world. Though in many countries explicit advertising in media is banned, tobacco companies found the way to heavily advertise products at the point of sale (POS). The shift from traditional forms of advertising to "innovative" ways is evident for USA: from 87 % of traditional promotion/advertising in 1986 to 10 % in 1996 (Chaloupka and Warner 2000). According to Ribisl (2011), reporting data of FTC out of $12.49 billion of advertising expenditure for USA in 2006 about 85.8 % were spent in POS.

[17] The discussion is centered on the "internal" nature of families such that mother's smoke affecting child cannot be considered an external effect.

[18] Viscusi (2003) harshly criticize the imperfect rationality approach, claiming that consumers are well informed and often *overestimate* the true risks due to smoking.

[19] If the above counterargument is accepted current smokers pay for health care of other smokers, implying a forced solidarity. See also Viscusi (2003).

The most common forms of advertising are:

- Price discounts: Are paid to retailers or wholesalers in order to reduce prices to consumers, and include off-invoice discounts, buy downs, voluntary price reductions, and trade programs. It is by far the most relevant advertising activity.
- Promotional allowances to retailers/wholesalers: Payments made to retailers or wholesalers to facilitate the sale or placement of own products (volume rebates, incentive payments, payments for stocking, shelving, displaying and merchandasing).
- POS advertising/promotion: Posted in retail outlets.
- Direct mail advertising: When promotion, without sample distribution, is sent directly to consumers.
- Internet advertising: Either on proprietary Website or on sites different from company Web pages.
- Free samples: Distribution either of products for direct consumer testing or evaluation, or distribution of coupons for free tobacco products.
- Coupons: Customers can obtain reductions in prices of tobacco goods and coupons are redeemed at the point-of-sale or by mail (a payment is associated to their use).
- Specialty items distribution: Distribution of items different from cigarettes (sunglasses, key chains, calendars, sporting goods, T-shirts, caps, and other clothing) either reporting the logo, name, part of the package of a brand (branded), or not (unbranded).
- Retail value-added bonus cigarettes/non cigarettes: Promotions involving free tobacco products (ex. buy two get one more free).
- Endorsements and testimonials: All expenditures made to procure tobacco use (mention/representation of a product/company),in any situation (motions,…) in which this may come to the public's attention.
- Sponsorships: Mainly sponsoring of sport and sporting events.
- Public entertainment events: Events in which the name or logo or an image of a tobacco product is referred or displayed.
- Newspaper/magazines.
- Outdoor advertising: mainly billboard.
- All other forms: Radio–television advertising, audiovisual, advertising by telephone, on public/private transports, etc.

The breakdown of US expenditures for 2005, taken from Davis et al. (2008) is illustrated in Table 14.3.

Other forms of advertising comprise indirect advertising, used when partial or total bans are in place, and consisting in sharing the brand name with nontobacco products such as the lance of another line of products (clothes), called with the name of the brand to publicize. Moreover, packaging is one of the best ways to attract consumer's attention and is not considered as advertising. Finally, last frontier of advertising is "viral advertising": "It is described as the situation in which 'the advertiser creates an environment in which the idea can replicate and spread. It's the virus that does the work, not the marketer.'… Examples might include paying teens to talk to their friends about a product or to infiltrate a chat room, commissioning

Table 14.3 Cigarette advertising and Expenditures in promotional activities (USA, 2005, millions of dollars)

Advertising medium/promotinoal activity[a]	Expenditures Unadjusted ($)	Adjusted ($)[b]	Percentage of total expenditures[c]
Newspapers	1.6	1.7	–
Magazines	44.8	46.2	–
Outdoor	9.8	10.1	–
Transit	0.0	0.0	–
Point of sale	182.2	188.1	1.4
Price discounts	9,776.1	10,091.5	74.6
Promotional allowances—retail	435.8	449.9	3.3
Promotional allowances—wholesalers	410.3	423.5	3.1
Promotional allowances—other	1.5	1.5	–
Sampling distriution	17.2	17.8	–
Specialty item distribution–branded	5.3	5.5	–
Speciality item distribution—nonbranded	225.3	232.6	1.7
Public entertainment—adult only	214.1	221.0	1.6
Public entertainment—general audience	0.15	0.2	–
Sponsorships	30.6	31.6	–
Direct mail	51.8	53.5	–
Endorsements and testimonials	0.0	0.0	–
Coupons	870.1	898.2	6.6
Retail value added—bonus cigarettes	725.0	748.4	5.5
Retail value added—noncigarette bonus	7.5	7.7	–
Company Website	2.7	2.8	–
Internet—other	0.0	0.0	–
Telephone	0.06	0.1	–
Other[d]	99.0	102.2	1.0
Total	13,111.0	13,533.9	100.0

[a] Definitions have been previously given
[b] Adjusted to 2006 dollars, using the consumer price index (all items)
[c] Figures are rounded to the nearest percentage point
[d] Expenditures for audiovisual are included in the "other" category to avoid disclosure of individual company data
"_" indicates values less than 1 %

footpath graffiti, or creating Websites or sponsoring events that support a product but without overt brand imagery." (Davis et al. 2008).

The economics of advertising focuses on the critical issue: does advertising increase youth smoking, or it simply affects companies' market share?

The main claim of companies that advertising is a powerful tool in shifting consumption across brands is confirmed, and youth seem to be more influenced and more prone to shift.

The direct ways in which advertising could increase consumption are:

- Suggesting to experiment, directed to children and young adults (hooking them).
- Reducing smokers' willingness to quit.
- Stimulating current smokers to increase daily consumption.
- Inducing former smokers to resume smoking habits.

The indirect ways are:

- Media dependent on tobacco advertising are silent on adverse health consequences.[20]
- Advertising' contribution to social environment perceiving smoke as socially acceptable.
- Institutions dependent on tobacco support create political opposition to tobacco control.

The first strand of evidence, that we do not summarize, is of sociological character, and is based mainly on experimental studies on the relationship between advertising and (1) the identification of adolescent needs such as peer acceptance, rebelliousness, risk-taking, and stress relief and (2) adolescents' self-images and their perceptions of smokers.

The conclusiveness of the results of econometric studies, based either on cross-sectional data or on longitudinal data, is influenced by the difficulty of the task: the main methodological point, if we want to judge the elasticity of consumption to advertising exposure, is how to measure "exposure": (1) absolute level of cigarette advertising or ratio of cigarettes' advertising to total advertising, (2) external measures or self-reported exposure, and (3) attitudes, belief on advertising or on its effects. Moreover endogeneity issues in cigarettes advertising are raised,[21] a "stock" effect, due to cumulative effect of advertising, could emerge, studies may fail to distinguish advertising from promotion effects, and there could be an omitted variable bias (if we disregard, for example, counteradvertising or social attitudes).

With respect to increased consumption we have evidence that[22]:

- Youth watching more television, and exposed more to advertising in television, increase their tobacco consumption.
- Youth exposure to magazine, in-store, and direct mail advertising is conducive to experimenting more smoking.
- Lagged cigarettes advertising has positive but small (and probably declining in time) impact on consumption. This confirms that longitudinal studies, in which today's consumption is influenced by past advertising are more powerful than cross-sectional studies in detecting causality effects.[23]

An indirect proof of the efficacy of advertising comes from the analysis of the effects of bans to advertising on smoking. Cross-country evidence gives support to

---

[20] There is evidence that magazine's coverage of smoking hazards is inversely linked to the share of advertising revenue coming from cigarettes (Warner 1985).

[21] Those who smoke or are interested in smoking pay more attention to advertising and are more influenced by advertising.

[22] For a survey of results see: Davis et al. 2008; see also Slater et al. 2007.

[23] Longitudinal studies are not without drawbacks, such as the failure to take account of individuals dropped from the sample, that can be non-randomly distributed between smokers and nonsmokers, and the possibility of spurious effects due to omitted variables influencing both advertising and consumption.

the effect of reduction of smoking if there is a ban (complete bans can reduce consumption of about 6 %): the main methodological point is that advertising restrictions and social–cultural differences can be correlated, so that conclusions are not reliable because of multicollinearity. Ex post evidence after bans in given countries is mixed and the possible contemporary decline in antismoking campaigns, because of fairness argument, can muddle interpretation of results. In Germany, for example (Anger et al. 2011), after bans of 2007–2008, the average smoking behavior of the population did not change, but a segment of population, composed by individuals that go out more often to bars and restaurants, became less likely to smoke and smoked less.

14.2.8 Market Diversification and Emerging Markets

As demand for cigarettes is declining in advanced countries and increasing in low-income countries, companies need to adapt to changing environment. This can be bone by diversifying products, in order to meet requirements of both mature markets and emerging markets.

We already spoke of another kind of product diversification, used as a marketing strategy, by launching clothing and other product that share the brand name and are used as an advertising device. In the same line is the diversification of production in other branches. According to Kumar et al. (2005), the Indian Tobacco Company (ITC) has transformed itself from a leading cigarette manufacturer to an umbrella group that offers a diversified product mix (hotels, confectionery and biscuits, information technology) to enhance its brand image (marketing itself as a company taking seriously its social responsibility) and reduce dependency on tobacco related products (though it still earns 80 % of revenues from selling cigarettes and other tobacco-related products).

In advanced markets, facing bans and restrictions imposed on cigarettes, companies are following two distinct strands. The first, probably intended as a pure marketing strategy to improve the respectability of companies, is the unlikely quest for a "safe cigarette." Some companies studied cigarettes that heat but do not burn tobacco, including products such as Reynolds' Eclipse and Philip Morris' Accord cigarettes. Other products contain modified tobacco that had been grown partially eliminating dangerous chemical components. The second, apparently contrasting their business, consists in an entire line of products overtly targeted to the minority of smokers (about 3 % in the USA) that each year try to give up smoking: nicotine gum and patches or aerosol-based nicotine: according to Aguinaga Bialous and Peeters 2012 "tobacco companies seem to be reframing their business as maintaining nicotine addiction through other products."

Price diversification is a practice that is common and is eased by what illustrated on tax components of prices: in high-income countries the tax component being higher leads to higher prices while in low-income countries the reduced tax component permits to keep prices low and to gain consumers among low-income people.

Table 14.4 Major segments, brands and advertising campaign in Mumbai, India

Segment/brand	Advertisment description	Advertised in higher/lower SES area	Present in print
Super premium			
ITC Insignia Cost Rs. 100 for 20	"Where quality touches infinity," "redefine perfection"	Higher	*India Today, Business Today*
Premium			
ITC Wills Classic/Mild Filter: King 70–74 mm. Cost Rs. 60 for 20	"Discover a passion"	Higher	None
ITC Wills, Novy Cut Filter: <70 mm. Cost Rs. 46 for 20	"Made for each other"	Higher	None
ITC Wills Silk Cut Filter: Actech. Cost Rs. 46 for 20	"A blend so right a filter so fine"	Higher	None
ITC Gold Floke/Lights Filter: Regular 68 mm. Cost: Rs. 24 for 20	"It's Honeydew Smooth," "Smooth, exquisite, timeless. But then, all art is"	Higher and Lower	*The Week, Business India, India Today, Filmfore*
GPI Four Square Filter: Regular. 68 mm Cost: Rs. 24 for 20 Bingo[a]	"Man with the smooth edge"	Higher and Lower	*Outlook, Filmfare*
ITC Bristol	"Rise to the taste"	Higher and Lower	None
GPI Red and White. Cost Rs. 14.50 for 10	Text in Hindi "Hum red and white peene walon ki baat hi kuch aur hai"	Higher and Lower	Stardust film magazine
VST Charms	"The taste that sets you free"	Lower	
GTC Platinum. Cost: Rs. 17.50 for 10	"Smoother than gold" Launched in 4/03	None	*Mumbai Mid Day insert*

US$1 = approximately Rs. 45

GPI Godfrey Philips India, Ltd, *GTC* Golden Tobacco Company, *ITC* Indian Tobacco Company, *VST* Vazir Sultan Tobacco Company

[a]Smaller plain segment cigarettes that compete in the bidi (hand rolled cigarettes) segment

More interesting is price and quality segmentation. The cigarette market is highly segmented, including at least three big segments: high price, medium price, and low price cigarettes. The high price is limited to a minority of smokers, but it is a high yield segment for companies: it includes upper premium and premium quality cigarettes. The others have wider diffusion but guarantee lower unit margins to companies. There is no geographical concentration of high-quality tobacco leaf in advanced countries, though in some big markets such as China the quality of tobacco is often poor. The marketing strategies are quite distinct for each segment. We report a table from Bansal et al. (2005). The segmentation targets different socioeconomic groups in Mumbai[24] (Table 14.4).

[24]In India low-income segment usually consumes other products, such as Bidi.

In low-income countries, moreover, low-quality high-tar, high-nicotine cigarettes, banned elsewere, are still sold, because of low prices and lack of regulations.

The final issue is globalization of production, involving both concentration of owners in order to better compete on the global market and delocalization of factories, from historical sites in advanced countries to cheaper offshore destinations. Concentration of property has witnessed a speedup in the new Century: mergers and acquisition are both part of the strategy; as an example of the first, the most important have been the mergers between BAT an Rothmans in 1999 and BAT's owned Brown and Williamson and Reynolds Tobacco Holding on the US market; among the acquisitions can be cited Japan Tobacco International's acquisition of Gallaher in 2007 and Imperial Tobacco's acquisition of Reemtsma in 2002 and of Altadis and Commonwealth in 2007, (Aguinaga Bialous and Peeters 2012)

Offshoring of factories was the case, for example, for British American Tobacco (BAT) who closed partially or completely factories in UK and activated new productions in Korea and Singapore. This creates first of all resistances because of job losses in origin countries. The balance is not always positive for destination countries: companies often exploit loopholes in regulations and controls in less advanced countries to locate there productions highly polluting such as the low-nicotine cigarettes. Moreover, being the projections of consumption growth pointing to the faster increase or lower decrease in medium–low income countries, the strategic location of factories in such countries may permit to lower transport costs and may gain more approval by local policy-makers and general public: this, in turn, can allow a more soft tobacco control attitude. The only constraint is to take account of riskiness of countries: Philip Morris int. for example chose to locate production mainly in center and South America and in Eastern and Southern Europe, with a plant in Africa and a few others in Asia.

14.3 Caring for Smoking-Related Illnesses

It is well recognized that tobacco consumption is the leading cause of preventable deaths in the majority of high-income nations and increasingly in low- and middle-income nations (Jha and Chaloupka 1999), and that it causes disability and productivity losses because of premature deaths (Office of the Surgeon General (US) and Office on Smoking and Health (US) 2004). Economic damages caused by smoking account for $200 billion and are based on the costs to treat tobacco-related illnesses and the indirect costs associated with disability (American Heart Association 2001).

One way to document and assess the adverse health effects of smoking on the societal level is to translate smoking-caused illnesses, premature mortality, and productivity losses into economic terms (Sung et al. 2006).

The economic burden of smoking comprises three main components:

- Direct medical costs of treating smoking-related diseases.
- Indirect morbidity costs of smoking.
- Indirect mortality costs of premature deaths caused by smoking related diseases.

The first component is mainly concerning with the costs sustained by the healthcare system for treating smoking-related illnesses, while the other two refer to a societal perspective.

Net costs of smoking in a lifetime perspective and, hence, the economic interests in antismoking policies have been questioned. It has been proposed that the health-related costs of smoking are balanced by smaller expenditure due to shorter life expectancy. In this perspective Barendregt et al. (1997) reported that, if people stopped smoking, there would be savings in healthcare costs, but only in the short term. Eventually, smoking cessation would lead to increased healthcare costs, because of the reduced mortality due to smoking cessation, which would create new possibilities for morbidity from other diseases in the years of life gained. Rasmussen et al. (2004) replied to this theory by affirming that the study by Barendregt did not include indirect costs related to smoking, i.e., value of lost productivity.

Here some general data concerning healthcare costs attributable to smoking are reported.

Every year in United States (USA) 443,000 deaths are estimated as a result of cigarette smoking and exposure to second-hand smoke. These deaths result in terms of costs for the nation approximately $97 billion in lost productivity and $96 billion in healthcare costs (CDC 2008, 2010).

A study carried out by Zhang et al. (1999) showed that in the USA in 1993, smoking-related diseases accounted for 9.4 % of Medicare expenditures—$14.2 billion, with considerable variation among States. Smoking-related illnesses accounted for 11.4 % of Medicare expenditures for hospital care, 11.3 % of nursing home care, 5.9 % of home health care, and 5.6 % of ambulatory care.

A successive review of all published studies on the medical costs of smoking in the USA reported that in 1999 at least 6–8 % of annual personal health expenditures, and quite possibly considerably more, were devoted to treating diseases caused by smoking. In particular this percentage represents a solid estimate of expenditures directly related to the three most important smoking-related diseases: lung cancer, heart disease, and chronic obstructive pulmonary disease (COPD) (Warner et al. 1999).

In a recent cross-sectional study smoking has been showed to be a very significant predictor of higer medical costs: compared with never smokers current smokers had 16 %, former smokers had 15 % and recent former smokes had 32 % higher median costs (Bland et al. 2009).

In United Kingdom (UK) the cost of smoking to the NHS, as a proportion of the total NHS budget, has not changed substantially since the early 1990s. In particular, as reported in a systematic review by Allender et al., in 2005 the estimated number of deaths attributable to smoking was 109164 (19 % of all deaths), smoking was directly responsible for 12 % of disability-adjusted life years lost (DALYL) in 2002, and the direct cost to the NHS was £5.2 billion in 2005–2006 (Allender et al. 2009).

In Taiwan in 2001, 191,313 years of life expectancy lost (YLEL) were attributable to major smoking-related diseases, with an average of about 3.6 YLEL per patient (Chung et al. 2007).

According to Sung et al., in 2000 the economic costs of smoking in China amounted to $25.43 per smoker (> age 35) and $5.0 billion (measured in 2000, US$)

in total, of which direct costs were $1.7 billion (34 % of the total), indirect morbidity costs were $0.4 billion (8 %), and indirect mortality costs were $2.9 billion (58 %). The direct costs of smoking accounted for 3.1 % of China's national health expenditures in 2000 (Sung et al. 2006).

Here an overview of scientific literature available about smoking-related illnesses economic costs is given (Table 14.5).

Rice et al. examined the direct and indirect costs of smoking in the USA in 1984 using a prevalence-based approach (i.e., they examined the current annual costs of past smoking practices). They focused on neoplasms and diseases of the circulatory and respiratory system and recognized that, even in smokers, only a portion of these illnesses can be attributed to smoking. Using a human capital approach to calculate the value of lost productivity, they concluded that the total economic costs of smoking were $38.6 billion; direct medical costs accounted for $14.4 billion (37 %), morbidity costs for $7.46 billion (19 %), and mortality costs for $16.8 billion (44 %). That is, smoking was associated with a large net cost to society (Rice et al. 1986; Goodwin and Shepherd 1998).

Moreover, Zaher et al. (2004) conducted an evaluation of the literature published from 1992 to 2000 in order to more specifically assess the burden of COPD produced by smoking. The economic US smoking attributable costs were $26.0 billion coronary heart disease (CHD), $24.9 billion COPD, and $9.0 billion stroke; more specifically the hospitalizations were 520,000 COPD, 460,000 CHD, and 183,000 stroke.

Kahende et al. (2007) examined the 1996–2001 period cost of treating the major smoking-related diseases in the USA too. The researchers found that expenditures were higher for all illnesses in the first year; ischemic heart disease was the main cause of medical expenditure for both 1-year ($263 million) and 2-year ($152 million), followed by COPD, cerebrovascular disease, and lung cancer.

A study realized in Taiwan by Chung et al. (2007) showed that in 2001 in all, COPD, strokes, oral cancer, and lung cancer in males accounted for about 68 % of the total YLEL and for about 81 % of the total lifetime medical costs. The COPD alone accounted for 16.7 % of the total YLEL and 42.4 % of the total lifetime medical costs, essentially as a result of its high incidence rate relative to other diseases.

Ross et al. (2007) reported that in 2005 the total costs of smoking-attributable inpatient health care reached at least 1,161,829 million Vietnamese dollars ($VN) (or $US 77.5 million). In particular the healthcare expenditure related to COPD treatment accounts for $VN 1,033,541 million (or $US 68.9 million) per year, followed by lung cancer ($VN 78,143 million, or $US5.2 million per year) and ischemic disease ($VN 50,145 million, or $US 3.3 million per year).

Leartsakulpanitch et al. (2007) estimated the direct out-of-pocket medical costs of treating major diseases attributable to smoking in Thailand in 2006. The number of cases attributable to smoking in 2006 was 5,299 for lung cancer, 624,309 for COPD, and 52,605 for CHD. The out-of-pocket expenditures for treatment were 368.49 million baht for lung cancer, 7,714.88 million baht for COPD, and 1,773.65 million baht for CHD. Total smoking-attributable out-of-pocket medical costs amounted to 9,857.02 million baht, 0.48 % of gross domestic product (GDP) in 2006.

Table 14.5 Smoking-related illnesses economic costs

Author	Year	Country	Setting	Main results
Rice et al.	1986	USA	1984 direct and indirect costs of smoking	The total economic costs of smoking accounted for $38.6 billion. In particular, the direct medical costs accounted for $14.4 billion (37 %), the morbidity costs for $7.46 billion (19 %) and the mortality costs for $16.8 billion (44 %)
Zaher et al.	2004	USA	1992–2000 economic US smoking attributable costs	The economic US smoking attributable costs amounted to $26.0 billion CHD, $24.9 billion COPD and $9.0 billion stroke
Kahende et al.	2007	USA	1996–2001 cost of treating the major smoking-related diseases	Expenditures were higher for all illnesses in the first year; ischemic heart disease was the main cause of medical expenditure for both 1 year ($263 million) and 2 year ($152 million), followed by COPD, cerebrovascular disease and lung cancer
Chung et al.	2007	Taiwan	2001 YLEL and lifetime medical costs related to COPD, strokes, oral cancer and lung cancer in males	COPD, strokes, oral cancer and lung cancer in males accounted for about 68 % of the total YLEL and for about 81 % of the total lifetime medical costs. The COPD alone accounted for 16.7 % of the total YLEL and 42.4 % of the total lifetime medical costs
Ross et al.	2007	Vietnam	2005 total costs of smoking-attributable inpatient health care	The total costs of smoking-attributable inpatient health care reached at least 1161829 million Vietnamese dollars ($VN) (or $US 77.5 million). In particular the healthcare expenditure related to COPD treatment accounted for $VN 1033541 million (or $US 68.9 million) per year, followed by lung cancer ($VN 78143 million, or $US5.2 million per year) and ischemic disease ($VN 50145 million, or $US 3.3 million per year)
Leartsakulpanitch et al.	2007	Thailand	2006 direct out-of-pocket medical costs of treating major diseases attributable to smoking	The out-of-pocket expenditures for treatment were 368.49 million baht (7.607 million €, currency 31-12-2005 of Banca d'Italia) for lung cancer, 7,714.88 million baht (159.267 million €) for COPD, and 1,773.65 million baht (36.615 million €) for CHD. Total smoking-attributable out-of-pocket medical costs amounted to 9,857.02 million baht (203.861 million €), 0.48 % of gross domestic product (GDP) in 2006
Sgambato et al.	1997	Italy	1997 costs related to hospitalization and lost work days due to smoking related illnesses.	The overall hospital costs were 2.016 billion lire (1.041 billion €s). The disease mainly impacting on the overall resources allocated to hospital treatment of smoking related illnesses was ischemic heart disease (treatment cost of more than 557 billion lire). At national level, the total putative direct costs amounted to 2.504 billion lire (1.293 billion €). The working days lost because of smoking were quantified as amounting to 1.333.588. The overall loss of productivity due to smoking was assessed in 51.9 billion lire, and the diseases most affecting it were ischemic heart disease (6.9 billion lire) and cerebrovascular disease (6.2 billion lire)

CHD coronary heart disease, *COPD* chronic obstructive pulmonary disease, *YLEL* total years of life expectancy lost

Box 14.1 Comparisons of Black and White Smoking Attributable Mortality

During 2000–2004 in Missouri, smoking caused 9,600 deaths, 132,000 Years of Potential Life Lost (YPLL), $2.4 billion in productivity losses, and $2.2 billion in smoking-related healthcare expenditures annually. A difference was also detected for races: black smokers had smoking-attributable YPLL 18 % higher than whites ones (Kayani et al. 2007). A similar outcome has been investigated by Rivo et al. (Rivo et al. 1989) concerning the racial differences in Columbia: of the estimated 3535 YPLL directly due to smoking 66 % were accounted for by black men, 25 % by black women, 7 % by white men, and 2 % by white women, with a great disproportion in smoking-attributable mortality between black residents, especially black men, and white residents.

An Italian study performed by Sgambato et al. estimated the 1997 total costs (medical and social) due to smoking-related illnesses. Costs related to hospitalization and lost work days were quantified. The overall hospital costs were 2.016 billion lire (1.041 billion €). The disease mainly impacting on the overall resources allocated to hospital treatment of smoking related illnesses was ischemic heart disease with a treatment cost of more than 557 billion lire. At national level, the total putative direct costs amounted to 2.504 billion lire (1.293 billion €). The working days lost because of smoking were quantified as amounting to 1.333.588. The overall loss of productivity due to smoking was assessed in 51.9 billion lire, and the diseases most affecting it were ischemic heart disease (6.9 billion lire) and cerebrovascular disease (6.2 billion lire) (Sgambato et al. 2001).

Smoking places tremendous financial and health burdens upon both society and individuals.

Treatment for smoking-related diseases is expensive and preventing these diseases could provide immediate short-term financial returns. Additionally, tobacco treatments programs could produce substantial saving in the long term, along with health and quality of life benefits (Kahende et al. 2007) (Box 14.1).

References

Abay, C., Miran, B., & Gunden, C. (2004). An analysis of input use efficiency in tobacco production with respect to sustainability: The case study of Turkey. *Journal of Sustainable Agriculture, 24*(3), 123–126.

Aguinaga Bialous, S., & Peeters, S. (2012). A brief overview of the tobacco industry in the last 20 years. *Tobacco Control, 21*, 92–94.

Allen, R. C. (1993). *The false dilemma: The impact of tobacco control policy on employment in Canada*. Ottawa, ON: National Campaign for Action on Tobacco.

Allender, S., Balakrishnan, R., Scarborough, P., et al. (2009). The burden of smoking-related ill health in the UK. *Tobacco Control, 18*(4), 262–267.

American Heart Association. (2001). *International cardiovascular disease statistics: Biostatistical fact sheets*. Dallas, TX: American Heart Association.

Anger, S., Kvasnicka, M., & Siedler, T. (2011). One last puff? Public smoking bans and smoking behavior. *Journal of Health Economics, 30*, 591–601.

ASH Fact Sheets. (2009). *Tobacco and the environment*. Retrieved from http://www.ash.org.uk/files/documents/ASH_127.pdf

Bansal, R., John, S., & Ling, P. (2005). Cigarette advertising in Mumbai, India: Targeting different socioeconomic groups, women and youth. *Tobacco Control, 14*, 201–206.

Barendregt, J. J., Bonneux, L., & van der Maas, P. J. (1997). The health care costs of smoking. *The New England Journal of Medicine, 337*(15), 1052–1057.

Becker, G. S., & Murphy, K. M. (1988). A theory of rational addiction. *Journal of Political Economy, 96*(4), 675–700.

Bland, P. C., An, L., Foldes, S. S., et al. (2009). Modifiable health behaviors and short-term medical costs among health plan members. *American Journal of Health Promotion, 23*(4), 265–273.

Buck, D., Godfrey, C., Raw, M., & Sutton, M. (1995). *Tobacco and jobs*. York, England: Society for the Study of Addiction and the Centre for Health Economics, University of York.

CDC. (2008). Smoking-attributable mortality, years of potential life lost, and productivity losses-United States, 2000–2004. *Morbidity and Mortality Weekly Report, 57*, 1226–1228.

Centers for Disease Control and Prevention. (2010). Racial disparities in smoking-attributable mortality and years of potential life lost—Missouri, 2003–2007. *Morbidity and Mortality Weekly Report, 59*(46), 1518–1522.

Central Statistic Office. (2008). *Agricultural cost of production survey 2005 (Acop)*. Republic of Mauritius, Ministry of Finance and Economic Development.

Chaloupka, F. (1998). *The impact of proposed cigarette price increases (Policy analysis No. 9), Health Sciences Analysis Project*. Washington: Advocacy Institute.

Chaloupka, F., & Warner, K. (2000). The economics of smoking. In A. Culyer & J. Newhouse (Eds.), *Handbook of health economics*. Elsevier: Netherlands.

Chaloupka, F., Yurekli, A., & Fong, G. (2012). Tobacco taxes as a tobacco control strategy. *Tobacco Control, 21*, 172–180.

Chung, C. W., Wang, J. D., Yu, C. F., et al. (2007). Lifetime medical expenditure and life expectancy lost attributable to smoking through major smoking related diseases in Taiwan. *Tobacco Control, 16*, 394–399.

Datamonitor. (2011). *Global tobacco*. Retrieved from http://www.datamonitor.com

Davis, R., Gilpin, E., et al. (Eds.). (2008). *The role of the media in promoting and reducing tobacco use*. Washington, DC: National Cancer Institute (US Dep of Health).

Gale, F. (1998). *Economic structure of tobacco-growing regions. Tobacco situation and outlook* (pp. 40–47). U.S. Department of Agriculture, Economic Research Service, TBS-241.

Geist, H. (1999). Global assessment of deforestation related to tobacco farming. *Tobacco Control, 8*, 18–28.

Goodwin, P., & Shepherd, F. A. (1998). Economic issues in lung cancer: A review. *Journal of Clinical Oncology, 16*, 3900–3912.

Harris, B. (2011). The intractable cigarette 'filter problem'. *Tobacco Control, 20*(Suppl. I), i10–i16.

Health Economics Consulting Group. (2009). *Cost of tobacco litter in San Francisco*. Health Economics Consulting Group. Retrieved from http://www.sfenvironment.org/our_programs/program_info.html?ssi=3

Hu, T., Mao, Z., Ong, M., et al. (2006). China at the crossroad: The economics of tobacco and health. *Tobacco Control, 15*(Suppl I), i37–i41.

Jha, P., & Chaloupka, F. J. (1999). *Curbing the epidemic: Governments and the economics of tobacco control*. Washington, DC: World Bank.

Jiang, H., Mao, Z., & Hu, T. W. (2004). An analysis of costs and revenue of tobacco leaf production. *Rural Economy (in Chinese), 6*, 46–48.

Joossens, L., & Raw, M. (2012). From cigarette smuggling to illicit tobacco trade. *Tobacco Control, 21*, 230–234.

Kahende, J. W., Woollery, T. A., & Lee, C. W. (2007). Assessing medical expenditures on 4 smoking-related diseases, 1996–2001. *American Journal of Health Behavior, 31*(6), 602–611.
Kayani, N., Yun, S., & Zhu, B. P. (2007). The health and economic burden of smoking in Missouri, 2000–2004. *Missouri Medicine, 104*, 265–269.
Kostova, D., Ross, H., Bleker, E., & Markovitz, S. (2011). Is youth smoking responsive to cigarette price? Evidence from low- and middle-income countries. *Tobacco Control, 20*, 419–424.
Kumar, K., & Dilipan, A., et al. *ITC: The Indian Tobacco major's diversification strategies for market leadership*. Retrieved from http://www.ibscdc.org/Case_Studies/Strategy/Diversification%20 Strategies/DIS0006.htm
Leartsakulpanitch, J., Nganthavee, W., & Salole, E. (2007). The economic burden of smoking-related disease in Thailand: A prevalence-based analysis. *Journal of the Medical Association of Thailand, 90*(9), 1925–1929.
Lecours, N., Almeida, G., Abdallah, J., & Novotny, T. (2010). Environmental health impacts of tobacco farming: A review of the literature. *Tobacco Control, 21*, 191–196.
MacKay, J., & Eriksen, M. (2002). *The tobacco atlas*. Geneva: WHO.
Marah, M., & Novotny, T. (2011). Geographic patterns of cigarette butt waste in the urban environment. *Tobacco Control, 20*(Suppl. I), i42–i44.
Moore, M. J. (1996). Death and tobacco taxes. *The RAND Journal of Economics, 27*(2), 415–428.
Non-smokers Rights Association. (2010). *The tobacco industry's negative impact on environment*. Retrieved from http://www.nsra-adnf.ca/cms/file/pdf/factsheet.pdf
Novotny, T., & Zhao, F. (1999). Consumption and production waste: Another externality of tobacco use. *Tobacco Control, 8*, 75–80.
Ocean Conservancy. (2009). *Guide to marine debris and the international coastal cleanup*. Retrieved from http://www.oceanconservancy.org/site/DocServer/ICCmarineDebrisGuideReadOnly.pdf?docID=5441
Office of the Surgeon General (US) and Office on Smoking and Health (US). (2004). *The health consequences of smoking: A report of the Surgeon General*. Atlanta (GA): Centers for Disease Control and Prevention (US). Retrieved from http://www.ncbi.nlm.nih.gov/books/NBK44695/
Philip Morris International Inc. (2012). *The cost breakdown of making cigarettes*. Presentation to Investors.
Rasmussen, S. R., Prescott, E., Søresen, T. I. A., et al. (2004). The total lifetime costs of smoking. *European Journal of Public Health, 14*, 95–100.
Ribisl, K. (2011, Febrauary). *Combating price discounting for tobacco products: Background an strategies*. Presentation to California Tobacco Control Regional Forum, San José CA.
Rice, D. P., Hodgson, T. A., Sinsheimer, P., et al. (1986). The economic costs of the health effects of smoking 1984. *The Milbank Quarterly, 64*, 489–547.
Rivo, M. L., Kofie, V., Schwartz, E., et al. (1989). Comparisons of black and white smoking attributable mortality, morbidity, and economic costs in the District of Columbia. *Journal of the National Medical Association, 11*, 1125–1130.
Ross, H., Trung, D. V., & Phu, V. X. (2007). The costs of smoking in Vietnam: The case of inpatient care. *Tobacco Control, 16*, 405–409.
Sauer, J., & Abdallah, J. (2007). Forest diversity, tobacco production and resource management in Tanzania. *Forest Policy and Economics, 9*, 421–439.
Sgambato, A., Cicchetti, A., Papa, A., et al. (2001, November). Analysis of economic and social impact of smoking related illnesses in Italy. *Osservatorio sul Tabacco*. Accessed May, 2012, from http://www.focuseventi.it/archivio/Atti/documenti_fumo_2011.pdf
Slater, S., Chaloupka, F., et al. (2007). The impact of retail cigarette marketing practice on youth smoking uptake. *Archives of Pediatrics and Adolescent Medicine, 161*, 440–445.
Smith, E., & Novotny, T. (2011). Whose butt is it? Tobacco industry research about smokers and cigarette butt waste. *Tobacco Control, 20*(Suppl. I), i2–i9.
Sung, H. Y., Wang, L., Jin, S., et al. (2006). Economic burden of smoking in China, 2000. *Tobacco Control, 15*(Suppl I), 5–11.
Tenn, S., Herman, D., & Wendling, B. (2010). The role of education in the production of health: An empirical analysis of smoking behavior. *Journal of Health Economics, 29*, 404–417.

Viscusi, W. K. The new cigarette paternalism. *Regulation 2002–2003*, 58–64.
Warner, K. E. (1985). Cigarette advertising and media coverage of smoking and health. *The New England Journal of Medicine, 312*, 384–388.
Warner, K. E., & Fulton, G. A. (1994). The economic implications of tobacco product sales in a nontobacco state. *Journal of the American Medical Association, 271*(10), 771–776.
Warner, K. E., Fulton, G. A., Nicolas, P., & Grimes, D. R. (1996). Employment implications of declining tobacco product sales for the regional economies of the United States. *Journal of the American Medical Association, 275*, 1241–1246.
Warner, E., Hodgson, T. A., & Carroll, C. E. (1999). Medical costs of smoking in the United States: Estimates, their validity, and their implications. *Tobacco Control, 8*, 290–300.
Zaher, C., Halbert, R., Dubois, R., et al. (2004). Smoking-related diseases: The importance of COPD. *The International Journal of Tuberculosis and Lung Disease, 8*(12), 1423–1428.
Zhang, X., Miller, L., Max, W., et al. (1999). Cost of smoking to the medicare program, 1993. *Health Care Financing Review, 20*(4), 179–196.

ERRATUM

Smoking Prevention and Cessation

Giuseppe La Torre

G. La Torre, *Smoking Prevention and Cessation*, DOI: 10.1007/978-1-4614-7046-5,

---

DOI 10.1007/978-1-4614-7046-5_15

The publisher regrets that in the print and online versions of this book the Foreword and the Preface was omitted from the Frontmatter. Included on the following pages are the Foreword and the Preface.

The online version of the book can be bound at http://dx.doi.org/10.1007/978-1-4614-7046-5

Foreword

With 650,000 estimated deaths in Europe and 443,000 in the USA, smoking is by far the leading cause of death in the population of developed countries. Furthermore, the global burden of cancer is expected to grow due to dramatic increases in smoking habits in less developed countries (Oppeltz and Jatoi 2011), thereby producing large disparities in cancer-related mortality rates in different geographical areas (Kanavos 2006).

As extensively discussed in this volume, smoking is associated with a variety of chronic degenerative diseases, and the fraction of deaths attributable to smoking has been estimated to be around 30% for all cancers, 85–90% for lung cancer, 50–70% for aerodigestive tract cancers, in synergism with alcohol, 75–80% for chronic obstructive pulmonary diseases (COPD), such as emphysema and chronic bronchitis, and 30% for cardiovascular and cerebrovascular diseases, in synergy with other risk factors (De Flora and Bartsch 2012). In particular, according to the International Agency for Research on Cancer (IARC), there is evidence for a causal association of CS with cancers affecting (a) the respiratory system (nasal cavity and paranasal sinuses; nasopharynx, oropharynx, and hypopharynx; larynx and lung), (b) the urinary tract (kidney pelvis, ureter, and bladder), (c) the digestive system (oral cavity, oesophagus, stomach, colon-rectum, liver, and pancreas), (d) the reproductive tract (ovary and uterine cervix), and (e) the hematopoietic system (myeloid leukemia) (International Agency for Research on Cancer 2012).

Understanding the mechanisms of action of tobacco smoke is difficult because combustion of tobacco leaves generates more than 5,000 identified chemical compounds, 73 of which have been evaluated by IARC to be carcinogenic in humans and/or experimental animals (Hecht 2012). Accordingly, multiple mechanisms are expected to contribute to the carcinogenicity of this complex mixture. These mechanisms are nowadays investigated in depth, also by exploring molecular end-points at the level of DNA (genome), microRNA (miRNome), gene expression (transcriptome), and protein expression (proteome) (De Flora and Bartsch 2012; Izzotti et al. 2009).

The obvious approach to the prevention of smoking-related diseases is to refrain from smoking, to quit smoking, and to avoid passive exposures to environmental tobacco smoke. Epidemiological studies have demonstrated, on a large scale, that a decrease in the consumption of cigarettes is successful in attenuating the epidemic of lung cancer in the population of several countries (De Flora et al. 2005). Chemoprevention by means of dietary and/or pharmacological agents provides a complementary strategy, which finds specific targets in addicted current smokers who are unable to quit smoking and especially in ex-smokers and involuntary smokers.

The present volume is a compendium that embraces a number of issues related to smoking cessation and prevention of smoking-related diseases. It gives a global vision of smoking habits worldwide and analyzes the crucial problems of genetic determinants, smoking initiation, and nicotine dependence. The volume includes an accurate overview of the epidemiology of smoking-related diseases and deals with a detailed analysis of smoking prevention strategies by highlighting the basic principles of smoking cessation techniques at different levels and with various targets. Giuseppe La Torre, who is Associate Professor at the "La Sapienza" University of Rome, made a great job by working as an editor and coordinator of the volume. He coauthored all chapters together with other experts. The result is a comprehensive and detailed treatise providing the state of the art on the health effects and the prevention strategies towards the most widespread plague affecting human health in today's world.

Silvio De Flora
Genoa, Italy
E-mail: sdf@unige.it

References

De Flora, S., & Bartsch, H. (2012). Genomic and post-genomic effects of cigarette smoke: Mechanisms and implications for risk assessment and prevention strategies. *International Journal of Cancer, 131*, 2721–2723.

De Flora, S., Quaglia, A., Bennicelli, C., & Vercelli, M. (2005). The epidemiological revolution of the 20th century. *FASEB Journal, 19*, 892–897.

Hecht, S. S. (2012). Lung carcinogenesis by tobacco smoke. *International Journal of Cancer, 131*, 2724–2732.

International Agency for Research on Cancer. (2012). *A review of human carcinogens: Personal habits and indoor combustions. IARC monographs on the evaluation of the carcinogenic risks to humans* (Vol. 100, part E). Lyon: IARC.

Izzotti, A., Calin, G. A., Arrigo, P., Steele, V. E., Croce, C. M., & De Flora, S. (2009). Downregulation of microRNA expression in the lungs of rats exposed to cigarette smoke. *FASEB Journal, 23*, 806–812.

Kanavos, P. (2006). The raising burden of cancer in the developing world. *Annals of Oncology, 17*, viii15–viii23.

Oppeltz, R. F., & Jatoi, I. (2011). Tobacco and the escalating global cancer burden. *Journal of Oncology, 2011*, 408104. doi:10.1155/2011/408104.

Preface

The idea behind this book has at least two roots, one in the past and the other more recent.

The oldest one is concerning the meeting I had to decide the title of my thesis to become a medical doctor. In 1989 Prof. Bruno Angelillo proposed to me to be involved in a research project, carried out by the Institute of Hygiene at the University of Naples, on the determination of urinary cotinine levels in children. The results of this research were astonishing: children of parents who were heavy smokers were comparable to light smokers, as concerning that of nicotine levels. The reason? They were passive smokers!

The more recent one is concerning my research activity on tobacco smoking that covers some important issues in this field, including smoking prevention among children and adolescents; smoking habits in particular settings (health professionals, medical students, general population, people with chronic diseases, patients with cancers); the association between smoking and gastric and pancreatic cancer, acne vulgaris, and erectile dysfunction; the impact of tobacco package health warnings with pictures on smoking cessation and prevention. But the main reason why I and my collaborators decided to start thinking about and writing this book is related to the fact that many health professionals paradoxically are smokers, despite the fact that they must play a key role in tobacco smoking prevention and control. At the international level there are very few examples of development of a curriculum at the undergraduate level on smoking prevention and cessation programs in bio-medical faculties. In a workshop recently organized by the European Public Health Association (EUPHA), the situation at the School of Medicine level in four WHO European country regions (Finland, Italy, Portugal, and Turkey) was presented. It was shown that at the national level in Italy, there is no formal course concerning tobacco smoking prevention and control among the curriculum of Medical students. A focus group with some of them revealed that the following issues could be covered in such a course: (a) nicotine addiction; (b) epidemiology of tobacco smoking-related pathologies; (c) motivation for starting smoking; (d) economic aspects; and (e) skills for treating a smoker who wants to quit.

In Portugal (Lisbon), there is an Environmental Health optional module available for Medical students in the second and third years at the Lisbon Faculty of Medicine. Tobacco consumption is one of the most relevant topics included in the course, in which some field work is usually developed. Among the optional curriculum there is another course for the fourth-year students aiming to build capacity in helping future patients to quit. Moreover, for students in the fourth and fifth years, a specific optional training activity is available, consisting of Research Community Projects that address the evaluation of tobacco consumption and related pathologies.

In Turkey (Ankara), Tobacco Control Classes have been developed since 2002, using a small-group discussion method. Medical students are distributed into up to 20 small groups, within which 10 hours of discussion are scheduled (five at the first class and five at the third class). The aim of the first year's program is to increase the level of awareness of the newly enrolled medical students, through the discussion of basic concepts regarding tobacco and tobacco use and its effects on health in general, and its effects on the economy of the single person and of the country. During the third year, there are more detailed discussions regarding health hazards of tobacco use and ways of protecting people from tobacco use (also concerning secondhand smoking).

In Finland, an Internet-based tobacco cessation model course has been developed and is currently in use. This course can be tailored for use in both undergraduate and specialist training and as a tool in continuous professional education of all health professionals. It includes short multi-professional video clips as well as theoretical knowledge on smoking cessation counseling in different settings, offering a comprehensive and multi-professional national standard for smoking cessation training. The course can be adjusted to be completely Internet-based or to include a half day multi-professional seminar with group discussions, role-play exercises, case studies, and lectures.

So, this book tries to consider all the elements that can help the health professional and the biomedical student to understand the tobacco smoking world and to develop skills to face a smoker, whether a patient or not, in order to give the right advice, as well as a nonsmoker with the aim to sustain smoking prevention in the right setting.

Chapter 1 has the goal to introduce the reader to the world of tobacco smoking, the role of nicotine in inducing a nicotine addiction, as well as to be confident with some tools in measuring nicotine dependence and motivation to quit. The role of tobacco smoking as cause of many diseases is now well established, from the scientific point of view. It is well recognized that tobacco consumption is the leading cause of preventable deaths in the majority of high-income nations and increasingly in low- and middle-income nations and that it causes disability and productivity losses because of premature deaths. Nevertheless, it is a common experience to see smokers in different settings. Smokers smoke even if for most of them it is dangerous for their health. Why?

This book wants to give answers to this question and to give the best available evidence concerning smoking prevention and cessation strategies, first of all recognizing that tobacco smoking is a disease for many smokers (International Classification of Disease 10th revision: F17Nicotine dependence).

Chapter 2 underlines how cigarette smoking is the most common mode of tobacco consumption in many countries and the single most preventable cause of death in the world today. Tobacco use is responsible each year for nearly six million deaths, and exposure to tobacco smoke in the environment, defined as "passive smoking" or "secondhand smoking" (SHS), is an important cause of mortality and morbidity worldwide.

The global prevalence of smoking any form of tobacco, in 2006, was higher for men (41.1%) than for women (8.9%) and males accounted for 80% of all smokers. Women's smoking prevalence rates are projected to rise, especially in many low- and- middle-income countries. Smoking behavior is usually established during adolescence, and adolescent smokers vastly underestimate the addictive potential of nicotine.

Chapter 3 concerns smoking-related diseases epidemiology. World Health Organization (WHO) ranks smoking consumption as the first leading cause of the global burden of disease in industrialized countries, and it continues to kill more than 600,000 nonsmokers who die from passive exposure to tobacco smoke. Tobacco-attributable mortality is projected to increase from three million deaths in 1990 to 8.4 million deaths by 2020: longevity has been improving rapidly for nonsmokers, but not for men who continue smoking cigarettes.

Cigarette smoke contains about 4,000 chemical agents that are known to be poisonous and toxic to the human body. This chapter describes the epidemiology of cigarette smoking-related diseases focusing on cardiovascular diseases, main smoking-related cancers, and other diseases less frequent but still related to cigarette smoking such as acne, Sudden Infant Death Syndrome (SIDS), maculopathy, smoking-related allergy, and early menopause. For each disease the epidemiology and the scientific evidence will be presented and discussed.

In Chapter 5 classic determinants of smoking initiation are considered: family, peer, society, and personal characteristics. In the family smoking is involved in both parental and sibling relations, through genetic and psychological pathway or indirectly by preventing friendship formation with smoking peers. Peer influence has been indicated as one of the most important determinant on smoking initiation. Selection and socialization are two main concepts used to explain peer role. At societal level, gender and socioeconomic status have been found associated with smoking initiation. Finally, personal characteristics are considered: the personality differences between smokers and nonsmokers are usually small, but they are important if one considers the large number of people who smoke: neuroticism, poor control, anger, and the levels of extraversion are involved.

Smoking prevention is the main theme of Chapter 6. Youth is a crucial moment for tobacco-related behaviors. The earlier a kid first tries smoking, the higher his or her chances of ultimately becoming a regular smoker, of experiencing a range of risk factors and health problems in adulthood, and of progressing to addiction to other harmful substances. Mass media campaigns intended to reduce tobacco initiation use brief, recurring messages to inform and motivate individuals to remain tobacco free. Other interventions such as school-based programs, laws, or parents' education can be also useful in reaching such a goal. The aim of this chapter is to help the reader get familiar with the main community interventions for preventing smoking in young. The first part of this chapter covers school-based smoking prevention interventions; the second and the third parts involve the workplace and the law in smoking prevention interventions, whereas the final part is concerned with the role of health communication in preventing smoking habits in youth.

How to tackle smoking at the population level is the general context of Chapter 8. Given the tobacco epidemic as a global challenge demanding concerted global and national action, the answer was the World Health Organization's Framework Convention on Tobacco Control (WHO FCTC), adopted in 2003. Regarding legislation on tobacco, in Europe it is based on two fundamental laws: one is the Directive on Tobacco Controls, dated 2001, which concerns the manufacture, presentation, and sale of tobacco products, in particular the use of warnings on packets and the prohibition of descriptions such as "mild" or "light," and the other is the Directive on Tobacco Advertising, published in 2003, that bans tobacco advertising in the print media, on radio, and over the Internet and at international sports events in Europe. Currently, 29 countries and jurisdictions have implemented policies on warnings of tobacco packages, and several studies were performed to evaluate the impact before and after the introduction.

The big issue of smoking among health professionals is the leading theme of Chapter 9. Tobacco smoking can be considered an old and a new challenge for public health and is both a matter of personal health and a public health concern for healthcare providers.

Healthcare professionals have an important role to play both as advisers—influencing smoking cessation—and as role models. Studies have shown that patients are often responsive to counseling received from healthcare professionals.

Healthcare workers and staff attitudes towards smoking have been shown to be important in determining the effectiveness of workplace smoking policies and nurses who smoke should set an example by quitting smoking both for themselves and their patients

Healthcare professionals, nurses, and medical doctor who smoke downplay their role in patient education and tend to show a more negative attitude towards patients. Moreover, it has been proposed that before nurses can serve as role models for positive health behaviors, they must incorporate these behaviors into their own personal lifestyles.

Among health professionals the prevalence of tobacco smoke is extremely high, more than other professional categories, and this could be partly attributed to a low weight that tobacco smoking has in the medical curriculum of future physicians, which will contribute in a determinant way to healthy choices of their patients. In order to realize that, medical students need to be adequately trained with the aim of acquiring competencies and skills that help patients to prevent tobacco smoking and to increase smoking cessation, through a program oriented to specific issues related to the potential harm of tobacco products.

The aim of Chapter 10 is to give an overview on the basic smoking cessation techniques, including counseling and use of first-line medications as recommended by the Clinical Practice guidelines.

This chapter, then, addresses three basic principles of smoking cessation: (a) TransTheoretical approach Model (TTM) of behavior change, (b) counseling, and (c) pharmacotherapy. The TTM identifies that the smoker can progress through five stages of change (Precontemplation, Contemplation, Preparation, Action, Maintenance) an individual passes through with the aim of changing an established behavior. The stage of change is a variable that involves past behavior and behavioral intention to characterize an individual's readiness to change. Counseling (individual and group counseling) and pharmacotherapies (nicotine replacement therapy, bupropion, varenicline) are explained and discussed extensively. Furthermore, since Advice and Assistance by physicians have an important role in helping smokers to quit, the so-called "minimal intervention" is described. The minimal intervention aims to create or strengthen motivation to stop smoking. It is rapid and effective and is based on the model of the five "As": Ask, Advice, Assess, Assist, Arrange.

Chapter 11 deals with smoking cessation among different settings. This chapter aims to address the role and the efficacy of smoking cessation interventions among different settings and concerning health professionals as well as workplace. By reading it the reader will be able to understand how smoking cessation interventions work in different settings, understand how smoking cessation interventions among healthcare personnel can play a fundamental role in supporting similar policies addressed to the general public, and learn what strategies have been adopted in real healthcare settings to promote smoking cessation.

Media and smoking cessation is the subject of Chapter 12. Quitting tobacco is not easy as tobacco dependence is a cluster of behavioral, cognitive, and physiological phenomena. The Easy way method, in fact, is based on the contrary on psychological mechanisms of smoking desire and also on the use of techniques borrowed from cognitive psychology. But the method described in the books "The Easy Way to Stop Smoking" written by Allen Carr was never tested in controlled trials. Through an examination of the conceptual bases of persuasion, the World Wide Web has many of the characteristics necessary for persuasive communication. The Internet, in fact, has opened up new possibilities in public health. The web is a promising channel to reach a large number of smokers. Substantial numbers of smokers from numerous countries seek Web-based smoking cessation resources and add to the growing support for Web-assisted tobacco interventions as an additional tool to address the need for global smoking cessation efforts.

A review of the ethical aspects of tobacco smoking is the content of Chapter 13. Philosophically, smoking has long been regarded as a paradigmatically private-regarding vice, best treated as such. Folk wisdom has long held tobacco smoking to be unhealthy and it actually is axiomatic that tobacco smoking is hazardous to health and that it is a merely private-regarding vice, harming only smokers themselves, is challenged by evidence of the harmful effects of "passive smoking."

Smokers and nonsmokers all have rights. Nonsmokers and employers are becoming less tolerant of smokers. Nonsmokers are speaking up their rights and demanding protection from smoke hazard. As the Surgeon General stated in the 1986 report: "the right of smokers to smoke ends where their behaviour affects the health and well-being of others." Three subtypes of individual rights can be distinguished: *the right to life, liberty, and use of private property*, and all three aspects of individual rights are central to efforts to control *environmental tobacco smoke* (ETS).

There are four main principles of bioethics that apply to tobacco control: autonomy, beneficence, non-maleficence, and justice. Persons are deemed to have autonomy on the basis of their nature as rational and moral beings. Preservation of individual autonomy requires both information about a health risk behavior and voluntary choice (that is, without nicotine addiction).

Beneficence is the obligation for national governments to promote public well-being, and non-maleficence refers to the obligation of governments to avoid harm (embodied, for example, in the "Precautionary principle," by which a government may preclude population exposure to a likely hazard even without absolute proof of the hazard). The principle of justice requires the fair and equitable distribution of social goods and, accordingly, the fair and equitable distribution of social and biological burdens.

Therefore, the central question is: Should political intervention in a private affair as basic as tobacco smoking in enclosed public spaces be justified in the name of public health protection?

Thus, without doubt, public health protection (primarily concerned with the health of the entire population, rather than the health of individuals) is the critical mass of the general governmental tobacco smoking discouragement policy or the burgeoning global wave of tobacco smoking proscription in enclosed public spaces, which is arguably buoyed by the 2005 World Health Organizations' Framework Convention on Tobacco Control.

Finally, Chapter 14 deals with the economic issues related to tobacco smoking. It causes disability and productivity losses because of premature deaths. Economic damages caused by smoking—based on both direct and indirect costs—account for $200 billion. The largest number of publications available about smoking-related illnesses economic costs dates back to the 1980s–1990s. They show that smoking places tremendous financial and health burdens upon both society and individuals.

Treatment for smoking-related diseases is expensive and preventing these diseases could provide immediate short-term financial returns. Additionally, tobacco treatment programs could produce substantial savings in the long term, along with health and quality of life benefits.

Hoping these ways of considering smoking cessation and prevention issues will be helpful for the reader, I wish you a good reading.

November 2012 Giuseppe La Torre

Appendix

G. La Torre, *Smoking Prevention and Cessation*, DOI 10.1007/978-1-4614-7046-5,

Area harvested (Ha)

	1990		2000		2010		% Increase 1990–2000	% Increase 2000–2010
Albania	24,000		5,700		1,200		−76.25	−78.94736842
Algeria	2,900		6,450		4,700	Im	122.4137931	−27.13178295
Angola	3,926	Im	3,473	Im	4,200	F	−11.53846154	20.93291103
Argentina	43,931		59,612		75,200	Im	35.69461201	26.1490975
Armenia			2,528		290	Im		−88.52848101
Australia	5,063		3,185		1,450	F	−37.09263283	−54.47409733
Austria	235		111		0	F	−52.76595745	−100
Azerbaijan			8,177		1,351			−83.47804818
Bangladesh	45,070		31,161		38,270		−30.86088307	22.81377363
Belgium			400		80	F		−80
Belgium–Luxembourg	444						−100	
Benin	432		1,007		140	Im	133.1018519	−86.09731877
Bhutan	100	F	110	Im	110	Im	10	0
Bolivia (Plurinational State of)	1,060		1,060		920	Im	0	−13.20754717
Bosnia and Herzegovina			3,204	a	1,461			−54.40074906
Brazil	274,098		309,989		446,361		13.09422177	43.99252877
Bulgaria	52,897		28,523		25,161		−46.0782275	−11.78697893
Burkina Faso	1,969	Im	1,000	F	1,000	Im	−49.21279837	0
Burundi	4,227	Im	705	a	1,497	F	−83.32150461	112.3404255
Cambodia	15,600		9,669		10,062		−38.01923077	4.064536146
Cameroon	210		3,400	a	4,500	F	1519.047619	32.35294118
Canada	29,342		23,800		15,600	Im	−18.88760139	−34.45378151
Central African Republic	625		750	a	715	F	20	−4.666666667
Chad	122	Im	145	a	221	F	18.85245902	52.4137931
Chile	4,480		3,508		2,509		−21.69642857	−28.47776511
China	1,600,200		1,441,537		1,345,703		−9.9151981	−6.648043026
Colombia	19,910		14,692		12,900	Im	−26.20793571	−12.19711408

Congo	300	F	600	F	950	F	100	58.33333333
Costa Rica	938		117		50		−87.52665245	−57.26495726
Côte d'Ivoire	12,000	F	20,000	a	17,000	Im	66.66666667	−15
Croatia			5,678		4,119			−27.456851
Cuba	53,171		45,323		20,256		−14.75992552	−55.30745979
Cyprus	101		76		70	Im	−24.75247525	−7.894736842
Czechoslovakia	3,276						−100	
Democratic People's Republic of Korea	35,593	Im	44,000	F	51,800	Im	23.61981288	17.72727273
Democratic Republic of the Congo	5,590		7,958		7,700	Im	42.36135957	−3.242020608
Dominican Republic	14,830		13,250	F	6,400	F	−10.65407957	−51.69811321
Ecuador	1,040		4,174		4,000	Im	301.3461538	−4.168663153
El Salvador	562	a	580	F	790	Im	3.202846975	36.20689655
Ethiopia			4,700	F	6,224	F		32.42553191
Ethiopia PDR	5,600	F					−100	
Fiji	220		300	F	650	F	36.36363636	116.6666667
France	10,785		9,282		7,245		−13.93602225	−21.94570136
Georgia			1,801		700	Im		−61.13270405
Germany	5,502		4,576		2,356		−16.83024355	−48.51398601
Ghana	4,000	a	3,950	a	5,700	Im	−1.25	44.30379747
Greece	78,796		61,000		15,600		−22.58490279	−74.42622951
Guatemala	9,908		8,374	a	8,500	Im	−15.48243843	1.504657273
Guinea	1,969	Im	3,470	Im	2,100	Im	76.23158964	−39.48126801
Guyana	100	a	91	Im	120	Im	−9	31.86813187
Haiti	540	F	400		420	Im	−25.92592593	5
Honduras	7,200		11,214		4,300	Im	55.75	−61.65507401
Hungary	8,672		5,764		5,300		−33.53321033	−8.049965302
India	413,100		433,400		459,600	Im	4.914064391	6.045223812
Indonesia	235,866		168,300		251,300	Im	−28.64592608	49.31669638
Iran (Islamic Republic of)	16,922		19,685		9,586		16.32785723	−51.30302261

(continued)

Area harvested (Ha)	1990		2000		2010		% Increase 1990–2000	% Increase 2000–2010
Iraq	5,125		2,400	[a]	2,300	Im	−53.17073171	−4.166666667
Israel	208		0	F	0	F	−100	
Italy	87,707		38,788		21,600	Im	−55.77547972	−44.31267402
Jamaica	1,175	[a]	1,163	Im	1,100	Im	−1.021276596	−5.417024936
Japan	30,000		23,991		15,000		−20.03	−37.47655371
Jordan	3,422		3,069		2,600	Im	−10.31560491	−15.28185077
Kazakhstan			8,900		1,600			−82.02247191
Kenya	4,500	F	14,160		23,000	F	214.6666667	62.42937853
Kyrgyzstan			14,465		4,000			−72.34704459
Lao People's Democratic Republic	11,665		6,700		6,500	Im	−42.56322332	−2.985074627
Lebanon	1,515		8,726		8,200	Im	475.9735974	−6.027962411
Libya	480	F	666	Im	700	F	38.75	5.105105105
Madagascar	3,650		2,807		2,720	F	−23.09589041	−3.099394371
Malawi	100,110	[a]	118,752		180,600	Im	18.62151633	52.08164915
Malaysia	10,168		9,129		15,700	Im	−10.21833202	71.97940629
Mali	541	Im	372		1,100	Im	−31.23844732	195.6989247
Mauritius	631		397		210		−37.08399366	−47.10327456
Mexico	21,722		22,674		4,004		4.382653531	−82.34100732
Montenegro					125			
Morocco	5,835		4,570		800	F	−21.67952014	−82.49452954
Mozambique	2,853	Im	9,000	F	59,200	Im	215.4574132	557.7777778
Myanmar	30,400		33,185		14,100	Im	9.161184211	−57.51092361
Nepal	7,610		4,283		2,534		−43.71879106	−40.83586271
New Zealand	450	F	0	F	0	F	−100	
Nicaragua	840		934		1,848		11.19047619	97.85867238
Niger	1,378	Im	6,200	F	750	Im	349.9274311	−87.90322581

Nigeria	22,000	F	37,000		19,400	Im	68.18181818	−47.56756757
Occupied Palestinian Territory		M	283		420	Im		48.40989399
Oman	409		270		260	Im	−33.98533007	−3.703703704
Pakistan	40,911		56,400		55,800		37.86023319	−1.063829787
Panama	1,083		1,100	F	1,500	Im	1.569713758	36.36363636
Paraguay	4,300	[a]	3,235		2,953		−24.76744186	−8.717156105
Peru	2,375	Im	4,900	F	503		106.3157895	−89.73469388
Philippines	63,335		41,051		29,706		−35.18433725	−27.63635478
Poland	27,527		14,057		15,500		−48.93377411	10.26534823
Portugal	2,262		2,118		300		−6.366047745	−85.83569405
Puerto Rico	9		2	F	2	F	−77.77777778	0
Republic of Korea	31,329		24,300		14,000	Im	−22.43608159	−42.38683128
Republic of Moldova			23,537		4,431			−81.17432128
Réunion	65		24	Im	29	F	−63.07692308	20.83333333
Romania	16,800		11,300		1,532		−32.73809524	−86.44247788
Russian Federation			1,840		3			−99.83695652
Rwanda	2,500	F	3,634	Im	4,459	F	45.36	22.70225647
Saint Vincent and the Grenadines	28	Im	50	Im	70	Im	78.57142857	40
Samoa	45	Im	40	F	50	F	−11.11111111	25
Serbia					5,828			
Serbia and Montenegro			9,858					−100
Sierra Leone	600		40		48	F	−93.33333333	20
Singapore	6	F	0	F	0	F	−100	
Slovakia			1,134		3			−99.73544974
Solomon Islands	104	Im	100	[a]	100	F	−3.846153846	0
Somalia	317	Im	250	F	344	F	−21.13564669	37.6
South Africa	25,000		15,600		3,950		−37.6	−74.67948718
Spain	21,093		14,078		10,600		−33.25747878	−24.70521381
Sri Lanka	8,920	[a]	4,480		2,560		−49.77578475	−42.85714286

(continued)

Area harvested (Ha)								
	1990		2000		2010		% Increase 1990–2000	% Increase 2000–2010
Swaziland	76		194		310	F	155.2631579	59.79381443
Switzerland	670		681		543		1.641791045	−20.26431718
Syrian Arab Republic	12,800		18,100		10,300		41.40625	−43.09392265
Tajikistan			3,702		90	Im		−97.56888169
Thailand	63,095	[a]	31,363		30,641		−50.2924162	−2.302075694
The former Yugoslav Republic of Macedonia			22,785		20,300			−10.906298
Togo	3,937	Im	4,000	[a]	4,100	Im	1.6002032	2.5
Trinidad and Tobago	48		60	F	130	Im	25	116.6666667
Tunisia	5,395		3,231		1,300	Im	−40.11121409	−59.76477871
Turkey	320,236		236,569		80,977		−26.12666908	−65.77024039
Turkmenistan			1,600	[a]	900	Im		−43.75
Uganda	4,280		13,712	Im	13,800	Im	220.3738318	0.641773629
Ukraine			3,600		280			−92.22222222
United Arab Emirates	82		52		40	Im	−36.58536585	−23.07692308
United Republic of Tanzania	20,574		44,000	F	43,000	F	113.8621561	−2.272727273
United States of America	296,760		189,970		136,561		−35.98530799	−28.11443912
Uruguay	845		830	F	800	Im	−1.775147929	−3.614457831
USSR	107,000						−100	
Uzbekistan			6,700	[a]	3,700	Im		−44.7761194
Venezuela (Bolivarian Republic of)	9,009		5,362		3,300	Im	−40.48174048	−38.45580007
Viet Nam	26,478		24,400		31,484		−7.848024775	29.03278689
Yemen	3,706		5,347		10,341		44.27954668	93.3981672
Yugoslav SFR	45,559						−100	
Zambia	5,071		9,000	F	59,988		77.47978702	566.5333333
Zimbabwe	60,103		90,769		94,175		51.02241153	3.752382421

[a]Unofficial figure

F FAO estimate, *Im* FAO data based on imputation methodology, *M* Data not available

% Increases in the last two columns are authors' calculations. Often a −100 % increase means that the Country is no longer a political entity

Yield (Hg/Ha)	1990		2000		2010		% Increase 1990–2000	% Increase 2000–2010
Albania	5,875	Fc	10,877	Fc	14,167	Fc	85.14042553	30.24731084
Algeria	12,338	Fc	11,090	Fc	16,809	Fc	−10.11509159	51.56898106
Angola	10,188	Fc	9,502	Fc	13,333	Fc	−6.733411857	40.31782783
Argentina	15,396	Fc	19,209	Fc	16,396	Fc	24.76617303	−14.64417721
Armenia			18,105	Fc	32,069	Fc		77.12786523
Australia	24,292	Fc	24,370	Fc	29,759	Fc	0.321093364	22.113254
Austria	17,787	Fc	20,721	Fc			16.49519312	−100
Azerbaijan			21,106	Fc	24,004	Fc		13.73069269
Bangladesh	8,387	Fc	11,232	Fc	14,447	Fc	33.92154525	28.6235755
Belgium			30,000	Fc	25,000	Fc		−16.66666667
Belgium–Luxembourg	33,604	Fc					−100	
Benin	5,949	Fc	6,743	Fc	7,143	Fc	13.34678097	5.93207771
Bhutan	14,000	Fc	13,091	Fc	13,636	Fc	−6.492857143	4.163165534
Bolivia (Plurinational State of)	8,821	Fc	9,198	Fc	13,043	Fc	4.273891849	41.80256578
Bosnia and Herzegovina			10,228	Fc	12,690	Fc		24.07117716
Brazil	16,253	Fc	18,660	Fc	17,496	Fc	14.80957362	−6.237942122
Bulgaria	14,470	Fc	11,323	Fc	16,317	Fc	−21.74844506	44.10491919
Burkina Faso	4,683	Fc	5,000	Fc	9,700	Fc	6.769165065	94
Burundi	9,463	Fc	10,809	Fc	9,352	Fc	14.22381908	−13.47950782
Cambodia	5,000	Fc	7,927	Fc	14,535	Fc	58.54	83.36066608
Cameroon	7,381	Fc	13,824	Fc	17,778	Fc	87.29169489	28.60243056
Canada	21,490	Fc	22,273	Fc	25,769	Fc	3.643555142	15.69613433
Central African Republic	8,016	Fc	8,693	Fc	9,091	Fc	8.445608782	4.578396411
Chad	15,000	Fc	12,690	Fc	10,407	Fc	−15.4	−17.99054374
Chile	32,170	Fc	29,991	Fc	31,684	Fc	−6.773391358	5.645026841

(continued)

Yield (Hg/Ha)								
	1990	2000	2010				% Increase 1990–2000	% Increase 2000–2010
China	16,533	Fc	17,786	Fc	22,336	Fc	7.57878183	25.58191836
Colombia	16,569	Fc	18,899	Fc	14,884	Fc	14.0624057	−21.24451029
Congo	4,267	Fc	3,333	Fc	4,421	Fc	−21.88891493	32.64326433
Costa Rica	18,305	Fc	15,983	Fc	15,800	Fc	−12.68505873	−1.144966527
Côte d'Ivoire	4,500	Fc	5,100	Fc	7,294	Fc	13.33333333	43.01960784
Croatia			17,108	Fc	20,614	Fc		20.49333645
Cuba	6,983	Fc	7,113	Fc	10,120	Fc	1.861664041	42.27470828
Cyprus	33,960	Fc	49,211	Fc	37,143	Fc	44.90871614	−24.52297251
Czechoslovakia	15,174	Fc					−100	
Democratic People's Republic of Korea	18,262	Fc	14,318	Fc	15,154	Fc	−21.5967583	5.838804302
Democratic Republic of the Congo	5,188	Fc	5,290	Fc	5,195	Fc	1.966075559	−1.79584121
Dominican Republic	12,359	Fc	13,003	Fc	10,964	Fc	5.210777571	−15.68099669
Ecuador	24,548	Fc	12,171	Fc	18,500	Fc	−50.41958612	52.0006573
El Salvador	13,167	Fc	18,103	Fc	16,456	Fc	37.48765854	−9.097939568
Ethiopia			7,021	Fc	9,158	Fc		30.43725965
Ethiopia PDR	7,143	Fc					−100	
Fiji	10,909	Fc	10,433	Fc	5,277	Fc	−4.363369695	−49.42010927
France	25,621	Fc	27,205	Fc	25,435	Fc	6.182428477	−6.506156956
Georgia			10,300	Fc	1,286	Fc		−87.51456311
Germany	18,977	Fc	24,006	Fc	25,976	Fc	26.50050061	8.206281763
Ghana	3,825	Fc	3,418	Fc	8,772	Fc	−10.64052288	156.6413107
Greece	17,220	Fc	22,392	Fc	14,103	Fc	30.03484321	−37.01768489
Guatemala	11,255	Fc	22,247	Fc	21,647	Fc	97.66326077	−2.696992853
Guinea	10,198	Fc	11,098	Fc	16,667	Fc	8.825259855	50.18021265
Guyana	10,000	Fc	9,890	Fc	6,667	Fc	−1.1	−32.58847321

Haiti	12,963	Fc	13,750	Fc	10,714	Fc	6.071125511	−22.08
Honduras	7,219	Fc	4,490	Fc	13,256	Fc	−37.80301981	195.233853
Hungary	15,663	Fc	18,190	Fc	14,717	Fc	16.13356317	−19.09290819
India	13,353	Fc	11,998	Fc	16,438	Fc	−10.14753239	37.00616769
Indonesia	6,632	Fc	8,681	Fc	7,760	Fc	30.89565742	−10.6093768
Iran (Islamic Republic of)	11,492	Fc	10,658	Fc	14,756	Fc	−7.257222416	38.44999062
Iraq	8,585	Fc	9,375	Fc	9,565	Fc	9.20209668	2.026666667
Israel	7,212	Fc					−100	
Italy	24,496	Fc	33,499	Fc	45,000	Fc	36.75293926	34.33236813
Jamaica	19,906	Fc	16,509	Fc	12,727	Fc	−17.06520647	−22.90871646
Japan	26,833	Fc	25,344	Fc	19,533	Fc	−5.549137256	−22.92850379
Jordan	8,457	Fc	8,693	Fc	7,692	Fc	2.790587679	−11.51501208
Kazakhstan			18,157	Fc	20,063	Fc		10.49732885
Kenya	19,556	Fc	12,684	Fc	6,155	Fc	−35.14011045	−51.47429833
Kyrgyzstan			23,929	Fc	24,750	Fc		3.430983326
Lao People's Democratic Republic	29,258	Fc	59,591	Fc	44,769	Fc	103.6742088	−24.87288349
Lebanon	11,188	Fc	12,377	Fc	11,341	Fc	10.62745799	−8.370364386
Libya	26,042	Fc	22,523	Fc	21,429	Fc	−13.51278704	−4.857257026
Madagascar	10,959	Fc	7,852	Fc	8,824	Fc	−28.35112693	12.37901172
Malawi	10,092	Fc	8,309	Fc	11,905	Fc	−17.66745937	43.27837285
Malaysia	9,986	Fc	7,856	Fc	9,682	Fc	−21.32986181	23.24338086
Mali	8,706	Fc	11,989	Fc	15,455	Fc	37.70962555	28.90983401
Mauritius	12,662	Fc	14,181	Fc	13,429	Fc	11.99652504	−5.302870037
Mexico	15,625	Fc	19,919	Fc	17,440	Fc	27.4816	−12.44540389
Montenegro					21,600	Fc		
Morocco	12,490	Fc	11,670	Fc	28,125	Fc	−6.565252202	141.0025707
Mozambique	10,515	Fc	10,522	Fc	14,527	Fc	0.066571564	38.06310587
Myanmar	13,158	Fc	15,338	Fc	14,326	Fc	16.56786746	−6.597991916

(continued)

Yield (Hg/Ha)								
	1990	2000	2010				% Increase 1990–2000	% Increase 2000–2010
Nepal	8,673	Fc	8,893	Fc	9,830	Fc	2.536607863	10.53637693
New Zealand	18,333	Fc					−100	
Nicaragua	14,940	Fc	15,835	Fc	16,229	Fc	5.990629183	2.488159141
Niger	7,039	Fc	7,132	Fc	14,667	Fc	1.321210399	105.6505889
Nigeria	4,091	Fc	5,946	Fc	8,866	Fc	45.34343681	49.10864447
Occupied Palestinian Territory			6,749	Fc	8,095	Fc		19.94369536
Oman	48,900	Fc	48,148	Fc	50,000	Fc	−1.537832311	3.846473374
Pakistan	16,645	Fc	19,096	Fc	21,384	Fc	14.72514269	11.98156682
Panama	18,116	Fc	16,364	Fc	16,000	Fc	−9.671009053	−2.224395013
Paraguay	18,091	Fc	13,867	Fc	21,470	Fc	−23.34862639	54.82800894
Peru	13,053	Fc	24,998	Fc	138,439	Fc	91.51152992	453.800304
Philippines	12,903	Fc	12,053	Fc	13,644	Fc	−6.587615283	13.20003319
Poland	21,434	Fc	21,018	Fc	20,267	Fc	−1.940841653	−3.573127795
Portugal	21,711	Fc	28,966	Fc	33,333	Fc	33.41624062	15.07629635
Puerto Rico	11,111	Fc	10,000	Fc	10,000	Fc	−9.999099991	0
Republic of Korea	22,367	Fc	28,065	Fc	29,357	Fc	25.47503018	4.603598789
Republic of Moldova			10,752	Fc	17,174	Fc		59.72842262
Réunion	16,615	Fc	9,167	Fc	13,793	Fc	−44.82696359	50.4636195
Romania	8,452	Fc	9,646	Fc	19,393	Fc	14.12683389	101.0470661
Russian Federation			7,826	Fc	10,000	Fc		27.77919755
Rwanda	13,600	Fc	10,457	Fc	16,820	Fc	−23.11029412	60.84919193
Saint Vincent and the Grenadines	14,286	Fc	17,200	Fc	11,429	Fc	20.39759205	−33.55232558
Samoa	32,222	Fc	35,000	Fc	41,400	Fc	8.621438769	18.28571429
Serbia					17,914	Fc		
Serbia and Montenegro			11,504	Fc				−100

Sierra Leone	10,833	Fc	5,000	Fc	6,250	Fc	−53.84473368	25
Singapore	21,667	Fc					−100	
Slovakia			16,490	Fc	3,333	Fc		−79.78775015
Solomon Islands	8,173	Fc	8,500	Fc	8,800	Fc	4.000978833	3.529411765
Somalia	4,038	Fc	4,000	Fc	6,105	Fc	−0.941059931	52.625
South Africa	10,960	Fc	19,038	Fc	28,190	Fc	73.70437956	48.0722765
Spain	20,470	Fc	30,479	Fc	30,472	Fc	48.89594529	−0.022966633
Sri Lanka	11,586	Fc	12,054	Fc	16,406	Fc	4.039357846	36.10419778
Swaziland	3,026	Fc	3,660	Fc	4,516	Fc	20.95175149	23.38797814
Switzerland	16,507	Fc	17,357	Fc	21,786	Fc	5.149330587	25.51708245
Syrian Arab Republic	10,234	Fc	14,427	Fc	18,932	Fc	40.97127223	31.22617315
Tajikistan			19,411	Fc	18,889	Fc		−2.689196847
Thailand	11,010	Fc	19,330	Fc	19,227	Fc	75.56766576	−0.532850491
The former Yugoslav Republic of Macedonia			9,732	Fc	14,916	Fc		53.2675709
Togo	5,080	Fc	4,500	Fc	8,293	Fc	−11.41732283	84.28888889
Trinidad and Tobago	21,042	Fc	15,000	Fc	11,538	Fc	−28.71400057	−23.08
Tunisia	12,604	Fc	10,634	Fc	13,077	Fc	−15.62995874	22.97348129
Turkey	9,243	Fc	8,466	Fc	6,792	Fc	−8.406361571	−19.77321049
Turkmenistan			20,125	Fc	22,222	Fc		10.41987578
Uganda	7,762	Fc	16,655	Fc	18,623	Fc	114.5709869	11.81627139
Ukraine			8,333	Fc	11,071	Fc		32.85731429
United Arab Emirates	101,829	Fc	126,923	Fc	210,000	Fc	24.64327451	65.45464573
United Republic of Tanzania	8,000	Fc	5,996	Fc	15,116	Fc	−25.05	152.1014009
United States of America	24,859	Fc	25,149	Fc	23,878	Fc	1.166579508	−5.053878882
Uruguay	22,012	Fc	33,735	Fc	31,250	Fc	53.25731419	−7.366236846
USSR	26,469	Fc					−100	
Uzbekistan			28,358	Fc	30,000	Fc		5.790253191

(continued)

Yield (Hg/Ha)

	1990	2000	2010				% Increase 1990–2000	% Increase 2000–2010
Venezuela (Bolivarian Republic of)	16,151	Fc	16,328	Fc	13,939	Fc	1.095907374	−14.63130818
Viet Nam	8,243	Fc	11,107	Fc	17,955	Fc	34.74463181	61.65481228
Yemen	18,292	Fc	21,719	Fc	22,414	Fc	18.73496611	3.199963166
Yugoslav SFR	10,036	Fc					−100	
Zambia	8,677	Fc	10,592	Fc	14,953	Fc	22.06983981	41.17258308
Zimbabwe	21,695	Fc	25,089	Fc	11,652	Fc	15.64415764	−53.55733588

[ ] = Official data
Fc = Calculated data
FAOSTAT, © FAO Statistics Division 2012, 16 March 2012
% Increases in the last two columns are authors' calculations. Often a −100 % increase means that the Country is no longer a political entity

Production (tons)

	1990		2000		2010		% Increase 1990–2000	% Increase 2000–2010
Albania	14,100		6,200		1,700		−56.02836879	−72.58064516
Algeria	3,578		7,153		7,900	Im	99.91615428	10.4431707
Angola	4,000	a	3,300	a	5,600	F	−17.5	69.6969697
Argentina	67,634		114,509		123,300	Im	69.3068575	7.677125815
Armenia			4,577		930	Im		−79.68101376
Australia	12,299		7,762		4,315	F	−36.88917798	−44.40865756
Austria	418		230	F	0	F	−44.97607656	−100
Azerbaijan			17,258		3,243			−81.2087148
Bangladesh	37,800		35,000		55,288		−7.407407407	57.96571429
Belgium			1,200		200			−83.33333333
Belgium–Luxembourg	1,492						−100	
Benin	257		679		100	F	164.2023346	−85.2724595
Bhutan	140	F	144	Im	150	Im	2.857142857	4.166666667
Bolivia (Plurinational State of)	935		975		1,200	Im	4.278074866	23.07692308
Bosnia and Herzegovina			3,277	a	1,854			−43.42386329
Brazil	445,489		578,451		780,942		29.84630372	35.00573082
Bulgaria	76,542		32,296		41,056		−57.80617177	27.12410206
Burkina Faso	922		500	F	970	Im	−45.77006508	94
Burundi	4,000		762		1,400	Im	−80.95	83.72703412
Cambodia	7,800		7,665		14,625		−1.730769231	90.80234834
Cameroon	155		4,700	a	8,000	F	2932.258065	70.21276596
Canada	63,057		53,010		40,200	Im	−15.93320329	−24.16525184
Central African Republic	501		652		650	F	30.13972056	−0.306748466
Chad	183	Im	184	a	230	Im	0.546448087	25
Chile	14,412		10,521		7,950		−26.99833472	−24.4368406
China	2,645,608		2,563,850		3,005,753		−3.090329331	17.23591474
Colombia	32,989		27,767		19,200	Im	−15.82951893	−30.85317103

(continued)

Production (tons)								
	1990		2000		2010		% Increase 1990–2000	% Increase 2000–2010
Congo	128		200	F	420	F	56.25	110
Costa Rica	1,717		187		79		−89.10891089	−57.7540107
Côte d'Ivoire	5,400		10,200	a	12,400	Im	88.88888889	21.56862745
Croatia			9,714		8,491			−12.59007618
Cuba	37,129		32,237		20,500		−13.17568477	−36.40847473
Cyprus	343		374		260	Im	9.037900875	−30.48128342
Czechoslovakia	4,971						−100	
Democratic People's Republic of Korea	65,000	F	63,000	F	78,500	Im	−3.076923077	24.6031746
Democratic Republic of the Congo	2,900		4,210		4,000	F	45.17241379	−4.988123515
Dominican Republic	18,328		17,229		7,017		−5.99628983	−59.27215741
Ecuador	2,553		5,080		7,400	Im	98.98159029	45.66929134
El Salvador	740	a	1,050	F	1,300	Im	41.89189189	23.80952381
Ethiopia			3,300	F	5,700	Im		72.72727273
Ethiopia PDR	4,000	a					−100	
Fiji	240		313		343	F	30.41666667	9.584664537
France	27,632		25,252		18,428		−8.613202085	−27.02360209
Georgia			1,855		90	Im		−95.14824798
Germany	10,441		10,985		6,120	F	5.210228905	−44.287665
Ghana	1,530		1,350	a	5,000	Im	−11.76470588	270.3703704
Greece	135,685		136,593		22,000		0.669197037	−83.89375737
Guatemala	11,151		18,630	a	18,400	Im	67.07021792	−1.234567901
Guinea	2,008	Im	3,851	Im	3,500	Im	91.78286853	−9.11451571
Guyana	100	a	90	a	80	Im	−10	−11.11111111
Haiti	700	F	550		450	Im	−21.42857143	−18.18181818
Honduras	5,198		5,035		5,700	Im	−3.13582147	13.20754717
Hungary	13,583		10,485		7,800		−22.80792167	−25.60801144
India	551,600		520,000		755,500	Im	−5.728788978	45.28846154
Indonesia	156,432		146,100		195,000	Im	−6.604786744	33.47022587

Iran (Islamic Republic of)	19,446		20,980		14,145		7.888511776	−32.57864633
Iraq	4,400		2,250	[a]	2,200	Im	−48.86363636	−2.222222222
Israel	150		0	F	0	F	−100	
Italy	214,851		129,937		97,200	Im	−39.52227358	−25.19451734
Jamaica	2,339	[a]	1,920	Im	1,400	Im	−17.91363831	−27.08333333
Japan	80,500		60,803		29,300		−24.46832298	−51.81158824
Jordan	2,894		2,668		2,000	Im	−7.809260539	−25.03748126
Kazakhstan			16,160		3,210			−80.13613861
Kenya	8,800	[a]	17,960		14,156		104.0909091	−21.18040089
Kyrgyzstan			34,613		9,900			−71.39802964
Lao People's Democratic Republic	34,130	[a]	39,926		29,100	Im	16.98212716	−27.11516305
Lebanon	1,695		10,800		9,300	Im	537.1681416	−13.88888889
Libya	1,250	F	1,500	[a]	1,500	F	20	0
Madagascar	4,000		2,204		2,400	Im	−44.9	8.89292196
Malawi	101,028		98,675		215,000	F	−2.329057291	117.8870028
Malaysia	10,154		7,172		15,200	Im	−29.36773685	111.935304
Mali	471		446		1,700	Im	−5.307855626	281.1659193
Mauritius	799		563		282		−29.53692115	−49.91119005
Mexico	33,941		45,164		6,983		33.06620312	−84.53857054
Montenegro					270			
Morocco	7,288		5,333		2,250	F	−26.82491767	−57.80986312
Mozambique	3,000	[a]	9,470		86,000	Im	215.6666667	808.1309398
Myanmar	40,000		50,900		20,200	Im	27.25	−60.31434185
Nepal	6,600		3,809		2,491		−42.28787879	−34.60225781
New Zealand	825		0	F	0	F	−100	
Nicaragua	1,255		1,479		2,999		17.84860558	102.7721433
Niger	970	F	4,422		1,100	Im	355.8762887	−75.12437811
Nigeria	9,000	[a]	22,000		17,200	Im	144.4444444	−21.81818182
Occupied Palestinian Territory		M	191		340	Im		78.0104712

(continued)

Production (tons)								
	1990		2000		2010		% Increase 1990–2000	% Increase 2000–2010
Oman	2,000		1,300		1,300	Im	−35	0
Pakistan	68,096		107,700		119,323		58.15906955	10.79201486
Panama	1,962		1,800	F	2,400	Im	−8.256880734	33.33333333
Paraguay	7,779		4,486		6,340		−42.33191927	41.3285778
Peru	3,100	a	12,249		6,964		295.1290323	−43.1463793
Philippines	81,722		49,479		40,530		−39.45449206	−18.08646092
Poland	59,000		29,545		31,414		−49.92372881	6.325943476
Portugal	4,911		6,135		1,000		24.92364081	−83.7000815
Puerto Rico	10		2	F	2	F	−80	0
Republic of Korea	70,073		68,198		41,100	Im	−2.675780971	−39.73430306
Republic of Moldova			25,306		7,610			−69.9280803
Réunion	108		22	Im	40	Im	−79.62962963	81.81818182
Romania	14,200		10,900		2,971		−23.23943662	−72.74311927
Russian Federation			1,440		3			−99.79166667
Rwanda	3,400	F	3,800	F	7,500	Im	11.76470588	97.36842105
Saint Vincent and the Grenadines	40		86	Im	80	Im	115	−6.976744186
Samoa	145	F	140	F	207	F	−3.448275862	47.85714286
Serbia					10,440			
Serbia and Montenegro			11,341					−100
Sierra Leone	650		20		30	Im	−96.92307692	50
Singapore	13	Im	0	F	0	F	−100	
Slovakia			1,870		1			−99.94652406
Solomon Islands	85	a	85	a	88	F	0	3.529411765
Somalia	128	Im	100	F	210	Im	−21.875	110
South Africa	27,400		29,700		11,135		8.394160584	−62.50841751
Spain	43,178		42,908		32,300		−0.625318449	−24.72266244
Sri Lanka	10,335	a	5,400		4,200		−47.75036284	−22.22222222
Swaziland	23		71		140	Im	208.6956522	97.18309859

Switzerland	1,106		1,182		1,183		6.871609403	0.084602369
Syrian Arab Republic	13,100		26,112		19,500		99.32824427	−25.32169118
Tajikistan			7,186		170	Im		−97.6342889
Thailand	69,469	a	60,624		58,912		−12.73229786	−2.823964107
The former Yugoslav Republic of Macedonia			22,175		30,280			36.55016911
Togo	2,000	a	1,800	a	3,400	Im	−10	88.88888889
Trinidad and Tobago	101		90	F	150	Im	−10.89108911	66.66666667
Tunisia	6,800		3,436		1,700	Im	−49.47058824	−50.52386496
Turkey	296,008		200,280		55,000		−32.3396665	−72.53844618
Turkmenistan			3,220	a	2,000	Im		−37.88819876
Uganda	3,322		22,837		25,700	Im	587.4473209	12.53667294
Ukraine			3,000		310			−89.66666667
United Arab Emirates	835		660		840	Im	−20.95808383	27.27272727
United Republic of Tanzania	16,459		26,384		65,000	F	60.30135488	146.3614312
United States of America	737,710		477,753		326,080		−35.2383728	−31.74715805
Uruguay	1,860		2,800	F	2,500	Im	50.53763441	−10.71428571
USSR	283,214						−100	
Uzbekistan			19,000	a	11,100	Im		−41.57894737
Venezuela (Bolivarian Republic of)	14,550		8,755		4,600	Im	−39.82817869	−47.45859509
Viet Nam	21,827		27,100		56,530		24.15815275	108.597786
Wallis and Futuna Islands	18	Im	12	Im	7	F	−33.33333333	−41.66666667
Yemen	6,779		11,613		23,178		71.30845257	99.58667011
Yugoslav SFR	45,721						−100	
Zambia	4,400		9,533		89,700	Im	116.6590909	840.941991
Zimbabwe	130,394		227,726		109,737		74.64453886	−51.81182649

[a]Unofficial figure
[ ] = Official data
F FAO estimate, *Im* FAO data based on imputation methodology, *M* Data not available
FAOSTAT, © FAO Statistics Division 2012, 16 March 2012
% Increases in the last two columns are authors' calculations. Often a −100 % increase means that the Country is no longer a political entity

Gross production value (constant 2004–2006 million US$) (USD)					
	1990	2000	2010	% Increase 1990–2000	% Increase 2000–2010
Albania	55	24	7	−56.36363636	−70.83333333
Algeria	1	2	2	100	0
Argentina	112	189	203	68.75	7.407407407
Armenia		5	1		−80
Australia	68	43	24	−36.76470588	−44.18604651
Austria	1	0		−100	
Azerbaijan		14	3		−78.57142857
Bangladesh	21	19	31	−9.523809524	63.15789474
Belgium		2	0		−100
Bhutan	1	1	1	0	0
Bolivia (Plurinational State of)	1	1	1	0	0
Bosnia and Herzegovina		5	3		−40
Brazil	550	714	963	29.81818182	34.87394958
Bulgaria	135	57	72	−57.77777778	26.31578947
Burkina Faso	1	0	1	−100	
Burundi	18	4	6	−77.77777778	50
Cambodia	15	15	28	0	86.66666667
Cameroon	0	7	12		71.42857143
Canada	248	209	158	−15.72580645	−24.40191388
Chile	25	18	14	−28	−22.22222222
China	3,230	3,130	3,669	−3.095975232	17.22044728
Colombia	24	20	14	−16.66666667	−30
Congo	0	0	1		
Costa Rica	2	0	0	−100	
Côte d'Ivoire	2	5	6	150	20
Croatia		22	19		−13.63636364
Cyprus	1	1	1	0	0
Dominican Republic	28	26	11	−7.142857143	−57.69230769
Ecuador	3	6	9	100	50
El Salvador	3	4	4	33.33333333	0
Ethiopia		2	4		100
France	24	22	16	−8.333333333	−27.27272727
Georgia		6	0		−100
Germany	26	27	15	3.846153846	−44.44444444
Ghana	3	3	11	0	266.6666667
Greece	216	217	35	0.462962963	−83.87096774
Guinea	4	8	7	100	−12.5
Honduras	22	22	25	0	13.63636364
Hungary	11	8	6	−27.27272727	−25
India	447	421	612	−5.81655481	45.36817102
Indonesia	180	168	224	−6.666666667	33.33333333
Iran (Islamic Republic of)	20	22	15	10	−31.81818182
Italy	787	476	356	−39.51715375	−25.21008403

(continued)

Gross production value (constant 2004–2006 million US$) (USD)					
	1990	2000	2010	% Increase 1990–2000	% Increase 2000–2010
Jamaica	3	3	2	0	−33.33333333
Japan	1,370	1,035	499	−24.45255474	−51.78743961
Jordan	3	3	2	0	−33.33333333
Kazakhstan		21	4		−80.95238095
Kenya	9	18	14	100	−22.22222222
Kyrgyzstan		18	5		−72.22222222
Lao People's Democratic Republic	31	36	26	16.12903226	−27.77777778
Lebanon	11	73	63	563.6363636	−13.69863014
Madagascar	2	1	1	−50	0
Malawi	97	94	205	−3.092783505	118.0851064
Malaysia	43	30	64	−30.23255814	113.3333333
Mali	0	0	1		
Mauritius	3	2	1	−33.33333333	−50
Mexico	55	73	11	32.72727273	−84.93150685
Morocco	10	7	3	−30	−57.14285714
Mozambique	5	15	136	200	806.6666667
Nepal	3	2	1	−33.33333333	−50
Nicaragua	5	6	12	20	100
Niger	0	2	0		−100
Nigeria	75	183	143	144	−21.8579235
Pakistan	51	81	89	58.82352941	9.87654321
Panama	4	4	5	0	25
Paraguay	6	3	5	−50	66.66666667
Peru	3	12	7	300	−41.66666667
Philippines	103	62	51	−39.80582524	−17.74193548
Poland	58	29	31	−50	6.896551724
Portugal	3	4	1	33.33333333	−75
Puerto Rico	0	0	0		
Republic of Korea	495	482	290	−2.626262626	−39.8340249
Republic of Moldova		20	6		−70
Romania	15	11	3	−26.66666667	−72.72727273
Russian Federation		8	0		−100
Rwanda	1	1	3	0	200
Serbia			18		
Serbia and Montenegro		14			−100
Singapore	0				
Slovakia		3	0		−100
South Africa	71	77	29	8.450704225	−62.33766234
Spain	28	28	21	0	−25
Sri Lanka	85	44	34	−48.23529412	−22.72727273
Switzerland	13	14	14	7.692307692	0
Tajikistan		2	0		−100
Thailand	7	6	6	−14.28571429	0

(continued)

Gross production value (constant 2004–2006 million US$) (USD)					
	1990	2000	2010	% Increase 1990–2000	% Increase 2000–2010
The former Yugoslav Republic of Macedonia		23	31		34.7826087
Togo	2	2	3	0	50
Trinidad and Tobago	1	1	1	0	0
Tunisia	8	4	2	–50	–50
Turkey	984	666	183	–32.31707317	–72.52252252
Turkmenistan		18	11		–38.88888889
Ukraine		3	0		–100
United States of America	2,868	1,858	1,268	–35.21617852	–31.75457481
Uruguay	4	6	5	50	–16.66666667
Venezuela (Bolivarian Republic of)	20	12	6	–40	–50
Viet Nam	40	50	104	25	108
Yemen	17	30	59	76.47058824	96.66666667

FAOSTAT, © FAO Statistics Division 2012, 16 March 2012

% Increases in the last two columns are authors' calculations. Often a –100 % increase means that the Country is no longer a political entity

Producer price (US $/ton) (USD)								
	1991		2000		2009		% Increase 1990–2000	% Increase 2000–2009
Albania	478.4	F	2679.0		3012.5		459.9916388	12.44867488
Algeria	849.9	F	192.5	F	305.1	F	–77.3502765	58.49350649
Armenia			915.6		175.1			–80.87592835
Australia	4817.1		3629.3		7175.0	F	–24.65798925	97.6965255
Austria	4696.8		989.7		1395.6	F	–78.92820644	41.01242801
Azerbaijan			516.3		987.7			91.30350571
Bangladesh	423.5	F	578.4		844.6	F	36.57615112	46.02351314
Belgium			2557.5	F	1861.7			–27.20625611
Bolivia (Plurinational State of)	1137.2		1200.4		2239.8		5.557509673	86.58780407
Bosnia and Herzegovina			1171.5		1740.0			48.52752881
Brazil	697.9	a	963.3	a	2937.5		38.02837083	204.9413475
Bulgaria	359.0	F	1307.4		2372.9		264.178273	81.49762888
Burkina Faso	1907.1	F	881.6	F	1488.6	F	–53.77274396	68.85208711
Burundi	606.0		604.0	a	10037.1	F	–0.330033003	1561.771523
Cambodia	2299.5	F	2017.8		1993.3	F	–12.25048924	–1.214193676
Cameroon	1651.4	F	2106.8		1559.8	F	27.57660167	–25.96354661
Canada	3716.5		3259.0		4473.7		–12.30996906	37.27216938
Chile	761.3		1679.3		2256.3	F	120.5832129	34.35955458
China	524.7		714.5	a	1711.6		36.17305127	139.5521344
Costa Rica	2622.2		1492.2	F	1652.8	F	–43.09358554	10.76263235

(continued)

Producer price (US $/ton) (USD)								
	1991		2000		2009		% Increase 1990–2000	% Increase 2000–2009
Côte d'Ivoire	620.3		393.3		534.4	F	−36.59519587	35.87592169
Croatia			1399.3		1677.0			19.8456371
Cyprus	2956.3		2361.8		4462.9	F	−20.10959646	88.96180879
Dominican Republic	1134.2		2085.1		2328.2		83.83882913	11.65891324
El Salvador	2906.4		2673.7	F	4366.3	F	−8.006468483	63.30553166
France	636.3		562.2		1811.1		−11.64545026	222.1451441
Georgia			3841.3	F	1476.5	F		−61.56249186
Germany	4615.3		1834.3		2486.1		−60.2561047	35.53399117
Ghana	1084.7		594.4	F	2752.9	F	−45.20143819	363.1393001
Greece	4668.4		1093.4		2548.1	F	−76.57869934	133.0437168
Guinea	733.8		2495.4	F	2713.2	F	240.0654129	8.72805963
Honduras	1458.2		4993.5		12856.2	F	242.4427376	157.4586963
Hungary	1432.0		1010.2		441.8	F	−29.45530726	−56.26608592
India	704.0		635.6		889.7	F	−9.715909091	39.97797357
Indonesia	1505.5		580.5	F	1253.9		−61.4413816	116.0034453
Iran (Islamic Republic of)	16405.4	F	2234.4		2888.5		−86.38009436	29.27407805
Italy	3351.2		3085.4	F			−7.931487228	−100
Japan	14104.7		17482.4		20984.5		23.9473367	20.03214662
Jordan	1175.0		932.3	F	1311.0	F	−20.65531915	40.61997211
Kazakhstan			997.9	F	1712.4			71.60036076
Kenya	752.5	F	873.7	F	1396.8		16.10631229	59.87180955
Kyrgyzstan			390.9		893.9			128.6774111
Lebanon	1310.6	F	5870.6		7473.8	F	347.9322448	27.30896331
Madagascar	427.7		664.9		690.7	F	55.45943418	3.880282749
Malawi	981.0		542.0	F	1325.4	F	−44.75025484	144.5387454
Malaysia	4658.1	F	3628.9		5212.5	F	−22.09484554	43.63856816
Mali	914.3		459.3		493.7	F	−49.76484742	7.489658175
Mauritius	3536.2		2754.0		5104.0		−22.1197896	85.33042847
Mexico	917.0		1380.6		1803.9		50.5561614	30.66058236
Morocco	1148.6		1129.3		1581.1	F	−1.68030646	40.00708403
Mozambique	1348.1	F	852.4		1823.1	F	−36.77026927	113.8784608
Nepal	791.9	F	636.0	F	535.4	F	−19.68682915	−15.81761006
New Zealand	3807.3						−100	
Nicaragua	6108.7	F	4869.5		6251.7		−20.28582186	28.38484444
Niger	587.3	F	244.4		463.2	F	−58.38583348	89.52536825
Paraguay	600.7	F	631.0		1263.9	F	5.044115199	100.3011094
Peru	75.5	F	538.7		720.9		613.5099338	33.82216447
Philippines	1080.1		810.0		1932.2		−25.0069438	138.5432099
Poland	1058.1		1178.8		1315.5		11.40723939	11.59653885
Portugal	4193.9		418.6		1252.5		−90.01883688	199.2116579
Puerto Rico	11464.0		9837.2	F	8703.7	F	−14.19050942	−11.52258773

(continued)

Producer price (US $/ton) (USD)								
	1991		2000		2009		% Increase 1990–2000	% Increase 2000–2009
Republic of Korea	5454.4		4969.2		6877.1		−8.895570549	38.39451018
Republic of Moldova			588.0		1700.6			189.2176871
Romania	725.6		856.3		1019.8	F	18.01267916	19.09377555
Russian Federation			4460.0	F	5348.9	F		19.93049327
Rwanda	600.6	F	541.4	F	507.1	F	−9.856809857	−6.335426672
Serbia								
Serbia and Montenegro			959.9					−100
Slovakia			1065.3		1534.9			44.0814794
South Africa	3836.9		2123.7		3282.0		−44.65062941	54.54160192
Spain	3487.0		2833.6		1321.7		−18.73817035	−53.35615471
Sri Lanka	10243.8	F	7282.6		13008.9	F	−28.90724145	78.62988493
Switzerland	10397.5		9012.1		13888.9		−13.32435682	54.11391352
Tajikistan			194.1	F	485.4			150.0772798
Thailand	171.2	F	73.0		378.2		−57.35981308	418.0821918
The former Yugoslav Republic of Macedonia			121.8		4250.3			3389.573071
Trinidad and Tobago	3505.9		9866.8	F	6983.9	F	181.4341539	−29.21818624
Tunisia	919.3		903.2		1229.6		−1.751332536	36.13817538
Turkey	2945.1		2773.5		4270.3		−5.826627279	53.96791058
Ukraine			576.1		2291.4			297.7434473
United States of America	3904.0		4211.0		4012.0		7.863729508	−4.725718357
Venezuela (Bolivarian Republic of)	2911.6		1352.2	F	3028.1	F	−53.55818107	123.9387665
Yemen	1353.3		1391.3		3285.1		2.807950935	136.1173004

[a]Unofficial figure

[ ] = Official data

F FAO estimate

FAOSTAT, © FAO Statistics Division 2012, 16 March 2012

% Increases in the last two columns are authors' calculations. Often a −100 % increase means that the Country is no longer a political entity

Commodity-by-industry direct requirements, after redefinitions (in producers' prices)			
Bureau of economic analysis			
2002			
	Commodities/Industries	111910	3122A0
IO code	Name	Tobacco farming	Tob. product manufacturing
1111A0	Oilseed farming	0.0044056	0
1111B0	Grain farming	0.0385902	0
111200	Vegetable and melon farming	0	0
111335	Tree nut farming	0	0
1113A0	Fruit farming	0	0
111400	Greenhouse, nursery, and floriculture production	0	0
111910	Tobacco farming	0.0487884	0.0398043
111920	Cotton farming	0	0
1119A0	Sugarcane and sugar beet farming	0	0
1119B0	All other crop farming	0.0008974	0
112120	Dairy cattle and milk production	0	0
1121A0	Cattle ranching and farming	0	0
112300	Poultry and egg production	0	0
112A00	Animal production, except cattle and poultry and eggs	0.0309211	0
113300	Logging	0	0
113A00	Forest nurseries, forest products, and timber tracts	0	0
114100	Fishing	0	0
114200	Hunting and trapping	0	0
115000	Support activities for agriculture and forestry	0.0883577	0
211000	Oil and gas extraction	0	0.0000042
212100	Coal mining	0	0.0001222
212210	Iron ore mining	0	0
212230	Copper, nickel, lead, and zinc mining	0	0
2122A0	Gold, silver, and other metal ore mining	0	0
212310	Stone mining and quarrying	0.0022028	0
212320	Sand, gravel, clay, and ceramic and refractory minerals mining and quarrying	0	0
212390	Other nonmetallic mineral mining and quarrying	0	0
213111	Drilling oil and gas wells	0	0
213112	Support activities for oil and gas operations	0	0
21311A	Support activities for other mining	0	0
221100	Electric power generation, transmission, and distribution	0.0271681	0.0025156
221200	Natural gas distribution	0.003753	0.0014263
221300	Water, sewage, and other systems	0.0012238	0.0000379
230101	Nonresidential commercial and health-care structures	0	0
230102	Nonresidential manufacturing structures	0	0
230103	Other nonresidential structures	0	0
230201	Residential permanent site single- and multi family structures	0	0

(continued)

Commodity-by-industry direct requirements, after redefinitions (in producers' prices)			
Bureau of economic analysis			
2002			
	Commodities/Industries	111910	3122A0
IO code	Name	Tobacco farming	Tob. product manufacturing
230202	Other residential structures	0	0
230301	Nonresidential maintenance and repair	0.0110141	0.0002802
230302	Residential maintenance and repair	0	0
311111	Dog and cat food manufacturing	0	0
311119	Other animal food manufacturing	0	0
311210	Flour milling and malt manufacturing	0	0
311221	Wet corn milling	0	0
311225	Fats and oils refining and blending	0	0
31122A	Soybean and other oilseed processing	0	0.0008448
311230	Breakfast cereal manufacturing	0	0
311313	Beet sugar manufacturing	0	0
31131A	Sugar cane mills and refining	0	0
311320	Chocolate and confectionery manufacturing from cacao beans	0	0
311330	Confectionery manufacturing from purchased chocolate	0	0
311340	Nonchocolate confectionery manufacturing	0	0
311410	Frozen food manufacturing	0	0
311420	Fruit and vegetable canning, pickling, and drying	0	0
311513	Cheese manufacturing	0	0
311514	Dry, condensed, and evaporated dairy product manufacturing	0	0
31151A	Fluid milk and butter manufacturing	0	0
311520	Ice cream and frozen dessert manufacturing	0	0
311615	Poultry processing	0	0
31161A	Animal (except poultry) slaughtering, rendering, and processing	0	0
311700	Seafood product preparation and packaging	0	0
311810	Bread and bakery product manufacturing	0	0
311820	Cookie, cracker, and pasta manufacturing	0	0
311830	Tortilla manufacturing	0	0
311910	Snack food manufacturing	0	0
311920	Coffee and tea manufacturing	0	0
311930	Flavoring syrup and concentrate manufacturing	0	0
311940	Seasoning and dressing manufacturing	0	0
311990	All other food manufacturing	0	0
312110	Soft drink and ice manufacturing	0	0
312120	Breweries	0	0
312130	Wineries	0	0
312140	Distilleries	0	0
3122A0	Tobacco product manufacturing	0	0.0556266

(continued)

Commodity-by-industry direct requirements, after redefinitions (in producers' prices)			
Bureau of economic analysis			
2002			
	Commodities/Industries	111910	3122A0
IO code	Name	Tobacco farming	Tob. product manufacturing
313100	Fiber, yarn, and thread mills	0	0
313210	Broadwoven fabric mills	0	0
313220	Narrow fabric mills and schiffli machine embroidery	0	0
313230	Nonwoven fabric mills	0	0.001401
313240	Knit fabric mills	0	0
313310	Textile and fabric finishing mills	0	0.0004593
313320	Fabric coating mills	0	0
314110	Carpet and rug mills	0	0
314120	Curtain and linen mills	0	0
314910	Textile bag and canvas mills	0	0
314990	All other textile product mills	0	0.0009439
315100	Apparel knitting mills	0	0
315210	Cut and sew apparel contractors	0	0
315220	Men's and boys' cut and sew apparel manufacturing	0	0
315230	Women's and girls' cut and sew apparel manufacturing	0	0
315290	Other cut and sew apparel manufacturing	0	0
315900	Apparel accessories and other apparel manufacturing	0	0
316100	Leather and hide tanning and finishing	0	0
316200	Footwear manufacturing	0	0
316900	Other leather and allied product manufacturing	0	0
321100	Sawmills and wood preservation	0	0.0025324
321219	Reconstituted wood product manufacturing	0	0
32121A	Veneer and plywood manufacturing	0	0
32121B	Engineered wood member and truss manufacturing	0	0
321910	Wood windows and doors and millwork	0	0
321920	Wood container and pallet manufacturing	0	0
321991	Manufactured home (mobile home) manufacturing	0	0
321992	Prefabricated wood building manufacturing	0	0
321999	All other miscellaneous wood product manufacturing	0.0003263	0
322110	Pulp mills	0	0
322120	Paper mills	0	0.0000253
322130	Paperboard Mills	0	0.001755
322210	Paperboard container manufacturing	0	0.0269548
32222A	Coated and laminated paper, packaging paper, and plastics film manufacturing	0	0.0000169
32222B	All other paper bag and coated and treated paper manufacturing	0	0
322230	Stationery product manufacturing	0.0000816	0
322291	Sanitary paper product manufacturing	0.0000816	0
322299	All other converted paper product manufacturing	0	0

(continued)

Commodity-by-industry direct requirements, after redefinitions (in producers' prices)			
Bureau of economic analysis			
2002			
	Commodities/Industries	111910	3122A0
IO code	Name	Tobacco farming	Tob. product manufacturing
323110	Printing	0.0003263	0.0007943
323120	Support activities for printing	0	0
324110	Petroleum refineries	0.0584972	0.0025071
324121	Asphalt paving mixture and block manufacturing	0	0
324122	Asphalt shingle and coating materials manufacturing	0	0
324191	Petroleum lubricating oil and grease manufacturing	0	0.0001391
324199	All other petroleum and coal products manufacturing	0	0
325110	Petrochemical manufacturing	0	0
325120	Industrial gas manufacturing	0	0
325130	Synthetic dye and pigment manufacturing	0	0
325181	Alkalies and chlorine manufacturing	0	0
325182	Carbon black manufacturing	0	0
325188	All other basic inorganic chemical manufacturing	0.0079138	0
325190	Other basic organic chemical manufacturing	0	0.000059
325211	Plastics material and resin manufacturing	0	0
325212	Synthetic rubber manufacturing	0	0
325220	Artificial and synthetic fibers and filaments manufacturing	0	0.0131782
325310	Fertilizer manufacturing	0.023252	0
325320	Pesticide and other agricultural chemical manufacturing	0.0503386	0
325411	Medicinal and botanical manufacturing	0	0
325412	Pharmaceutical preparation manufacturing	0	0
325413	In vitro diagnostic substance manufacturing	0	0
325414	Biological product (except diagnostic) manufacturing	0	0
325510	Paint and coating manufacturing	0	0
325520	Adhesive manufacturing	0	0
325610	Soap and cleaning compound manufacturing	0	0.0040662
325620	Toilet preparation manufacturing	0	0
325910	Printing ink manufacturing	0	0
3259A0	All other chemical product and preparation manufacturing	0.000979	0.001203
326110	Plastics packaging materials and unlaminated film and sheet manufacturing	0.0016317	0
326121	Unlaminated plastics profile shape manufacturing	0	0.0009586
326122	Plastic pipe and pipe-fitting manufacturing	0	0
326130	Laminated plastics plate, sheet (except packaging), and shape manufacturing	0	0.0001896

(continued)

Commodity-by-industry direct requirements, after redefinitions (in producers' prices)			
Bureau of economic analysis			
2002			
	Commodities/Industries	111910	3122A0
IO code	Name	Tobacco farming	Tob. product manufacturing
326140	Polystyrene foam product manufacturing	0	0
326150	Urethane and other foam product (except polystyrene) manufacturing	0	0
326160	Plastics bottle manufacturing	0	0
32619A	Other plastics product manufacturing	0.0035082	0.0000969
326210	Tire manufacturing	0.0068532	0
326220	Rubber and plastics hoses and belting manufacturing	0.0005711	0
326290	Other rubber product manufacturing	0	0
32711A	Pottery, ceramics, and plumbing fixture manufacturing	0	0
32712A	Brick, tile, and other structural clay product manufacturing	0	0.0003582
32712B	Clay and nonclay refractory manufacturing	0	0
327211	Flat glass manufacturing	0	0
327212	Other pressed and blown glass and glassware manufacturing	0	0.0005393
327213	Glass container manufacturing	0	0
327215	Glass product manufacturing made of purchased glass	0	0
327310	Cement manufacturing	0	0
327320	Ready-mix concrete manufacturing	0	0
327330	Concrete pipe, brick and block manufacturing	0	0
327390	Other concrete product manufacturing	0	0
3274A0	Lime and gypsum product manufacturing	0	0
327910	Abrasive product manufacturing	0	0
327991	Cut stone and stone product manufacturing	0	0
327992	Ground or treated mineral and earth manufacturing	0	0
327993	Mineral wool manufacturing	0	0.0004951
327999	Miscellaneous nonmetallic mineral products	0	0
331510	Ferrous metal foundries	0	0
331520	Nonferrous metal foundries	0	0
331110	Iron and steel mills and ferroalloy manufacturing	0	0.0007943
331200	Steel product manufacturing from purchased steel	0.0004079	0
331314	Secondary smelting and alloying of aluminum	0	0
33131A	Alumina refining and primary aluminum production	0	0.0002907
33131B	Aluminum product manufacturing from purchased aluminum	0	0
331411	Primary smelting and refining of copper	0	0.0004972
331419	Primary smelting and refining of nonferrous metal (except copper and aluminum)	0	0

(continued)

Commodity-by-industry direct requirements, after redefinitions (in producers' prices)			
Bureau of economic analysis			
2002			
	Commodities/Industries	111910	3122A0
IO code	Name	Tobacco farming	Tob. product manufacturing
331420	Copper rolling, drawing, extruding, and alloying	0	0
331490	Nonferrous metal (except copper and aluminum) rolling, drawing, extruding, and alloying	0	0
332114	Custom roll forming	0	0
33211A	All other forging, stamping, and sintering	0	0
33211B	Crown and closure manufacturing and metal stamping	0	0
33221A	Cutlery, utensil, pot, and pan manufacturing	0	0
33221B	Handtool manufacturing	0.0029371	0
332310	Plate work and fabricated structural product manufacturing	0.0004079	0
332320	Ornamental and architectural metal products manufacturing	0	0
332410	Power boiler and heat exchanger manufacturing	0	0
332420	Metal tank (heavy gauge) manufacturing	0	0
332430	Metal can, box, and other metal container (light gauge) manufacturing	0	0.0086696
33299A	Ammunition manufacturing	0	0
33299B	Arms, ordnance, and accessories manufacturing	0	0
332500	Hardware manufacturing	0	0
332600	Spring and wire product manufacturing	0	0
332710	Machine shops	0.0003263	0.0006384
332720	Turned product and screw, nut, and bolt manufacturing	0	0
332800	Coating, engraving, heat treating, and allied activities	0	0.0008343
332913	Plumbing, fixture fitting, and trim manufacturing	0	0
33291A	Valve and fittings other than plumbing	0	0.0021089
332991	Ball and roller bearing manufacturing	0	0
332996	Fabricated pipe and pipe-fitting manufacturing	0	0
33299C	Other fabricated metal manufacturing	0.000979	0.0011588
333111	Farm machinery and equipment manufacturing	0.0133801	0
333112	Lawn and garden equipment manufacturing	0	0
333120	Construction machinery manufacturing	0	0
333130	Mining and oil and gas field machinery manufacturing	0	0
333220	Plastics and rubber industry machinery manufacturing	0	0
333295	Semiconductor machinery manufacturing	0	0
33329A	Other industrial machinery manufacturing	0	0
333314	Optical instrument and lens manufacturing	0	0

(continued)

Commodity-by-industry direct requirements, after redefinitions (in producers' prices)			
Bureau of economic analysis			
2002			
	Commodities/Industries	111910	3122A0
IO code	Name	Tobacco farming	Tob. product manufacturing
333315	Photographic and photocopying equipment manufacturing	0	0
333319	Other commercial and service industry machinery manufacturing	0	0
33331A	Vending, commercial, industrial, and office machinery manufacturing	0	0
333414	Heating equipment, except warm air furnaces	0	0
333415	Air conditioning, refrigeration, and warm air heating equipment manufacturing	0	0.0008701
33341A	Air purification and ventilation equipment manufacturing	0	0
333511	Industrial mold manufacturing	0	0
333514	Special tool, die, jig, and fixture manufacturing	0	0
333515	Cutting tool and machine tool accessory manufacturing	0	0
33351A	Metal cutting and forming machine tool manufacturing	0	0
33351B	Rolling mill and other metalworking machinery manufacturing	0	0
333611	Turbine and turbine generator set units manufacturing	0	0
333612	Speed changer, industrial high-speed drive, and gear manufacturing	0	0.0010913
333613	Mechanical power transmission equipment manufacturing	0	0.0012978
333618	Other engine equipment manufacturing	0	0.000295
333911	Pump and pumping equipment manufacturing	0	0
333912	Air and gas compressor manufacturing	0	0
333920	Material handling equipment manufacturing	0.0013054	0.000099
333991	Power-driven handtool manufacturing	0.0004079	0
333993	Packaging machinery manufacturing	0	0
333994	Industrial process furnace and oven manufacturing	0	0
33399A	Other general purpose machinery manufacturing	0.0024476	0
33399B	Fluid power process machinery	0	0
334111	Electronic computer manufacturing	0	0
334112	Computer storage device manufacturing	0	0
33411A	Computer terminals and other computer peripheral equipment manufacturing	0	0
334411	Electron tube manufacturing	0	0
334412	Bare printed circuit board manufacturing	0	0

(continued)

Commodity-by-industry direct requirements, after redefinitions (in producers' prices)			
Bureau of economic analysis			
2002			
	Commodities/Industries	111910	3122A0
IO code	Name	Tobacco farming	Tob. product manufacturing
334413	Semiconductor and related device manufacturing	0	0
334417	Electronic connector manufacturing	0	0
334418	Printed circuit assembly (electronic assembly) manufacturing	0	0.0004698
334419	Other electronic component manufacturing	0	0.0003813
33441A	Electronic capacitor, resistor, coil, transformer, and other inductor manufacturing	0	0
334510	Electromedical and electrotherapeutic apparatus manufacturing	0	0
334511	Search, detection, and navigation instruments manufacturing	0	0
334512	Automatic environmental control manufacturing	0	0
334513	Industrial process variable instruments manufacturing	0	0
334514	Totalizing fluid meters and counting devices manufacturing	0	0
334515	Electricity and signal testing instruments manufacturing	0	0
334516	Analytical laboratory instrument manufacturing	0	0
334517	Irradiation apparatus manufacturing	0	0
33451A	Other measuring and controlling device manufacturing	0	0.0009755
334613	Magnetic and optical recording media manufacturing	0	0
33461A	Software, audio, and video media reproducing	0	0.0016665
334210	Telephone apparatus manufacturing	0	0
334220	Broadcast and wireless communications equipment	0	0
334290	Other communications equipment manufacturing	0	0
334300	Audio and video equipment manufacturing	0	0
335110	Electric lamp bulb and part manufacturing	0.0008159	0
335120	Lighting fixture manufacturing	0	0.0010155
335210	Small electrical appliance manufacturing	0	0
335221	Household cooking appliance manufacturing	0	0
335222	Household refrigerator and home freezer manufacturing	0	0
335224	Household laundry equipment manufacturing	0	0
335228	Other major household appliance manufacturing	0	0
335311	Power, distribution, and specialty transformer manufacturing	0	0
335312	Motor and generator manufacturing	0.0004895	0
335313	Switchgear and switchboard apparatus manufacturing	0	0

(continued)

Commodity-by-industry direct requirements, after redefinitions (in producers' prices)			
Bureau of economic analysis			
2002			
	Commodities/Industries	111910	3122A0
IO code	Name	Tobacco farming	Tob. product manufacturing
335314	Relay and industrial control manufacturing	0	0
335911	Storage battery manufacturing	0.0035898	0.0014495
335912	Primary battery manufacturing	0	0
335920	Communication and energy wire and cable manufacturing	0	0
335930	Wiring device manufacturing	0	0
335991	Carbon and graphite product manufacturing	0	0.000512
335999	All other miscellaneous electrical equipment and component manufacturing	0	0
336111	Automobile manufacturing	0	0
336112	Light truck and utility vehicle manufacturing	0	0
336120	Heavy duty truck manufacturing	0	0
336411	Aircraft manufacturing	0	0
336412	Aircraft engine and engine parts manufacturing	0	0
336413	Other aircraft parts and auxiliary equipment manufacturing	0	0
336414	Guided missile and space vehicle manufacturing	0	0
33641A	Propulsion units and parts for space vehicles and guided missiles	0	0
336211	Motor vehicle body manufacturing	0	0
336212	Truck trailer manufacturing	0	0
336213	Motor home manufacturing	0	0
336214	Travel trailer and camper manufacturing	0	0
336300	Motor vehicle parts manufacturing	0.0084034	0.0027852
336500	Railroad rolling stock manufacturing	0	0
336611	Ship building and repairing	0	0
336612	Boat building	0	0
336991	Motorcycle, bicycle, and parts manufacturing	0	0
336992	Military armored vehicle, tank, and tank component manufacturing	0	0
336999	All other transportation equipment manufacturing	0	0
337110	Wood kitchen cabinet and countertop manufacturing	0	0
337121	Upholstered household furniture manufacturing	0	0
337122	Nonupholstered wood household furniture manufacturing	0	0
337127	Institutional furniture manufacturing	0	0
33712A	Metal and other household furniture (except wood) manufacturing/1/	0	0
337212	Office furniture and custom architectural woodwork and millwork manufacturing/1/	0	0

(continued)

Commodity-by-industry direct requirements, after redefinitions (in producers' prices)

Bureau of economic analysis

2002

	Commodities/Industries	111910	3122A0
IO code	Name	Tobacco farming	Tob. product manufacturing
337215	Showcase, partition, shelving, and locker manufacturing	0	0
33721A	Wood television, radio, and sewing machine cabinet manufacturing/1/	0	0
337910	Mattress manufacturing	0	0
337920	Blind and shade manufacturing	0	0
339111	Laboratory apparatus and furniture manufacturing	0	0
339112	Surgical and medical instrument manufacturing	0	0
339113	Surgical appliance and supplies manufacturing	0	0
339114	Dental equipment and supplies manufacturing	0	0
339115	Ophthalmic goods manufacturing	0	0
339116	Dental laboratories	0	0
339910	Jewelry and silverware manufacturing	0	0
339920	Sporting and athletic goods manufacturing	0	0
339930	Doll, toy, and game manufacturing	0	0
339940	Office supplies (except paper) manufacturing	0.0000816	0
339950	Sign manufacturing	0	0
339991	Gasket, packing, and sealing device manufacturing	0	0
339992	Musical instrument manufacturing	0	0
339994	Broom, brush, and mop manufacturing	0.000979	0
33999A	All other miscellaneous manufacturing	0.0002448	0.0004698
420000	Wholesale trade	0.0370401	0.0177901
4A0000	Retail trade	0.0014685	0.0000169
481000	Air transportation	0.0008159	0.0004172
482000	Rail transportation	0.0016317	0.0003202
483000	Water transportation	0.0004079	0.0001707
484000	Truck transportation	0.0087297	0.0064005
485000	Transit and ground passenger transportation	0	0.0000253
486000	Pipeline transportation	0	0.0000822
48A000	Scenic and sightseeing transportation and support activities for transportation	0	0
492000	Couriers and messengers	0	0
493000	Warehousing and storage	0.0258628	0.0004593
511110	Newspaper publishers	0	0
511120	Periodical publishers	0.0003263	0
511130	Book publishers	0	0
5111A0	Directory, mailing list, and other publishers	0	0
511200	Software publishers	0	0
512100	Motion picture and video industries	0	0
512200	Sound recording industries	0	0
515100	Radio and television broadcasting	0	0

(continued)

Commodity-by-industry direct requirements, after redefinitions (in producers' prices)			
Bureau of economic analysis			
2002			
	Commodities/Industries	111910	3122A0
IO code	Name	Tobacco farming	Tob. product manufacturing
515200	Cable and other subscription programming	0	0
516110	Internet Publishing and Broadcasting	0	0
517000	Telecommunications	0.0019581	0.0002065
518100	Internet service providers and web search portals	0.0008159	0.0000295
518200	Data processing, hosting, and related services	0	0.0003097
519100	Other information services	0	0
523000	Securities, commodity contracts, investments, and related activities	0.0054663	0.0000822
524100	Insurance carriers	−0.0547442	0.0000126
524200	Insurance agencies, brokerages, and related activities	0	0
525000	Funds, trusts, and other financial vehicles	0	0
522A00	Nondepository credit intermediation and related activities	0.0005711	0.0000421
52A000	Monetary authorities and depository credit intermediation	0.0741617	0.0002423
531000	Real estate	0.1776128	0.0006363
532100	Automotive equipment rental and leasing	0.0051399	0.0004108
532400	Commercial and industrial machinery and equipment rental and leasing	0.003345	0.000217
532230	Video tape and disc rental	0	0
532A00	General and consumer goods rental except video tapes and discs	0	0.0000316
533000	Lessors of nonfinancial intangible assets	0.0024476	0.001854
S00800	Owner-occupied dwellings	0	0
541100	Legal services	0.0230073	0.0003687
541200	Accounting, tax preparation, bookkeeping, and payroll services	0.0096272	0.0002739
541300	Architectural, engineering, and related services	0.001387	0.0002886
541400	Specialized design services	0.0004079	0.0000253
541511	Custom computer programming services	0	0.000236
541512	Computer systems design services	0.0016317	0.0000527
54151A	Other computer related services, including facilities management	0.0065269	0.0001096
541610	Management, scientific, and technical consulting services	0.000979	0.000788
5416A0	Environmental and other technical consulting services	0	0.0000948
541700	Scientific research and development services	0	0.0021258
541800	Advertising and related services	0.0006527	0.0008406
541920	Photographic services	0	0

(continued)

Commodity-by-industry direct requirements, after redefinitions (in producers' prices)			
Bureau of economic analysis			
2002			
	Commodities/Industries	111910	3122A0
IO code	Name	Tobacco farming	Tob. product manufacturing
541940	Veterinary services	0	0
5419A0	All other miscellaneous professional, scientific, and technical services	0	0.0002676
550000	Management of companies and enterprises	0	0.0281093
561300	Employment services	0.0008974	0.000257
561500	Travel arrangement and reservation services	0	0
561100	Office administrative services	0.0007343	0.0000864
561200	Facilities support services	0	0.0000105
561400	Business support services	0.000979	0.0001643
561600	Investigation and security services	0	0.0000358
561700	Services to buildings and dwellings	0.0043241	0.0002612
561900	Other support services	0	0.0000232
562000	Waste management and remediation services	0	0.000099
611100	Elementary and secondary schools	0	0
611A00	Junior colleges, colleges, universities, and professional schools	0.0032634	0
611B00	Other educational services	0	0
621600	Home health care services	0	0
621A00	Offices of physicians, dentists, and other health practitioners	0	0
621B00	Medical and diagnostic labs and outpatient and other ambulatory care services	0	0
622000	Hospitals	0	0
623000	Nursing and residential care facilities	0	0
624200	Community food, housing, and other relief services, including rehabilitation services	0	0
624400	Child day care services	0	0
624A00	Individual and family services	0	0
713940	Fitness and recreational sports centers	0	0.0000084
713950	Bowling centers	0	0
713A00	Amusement parks, arcades, and gambling industries	0	0
713B00	Other amusement and recreation industries	0	0.0000042
711100	Performing arts companies	0	0
711200	Spectator sports	0	0.0000084
711500	Independent artists, writers, and performers	0	0.0000316
711A00	Promoters of performing arts and sports and agents for public figures	0.0002448	0.0000084
712000	Museums, historical sites, zoos, and parks	0	0
7211A0	Hotels and motels, including casino hotels	0.0001632	0.0000969
721A00	Other accommodations	0	0

(continued)

Commodity-by-industry direct requirements, after redefinitions (in producers' prices)			
Bureau of economic analysis			
2002			
	Commodities/Industries	111910	3122A0
IO code	Name	Tobacco farming	Tob. product manufacturing
722000	Food services and drinking places	0.0006527	0.0002065
811192	Car washes	0	0.0000063
8111A0	Automotive repair and maintenance, except car washes	0.0038345	0.0001685
811200	Electronic and precision equipment repair and maintenance	0.0011422	0.0001032
811300	Commercial and industrial machinery and equipment repair and maintenance	0.0002448	0.0001496
811400	Personal and household goods repair and maintenance	0	0.0000358
812100	Personal care services	0	0
812200	Death care services	0	0
812300	Dry cleaning and laundry services	0	0
812900	Other personal services	0	0
813100	Religious organizations	0	0
813A00	Grantmaking, giving, and social advocacy organizations	0	0
813B00	Civic, social, professional, and similar organizations	0.0017133	0.0000358
814000	Private households	0	0
491000	Postal service	0.0004895	0
S00101	Federal electric utilities	0	0
S00102	Other Federal Government enterprises	0	0
S00201	State and local government passenger transit	0	0
S00202	State and local government electric utilities	0	0
S00203	Other state and local government enterprises	0	0.0000295
S00500	General Federal defense government services	0	0
S00600	General Federal nondefense government services	0	0
S00700	General state and local government services	0	0
S00401	Scrap	0	0
S00402	Used and secondhand goods	0	0
S00300	Noncomparable imports	0	0.0011545
S00900	Rest of the world adjustment	0	0
V00100	Compensation of employees	0.1600718	0.0391386
V00200	Taxes on production and imports, less subsidies	0.0329608	0.1717403
V00300	Gross operating surplus	0.0021212	0.5350924
	Total	1	1

The 1992 and 1997 benchmark files available on this page do not reflect the 1999 and 2003 comprehensive revision of the NIPAs, respectively
Selected data with zero values are not shown
Detail may not add to total due to rounding

Import value ($1,000)

Country	Item	1990		2000		2009		% Increase 2009–1990
Afghanistan	Cigarettes	8,600		13,000	F	48,071		458.9651163
Afghanistan	Tob. prod. nes.	0		0	F	1,828		
Afghanistan	Tob. unmanuf.	0		0	F	0	[a]	
Albania	Cigarettes	550	[a]	21,622		84,559		15274.36364
Albania	Cigars cheroots	0	M	805		77		
Albania	Tob. prod. nes.	0	M	30		48		
Albania	Tob. unmanuf.	9,000	[a]	0		29	F	−99.67777778
Algeria	Cigarettes	24		0		80,309		334520.8333
Algeria	Cigars cheroots	11		0		0	F	−100
Algeria	Tob. prod. nes.	1,152		0		64,750		5520.659722
Algeria	Tob. unmanuf.	10,714		35,651		56,011		422.7832742
American Samoa	Cigarettes	1,963		390	F	6	F	−99.69434539
American Samoa	Cigars cheroots	0		0	F	1	F	
American Samoa	Tob. prod. nes.	0		0	F	1	F	
American Samoa	Tob. unmanuf.	23		0	F	0	F	−100
Angola	Cigarettes	4,400	F	21,000	[a]	17,404	R	295.5454545
Angola	Cigars cheroots	0		0	F	110	R	
Angola	Tob. prod. nes.	0		0	F	1,574	F	
Angola	Tob. unmanuf.	7,000	F	210	[a]	4,224	R	−39.65714286
Antigua and Barbuda	Cigarettes	1,000	F	264	[a]	1,019	R	1.9
Antigua and Barbuda	Cigars cheroots	0	F	15	[a]	11	F	
Antigua and Barbuda	Tob. prod. nes.	0		6	F	25	F	
Antigua and Barbuda	Tob. unmanuf.	0		220	F	6	F	
Argentina	Cigarettes	69		800		223		223.1884058
Argentina	Cigars cheroots	201		3,012		2,939		1362.189055
Argentina	Tob. prod. nes.	870		2,720		26,722		2971.494253
Argentina	Tob. unmanuf.	2,003		6,987		14,285		613.1802297

Armenia	Cigarettes			17,160		53,368	
Armenia	Cigars cheroots			8		360	
Armenia	Tob. prod. nes.			166		18	
Armenia	Tob. unmanuf.			3,246		11,865	
Aruba	Cigarettes	0	M	1,197		28,918	
Aruba	Cigars cheroots	206		15,889		3,269	1486.893204
Aruba	Tob. prod. nes.	2,173		65	a	141	−93.51127474
Aruba	Tob. unmanuf.	180		1,952		2	−98.88888889
Australia	Cigarettes	12,503		39,803		61,170	389.2425818
Australia	Cigars cheroots	7,047		14,257		20,106	185.3128991
Australia	Tob. prod. nes.	8,363		11,160		36,946	341.7792658
Australia	Tob. unmanuf.	42,933		46,093		101,453	136.3054061
Austria	Cigarettes	6,775		27,400		276,834	3986.110701
Austria	Cigars cheroots	398		8,128		20,252	4988.442211
Austria	Tob. prod. nes.	4,770		10,812		14,414	202.1802935
Austria	Tob. unmanuf.	40,416		57,270		49,880	23.41646873
Azerbaijan	Cigarettes			2,654		217,619	
Azerbaijan	Cigars cheroots			0	F	74	
Azerbaijan	Tob. prod. nes.			0	a	610	
Azerbaijan	Tob. unmanuf.			726		4,410	
Bahamas	Cigarettes	2,967		2,643		4,077	37.41152679
Bahamas	Cigars cheroots	399		152		488	22.30576441
Bahamas	Tob. prod. nes.	119		48		46	−61.34453782
Bahamas	Tob. unmanuf.	226		600		115	−49.11504425
Bahrain	Cigarettes	19,000	a	22,725		37,187	95.72105263
Bahrain	Cigars cheroots	250	a	323		758	203.2
Bahrain	Tob. prod. nes.	60	a	432		1,033	1621.666667
Bahrain	Tob. unmanuf.	200	a	486		415	107.5

(continued)

Import value ($1,000)								
Country	Item	1990		2000		2009		% Increase 2009–1990
Bangladesh	Cigarettes	1,209		0	F	1,318	R	9.015715467
Bangladesh	Cigars cheroots	10		70	[a]	25	F	150
Bangladesh	Tob. prod. nes.	447		2,500	[a]	298	F	−33.33333333
Bangladesh	Tob. unmanuf.	2,789		12,000	F	9,200	R	229.867336
Barbados	Cigarettes	332		1,700	[a]	6,259		1785.240964
Barbados	Cigars cheroots	88		435	F	404		359.0909091
Barbados	Tob. prod. nes.	28		43	[a]	213		660.7142857
Barbados	Tob. unmanuf.	571		4	[a]	37		−93.52014011
Belarus	Cigarettes			56,219		11,989		
Belarus	Cigars cheroots			0	[a]	205		
Belarus	Tob. prod. nes.			3,500	F	52,871		
Belarus	Tob. unmanuf.			26,000	F	41,061		
Belgium	Cigarettes			201,343		392,792		
Belgium	Cigars cheroots			25,894		59,616		
Belgium	Tob. prod. nes.			143,017		154,235		
Belgium	Tob. unmanuf.			129,871		596,730		
Belgium–Luxembourg	Cigarettes	54,061						−100
Belgium–Luxembourg	Cigars cheroots	25,609						−100
Belgium–Luxembourg	Tob. prod. nes.	70,953						−100
Belgium–Luxembourg	Tob. unmanuf.	202,250						−100
Belize	Cigarettes	512		377		4,521	F	783.0078125
Belize	Cigars cheroots	5		85		28	F	460
Belize	Tob. prod. nes.	8		30		8	F	0
Belize	Tob. unmanuf.	338		689		87	R	−74.26035503
Benin	Cigarettes	9,000	F	60,000	F	9,266	R	2.955555556
Benin	Cigars cheroots	0	M	800	F	4	F	

Benin	Tob. prod. nes.	800	[a]	988		3,264	R	308
Benin	Tob. unmanuf.	650	[a]	0		327	F	−49.69230769
Bermuda	Cigarettes	2,270		1,900	F	587	R	−74.14096916
Bermuda	Cigars cheroots	640	F	1,900	F	143	R	−77.65625
Bermuda	Tob. prod. nes.	18	[a]	50	F	112	R	522.2222222
Bermuda	Tob. unmanuf.	0		0	M	0	M	
Bhutan	Cigarettes	2		148	F	49	F	2,350
Bhutan	Tob. prod. nes.	4		1	F	176	F	4,300
Bhutan	Tob. unmanuf.	0	M	1	F	1	F	
Bolivia (Plurinational State of)	Cigarettes	164		193		4,551		2,675
Bolivia (Plurinational State of)	Cigars cheroots	2		0		0	F	−100
Bolivia (Plurinational State of)	Tob. prod. nes.	875		12		2,328		166.0571429
Bolivia (Plurinational State of)	Tob. unmanuf.	1,667		2,896		2,008		20.45590882
Bosnia and Herzegovina	Cigarettes			24,800	F	91,351		
Bosnia and Herzegovina	Cigars cheroots			0	M	1		
Bosnia and Herzegovina	Tob. prod. nes.			0	M	1,473		
Bosnia and Herzegovina	Tob. unmanuf.			1,900	F	12,540		
Botswana	Cigarettes	16,756		14,147		40,772		143.3277632
Botswana	Cigars cheroots	2,409		4,373		6,074		152.1378165
Botswana	Tob. prod. nes.	494		2,063		2,861		479.1497976
Botswana	Tob. unmanuf.	117		428		2,613		2133.333333
Brazil	Cigarettes	5		1,943		437		8,640
Brazil	Cigars cheroots	0		1,422		1,383		
Brazil	Tob. prod. nes.	2,433		2,160		3,060		25.77065351
Brazil	Tob. unmanuf.	138		13,768		62,344		45076.81159
British Virgin Islands	Cigarettes	300	[a]	80	F	0	F	−100
British Virgin Islands	Cigars cheroots	0		0	F	0	F	
Brunei Darussalam	Cigarettes	28,500	[a]	13,000	F	15,735	R	−44.78947368

(continued)

Import value ($1,000)								
Country	Item	1990		2000		2009		% Increase 2009–1990
Brunei Darussalam	Cigars cheroots	40	a	1	a	81	F	102.5
Brunei Darussalam	Tob. prod. nes.	0		0	F	6	F	
Brunei Darussalam	Tob. unmanuf.	0		0	F	531	F	
Bulgaria	Cigarettes	13,533		1,400	F	77,642		473.7234907
Bulgaria	Cigars cheroots	463		38	F	1,787		285.9611231
Bulgaria	Tob. prod. nes.	0		2,800	F	4,105		
Bulgaria	Tob. unmanuf.	29,149		26,703		120,795		314.4052969
Burkina Faso	Cigarettes	2,157		243		134		−93.78766806
Burkina Faso	Cigars cheroots	0		0		0	a	
Burkina Faso	Tob. prod. nes.	470	a	9,048		34,342		7206.808511
Burkina Faso	Tob. unmanuf.	1,500	a	11,875		45		−97
Burundi	Cigarettes	0		3		110		
Burundi	Cigars cheroots	0	M	80		0		
Burundi	Tob. prod. nes.	0	M	3	F	0	F	
Burundi	Tob. unmanuf.	0		79		1,227		
Cambodia	Cigarettes	0	M	70,221		193,952	R	
Cambodia	Cigars cheroots	0	M	234		329	R	
Cambodia	Tob. prod. nes.	0		59		24,883	R	
Cambodia	Tob. unmanuf.	0		6,515		9,180	R	
Cameroon	Cigarettes	22		2,951		26,678		121163.6364
Cameroon	Cigars cheroots	5		0		0	F	−100
Cameroon	Tob. prod. nes.	16,322		0		0	F	−100
Cameroon	Tob. unmanuf.	7,211		7,269		227		−96.85203162
Canada	Cigarettes	4,743		12,096		10,821		128.1467426
Canada	Cigars cheroots	1,634		10,367		35,396		2066.21787
Canada	Tob. prod. nes.	9,900		15,934		21,099		113.1212121
Canada	Tob. unmanuf.	6,756		18,157		47,441		602.205447

Cape Verde	Cigarettes	7		1,071		2,325		33114.28571
Cape Verde	Tob. prod. nes.	0	M	0		1		
Cape Verde	Tob. unmanuf.	678		475		777		14.60176991
Cayman Islands	Cigarettes	1,556		690	F	2,522	R	62.08226221
Cayman Islands	Tob. prod. nes.	5		271	F	106	F	2,020
Central African Republic	Cigarettes	413		2,030		0	[a]	−100
Central African Republic	Cigars cheroots	6		10		0	F	−100
Central African Republic	Tob. prod. nes.	68		2,236		5,456		7923.529412
Central African Republic	Tob. unmanuf.	2,378		3,000	F	0	[a]	−100
Chad	Cigarettes	800	F	825	F	1	F	−99.875
Chad	Tob. prod. nes.	0		5,700	F	19,609	R	
Chad	Tob. unmanuf.	250	[a]	5	F	96	F	−61.6
Chile	Cigarettes	90		807		3,844		4171.111111
Chile	Cigars cheroots	4		61		174		4,250
Chile	Tob. prod. nes.	781		1,440		1,311		67.86171575
Chile	Tob. unmanuf.	4,256		8,111		11,333		166.2828947
China	Cigarettes	212,312		526,018		512,989		141.6203512
China	Cigars cheroots	184	[a]	1,145		2,318		1159.782609
China	Tob. prod. nes.	193		10,822		31,981		16470.46632
China	Tob. unmanuf.	108,712		190,255		806,504		641.8721024
China, Hong Kong SAR	Cigarettes	1,036,880		507,826		465,516		−55.10415863
China, Hong Kong SAR	Cigars cheroots	2,137		14,022		36,290		1598.175012
China, Hong Kong SAR	Tob. prod. nes.	7,180		4,762		11,483		59.93036212
China, Hong Kong SAR	Tob. unmanuf.	161,038		22,145		74,944		−53.46191582
China, Macao SAR	Cigarettes	41,506		34,380		51,797		24.79400569
China, Macao SAR	Cigars cheroots	74		2,607		16,258		21870.27027
China, Macao SAR	Tob. prod. nes.	34		7,492		18,530		54,400
China, Macao SAR	Tob. unmanuf.	92		103		130		41.30434783

(continued)

Import value ($1,000)								
Country	Item	1990		2000		2009		% Increase 2009–1990
Colombia	Cigarettes	97		34,093		12,822		13118.5567
Colombia	Cigars cheroots	0		35		56		
Colombia	Tob. prod. nes.	0		9		1,170		
Colombia	Tob. unmanuf.	240		6,648		3,128		1203.333333
Comoros	Cigarettes	200	a	433		377	F	88.5
Comoros	Tob. prod. nes.	0		0		57	R	
Comoros	Tob. unmanuf.	0		2		7	R	
Congo	Cigarettes	70		1	a	460		557.1428571
Congo	Cigars cheroots	2		1	F	9		350
Congo	Tob. prod. nes.	0		26	F	6,753		
Congo	Tob. unmanuf.	3,032		7,739		0	a	−100
Cook Islands	Cigarettes	145		110	F	759	R	423.4482759
Cook Islands	Cigars cheroots	0		1	F	2	F	
Cook Islands	Tob. prod. nes.	2		0	F	137	R	6,750
Costa Rica	Cigarettes	0		2,493		3,407		
Costa Rica	Cigars cheroots	0		47		8		
Costa Rica	Tob. prod. nes.	33		347		597		1709.090909
Costa Rica	Tob. unmanuf.	475		3,509		5,166		987.5789474
Côte d'Ivoire	Cigarettes	1,350	a	75		10,442		673.4814815
Côte d'Ivoire	Cigars cheroots	15	a	33		391		2506.666667
Côte d'Ivoire	Tob. prod. nes.	2,200	a	1,011		487		−77.86363636
Côte d'Ivoire	Tob. unmanuf.	16,047		23,660		77,014		379.9277123
Croatia	Cigarettes			381		34,909		
Croatia	Cigars cheroots			342		1,283		
Croatia	Tob. prod. nes.			10,590		4,353		
Croatia	Tob. unmanuf.			20,287		20,671		
Cuba	Cigarettes	0	M	3,105		78	R	

Cuba	Cigars cheroots	0	M	85		1,275	F	
Cuba	Tob. prod. nes.	0	M	169		121	R	
Cuba	Tob. unmanuf.	3,500	[a]	5,003		564	R	−83.88571429
Cyprus	Cigarettes	1,186		301,414		53,146		4381.112985
Cyprus	Cigars cheroots	835		11,035		8,514		919.6407186
Cyprus	Tob. prod. nes.	6,889		24,992		10,258		48.90404993
Cyprus	Tob. unmanuf.	5,233		7,000	F	0		−100
Czech Republic	Cigarettes			14,361		120,866		
Czech Republic	Cigars cheroots			2,671		8,657		
Czech Republic	Tob. prod. nes.			18,822		34,211		
Czech Republic	Tob. unmanuf.			66,233		69,083		
Czechoslovakia	Cigarettes	10,000	F					−100
Czechoslovakia	Cigars cheroots	130	F					−100
Czechoslovakia	Tob. prod. nes.	0	M					
Czechoslovakia	Tob. unmanuf.	42,146						−100
Democratic People’s Republic of Korea	Cigarettes	3,500	[a]	22,100	F	8,109	R	131.6857143
Democratic People’s Republic of Korea	Tob. unmanuf.	850	[a]	1,800	R	29,725	R	3397.058824
Democratic Republic of the Congo	Cigarettes	0		2,400	F	1,366	F	
Democratic Republic of the Congo	Cigars cheroots	0		159	R	1,271	R	
Democratic Republic of the Congo	Tob. prod. nes.	0		415	R	1,520	F	
Democratic Republic of the Congo	Tob. unmanuf.	1,600	[a]	950	F	806	R	−49.625
Denmark	Cigarettes	2,560		9,482		36,882		1340.703125
Denmark	Cigars cheroots	1,506		4,761		9,214		511.8193891
Denmark	Tob. prod. nes.	3,142		1,150		10,647		238.8605983
Denmark	Tob. unmanuf.	90,031		90,754		89,181		−0.944119248
Djibouti	Cigarettes	5,571		36,655	[a]	1,928	R	−65.39220966
Djibouti	Cigars cheroots	6		28	F	3	F	−50
Djibouti	Tob. prod. nes.	0		0	F	92	F	

(continued)

Import value ($1,000)								
Country	Item	1990		2000		2009		% Increase 2009–1990
Djibouti	Tob. unmanuf.	146		90	F	9,415	R	6348.630137
Dominica	Cigarettes	101		81		186	F	84.15841584
Dominica	Cigars cheroots	0	M	2		3	F	
Dominica	Tob. prod. nes.	0	M	0	M	0	F	
Dominica	Tob. unmanuf.	108		1		123	F	13.88888889
Dominican Republic	Cigarettes	270	a	630	F	3,496	F	1194.814815
Dominican Republic	Cigars cheroots	0		0	F	4,268	R	
Dominican Republic	Tob. prod. nes.	8	a	510	F	7,095	R	88587.5
Dominican Republic	Tob. unmanuf.	400	a	0	F	129,631	R	32307.75
Ecuador	Cigarettes	0		369		237		
Ecuador	Cigars cheroots	0	M	1		2	F	
Ecuador	Tob. prod. nes.	0		57		646		
Ecuador	Tob. unmanuf.	11		1,315		2,196		19863.63636
Egypt	Cigarettes	1,375		10		56,254		3991.2
Egypt	Cigars cheroots	133		43		187		40.60150376
Egypt	Tob. prod. nes.	0		92,516		162,957		
Egypt	Tob. unmanuf.	90,028		174,983		23,000		−74.45239259
El Salvador	Cigarettes	70	a	7,307		13,926		19794.28571
El Salvador	Cigars cheroots	0		244		132		
El Salvador	Tob. prod. nes.	978	a	85		2		−99.79550102
El Salvador	Tob. unmanuf.	598		179		123		−79.43143813
Equatorial Guinea	Tob. unmanuf.	0		0	F	0	F	
Estonia	Cigarettes			24,184		33,733		
Estonia	Cigars cheroots			92		1,591		
Estonia	Tob. prod. nes.			503		1,566		
Estonia	Tob. unmanuf.			16		2	F	
Ethiopia	Cigarettes			1,211		3,825		

Ethiopia	Cigars cheroots		26		187		
Ethiopia	Tob. prod. nes.		0	M	0	[a]	
Ethiopia	Tob. unmanuf.		1,488		8,265		
Ethiopia PDR	Cigarettes	284					−100
Ethiopia PDR	Cigars cheroots	6					−100
Ethiopia PDR	Tob. prod. nes.	46					−100
Ethiopia PDR	Tob. unmanuf.	1,870					−100
Faroe Islands	Cigarettes	1,268	2,800	F	2,597		104.8107256
Faroe Islands	Cigars cheroots	83	61	R	49		−40.96385542
Faroe Islands	Tob. prod. nes.	326	399	R	634		94.47852761
Faroe Islands	Tob. unmanuf.	0	49	R	7	F	
Fiji	Cigarettes	234	408		943		302.991453
Fiji	Cigars cheroots	35	50		85		142.8571429
Fiji	Tob. prod. nes.	10	24		94		840
Fiji	Tob. unmanuf.	1,416	537		156		−88.98305085
Finland	Cigarettes	1,236	24,263		100,717		8048.624595
Finland	Cigars cheroots	3,316	13,675		27,024		714.9577805
Finland	Tob. prod. nes.	9,801	14,052		16,675		70.13570044
Finland	Tob. unmanuf.	42,093	18,148		0	F	−100
France	Cigarettes	811,097	1,114,410		1,631,120		101.1004849
France	Cigars cheroots	94,697	127,627		217,725		129.9175264
France	Tob. prod. nes.	26,413	83,334		283,134		971.9494188
France	Tob. unmanuf.	115,862	129,296		177,052		52.81282906
French Polynesia	Cigarettes	1,559	1,506		2,614		67.67158435
French Polynesia	Cigars cheroots	27	19		17		−37.03703704
French Polynesia	Tob. prod. nes.	1,908	1,937		2,598		36.16352201
Gabon	Cigarettes	505	2,108		5,775	R	1043.564356
Gabon	Cigars cheroots	42	35		91	F	116.6666667

(continued)

Import value ($1,000)								
Country	Item	1990		2000		2009		% Increase 2009–1990
Gabon	Tob. prod. nes.	2,710		6,930		1,250	F	–53.87453875
Gabon	Tob. unmanuf.	335		218		18,253	R	5348.656716
Gambia	Cigarettes	3,000	a	2,679		3,337		11.23333333
Gambia	Cigars cheroots	0	M	49		4	F	
Gambia	Tob. prod. nes.	0		23		32		
Gambia	Tob. unmanuf.	2,800	F	118		103		–96.32142857
Georgia	Cigarettes			29,388		57,160		
Georgia	Cigars cheroots			3		265		
Georgia	Tob. prod. nes.			54		16,775		
Georgia	Tob. unmanuf.			4,225		5,111		
Germany	Cigarettes	141,810		406,245		904,899		538.1066215
Germany	Cigars cheroots	27,661		58,814		78,900		185.2391454
Germany	Tob. prod. nes.	137,111		188,598		378,023		175.705815
Germany	Tob. unmanuf.	683,275		896,848		981,898		43.70465771
Ghana	Cigarettes	0		26,939		8,387	F	
Ghana	Cigars cheroots	0		10		10	F	
Ghana	Tob. prod. nes.	0	M	1		2	R	
Ghana	Tob. unmanuf.	7,000	a	2,985		0	F	–100
Greece	Cigarettes	52,233		112,151		276,189		428.7634254
Greece	Cigars cheroots	1,386		7,574		25,514		1740.836941
Greece	Tob. prod. nes.	5,228		19,888		46,206		783.8179036
Greece	Tob. unmanuf.	51,348		128,224		210,651		310.2418789
Grenada	Cigarettes	93		388		1,359		1361.290323
Grenada	Cigars cheroots	0		21	F	16		
Grenada	Tob. prod. nes.	17		2	F	3		–82.35294118
Grenada	Tob. unmanuf.	48		65	F	21		–56.25

Guam	Cigarettes	9,000	F	963	R	0	F	−100
Guam	Cigars cheroots	70	F	20	F	0	F	−100
Guam	Tob. prod. nes.	0		42	F	0	F	
Guatemala	Cigarettes	0		2,408		9,323		
Guatemala	Cigars cheroots	68		45		218		220.5882353
Guatemala	Tob. prod. nes.	0	M	114		1,082		
Guatemala	Tob. unmanuf.	780		794		6,023		672.1794872
Guinea	Cigarettes	3,450		22,877		33,279	F	864.6086957
Guinea	Cigars cheroots	0	M	146		8	F	
Guinea	Tob. prod. nes.	1,500	[a]	5		7	F	−99.53333333
Guinea	Tob. unmanuf.	140	F	510		0	F	−100
Guinea–Bissau	Cigarettes	140	[a]	780	F	3,212	R	2194.285714
Guinea–Bissau	Cigars cheroots	0		0	F	0	F	
Guinea–Bissau	Tob. prod. nes.	0		220	F	0	F	
Guinea–Bissau	Tob. unmanuf.	0		250	F	394	F	
Guyana	Cigarettes	680	[a]	3,244		5,092	R	648.8235294
Guyana	Cigars cheroots	0		0		87	R	
Guyana	Tob. prod. nes.	0		0	F	56	R	
Guyana	Tob. unmanuf.	750	F	0		241	F	−67.86666667
Haiti	Cigarettes	1,100	[a]	1,480	[a]	172	R	−84.36363636
Haiti	Tob. prod. nes.	0		90	[a]	160	R	
Haiti	Tob. unmanuf.	430	[a]	1,200	[a]	1,973	R	358.8372093
Honduras	Cigarettes	330	F	723		3,509		963.3333333
Honduras	Cigars cheroots	0		1,026		1,190		
Honduras	Tob. prod. nes.	0		251		338		
Honduras	Tob. unmanuf.	3,000	[a]	27,570		18,296		509.8666667
Hungary	Cigarettes	13,482		4,724		0	F	−100
Hungary	Cigars cheroots	154		520		0	F	−100

(continued)

Import value ($1,000)

Country	Item	1990		2000		2009		% Increase 2009–1990
Hungary	Tob. prod. nes.	123		3,847		21,959		17752.84553
Hungary	Tob. unmanuf.	13,834		29,973		29,242		111.3777649
Iceland	Cigarettes	9,558		12,383		15,911		66.46788031
Iceland	Cigars cheroots	1,551		1,234		1,607		3.610573823
Iceland	Tob. prod. nes.	242		272		356		47.10743802
Iceland	Tob. unmanuf.	75		0		0	F	−100
India	Cigarettes	850		601		10,385		1121.764706
India	Cigars cheroots	50		158		843		1,586
India	Tob. prod. nes.	0		14		5,044		
India	Tob. unmanuf.	68		3,897		7,804		11376.47059
Indonesia	Cigarettes	157		1,715		3,003		1812.738854
Indonesia	Cigars cheroots	0		93		871		
Indonesia	Tob. prod. nes.	5,101		47,052		71,724		1306.07724
Indonesia	Tob. unmanuf.	41,964		114,834		290,171		591.4760271
Iran (Islamic Republic of)	Cigarettes	120,000	F	162,000	F	233,117	R	94.26416667
Iran (Islamic Republic of)	Cigars cheroots	0		0		2,941	R	
Iran (Islamic Republic of)	Tob. prod. nes.	0		1,579		35,180	F	
Iran (Islamic Republic of)	Tob. prod. nes.	0		14,423		67,176	R	
Iraq	Cigarettes	75,000	F	0		177,995	R	137.3266667
Iraq	Cigars cheroots	0		0	F	793	F	
Iraq	Tob. prod. nes.	2,600	a	0	F	1,800	F	−30.76923077
Iraq	Tob. unmanuf.	55,000	F	11,000	F	34	F	−99.93818182
Ireland	Cigarettes	6,427		14,064		74,283		1055.795861
Ireland	Cigars cheroots	7,082		6,508		9,174		29.53967806
Ireland	Tob. prod. nes.	16,420		25,667		29,708		80.92570037
Ireland	Tob. unmanuf.	22,200		23,748		15,163		−31.6981982
Israel	Cigarettes	39,406		94,113		153,317		289.0701924

Israel	Cigars cheroots	321	2,043		1,787	456.6978193
Israel	Tob. prod. nes.	400	1,296		3,562	790.5
Israel	Tob. unmanuf.	23,145	16,416		6,301	−72.77597753
Italy	Cigarettes	918,004	1,118,740		2,951,660	221.5301894
Italy	Cigars cheroots	13,107	18,457		13,636	4.036011292
Italy	Tob. prod. nes.	8,545	22,280		44,707	423.1948508
Italy	Tob. unmanuf.	181,997	139,316		57,447	−68.43519399
Jamaica	Cigarettes	45	400	F	6,779	14964.44444
Jamaica	Cigars cheroots	35	0	F	143	308.5714286
Jamaica	Tob. prod. nes.	5	0	F	106	2,020
Jamaica	Tob. unmanuf.	5,041	2,500	[a]	53	−98.94862131
Japan	Cigarettes	1,034,540	2,361,590		3,279,620	217.012392
Japan	Cigars cheroots	2,072	6,866		9,289	348.3108108
Japan	Tob. prod. nes.	13,629	15,917		27,941	105.0113728
Japan	Tob. unmanuf.	449,602	519,549		400,572	−10.9052006
Jordan	Cigarettes	2,224	9,465		145	−93.48021583
Jordan	Cigars cheroots	524	91		14	−97.32824427
Jordan	Tob. prod. nes.	103	22,109		55,761	54036.8932
Jordan	Tob. unmanuf.	7,742	6,275		15,159	95.80211832
Kazakhstan	Cigarettes		5,129		95,951	
Kazakhstan	Cigars cheroots		23		421	
Kazakhstan	Tob. prod. nes.		9,544		16,144	
Kazakhstan	Tob. unmanuf.		29,354		52,086	
Kenya	Cigarettes	252	756		1,809	617.8571429
Kenya	Cigars cheroots	131	54		121	−7.633587786
Kenya	Tob. prod. nes.	22	17		239	986.3636364
Kenya	Tob. unmanuf.	0	5,614		37,147	
Kiribati	Cigarettes	0	750	[a]	639	

(continued)

Import value ($1,000)								
Country	Item	1990		2000		2009		% Increase 2009–1990
Kiribati	Cigars cheroots	0	M	35	[a]	2	F	
Kiribati	Tob. prod. nes.	440		1,300	F	2,188		397.2727273
Kuwait	Cigarettes	35,437		32,155		62,129	R	75.32240314
Kuwait	Cigars cheroots	202		112		179	R	−11.38613861
Kuwait	Tob. prod. nes.	1,191		2,658		391	F	−67.170445
Kuwait	Tob. unmanuf.	0	F	40		35	R	
Kyrgyzstan	Cigarettes			11,002		31,042	R	
Kyrgyzstan	Cigars cheroots			20		58	R	
Kyrgyzstan	Tob. prod. nes.			110		0	F	
Kyrgyzstan	Tob. unmanuf.			2,353		5,512	R	
Lao People's Democratic Republic	Cigarettes	0		14,697	[a]	5,249	R	
Lao People's Democratic Republic	Cigars cheroots	0		0	F	47	F	
Lao People's Democratic Republic	Tob. prod. nes.	0		847	[a]	318	F	
Lao People's Democratic Republic	Tob. unmanuf.	410	[a]	170	F	407	F	−0.731707317
Latvia	Cigarettes			39,588		57,752		
Latvia	Cigars cheroots			352		1,683		
Latvia	Tob. prod. nes.			466		624		
Latvia	Tob. unmanuf.			6,235		1,760		
Lebanon	Cigarettes	90,000	F	105,183		167,901		86.55666667
Lebanon	Cigars cheroots	1,850	[a]	321		5,548		199.8918919
Lebanon	Tob. prod. nes.	0		1,619		8,913		
Lebanon	Tob. unmanuf.	0	[a]	2,146		1,070		
Lesotho	Tob. prod. nes.	8,500	F	9,200	F	11,700	F	37.64705882
Liberia	Cigarettes	2,300	[a]	3,000	F	6,731	R	192.6521739
Liberia	Cigars cheroots	15	F	15	F	31	F	106.6666667
Liberia	Tob. prod. nes.	0		0	F	249	F	

Liberia	Tob. unmanuf.	650	[a]	1,550	F	1,194	R	83.69230769
Libya	Cigarettes	1,299		13,900	F	5,223	F	302.0785219
Libya	Cigars cheroots	17		18	[a]	11	F	−35.29411765
Libya	Tob. prod. nes.	74		2,900	F	3,959	F	5,250
Libya	Tob. unmanuf.	4,734		82,233		7,559	R	59.67469371
Lithuania	Cigarettes			10,518		49,467		
Lithuania	Cigars cheroots			95		8,152		
Lithuania	Tob. prod. nes.			19,493		23,871		
Lithuania	Tob. unmanuf.			5,142		58,436		
Luxembourg	Cigarettes			107,896		109,584		
Luxembourg	Cigars cheroots			8,086		11,552		
Luxembourg	Tob. prod. nes.			69,860		79,883		
Luxembourg	Tob. unmanuf.			13,340		32,675		
Madagascar	Cigarettes	313		226		480		53.35463259
Madagascar	Cigars cheroots	19		9		35		84.21052632
Madagascar	Tob. prod. nes.	1		0		829		82,800
Madagascar	Tob. unmanuf.	774		930		3,943		409.4315245
Malawi	Cigarettes	4		0		4,864		121,500
Malawi	Cigars cheroots	1		0		1		0
Malawi	Tob. prod. nes.	4		0		34		750
Malawi	Tob. unmanuf.	0		9,369		53,464		
Malaysia	Cigarettes	17,966		23,137		62,962		250.4508516
Malaysia	Cigars cheroots	351		1,381		18,949		5298.575499
Malaysia	Tob. prod. nes.	2,259		12,382		24,082		966.0469234
Malaysia	Tob. unmanuf.	30,030		96,063		206,143		586.4568765
Maldives	Cigarettes	7,000	[a]	3,100	F	13,235	R	89.07142857
Maldives	Cigars cheroots	0		7	[a]	230	F	
Maldives	Tob. prod. nes.	0	F	8	F	188	R	

(continued)

Import value ($1,000)

Country	Item	1990		2000		2009		% Increase 2009–1990
Maldives	Tob. unmanuf.	0		20	[a]	73	R	
Mali	Cigarettes	5,300	[a]	6,001		13,355	R	151.9811321
Mali	Cigars cheroots	0	M	0	M	8	F	
Mali	Tob. prod. nes.	860	[a]	203		5,658	R	557.9069767
Mali	Tob. unmanuf.	3,500	[a]	396		7	F	−99.8
Malta	Cigarettes	1,934		7,222		18,977		881.2306101
Malta	Cigars cheroots	419		768		677		61.575179
Malta	Tob. prod. nes.	4,224		13,175		769		−81.79450758
Malta	Tob. unmanuf.	3,003		166		42		−98.6013986
Mauritania	Cigarettes	1,400	[a]	13,286	[a]	16,264	R	1061.714286
Mauritania	Cigars cheroots	0		274	[a]	1	F	
Mauritania	Tob. prod. nes.	0		3	F	137	R	
Mauritania	Tob. unmanuf.	750	F	593	[a]	203	F	−72.93333333
Mauritius	Cigarettes	273		2,261		38,010		13823.07692
Mauritius	Cigars cheroots	60		236		390		550
Mauritius	Tob. prod. nes.	3		5		28		833.3333333
Mauritius	Tob. unmanuf.	159		130		0	F	−100
Mexico	Cigarettes	6		4,032		12,502		208266.6667
Mexico	Cigars cheroots	324		5,811		2,887		791.0493827
Mexico	Tob. prod. nes.	17		2,111		4,782		28029.41176
Mexico	Tob. unmanuf.	40,963		37,612		144,465		252.6719234
Mongolia	Cigarettes	0	M	9,173		33,977	R	
Mongolia	Cigars cheroots	0	M	10		34	F	
Mongolia	Tob. prod. nes.	40	[a]	1,192		3,559	R	8797.5
Montenegro	Cigarettes					28,148		
Montenegro	Cigars cheroots					270		
Montenegro	Tob. prod. nes.					3	F	

Montenegro	Tob. unmanuf.					88		
Morocco	Cigarettes	29,955		44,109		59,572		98.87164079
Morocco	Cigars cheroots	454		342		1,403		209.030837
Morocco	Tob. prod. nes.	154		491		5,548		3502.597403
Morocco	Tob. unmanuf.	13,173		12,907		53,306		304.6610491
Mozambique	Cigarettes	0		0	F	12,640	R	
Mozambique	Cigars cheroots	0		0	F	119	R	
Mozambique	Tob. prod. nes.	0		0	F	768	R	
Mozambique	Tob. unmanuf.	1,300	a	320	F	11,766	R	805.0769231
Myanmar	Cigarettes	33,000	a	17,400	F	8,483	R	−74.29393939
Myanmar	Tob. prod. nes.	0		17,600	F	14,900	F	
Myanmar	Tob. unmanuf.	0		1,250	F	1,659	R	
Namibia	Cigarettes	0	M	4,578		4,865	R	
Namibia	Cigars cheroots	0	M	136		55	R	
Namibia	Tob. prod. nes.	0	M	1,645		143	R	
Namibia	Tob. unmanuf.	0	M	654		32	F	
Nauru	Tob. prod. nes.	210	F	220	F	1	F	−99.52380952
Nepal	Cigarettes	60		713		727		1111.666667
Nepal	Cigars cheroots	0	M	0	M	0	a	
Nepal	Tob. prod. nes.	565		105		44		−92.21238938
Nepal	Tob. unmanuf.	7,710		8,664		18,540		140.4669261
Netherlands	Cigarettes	184,706		169,828		350,931		89.99436943
Netherlands	Cigars cheroots	82,847		93,620		189,248		128.4307217
Netherlands	Tob. prod. nes.	47,978		67,722		103,448		115.6154904
Netherlands	Tob. unmanuf.	436,567		748,181		763,764		74.94771707
Netherlands Antilles	Cigarettes	3,943		690	F	3,100	R	−21.37966016
Netherlands Antilles	Cigars cheroots	521		140	F	1,490	R	185.9884837
Netherlands Antilles	Tob. prod. nes.	149		830	F	1,345	R	802.6845638

(continued)

Import value ($1,000)								
Country	Item	1990		2000		2009		% Increase 2009–1990
Netherlands Antilles	Tob. unmanuf.	0		1,064	F	799	F	
New Caledonia	Cigarettes	0	M	6,500	F	11,367		
New Caledonia	Cigars cheroots	0	M	89	F	389		
New Caledonia	Tob. prod. nes.	7,000	[a]	5,500	F	2,259		−67.72857143
New Zealand	Cigarettes	582		3,893		32,433		5472.680412
New Zealand	Cigars cheroots	290		1,722		2,477		754.137931
New Zealand	Tob. prod. nes.	766		547		12,908		1585.117493
New Zealand	Tob. unmanuf.	14,092		12,765		7,137		−49.35424354
Nicaragua	Cigarettes	0		9,568		20,520		
Nicaragua	Cigars cheroots	60	F	4		3		−95
Nicaragua	Tob. prod. nes.	0		0		1		
Nicaragua	Tob. unmanuf.	65	F	246		10		−84.61538462
Niger	Cigarettes	11,078	[a]	9,947		39,568	R	257.1763856
Niger	Cigars cheroots	0		1		70	F	
Niger	Tob. prod. nes.	0		1		0	F	
Niger	Tob. unmanuf.	2		16		10	F	400
Nigeria	Cigarettes	483		16,389		19,172	R	3869.358178
Nigeria	Cigars cheroots	76		0		8,627	F	11251.31579
Nigeria	Tob. prod. nes.	1,146		13		50	R	−95.63699825
Nigeria	Tob. unmanuf.	9,290		7,303		45,485	R	389.6124865
Niue	Tob. prod. nes.	42	F	0	F	0	F	−100
Norfolk Island	Cigarettes	78		70	F	0	F	−100
Norfolk Island	Cigars cheroots	9		0	F	0	F	−100
Norfolk Island	Tob. prod. nes.	7		3	F	0	F	−100
Norway	Cigarettes	39,003		24,234		88,252		126.2697741
Norway	Cigars cheroots	2,850		3,289		4,975		74.56140351
Norway	Tob. prod. nes.	6,827		9,464		52,583		670.2211806

Norway	Tob. unmanuf.	25,043		19,269		0	[a]	−100
Occupied Palestinian Territory	Cigarettes	0	M	774	[a]	12,942	R	
Occupied Palestinian Territory	Tob. prod. nes.	0	M	159		113	F	
Occupied Palestinian Territory	Tob. unmanuf.	0	M	1,701		6,500	F	
Oman	Cigarettes	21,246		385,820		82,509		288.3507484
Oman	Cigars cheroots	170		45		659		287.6470588
Oman	Tob. prod. nes.	168		62		869		417.2619048
Oman	Tob. unmanuf.	150		3,801		11		−92.66666667
Pacific Islands Trust Territory	Cigarettes	1,300	F					−100
Pacific Islands Trust Territory	Cigars cheroots	0						
Pacific Islands Trust Territory	Tob. unmanuf.	0						
Pakistan	Cigarettes	38		119		439		1055.263158
Pakistan	Cigars cheroots	1		10		261		26,000
Pakistan	Tob. prod. nes.	11		82		87		690.9090909
Pakistan	Tob. unmanuf.	568		110		11,894		1994.014085
Panama	Cigarettes	2		4,412		7,531		376,450
Panama	Cigars cheroots	61		278		302		395.0819672
Panama	Tob. prod. nes.	1,302		15		42		−96.77419355
Panama	Tob. unmanuf.	660		118		73		−88.93939394
Papua New Guinea	Cigarettes	29		1		38	R	31.03448276
Papua New Guinea	Cigars cheroots	22		1		10	F	−54.54545455
Papua New Guinea	Tob. prod. nes.	1,837		2,710		6,087	R	231.3554709
Papua New Guinea	Tob. unmanuf.	3,313		95		352	R	−89.37518865
Paraguay	Cigarettes	23,399		95,554		26,312		12.44924997
Paraguay	Cigars cheroots	25		356		618		2,372
Paraguay	Tob. prod. nes.	239		15,545		6,230		2506.694561
Paraguay	Tob. unmanuf.	1,471		28,469		100,486		6731.135282
Peru	Cigarettes	0		5,534		27,643		

(continued)

Import value ($1,000)

Country	Item	1990		2000	2009		% Increase 2009–1990
Peru	Cigars cheroots	2		84	63		3,050
Peru	Tob. prod. nes.	0		4	14		
Peru	Tob. unmanuf.	561		3,286	3		−99.46524064
Philippines	Cigarettes	6,602		40,110	5,232		−20.75128749
Philippines	Cigars cheroots	20		762	171		755
Philippines	Tob. prod. nes.	2		214	1,163		58,050
Philippines	Tob. unmanuf.	60,715		109,848	192,892		217.7007329
Poland	Cigarettes	36,855		1,037	43,803		18.85225885
Poland	Cigars cheroots	0	M	394	3,132		
Poland	Tob. prod. nes.	0		9,519	63,340		
Poland	Tob. unmanuf.	32,303		79,952	328,830		917.9549887
Portugal	Cigarettes	1,396		17,647	40,618		2809.598854
Portugal	Cigars cheroots	668		4,362	13,588		1934.131737
Portugal	Tob. prod. nes.	238		19,450	28,476		11864.70588
Portugal	Tob. unmanuf.	27,611		58,757	30,381		10.03223353
Qatar	Cigarettes	13,195		15,472	26,107	R	97.8552482
Qatar	Cigars cheroots	102		48	272	R	166.6666667
Qatar	Tob. prod. nes.	850		101	691	R	−18.70588235
Qatar	Tob. unmanuf.	102		91	17	R	−83.33333333
Republic of Korea	Cigarettes	103,967		207,998	11,027		−89.39374994
Republic of Korea	Cigars cheroots	164		742	738		350
Republic of Korea	Tob. prod. nes.	37		6	91,966		248456.7568
Republic of Korea	Tob. unmanuf.	36,891		73,870	242,882		558.377382
Republic of Moldova	Cigarettes			48,012	76,539		
Republic of Moldova	Cigars cheroots			10	239		
Republic of Moldova	Tob. prod. nes.			214	1,007		

Republic of Moldova	Tob. unmanuf.			6,127		10,333		
Romania	Cigarettes	20,921		52,439		77,891		272.310119
Romania	Cigars cheroots	0		385		1,834		
Romania	Tob. prod. nes.	2,495		7,009		28,229		1031.422846
Romania	Tob. unmanuf.	6,016		68,991		154,063		2460.887633
Russian Federation	Cigarettes			163,743		114,745		
Russian Federation	Cigars cheroots			2,691		18,831		
Russian Federation	Tob. prod. nes.			40,401		40,613		
Russian Federation	Tob. unmanuf.			517,091		1,040,980		
Rwanda	Cigarettes	73		50	F	3,871		5202.739726
Rwanda	Cigars cheroots	0		0	F	20		
Rwanda	Tob. prod. nes.	0		0	F	93		
Rwanda	Tob. unmanuf.	1,435		1,300	F	952		−33.65853659
Saint Kitts and Nevis	Cigarettes	700	F	305		346	R	−50.57142857
Saint Kitts and Nevis	Cigars cheroots	0	M	0	M	130	F	
Saint Kitts and Nevis	Tob. unmanuf.	0	M	0		11	F	
Saint Lucia	Cigarettes	599		1,415		3,929	F	555.9265442
Saint Lucia	Cigars cheroots	23		25		142	F	517.3913043
Saint Lucia	Tob. prod. nes.	18		0		36	F	100
Saint Lucia	Tob. unmanuf.	130		34		97	R	−25.38461538
Saint Pierre and Miquelon	Cigarettes	590	[a]	0		787	R	33.38983051
Saint Pierre and Miquelon	Cigars cheroots	12	F	0		6	F	−50
Saint Pierre and Miquelon	Tob. prod. nes.	150	[a]	0		0	F	−100
Saint Vincent and the Grenadines	Cigarettes	241		716	F	1,195		395.8506224
Saint Vincent and the Grenadines	Cigars cheroots	0	M	0	M	12		
Saint Vincent and the Grenadines	Tob. prod. nes.	0	M	0	M	0		
Saint Vincent and the Grenadines	Tob. unmanuf.	64		73	F	60		−6.25
Samoa	Cigarettes	239		22	F	9	F	−96.23430962

(continued)

Import value ($1,000)								
Country	Item	1990		2000		2009		% Increase 2009–1990
Samoa	Cigars cheroots	0		0	F	0	F	
Samoa	Tob. prod. nes.	951		527		871	R	−8.412197687
Sao Tome and Principe	Cigarettes	150	[a]	29	[a]	151		0.666666667
Sao Tome and Principe	Cigars cheroots	0		0	F	0		
Sao Tome and Principe	Tob. prod. nes.	0		0	F	0	F	
Saudi Arabia	Cigarettes	261,259		298,800		513,490		96.54442526
Saudi Arabia	Cigars cheroots	549		439		321		−41.53005464
Saudi Arabia	Tob. prod. nes.	12,339		12,967		0	[a]	−100
Saudi Arabia	Tob. unmanuf.	3,380		998		6,307	F	86.59763314
Senegal	Cigarettes	1,334		9		2,198		64.76761619
Senegal	Cigars cheroots	33		0		179		442.4242424
Senegal	Tob. prod. nes.	105		34		1,689		1508.571429
Senegal	Tob. unmanuf.	20,030		21,786		43,508		117.2141787
Serbia	Cigarettes					48,655		
Serbia	Cigars cheroots					713		
Serbia	Tob. prod. nes.					870		
Serbia	Tob. unmanuf.					3,704		
Serbia and Montenegro	Cigarettes			19,797				
Serbia and Montenegro	Cigars cheroots			253				
Serbia and Montenegro	Tob. prod. nes.			49				
Serbia and Montenegro	Tob. unmanuf.			14,640				
Seychelles	Cigarettes	459		494		625	R	36.16557734
Seychelles	Cigars cheroots	17		99		4	F	−76.47058824
Seychelles	Tob. prod. nes.	25		14		0	F	−100
Seychelles	Tob. unmanuf.	441		92		212	R	−51.92743764
Sierra Leone	Cigarettes	210	F	6,381	[a]	7,855	R	3640.47619
Sierra Leone	Cigars cheroots	0	M	0	M	41	F	

Sierra Leone	Tob. prod. nes.	0	M	0	M	52	R	
Sierra Leone	Tob. unmanuf.	2,800	F	0	F	218	F	−92.21428571
Singapore	Cigarettes	432,877		594,714		394,899		−8.773392904
Singapore	Cigars cheroots	1,019		3,857		4,599		351.3248283
Singapore	Tob. prod. nes.	2,144		5,730		18,624		768.6567164
Singapore	Tob. unmanuf.	57,210		26,542		53,169		−7.063450446
Slovakia	Cigarettes			37,204		66,184		
Slovakia	Cigars cheroots			916		2,805		
Slovakia	Tob. prod. nes.			7,452		598		
Slovakia	Tob. unmanuf.			14,497		2,761		
Slovenia	Cigarettes			37,204		96,468		
Slovenia	Cigars cheroots			916		1,673		
Slovenia	Tob. prod. nes.			7,452		1,011		
Slovenia	Tob. unmanuf.			14,497		35		
Solomon Islands	Cigarettes	500	[a]	1,100	F	32	F	−93.6
Solomon Islands	Cigars cheroots	0		0	F	1	F	
Solomon Islands	Tob. prod. nes.	0		50	F	3,007	R	
Solomon Islands	Tob. unmanuf.	305		100	F	96	R	−68.52459016
Somalia	Tob. prod. nes.	1,500	F	500	F	138	F	−90.8
Somalia	Tob. unmanuf.	630	F	1,780		24	F	−96.19047619
South Africa	Cigarettes	11,267		2,331		19,932		76.9060087
South Africa	Cigars cheroots	1,592		2,504		3,550		122.9899497
South Africa	Tob. prod. nes.	887		929		20,942		2260.992108
South Africa	Tob. unmanuf.	40,857		42,730		191,453		368.5928972
Spain	Cigarettes	14,186		124,171		1,512,900		10564.73988
Spain	Cigars cheroots	8,601		50,910		137,661		1500.523195
Spain	Tob. prod. nes.	31,403		19,854		178,423		468.1718307
Spain	Tob. unmanuf.	318,114		301,667		145,172		−54.36478747

(continued)

Import value ($1,000)								
Country	Item	1990		2000		2009		% Increase 2009–1990
Sri Lanka	Cigarettes	1,800		5,345		889		–50.61111111
Sri Lanka	Cigars cheroots	10		39		592		5,820
Sri Lanka	Tob. prod. nes.	1		61		2,051		205,000
Sri Lanka	Tob. unmanuf.	3,101		44,098		39,238		1165.333763
Sudan	Cigarettes	6,000	F	99		26,917	R	348.6166667
Sudan	Cigars cheroots	0		0	M	240	R	
Sudan	Tob. prod. nes.	2,400	a	112	a	66	F	–97.25
Sudan	Tob. unmanuf.	600	F	11,954		12,930	R	2,055
Suriname	Cigarettes	44		12,300	F	491	F	1015.909091
Suriname	Cigars cheroots	15		1,015	F	827	R	5413.333333
Suriname	Tob. prod. nes.	518		86	a	85	F	–83.59073359
Suriname	Tob. unmanuf.	1,561		4,300	F	0	F	–100
Swaziland	Cigarettes	1,576	a	1,172		2,846	F	80.58375635
Swaziland	Cigars cheroots	254	a	123		29	F	–88.58267717
Swaziland	Tob. prod. nes.	0	M	917		18	F	
Swaziland	Tob. unmanuf.	48		47		3,051	F	6256.25
Sweden	Cigarettes	62,727		65,911		135,387		115.8352862
Sweden	Cigars cheroots	3,479		5,971		6,272		80.28169014
Sweden	Tob. prod. nes.	12,042		3,549		9,520		–20.94336489
Sweden	Tob. unmanuf.	50,926		30,918		15,503		–69.55778973
Switzerland	Cigarettes	6,425		2,679		15,525		141.6342412
Switzerland	Cigars cheroots	12,058		22,647		37,217		208.649859
Switzerland	Tob. prod. nes.	14,390		17,312		48,311		235.7261987
Switzerland	Tob. unmanuf.	148,006		189,483		267,381		80.65551397
Syrian Arab Republic	Cigarettes	0		8,397		132,458	R	
Syrian Arab Republic	Cigars cheroots	0		0	F	784	R	

Syrian Arab Republic	Tob. prod. nes.	0		1,822	F	12,084	F	
Syrian Arab Republic	Tob. unmanuf.	0		4,596		0	F	
Tajikistan	Cigarettes			30	F	1,600	F	
Tajikistan	Tob. unmanuf.			175	R	200	F	
Thailand	Cigarettes	9,728		63,334		80,801		730.6023849
Thailand	Cigars cheroots	448		937		1,480		230.3571429
Thailand	Tob. prod. nes.	181		179		710		292.2651934
Thailand	Tob. unmanuf.	55,989		57,762		23,625		−57.80421154
The former Yugoslav Republic of Macedonia	Cigarettes			1,659		8,401		
The former Yugoslav Republic of Macedonia	Cigars cheroots			9		107		
The former Yugoslav Republic of Macedonia	Tob. prod. nes.			701		120		
The former Yugoslav Republic of Macedonia	Tob. unmanuf.			14,429		9,662		
Timor–Leste	Cigarettes	330	F	500	F	91	F	−72.42424242
Togo	Cigarettes	24,713		6,254		13,752		−44.35317444
Togo	Cigars cheroots	30		2		8		−73.33333333
Togo	Tob. prod. nes.	177		0		0	F	−100
Togo	Tob. unmanuf.	172		0		0	[a]	−100
Tonga	Cigarettes	1,140		887		1,654	R	45.0877193
Tonga	Cigars cheroots	0	M	34		0	F	
Tonga	Tob. prod. nes.	248		548		321	R	29.43548387
Tonga	Tob. unmanuf.	0		8		101	R	
Trinidad and Tobago	Cigarettes	261		72		479		83.52490421
Trinidad and Tobago	Cigars cheroots	11		58		57		418.1818182
Trinidad and Tobago	Tob. prod. nes.	10		22		0		−100

(continued)

Import value ($1,000)

Country	Item	1990		2000		2009		% Increase 2009–1990
Trinidad and Tobago	Tob. unmanuf.	2,642		3,971		8,780		232.323997
Tunisia	Cigarettes	17,083		23,044		73,485		330.164491
Tunisia	Cigars cheroots	121		56		17		−85.95041322
Tunisia	Tob. prod. nes.	1,071		10,016		4,135		286.0877684
Tunisia	Tob. unmanuf.	10,905		14,524		58,197		433.6726272
Turkey	Cigarettes	312,810		9		27		−99.99136856
Turkey	Cigars cheroots	0		32		1,554		
Turkey	Tob. prod. nes.	2,956		42,502		108,359		3565.730717
Turkey	Tob. unmanuf.	21,429		308,183		289,876		1252.727612
Turkmenistan	Cigarettes			8,300	R	9,874	R	
Turkmenistan	Tob. unmanuf.			0	M	20	F	
Tuvalu	Cigarettes	40	F	15	F	220	R	450
Tuvalu	Tob. prod. nes.	50	[a]	80	F	106	R	112
Uganda	Cigarettes	0		896		11,784		
Uganda	Cigars cheroots	0		24		42		
Uganda	Tob. prod. nes.	0		2		58		
Uganda	Tob. unmanuf.	0		476		11		
Ukraine	Cigarettes			24,649		90,844		
Ukraine	Cigars cheroots			0	M	904		
Ukraine	Tob. prod. nes.			11,143		91,467		
Ukraine	Tob. unmanuf.			107,843		272,351		
United Arab Emirates	Cigarettes	62,272		267,000	F	198,170	F	218.2329137
United Arab Emirates	Cigars cheroots	1,800	[a]	670	F	3,436	R	90.88888889
United Arab Emirates	Tob. prod. nes.	3,000	[a]	20,700	F	5,106	F	70.2
United Arab Emirates	Tob. unmanuf.	316		1,100	F	1,101	F	248.4177215
United Kingdom	Cigarettes	135,729		77,327		245,652		80.98711403
United Kingdom	Cigars cheroots	49,251		32,495		44,924		−8.785608414

United Kingdom	Tob. prod. nes.	38,000		35,826		53,331		40.34473684
United Kingdom	Tob. unmanuf.	431,899		460,194		300,948		−30.31982014
United Republic of Tanzania	Cigarettes	2,800	a	388		903		−67.75
United Republic of Tanzania	Cigars cheroots	0		96		185		
United Republic of Tanzania	Tob. prod. nes.	0		129		8		
United Republic of Tanzania	Tob. unmanuf.	0		4,076		13,947		
United States of America	Cigarettes	55,199		269,741		187,425		239.5441946
United States of America	Cigars cheroots	50,068		281,006		453,016		804.80147
United States of America	Tob. prod. nes.	19,383		23,643		49,894		157.4111335
United States of America	Tob. unmanuf.	731,387		595,527		923,755		26.30180739
Uruguay	Cigarettes	80		20		841		951.25
Uruguay	Cigars cheroots	21		152		62		195.2380952
Uruguay	Tob. prod. nes.	169		6,160		3,854		2180.473373
Uruguay	Tob. unmanuf.	4,394		20,952		29,689		575.6713701
USSR	Cigarettes	824,378						−100
USSR	Cigars cheroots	3,268						−100
USSR	Tob. prod. nes.	5,300	F					−100
USSR	Tob. unmanuf.	140,935						−100
Uzbekistan	Cigarettes			4,100	a	7,367	R	
Uzbekistan	Tob. prod. nes.			0	M	0	M	
Uzbekistan	Tob. unmanuf.			3,870	F	19,270	R	
Vanuatu	Cigarettes	467		920	F	2,303		393.1477516
Vanuatu	Cigars cheroots	0		0	M	112		
Vanuatu	Tob. prod. nes.	191		100	F	49		−74.34554974
Venezuela (Bolivarian Republic of)	Cigarettes	477		724		493		3.354297694
Venezuela (Bolivarian Republic of)	Cigars cheroots	155		712		396		155.483871
Venezuela (Bolivarian Republic of)	Tob. prod. nes.	48		258		2,566		5245.833333
Venezuela (Bolivarian Republic of)	Tob. unmanuf.	216		10,966		14,801		6752.314815

(continued)

Import value ($1,000)								
Country	Item	1990		2000		2009		% Increase 2009–1990
Viet Nam	Cigarettes	700	[a]	455,300	F	351,155	R	50,065
Viet Nam	Tob. prod. nes.	90	[a]	26,700	F	25,227	R	27,930
Viet Nam	Tob. unmanuf.	2,500	[a]	21,297		124,713	R	4888.52
Yemen	Cigarettes	85		1,100	F	1,521		1689.411765
Yemen	Cigars cheroots	0		50	F	157		
Yemen	Tob. prod. nes.	30,000	[a]	2,751		27,845		−7.183333333
Yemen	Tob. unmanuf.	26,851		21,509		35,573		32.48296153
Yugoslav SFR	Cigarettes	31,670						−100
Yugoslav SFR	Cigars cheroots	18						−100
Yugoslav SFR	Tob. prod. nes.	87						−100
Yugoslav SFR	Tob. unmanuf.	34,348						−100
Zambia	Cigarettes	1		65		6,784		678,300
Zambia	Cigars cheroots	0		18		5		
Zambia	Tob. prod. nes.	2		5		1		−50
Zambia	Tob. unmanuf.	438		1		60		−86.30136986
Zimbabwe	Cigarettes	2		8,989		131		6,450
Zimbabwe	Cigars cheroots	18		15		2		−88.88888889
Zimbabwe	Tob. prod. nes.	0		131		3		
Zimbabwe	Tob. unmanuf.	4,222		12,150		32,902		679.2989105

[a]Unofficial figure
[ ]=Official data
F FAO estimate, *M* Data not available, *R* Estimated data using trading partners database
% Increase in the last column is authors' calculations. Often a −100% increase means that the Country is no longer a political entity

Export value ($1,000)

Country	Item	1990		2000		2009		% Increase 09–90
Afghanistan	Tob. prod. nes.	0		0	F	0	F	
Albania	Cigarettes	17,000	F	114		0	F	−100
Albania	Cigars cheroots	0	M	0		0	F	
Albania	Tob. prod. nes.	0	M	4,499		0	F	
Albania	Tob. unmanuf.	11,500	[a]	2,515		2,332		−79.72173913
Algeria	Cigarettes	0		0		0	F	
Algeria	Cigars cheroots	0	M	203		0	F	
Algeria	Tob. prod. nes.	0		265		48		
Algeria	Tob. unmanuf.	0		0		31		
Angola	Cigarettes	0		0	F	29	R	
Angola	Cigars cheroots	0		0	F	0	F	
Angola	Tob. prod. nes.	0		0	F	0	F	
Angola	Tob. unmanuf.	0		0	F	381	R	
Antigua and Barbuda	Cigarettes	0	M	0	M	18	F	
Argentina	Cigarettes	3,188		21,036		13,654		328.293601
Argentina	Cigars cheroots	0		0		888		
Argentina	Tob. prod. nes.	495		5,033		4,752		860
Argentina	Tob. unmanuf.	94,950		120,096		359,250		278.35703
Armenia	Cigarettes			1,272		7,182		
Armenia	Cigars cheroots			76	F	0	F	
Armenia	Tob. prod. nes.			69		603		
Armenia	Tob. unmanuf.			0		797		
Aruba	Cigarettes	0	M	94		26,226		
Aruba	Cigars cheroots	8,520		14,498		2,640		−69.01408451
Aruba	Tob. prod. nes.	0		0	F	4		

(continued)

Export value ($1,000)

Country	Item	1990		2000		2009		% Increase 09–90
Aruba	Tob. unmanuf.	0	M	1,119		0	F	
Australia	Cigarettes	8,203		24,255		74,090		803.2061441
Australia	Cigars cheroots	280		688		2,598		827.8571429
Australia	Tob. prod. nes.	4,725		6,166		25,470		439.047619
Australia	Tob. unmanuf.	453		848		458		1.103752759
Austria	Cigarettes	18,243		82,475		216,902		1088.960149
Austria	Cigars cheroots	519		505		1,424		174.3737958
Austria	Tob. prod. nes.	1,026		727		7,224		604.0935673
Austria	Tob. unmanuf.	4,442		2,079		328		−92.61593877
Azerbaijan	Cigarettes			1,866		1,216		
Azerbaijan	Cigars cheroots			0	F	0	F	
Azerbaijan	Tob. prod. nes.			4	F	65		
Azerbaijan	Tob. unmanuf.			8,827		3,960		
Bahamas	Cigarettes	0	M	260		703		
Bahamas	Cigars cheroots	0	M	894		536		
Bahamas	Tob. prod. nes.	0	M	165		1	F	
Bahamas	Tob. unmanuf.	0	M	30		0	[a]	
Bahrain	Cigarettes	2,500	F	0	M	3,047		21.88
Bahrain	Cigars cheroots	0		0	M	398		
Bahrain	Tob. prod. nes.	0		4		47		
Bahrain	Tob. unmanuf.	0		0		201		
Bangladesh	Cigarettes	60		421		679	R	1031.666667
Bangladesh	Cigars cheroots	60		0	F	71	F	18.33333333
Bangladesh	Tob. prod. nes.	125		60		79	F	−36.8
Bangladesh	Tob. unmanuf.	1,668		1,706		41,257	R	2373.441247
Barbados	Cigarettes	723		401	F	2,113		192.2544952
Barbados	Cigars cheroots	90		23	[a]	269		198.8888889

Barbados	Tob. prod. nes.	30		8	F	157		423.3333333
Barbados	Tob. unmanuf.	0		0	F	1		
Belarus	Cigarettes			40,000	F	343		
Belarus	Cigars cheroots			0	[a]	0	[a]	
Belarus	Tob. prod. nes.			0	M	50		
Belarus	Tob. unmanuf.			300	F	184		
Belgium	Cigarettes			167,098		80,718		
Belgium	Cigars cheroots			154,646		368,789		
Belgium	Tob. prod. nes.			74,398		276,619		
Belgium	Tob. unmanuf.			75,043		401,065		
Belgium–Luxembourg	Cigarettes	187,108						−100
Belgium–Luxembourg	Cigars cheroots	95,688						−100
Belgium–Luxembourg	Tob. prod. nes.	45,164						−100
Belgium–Luxembourg	Tob. unmanuf.	30,312						−100
Belize	Cigarettes	22		201		0	F	−100
Belize	Cigars cheroots	0	M	22	F	0	F	
Belize	Tob. unmanuf.	0		0	F	0	F	
Benin	Cigarettes	0		2,500	F	10,301	F	
Benin	Cigars cheroots	0	M	2,912		0	F	
Benin	Tob. prod. nes.	0		0		191	F	
Benin	Tob. unmanuf.	0		0		0	F	
Bermuda	Cigarettes	0		0	F	0	F	
Bolivia (Plurinational State of)	Cigarettes	1		1,689		25		2,400
Bolivia (Plurinational State of)	Tob. prod. nes.	0		0		2		
Bolivia (Plurinational State of)	Tob. unmanuf.	0		11		0	F	
Bosnia and Herzegovina	Cigarettes			0	M	11,694		
Bosnia and Herzegovina	Cigars cheroots			0	M	0	F	
Bosnia and Herzegovina	Tob. prod. nes.			0	M	5		

(continued)

Export value ($1,000)								
Country	Item	1990		2000		2009		% Increase 09–90
Bosnia and Herzegovina	Tob. unmanuf.			2,500	F	3,845		
Botswana	Cigarettes	16		45	F	7,150		44587.5
Botswana	Cigars cheroots	0		3		2	F	
Botswana	Tob. prod. nes.	5		22		257		5,040
Botswana	Tob. unmanuf.	3		21		110		3566.666667
Brazil	Cigarettes	5		5,787		14,208		284,060
Brazil	Cigars cheroots	57,606		350		577		−98.99836823
Brazil	Tob. prod. nes.	434		22,417		39,429		8985.023041
Brazil	Tob. unmanuf.	565,521		812,921		2,991,820		429.0378253
Brunei Darussalam	Cigarettes	0		0	F	0	F	
Brunei Darussalam	Tob. prod. nes.	0	M	0	M	3	F	
Bulgaria	Cigarettes	765,722		20,500	F	93,203		−87.82808905
Bulgaria	Cigars cheroots	0	M	0	F	17		
Bulgaria	Tob. prod. nes.	0	M	6,700	F	1,103		
Bulgaria	Tob. unmanuf.	165,936		45,855		288,172		73.66454537
Burkina Faso	Cigarettes	0		1,643		2,908		
Burkina Faso	Cigars cheroots	0	M	0	M	0	[a]	
Burkina Faso	Tob. prod. nes.	101	[a]	3		3	F	−97.02970297
Burkina Faso	Tob. unmanuf.	0		75		0	[a]	
Burundi	Cigarettes	0		73		1,437		
Burundi	Tob. unmanuf.	1,302		0		0		−100
Cambodia	Cigarettes	0	M	1,838		4,304	R	
Cambodia	Cigars cheroots	0	M	50		0	F	
Cambodia	Tob. prod. nes.	0		0	F	120	F	
Cambodia	Tob. unmanuf.	0		519		361	R	
Cameroon	Cigarettes	1,534		174		0	F	−100
Cameroon	Cigars cheroots	0		0		0	F	

Cameroon	Tob. prod. nes.	92		60		0	F	−100
Cameroon	Tob. unmanuf.	2,529		481		2,018		−20.20561487
Canada	Cigarettes	35,967		30,808		79,282		120.4298385
Canada	Cigars cheroots	269		223		605		124.9070632
Canada	Tob. prod. nes.	6,286		3,464		1,121		−82.16671969
Canada	Tob. unmanuf.	56,588		62,844		56,123		−0.821728988
Cape Verde	Cigarettes	0	M	19		0	F	
Central African Republic	Cigarettes	300	F	22		27		−91
Central African Republic	Cigars cheroots	0		0	F	0	F	
Central African Republic	Tob. prod. nes.	0	F	0	F	0	F	
Central African Republic	Tob. unmanuf.	37		3,300	F	0	F	−100
Chad	Cigarettes	0		0	F	0	F	
Chad	Tob. unmanuf.	0		0	F	27	F	
Chile	Cigarettes	216		8,916		31,605		14531.94444
Chile	Tob. prod. nes.	0		1,540		67		
Chile	Tob. unmanuf.	10,952		3,011		1,775		−83.79291454
China	Cigarettes	109,425		126,522		304,994		178.7242403
China	Cigars cheroots	3,312		0		125		−96.22584541
China	Tob. prod. nes.	226		25,187		65,130		28718.58407
China	Tob. unmanuf.	64,293		151,443		533,301		729.485325
China, Hong Kong SAR	Cigarettes	1,225,540		661,558		676,927		−44.76500155
China, Hong Kong SAR	Cigars cheroots	194		11,632		32,433		16618.04124
China, Hong Kong SAR	Tob. prod. nes.	313		6,458		6,245		1895.207668
China, Hong Kong SAR	Tob. unmanuf.	7,630		9,356		22,578		195.9108781
China, Macao SAR	Cigarettes	0		13,528		32,917		
China, Macao SAR	Cigars cheroots	0	M	8		213		
China, Macao SAR	Tob. prod. nes.	297		276		489		64.64646465
China, Macao SAR	Tob. unmanuf.	0		0		0	F	

(continued)

Export value ($1,000)

Country	Item	1990		2000		2009		% Increase 09–90
Colombia	Cigarettes	3,232		16,996		10,468		223.8861386
Colombia	Cigars cheroots	0		9		38		
Colombia	Tob. prod. nes.	31		0		3,209		10251.6129
Colombia	Tob. unmanuf.	23,337		17,996		18,076		−22.54360029
Comoros	Cigarettes	0	M	3	F	0	F	
Congo	Cigarettes	2		152	F	310		15,400
Congo	Cigars cheroots	0	M	0	M	0	M	
Congo	Tob. prod. nes.	0		0	F	0	[a]	
Congo	Tob. unmanuf.	0		0	F	0	[a]	
Cook Islands	Cigarettes	0		0	F	0	F	
Costa Rica	Cigarettes	0		1,295		23		
Costa Rica	Cigars cheroots	1,541		2,709		575		−62.68656716
Costa Rica	Tob. prod. nes.	0		18		11		
Costa Rica	Tob. unmanuf.	50	F	1,351		608		1,116
Côte d'Ivoire	Cigarettes	3,000	F	2,899		11,451		281.7
Côte d'Ivoire	Cigars cheroots	450	[a]	0		0	F	−100
Côte d'Ivoire	Tob. prod. nes.	0		4,362		35,030		
Côte d'Ivoire	Tob. unmanuf.	90	[a]	363		0	[a]	−100
Croatia	Cigarettes			65,212		88,485		
Croatia	Cigars cheroots			1		11	F	
Croatia	Tob. prod. nes.			559		166		
Croatia	Tob. unmanuf.			10,846		16,427		
Cuba	Cigarettes	10,000	F	5,987		2,969		−70.31
Cuba	Cigars cheroots	79,480	F	140,346		201,476		153.4927026
Cuba	Tob. prod. nes.	17	F	33		19	R	11.76470588
Cuba	Tob. unmanuf.	46,000	[a]	19,945		7,575		−83.5326087

Cyprus	Cigarettes	64,399		284,579		14,922		−76.82883275
Cyprus	Cigars cheroots	839		6,499		4,756		466.8653159
Cyprus	Tob. prod. nes.	653		970		12		−98.16232772
Cyprus	Tob. unmanuf.	74		1,753		0	F	−100
Czech Republic	Cigarettes			76,414		352,984		
Czech Republic	Cigars cheroots			14		363		
Czech Republic	Tob. prod. nes.			8,200		6,491		
Czech Republic	Tob. unmanuf.			53		4,663		
Czechoslovakia	Cigarettes	10						−100
Czechoslovakia	Tob. prod. nes.	0						
Czechoslovakia	Tob. unmanuf.	0						
Democratic People's Republic of Korea	Cigarettes	50	a	300	F	67	R	34
Democratic People's Republic of Korea	Tob. unmanuf.	55	a	2,800	F	0	F	−100
Democratic Republic of the Congo	Cigarettes	0		0	F	0	F	
Democratic Republic of the Congo	Cigars cheroots	0		0	F	0	F	
Democratic Republic of the Congo	Tob. prod. nes.	0		0	F	0	F	
Democratic Republic of the Congo	Tob. unmanuf.	500	a	480	a	19,995	R	3,899
Denmark	Cigarettes	78,604		100,253		144,099		83.32273167
Denmark	Cigars cheroots	18,206		20,990		39,053		114.5062067
Denmark	Tob. prod. nes.	22,372		38,465		125,411		460.5712498
Denmark	Tob. unmanuf.	5,307		13,379		7,824		47.42792538
Djibouti	Cigarettes	0		69	F	38	F	

(continued)

Export value ($1,000)

Country	Item	1990		2000		2009		% Increase 09–90
Dominica	Cigarettes	0	M	165		39	R	
Dominica	Tob. unmanuf.	0	M	0		0	F	
Dominican Republic	Cigars cheroots	2,464		245,000	[a]	275,531	R	11082.26461
Dominican Republic	Tob. prod. nes.	3,285		0	F	6,210	F	89.04109589
Dominican Republic	Tob. unmanuf.	16,163		24,215		783		−95.1556023
Ecuador	Cigarettes	2,027		959		999		−50.71534287
Ecuador	Cigars cheroots	0		298		1		
Ecuador	Tob. prod. nes.	0		180		357		
Ecuador	Tob. unmanuf.	2,251		7,760		38,329		1602.754331
Egypt	Cigarettes	986		0		1,543		56.49087221
Egypt	Cigars cheroots	0		0		625		
Egypt	Tob. prod. nes.	34		2,152		78,883		231908.8235
Egypt	Tob. unmanuf.	169		3,200	F	366		116.5680473
El Salvador	Cigarettes	0		50		11		
El Salvador	Cigars cheroots	0	M	0		19		
El Salvador	Tob. prod. nes.	4		0		0	F	−100
El Salvador	Tob. unmanuf.	193		9		0	[a]	−100
Estonia	Cigarettes			1,209		9,261		
Estonia	Cigars cheroots			47		638		
Estonia	Tob. prod. nes.			326		10		
Estonia	Tob. unmanuf.			0		0	F	
Ethiopia	Cigarettes			0	M	35		
Ethiopia	Cigars cheroots			0	M	205		
Ethiopia	Tob. unmanuf.			1		0	F	
Ethiopia PDR	Cigarettes	0						
Ethiopia PDR	Tob. prod. nes.	0						

Ethiopia PDR	Tob. unmanuf.	0						
Fiji	Cigarettes	140		167		258		84.28571429
Fiji	Cigars cheroots	0		0		2		
Fiji	Tob. prod. nes.	0		0		16		
Fiji	Tob. unmanuf.	0		0		0	F	
Finland	Cigarettes	16,671		6,372		2,260		−86.44352468
Finland	Cigars cheroots	83		59		102		22.89156627
Finland	Tob. prod. nes.	62		165		683		1001.612903
Finland	Tob. unmanuf.	811		77		0	F	−100
France	Cigarettes	81,085		227,750		363,638		348.4651908
France	Cigars cheroots	2,510		6,093		5,382		114.4223108
France	Tob. prod. nes.	51,676		119,214		204,790		296.296153
France	Tob. unmanuf.	47,412		74,776		205,785		334.0356872
French Polynesia	Cigarettes	0		0	F	0	F	
French Polynesia	Cigars cheroots	0	M	0	M	0	F	
French Polynesia	Tob. prod. nes.	0	M	3		0	F	
Gabon	Cigarettes	0	M	7,152		0	M	
Gabon	Cigars cheroots	0	M	0	M	0	F	
Gabon	Tob. prod. nes.	0	M	382		0	M	
Gabon	Tob. unmanuf.	0	M	4		845	F	
Gambia	Cigarettes	0	M	0		16		
Gambia	Tob. prod. nes.	0	M	0	M	1	F	
Gambia	Tob. unmanuf.	0	M	0		0	F	
Georgia	Cigarettes			1,259		9		
Georgia	Cigars cheroots			0	F	0	F	
Georgia	Tob. prod. nes.			4,082		0	F	
Georgia	Tob. unmanuf.			777		1		
Germany	Cigarettes	898,319		1,815,500		3,722,150		314.3461287

(continued)

Export value ($1,000)								
Country	Item	1990		2000		2009		% Increase 09–90
Germany	Cigars cheroots	21,661		52,167		106,554		391.9163474
Germany	Tob. prod. nes.	68,966		138,640		383,721		456.3915553
Germany	Tob. unmanuf.	54,451		229,612		335,292		515.7683054
Ghana	Cigarettes	0	M	9,000	F	0	F	
Ghana	Cigars cheroots	0	M	6		0	F	
Ghana	Tob. prod. nes.	0	M	0	M	0	F	
Ghana	Tob. unmanuf.	581		387		3,120	F	437.0051635
Greece	Cigarettes	24,116		162,993		171,822		612.4813402
Greece	Cigars cheroots	68		36		35		–48.52941176
Greece	Tob. prod. nes.	20		21,987		17,162		85,710
Greece	Tob. unmanuf.	311,722		247,115		380,313		22.00390091
Grenada	Cigarettes	0	M	0	M	0	[a]	
Grenada	Cigars cheroots	0	M	0	M	0	[a]	
Grenada	Tob. prod. nes.	0	M	0	M	0	[a]	
Guam	Cigarettes	1,000	F	0	F	0	F	–100
Guam	Cigars cheroots	0		0	F	0	F	
Guam	Tob. prod. nes.	0		0	F	0	F	
Guatemala	Cigarettes	0		6,572		14,453		
Guatemala	Cigars cheroots	2,078		438		524		–74.78344562
Guatemala	Tob. prod. nes.	0	M	83		9		
Guatemala	Tob. unmanuf.	20,998		42,758		52,384		149.4713782
Guinea	Cigarettes	0	M	27		1,071	F	
Guinea	Cigars cheroots	0	M	5		0	F	
Guinea	Tob. prod. nes.	0	M	0	M	0	M	
Guinea	Tob. unmanuf.	0	M	40		156	F	
Guinea–Bissau	Tob. unmanuf.	0		0	F	133	F	

Guyana	Cigarettes	0		0	F	65	F	
Guyana	Tob. prod. nes.	0	M	0	M	0	F	
Guyana	Tob. unmanuf.	0		0	F	0	F	
Haiti	Tob. unmanuf.	0	M	5	[a]	0	M	
Honduras	Cigarettes	0		7,488		27,204		
Honduras	Cigars cheroots	8,263		996		50,357		509.4275687
Honduras	Tob. prod. nes.	0		55		1,110		
Honduras	Tob. unmanuf.	1,980		7,298		9,312		370.3030303
Hungary	Cigarettes	14,420		0		36,993	F	156.5395284
Hungary	Cigars cheroots	0		0		0	[a]	
Hungary	Tob. prod. nes.	1,329		0		2,272		70.95560572
Hungary	Tob. unmanuf.	1,838		3,686		11,023		499.7279652
Iceland	Cigars cheroots	0	M	0		0	F	
Iceland	Tob. prod. nes.	0	M	0	M	0	F	
Iceland	Tob. unmanuf.	0	M	0		0	F	
India	Cigarettes	22,194		23,940		53,603		141.5202307
India	Cigars cheroots	7,441		1,488		8,109		8.977287999
India	Tob. prod. nes.	9,545		21,270		87,724		819.057098
India	Tob. unmanuf.	108,321		147,255		748,553		591.0506735
Indonesia	Cigarettes	65,950		139,723		382,666		480.2365428
Indonesia	Cigars cheroots	134		3,919		27,824		20664.1791
Indonesia	Tob. prod. nes.	101		6,047		12,489		12265.34653
Indonesia	Tob. unmanuf.	58,613		71,287		172,629		194.5233992
Iran (Islamic Republic of)	Cigarettes	0		0		201	F	
Iran (Islamic Republic of)	Tob. prod. nes.	0		0		19	F	
Iran (Islamic Republic of)	Tob. unmanuf.	0		2,519		3,348	R	
Iraq	Cigarettes	0		0	F	0	F	
Iraq	Tob. prod. nes.	0		0	F	40	F	

(continued)

Export value ($1,000)

Country	Item	1990		2000		2009		% Increase 09–90
Iraq	Tob. unmanuf.	0		0	F	299	F	
Ireland	Cigarettes	6,132		7,516		191		–96.88519243
Ireland	Cigars cheroots	3,886		6,371		2,792		–28.15234174
Ireland	Tob. prod. nes.	34,582		87,308		96,302		178.4743508
Ireland	Tob. unmanuf.	1,551		340		0	a	–100
Israel	Cigarettes	182		2,542		6		–96.7032967
Israel	Cigars cheroots	0		0		37		
Israel	Tob. prod. nes.	0		0		490		
Israel	Tob. unmanuf.	1		0		0	F	–100
Italy	Cigarettes	7,013		4,487		6,458		–7.913874234
Italy	Cigars cheroots	1,157		1,923		5,636		387.1218669
Italy	Tob. prod. nes.	223		364		292		30.94170404
Italy	Tob. unmanuf.	130,729		183,335		284,800		117.8552578
Jamaica	Cigarettes	268		240	F	11		–95.89552239
Jamaica	Cigars cheroots	5,871		17,000	F	10		–99.82967127
Jamaica	Tob. prod. nes.	349		0	F	0	a	–100
Jamaica	Tob. unmanuf.	404		500	F	183		–54.7029703
Japan	Cigarettes	97,688		166,735		278,679		185.2745475
Japan	Cigars cheroots	0		495		3		
Japan	Tob. prod. nes.	609		128		403		–33.82594417
Japan	Tob. unmanuf.	79		60		8,370		10494.93671
Jordan	Cigarettes	2,415		13,009		29,746		1131.718427
Jordan	Cigars cheroots	0	M	1		0	F	
Jordan	Tob. prod. nes.	0		87		4,444		
Jordan	Tob. unmanuf.	0		1,058		2,500		
Kazakhstan	Cigarettes			6,711		29,945		

Kazakhstan	Cigars cheroots			0		62	F	
Kazakhstan	Tob. prod. nes.			1,274		4		
Kazakhstan	Tob. unmanuf.			9,490		9,166		
Kenya	Cigarettes	418		20,405		85,770		20419.13876
Kenya	Cigars cheroots	9		0		24		166.6666667
Kenya	Tob. prod. nes.	2		425		251		12,450
Kenya	Tob. unmanuf.	150		7,654		50,121		33,314
Kuwait	Cigarettes	79		265		257		225.3164557
Kuwait	Cigars cheroots	0		29		12		
Kuwait	Tob. prod. nes.	72		19		19		−73.61111111
Kuwait	Tob. unmanuf.	0	F	0		0		
Kyrgyzstan	Cigarettes			1,046		523	F	
Kyrgyzstan	Cigars cheroots			542		0	F	
Kyrgyzstan	Tob. prod. nes.			1,211		1,100	F	
Kyrgyzstan	Tob. unmanuf.			30,172		14,085	R	
Latvia	Cigarettes			12,588		43,092		
Latvia	Cigars cheroots			0		1,152		
Latvia	Tob. prod. nes.			11		16		
Latvia	Tob. unmanuf.			140		2,752		
Lebanon	Cigarettes	0		1		393		
Lebanon	Cigars cheroots	0		34		1		
Lebanon	Tob. prod. nes.	0		0		266		
Lebanon	Tob. unmanuf.	2,800	F	20,206		18,576		563.4285714
Lesotho	Tob. prod. nes.	0	F	0	F	0	F	
Liberia	Cigarettes	0		0	F	0	F	
Liberia	Tob. prod. nes.	0		0	F	14	F	
Liberia	Tob. unmanuf.	0		0	F	141	F	
Libya	Cigarettes	0		0	F	158	F	

(continued)

Export value ($1,000)								
Country	Item	1990		2000		2009		% Increase 09–90
Libya	Tob. unmanuf.	0		0	F	0	F	
Lithuania	Cigarettes			23,707		165,756		
Lithuania	Cigars cheroots			0		2,268		
Lithuania	Tob. prod. nes.			0		20,194		
Lithuania	Tob. unmanuf.			1		0	[a]	
Luxembourg	Cigarettes			87,724		92,441		
Luxembourg	Cigars cheroots			2,609		7,259		
Luxembourg	Tob. prod. nes.			65,860		66,673		
Luxembourg	Tob. unmanuf.			15		4,125		
Madagascar	Cigarettes	71		11		3		−95.77464789
Madagascar	Cigars cheroots	6		0		56	F	833.3333333
Madagascar	Tob. prod. nes.	0		0		1	F	
Madagascar	Tob. unmanuf.	0		0		47		
Malawi	Cigarettes	39		0		0	F	−100
Malawi	Cigars cheroots	0	M	0		26		
Malawi	Tob. prod. nes.	0		0		0	F	
Malawi	Tob. unmanuf.	276,654		336,000	[a]	758,969		174.3387047
Malaysia	Cigarettes	6,008		141,469		171,027		2746.654461
Malaysia	Cigars cheroots	64		448		18,799		29273.4375
Malaysia	Tob. prod. nes.	1,927		58,934		92,309		4690.295797
Malaysia	Tob. unmanuf.	6		2,091		16,710		278,400
Maldives	Cigarettes	0	M	0	M	0	F	
Mali	Cigarettes	0		0		29	R	
Mali	Cigars cheroots	0	M	0	M	8	F	
Mali	Tob. prod. nes.	0		0		0	F	
Mali	Tob. unmanuf.	0		0		0	F	

Malta	Cigarettes	5,450		15,957		35		−99.35779817
Malta	Cigars cheroots	460		637		113		−75.43478261
Malta	Tob. prod. nes.	383		279		5		−98.69451697
Malta	Tob. unmanuf.	3,879		76		0	F	−100
Mauritania	Cigarettes	0		0	F	0	F	
Mauritius	Cigarettes	462		0		5,463		1082.467532
Mauritius	Cigars cheroots	0		0		3		
Mauritius	Tob. prod. nes.	0	M	0		0	[a]	
Mauritius	Tob. unmanuf.	0		0		1,381		
Mexico	Cigarettes	3,316		51,757		222,267		6602.864897
Mexico	Cigars cheroots	2,686		3,450		6,016		123.9761727
Mexico	Tob. prod. nes.	163		125		13,474		8166.257669
Mexico	Tob. unmanuf.	22,948		34,584		28,958		26.18964616
Mongolia	Cigarettes	0	M	92		50	F	
Mongolia	Cigars cheroots	0	M	0	M	0	F	
Montenegro	Tob. unmanuf.					974		
Morocco	Cigarettes	22		188		15,286		69381.81818
Morocco	Cigars cheroots	0		0		588		
Morocco	Tob. prod. nes.	82		14		246		200
Morocco	Tob. unmanuf.	0		0		1,524		
Mozambique	Cigarettes	0		0	F	7	F	
Mozambique	Tob. prod. nes.	0		0	M	42	R	
Mozambique	Tob. unmanuf.	0		0	F	123,648	R	
Myanmar	Cigarettes	0	M	150	F	953	F	
Myanmar	Cigars cheroots	0	M	0	F	0	F	
Myanmar	Tob. prod. nes.	0		0	F	0	F	
Myanmar	Tob. unmanuf.	0		0	F	560	F	
Namibia	Cigarettes	0	M	6,059		29	F	

(continued)

Export value ($1,000)								
Country	Item	1990		2000		2009		% Increase 09–90
Namibia	Cigars cheroots	0	M	22		5	F	
Namibia	Tob. prod. nes.	0	M	6		11	F	
Namibia	Tob. unmanuf.	0	M	49		1,345	F	
Nepal	Cigarettes	0	M	0	M	394		
Nepal	Cigars cheroots	0	M	0	M	1		
Nepal	Tob. prod. nes.	482		0		2		−99.58506224
Nepal	Tob. unmanuf.	53		45		22		−58.49056604
Netherlands	Cigarettes	1,463,660		2,081,210		3,088,130		110.9868412
Netherlands	Cigars cheroots	161,063		161,335		283,622		76.09382664
Netherlands	Tob. prod. nes.	184,808		221,769		616,462		233.5688931
Netherlands	Tob. unmanuf.	93,109		123,090		137,228		47.38424857
Netherlands Antilles	Tob. prod. nes.	0		0	M	0	M	
New Caledonia	Cigarettes	0	M	70	F	4		
New Caledonia	Cigars cheroots	0	M	2	F	2		
New Caledonia	Tob. prod. nes.	220	F	0	F	0	F	−100
New Zealand	Cigarettes	1,290		1,899		8,883		588.6046512
New Zealand	Cigars cheroots	602		103		21		−96.51162791
New Zealand	Tob. prod. nes.	294		941		6,933		2258.163265
New Zealand	Tob. unmanuf.	35		64		0	F	−100
Nicaragua	Cigarettes	0		16		4		
Nicaragua	Cigars cheroots	250	[a]	6,956		16,908		6663.2
Nicaragua	Tob. prod. nes.	0		654		370		
Nicaragua	Tob. unmanuf.	1,400	[a]	5,317		5,141		267.2142857
Niger	Cigarettes	6,585		8,738		7,754	F	17.75246773
Niger	Cigars cheroots	0	M	0		1	F	
Niger	Tob. prod. nes.	0		0		0	F	
Niger	Tob. unmanuf.	289		151		56	F	−80.62283737

Nigeria	Cigarettes	0		0		23,472	F	
Nigeria	Tob. unmanuf.	379		0		0	R	−100
Norway	Cigarettes	1,631		271		626		−61.61863887
Norway	Cigars cheroots	66		14		3		−95.45454545
Norway	Tob. prod. nes.	9,018		5,445		4,995		−44.61077844
Norway	Tob. unmanuf.	1,492		228		0	[a]	−100
Occupied Palestinian Territory	Tob. prod. nes.	0	M	10		15	F	
Occupied Palestinian Territory	Tob. unmanuf.	0		97	[a]	0	F	
Oman	Cigarettes	917		133,093		45,050		4812.758997
Oman	Cigars cheroots	0		0	F	2,563		
Oman	Tob. prod. nes.	0		3		21		
Oman	Tob. unmanuf.	871		717		551		−36.73938002
Pakistan	Cigarettes	8,360		202		311		−96.27990431
Pakistan	Cigars cheroots	0	M	3		116		
Pakistan	Tob. prod. nes.	1,269		327		309		−75.6501182
Pakistan	Tob. unmanuf.	360		5,568		11,482		3089.444444
Panama	Cigarettes	283		6		0	F	−100
Panama	Cigars cheroots	219		37,677		59		−73.05936073
Panama	Tob. prod. nes.	0		0		0	F	
Panama	Tob. unmanuf.	3,389		588		701		−79.31543228
Papua New Guinea	Cigarettes	81		0		61	F	−24.69135802
Papua New Guinea	Tob. prod. nes.	628		0		1	F	−99.84076433
Papua New Guinea	Tob. unmanuf.	312		0		0	F	−100
Paraguay	Cigarettes	0		15,254		21,015		
Paraguay	Cigars cheroots	0		84		0	F	
Paraguay	Tob. prod. nes.	0	M	22		2,382		
Paraguay	Tob. unmanuf.	5,685		3,673		8,153		43.41248901
Peru	Cigarettes	0	M	10,041		3		

(continued)

Export value ($1,000)

Country	Item	1990		2000		2009		% Increase 09–90
Peru	Cigars cheroots	0		0		125		
Peru	Tob. prod. nes.	0		0		0	F	
Peru	Tob. unmanuf.	60		546		6,687		11,045
Philippines	Cigarettes	27,553		15,053		79,657		189.1046347
Philippines	Cigars cheroots	915		1,618		1,070		16.93989071
Philippines	Tob. prod. nes.	86		2,601		28,477		33012.7907
Philippines	Tob. unmanuf.	20,426		18,959		96,849		374.1456967
Poland	Cigarettes	0		49,325		1,352,660		
Poland	Cigars cheroots	0	M	115		226		
Poland	Tob. prod. nes.	0	M	6,243		72,381		
Poland	Tob. unmanuf.	19,303		7,638		53,077		174.9676216
Portugal	Cigarettes	2,932		44,271		421,154		14264.05184
Portugal	Cigars cheroots	204		27		805		294.6078431
Portugal	Tob. prod. nes.	37		438		28,220		76170.27027
Portugal	Tob. unmanuf.	5,224		6,139		94,833		1715.333078
Qatar	Cigarettes	0		21		0	F	
Qatar	Cigars cheroots	0	M	121		0	F	
Qatar	Tob. prod. nes.	0	M	5		0	F	
Qatar	Tob. unmanuf.	0	M	0	M	0	F	
Republic of Korea	Cigarettes	3,564		36,854		466,990		13002.97419
Republic of Korea	Cigars cheroots	104		31		1,344		1192.307692
Republic of Korea	Tob. prod. nes.	1		429		2,570		256,900
Republic of Korea	Tob. unmanuf.	77,289		14,715		7,194		−90.69207779
Republic of Moldova	Cigarettes			1,216		4,790		
Republic of Moldova	Cigars cheroots			0		0		
Republic of Moldova	Tob. prod. nes.			521		124		

Republic of Moldova	Tob. unmanuf.			28,819		10,740		
Romania	Cigarettes	0		324		503,988		
Romania	Cigars cheroots	0	M	0		55		
Romania	Tob. prod. nes.	0		128		1,586		
Romania	Tob. unmanuf.	1,782		1,995		4,380		145.7912458
Russian Federation	Cigarettes			3,151		326,078		
Russian Federation	Cigars cheroots			16		23		
Russian Federation	Tob. prod. nes.			16,291		124,879		
Russian Federation	Tob. unmanuf.			18		16,533		
Rwanda	Cigarettes	0	M	0	M	0	F	
Rwanda	Cigars cheroots	0	M	0	M	16		
Rwanda	Tob. prod. nes.	0		0	F	0	[a]	
Saint Kitts and Nevis	Cigarettes	0	M	0	M	0	F	
Saint Lucia	Cigarettes	0		0		457	F	
Saint Lucia	Cigars cheroots	0	M	0	M	148	F	
Saint Lucia	Tob. prod. nes.	0	M	0	M	73	F	
Saint Lucia	Tob. unmanuf.	0	M	0	M	1	F	
Saint Vincent and the Grenadines	Cigars cheroots	0	M	0	M	0	F	
Saint Vincent and the Grenadines	Tob. unmanuf.	170		0	M	4		−97.64705882
Samoa	Cigarettes	196		170		15	F	−92.34693878
Samoa	Tob. prod. nes.	152		0	F	0	F	−100
Saudi Arabia	Cigarettes	2,815		1		21,802		674.4937833
Saudi Arabia	Cigars cheroots	41		0		3	F	−92.68292683
Saudi Arabia	Tob. prod. nes.	205		393		0	[a]	−100
Saudi Arabia	Tob. unmanuf.	196		0		4	F	−97.95918367
Senegal	Cigarettes	1,006		2,245		39,318		3808.349901
Senegal	Cigars cheroots	0		393		117		
Senegal	Tob. prod. nes.	180		357		22,556		12431.11111

(continued)

Export value ($1,000)

Country	Item	1990		2000		2009		% Increase 09–90
Senegal	Tob. unmanuf.	239		1,890		21,813		9026.778243
Serbia	Cigarettes					29,769		
Serbia	Cigars cheroots					2,924		
Serbia	Tob. prod. nes.					2,627		
Serbia	Tob. unmanuf.					20,753		
Serbia and Montenegro	Cigarettes			614				
Serbia and Montenegro	Cigars cheroots			0				
Serbia and Montenegro	Tob. prod. nes.			80				
Serbia and Montenegro	Tob. unmanuf.			1,956				
Seychelles	Cigarettes	58		65	F	618	F	965.5172414
Seychelles	Cigars cheroots	0		0		58	F	
Seychelles	Tob. unmanuf.	0	M	0	M	8	F	
Sierra Leone	Cigarettes	810	F	0	F	0	F	−100
Sierra Leone	Tob. unmanuf.	646		510	F	0	F	−100
Singapore	Cigarettes	457,027		670,312		446,514		−2.300301733
Singapore	Cigars cheroots	113		450		843		646.0176991
Singapore	Tob. prod. nes.	11,285		36,544		39,380		248.9587949
Singapore	Tob. unmanuf.	1,903		1,046		15,354		706.831319
Slovakia	Cigarettes			17,212		0	F	
Slovakia	Cigars cheroots			1,970		18	F	
Slovakia	Tob. prod. nes.			818		0	[a]	
Slovakia	Tob. unmanuf.			5,694		466		
Slovenia	Cigarettes			17,212		209		
Slovenia	Cigars cheroots			1,970		68		
Slovenia	Tob. prod. nes.			818		3	F	
Slovenia	Tob. unmanuf.			5,694		279		

Solomon Islands	Cigarettes	0	M	0	M	0	M	
Solomon Islands	Tob. prod. nes.	11		0	F	7	R	−36.36363636
Somalia	Tob. prod. nes.	0		0	F	0	F	
Somalia	Tob. unmanuf.	0		0	F	0	F	
South Africa	Cigarettes	2,357		79,043		80,551		3317.522274
South Africa	Cigars cheroots	76		58		162		113.1578947
South Africa	Tob. prod. nes.	403		1,114		102,638		25368.48635
South Africa	Tob. unmanuf.	14,225		29,669		40,396		183.9789104
Spain	Cigarettes	12,246		50,306		125,477		924.636616
Spain	Cigars cheroots	3,259		8,046		117,625		3509.235962
Spain	Tob. prod. nes.	178		354		20,359		11337.64045
Spain	Tob. unmanuf.	20,980		79,264		113,454		440.772164
Sri Lanka	Cigarettes	2,363		1,685		427		−81.92975032
Sri Lanka	Cigars cheroots	0		2		3,949		
Sri Lanka	Tob. prod. nes.	0		0		19,895		
Sri Lanka	Tob. unmanuf.	3,793		37,445		33,545		784.3923016
Sudan	Cigarettes	0	M	0	M	0	F	
Sudan	Tob. prod. nes.	0		146		89		
Sudan	Tob. unmanuf.	0		55	[a]	15		
Swaziland	Cigarettes	0	M	262		6	F	
Swaziland	Cigars cheroots	0	M	0		0	F	
Swaziland	Tob. prod. nes.	0	M	96		0	F	
Swaziland	Tob. unmanuf.	88		5		1	F	−98.86363636
Sweden	Cigarettes	2,524		8,491		11,699		363.5103011
Sweden	Cigars cheroots	3,428		1,001		655		−80.89264877
Sweden	Tob. prod. nes.	16,109		19,647		53,410		231.5537898
Sweden	Tob. unmanuf.	2,987		366		59		−98.02477402
Switzerland	Cigarettes	237,535		204,206		627,891		164.3362031

(continued)

Export value ($1,000)								
Country	Item	1990		2000		2009		% Increase 09–90
Switzerland	Cigars cheroots	2,522		4,864		9,612		281.1260904
Switzerland	Tob. prod. nes.	1,775		121,444		14,510		717.4647887
Switzerland	Tob. unmanuf.	47,122		32,924		15,325		−67.47803574
Syrian Arab Republic	Cigarettes	9,943		43	F	92	F	−99.07472594
Syrian Arab Republic	Cigars cheroots	42		0	F	0	F	−100
Syrian Arab Republic	Tob. prod. nes.	0		0		0	F	
Syrian Arab Republic	Tob. unmanuf.	11,952		1,782		1,662	R	−86.09437751
Tajikistan	Cigarettes			0	M	1	F	
Tajikistan	Tob. unmanuf.			5,804		370	F	
Thailand	Cigarettes	0		12,232		11,405		
Thailand	Cigars cheroots	0		0		9		
Thailand	Tob. prod. nes.	185		142		130		−29.72972973
Thailand	Tob. unmanuf.	72,047		58,743		81,366		12.93461213
The former Yugoslav Republic of Macedonia	Cigarettes			37,151		14,384		
The former Yugoslav Republic of Macedonia	Cigars cheroots			0		0	F	
The former Yugoslav Republic of Macedonia	Tob. prod. nes.			269		0	[a]	
The former Yugoslav Republic of Macedonia	Tob. unmanuf.			47,695		88,098		
Togo	Cigarettes	12		1,463		444		3,600
Togo	Cigars cheroots	0	M	0	M	15		
Togo	Tob. prod. nes.	0		0		0	F	
Togo	Tob. unmanuf.	0		0		0	F	
Tonga	Cigarettes	16		1		23	F	43.75
Trinidad and Tobago	Cigarettes	578		9,215		42,297		7217.820069

Trinidad and Tobago	Cigars cheroots	0		0		0	F	
Trinidad and Tobago	Tob. prod. nes.	7		1		20		185.7142857
Trinidad and Tobago	Tob. unmanuf.	0		2		1		
Tunisia	Cigarettes	12,540		22,284		31,720		152.9505582
Tunisia	Cigars cheroots	211		228		0	F	−100
Tunisia	Tob. prod. nes.	3,239		4,646		6,069		87.37264588
Tunisia	Tob. unmanuf.	1,577		233		645		−59.09955612
Turkey	Cigarettes	23,601		96,315		198,381		740.5618406
Turkey	Cigars cheroots	0		1		0	F	
Turkey	Tob. prod. nes.	267		26,739		67,604		25219.85019
Turkey	Tob. unmanuf.	418,491		368,363		491,087		17.34708751
Turkmenistan	Cigarettes			0	M	0	M	
Turkmenistan	Tob. unmanuf.			0	M	0	M	
Uganda	Cigarettes	0		588		5,800		
Uganda	Cigars cheroots	0		224		59		
Uganda	Tob. prod. nes.	0		0		49		
Uganda	Tob. unmanuf.	2,821		26,301		56,572		1905.38816
Ukraine	Cigarettes			66,614		159,845		
Ukraine	Cigars cheroots			0	M	0	[a]	
Ukraine	Tob. prod. nes.			4,313		31,410		
Ukraine	Tob. unmanuf.			6,037		11,136		
United Arab Emirates	Cigarettes	82,830	[a]	168,000	F	386,070	F	366.0992394
United Arab Emirates	Cigars cheroots	500	F	300	F	4,840	F	868
United Arab Emirates	Tob. prod. nes.	0	M	0	M	7,170	R	
United Arab Emirates	Tob. unmanuf.	127		250	[a]	3,438	F	2607.086614
United Kingdom	Cigarettes	1,044,080		1,531,840		407,410		−60.97904375
United Kingdom	Cigars cheroots	6,487		7,725		9,404		44.96685679
United Kingdom	Tob. prod. nes.	89,045		179,799		197,381		121.664327

(continued)

Export value ($1,000)								
Country	Item	1990		2000		2009		% Increase 09–90
United Kingdom	Tob. unmanuf.	28,445		25,694		14,469		–49.13341536
United Republic of Tanzania	Cigarettes	1,641		2,671		3,647		122.242535
United Republic of Tanzania	Cigars cheroots	0		85		1,445		
United Republic of Tanzania	Tob. prod. nes.	0		0		2,413		
United Republic of Tanzania	Tob. unmanuf.	12,881		49,060		90,365		601.5371477
United States of America	Cigarettes	4,766,550		3,328,430		453,209		–90.49188617
United States of America	Cigars cheroots	6,504		27,063		40,210		518.2349323
United States of America	Tob. prod. nes.	271,840		679,206		40,237		–85.1982784
United States of America	Tob. unmanuf.	1,469,800		1,234,640		1,163,470		–20.8416111
Uruguay	Cigarettes	555		59,018		22,102		3882.342342
Uruguay	Cigars cheroots	11		0		4	F	–63.63636364
Uruguay	Tob. prod. nes.	37		657		3,351		8956.756757
Uruguay	Tob. unmanuf.	64		0		10,415		16173.4375
USSR	Cigarettes	2,375						–100
USSR	Tob. prod. nes.	6,178						–100
USSR	Tob. unmanuf.	3,426						–100
Uzbekistan	Tob. prod. nes.			0	M	0	M	
Uzbekistan	Tob. unmanuf.			25,200	F	17,058	R	
Vanuatu	Cigarettes	0	M	0	M	744		
Vanuatu	Cigars cheroots	0	M	0	M	78		
Vanuatu	Tob. prod. nes.	0	M	0	M	60		
Venezuela (Bolivarian Republic of)	Cigarettes	37,704		29,882		33		–99.91247613
Venezuela (Bolivarian Republic of)	Cigars cheroots	0		47		0	F	
Venezuela (Bolivarian Republic of)	Tob. prod. nes.	59		15,568		6,075		10196.61017
Venezuela (Bolivarian Republic of)	Tob. unmanuf.	2,069		1,198		53		–97.43837603
Viet Nam	Cigarettes	0		2,900	F	19,491	F	

Viet Nam	Tob. unmanuf.	0		4,300	F	8,782	R	
Yemen	Cigarettes	4,674		2,600	F	24,349		420.9456568
Yemen	Cigars cheroots	0		0	F	23		
Yemen	Tob. prod. nes.	0		169		700		
Yemen	Tob. unmanuf.	2,487		23	F	244		−90.18898271
Yugoslav SFR	Cigarettes	24,010						−100
Yugoslav SFR	Cigars cheroots	129						−100
Yugoslav SFR	Tob. prod. nes.	405						−100
Yugoslav SFR	Tob. unmanuf.	35,535						−100
Zambia	Cigarettes	0		136		10		
Zambia	Cigars cheroots	0	M	0		1		
Zambia	Tob. prod. nes.	0	M	15		4,933		
Zambia	Tob. unmanuf.	4,259		9,532		84,688		1888.447992
Zimbabwe	Cigarettes	1,582		18,246		31,938		1918.836915
Zimbabwe	Cigars cheroots	3,978		8		1	F	−99.97486174
Zimbabwe	Tob. prod. nes.	473		10,956		2,478		423.8900634
Zimbabwe	Tob. unmanuf.	340,678		565,532		241,775		−29.03122597

[a]Unofficial figure

[ ] Official data

F FAO estimate, *M* Data not available, *R* Estimated data using trading partners database

FAOSTAT, © FAO Statistics Division 2012, 16 March 2012

% Increase in the last column is authors' calculations. Often a −100% increase means that the Country is no longer a political entity

Value of import, export, balance—cigarettes—2009—$1,000				
Countries	Item	2009 Imp	2009 Exp	Balance
Afghanistan	Cigarettes	48,071		–48,071
Albania	Cigarettes	84,559	0	–84,559
Algeria	Cigarettes	80,309	0	–80,309
American Samoa	Cigarettes	6		–6
Angola	Cigarettes	17,404	29	–17,375
Antigua and Barbuda	Cigarettes	1,019	18	–1,001
Argentina	Cigarettes	223	1,3654	13,431
Armenia	Cigarettes	53,368	7,182	–46,186
Aruba	Cigarettes	28,918	26,226	–2,692
Australia	Cigarettes	61,170	74,090	12,920
Austria	Cigarettes	276,834	216,902	–59,932
Azerbaijan	Cigarettes	217,619	1,216	–216,403
Bahamas	Cigarettes	4,077	703	–3,374
Bahrain	Cigarettes	37,187	3,047	–34,140
Bangladesh	Cigarettes	1,318	679	–639
Barbados	Cigarettes	6,259	2,113	–4,146
Belarus	Cigarettes	11,989	343	–11,646
Belgium	Cigarettes	392,792	80,718	–312,074
Belize	Cigarettes	4,521	0	–4,521
Benin	Cigarettes	9,266	10,301	1,035
Bermuda	Cigarettes	587	0	–587
Bhutan	Cigarettes	49		–49
Bolivia (Plurinational State of)	Cigarettes	4,551	25	–4,526
Bosnia and Herzegovina	Cigarettes	91,351	11,694	–79,657
Botswana	Cigarettes	40,772	7,150	–33,622
Brazil	Cigarettes	437	14,208	13,771
British Virgin Islands	Cigarettes	0		0
Brunei Darussalam	Cigarettes	15,735	0	–15,735
Bulgaria	Cigarettes	77,642	93,203	15,561
Burkina Faso	Cigarettes	134	2,908	2,774
Burundi	Cigarettes	110	1,437	1,327
Cambodia	Cigarettes	193,952	4,304	–189,648
Cameroon	Cigarettes	26,678	0	–26,678
Canada	Cigarettes	10,821	79,282	68,461
Cape Verde	Cigarettes	2,325	0	–2,325
Cayman Islands	Cigarettes	2,522		–2,522
Central African Republic	Cigarettes	0	27	27
Chad	Cigarettes	1	0	–1
Chile	Cigarettes	3,844	31,605	27,761
China	Cigarettes	512,989	304,994	–207,995
China, Hong Kong SAR	Cigarettes	465,516	676,927	211,411
China, Macao SAR	Cigarettes	51,797	32,917	–18,880
Colombia	Cigarettes	12,822	10,468	–2,354
Comoros	Cigarettes	377	0	–377
Congo	Cigarettes	460	310	–150

(continued)

Value of import, export, balance—cigarettes—2009—$1,000				
Countries	Item	2009 Imp	2009 Exp	Balance
Cook Islands	Cigarettes	759	0	–759
Costa Rica	Cigarettes	3,407	23	–3,384
Côte d'Ivoire	Cigarettes	10,442	11,451	1,009
Croatia	Cigarettes	34,909	88,485	53,576
Cuba	Cigarettes	78	2,969	2,891
Cyprus	Cigarettes	53,146	14,922	–38,224
Czech Republic	Cigarettes	120,866	352,984	232,118
Democratic People's Republic of Korea	Cigarettes	8,109	67	–8,042
Democratic Republic of the Congo	Cigarettes	1,366	0	–1,366
Denmark	Cigarettes	36,882	144,099	107,217
Djibouti	Cigarettes	1,928	38	–1,890
Dominica	Cigarettes	186	39	–147
Dominican Republic	Cigarettes	3,496		–3,496
Ecuador	Cigarettes	237	999	762
Egypt	Cigarettes	56,254	1,543	–54,711
El Salvador	Cigarettes	13,926	11	–13,915
Estonia	Cigarettes	33,733	9,261	–24,472
Ethiopia	Cigarettes	3,825	35	–3,790
EU(12)ex.int	Cigarettes	2,036,280	2,407,357	371,077
EU(15)ex.int	Cigarettes	1,998,591	2,205,917	207,326
EU(25)ex.int	Cigarettes	479,361	2,278,584	1,799,223
EU(27)ex.int	Cigarettes	28,323	2,272,462	2,244,139
Faroe Islands	Cigarettes	2,597		–2,597
Fiji	Cigarettes	943	258	–685
Finland	Cigarettes	100,717	2,260	–98,457
France	Cigarettes	1,631,120	363,638	–1,267,482
French Polynesia	Cigarettes	2,614	0	–2,614
Gabon	Cigarettes	5,775	0	–5,775
Gambia	Cigarettes	3,337	16	–3,321
Georgia	Cigarettes	57,160	9	–57,151
Germany	Cigarettes	904,899	3,722,150	2,817,251
Ghana	Cigarettes	8,387	0	–8,387
Greece	Cigarettes	276,189	171,822	–104,367
Grenada	Cigarettes	1,359	0	–1,359
Guam	Cigarettes	0	0	0
Guatemala	Cigarettes	9,323	14,453	5,130
Guinea	Cigarettes	33,279	1,071	–32,208
Guinea–Bissau	Cigarettes	3,212		–3,212
Guyana	Cigarettes	5,092	65	–5,027
Haiti	Cigarettes	172		–172
Honduras	Cigarettes	3,509	27,204	23,695
Hungary	Cigarettes	0	36,993	36,993
Iceland	Cigarettes	15,911		–15,911
India	Cigarettes	10,385	53,603	43,218
Indonesia	Cigarettes	3,003	382,666	379,663

(continued)

Value of import, export, balance—cigarettes—2009—$1,000				
Countries	Item	2009 Imp	2009 Exp	Balance
Iran (Islamic Republic of)	Cigarettes	233,117	201	−232,916
Iraq	Cigarettes	177,995	0	−177,995
Ireland	Cigarettes	74,283	191	−74,092
Israel	Cigarettes	153,317	6	−153,311
Italy	Cigarettes	2,951,660	6,458	−2,945,202
Jamaica	Cigarettes	6,779	11	−6,768
Japan	Cigarettes	3,279,620	278,679	−3,000,941
Jordan	Cigarettes	145	29,746	29,601
Kazakhstan	Cigarettes	95,951	29,945	−66,006
Kenya	Cigarettes	1,809	85,770	83,961
Kiribati	Cigarettes	639		−639
Kuwait	Cigarettes	62,129	257	−61,872
Kyrgyzstan	Cigarettes	31,042	523	−30,519
Lao People's Democratic Republic	Cigarettes	5,249		−5,249
Latvia	Cigarettes	57,752	43,092	−14,660
Lebanon	Cigarettes	167,901	393	−167,508
Liberia	Cigarettes	6,731	0	−6,731
Libya	Cigarettes	5,223	158	−5,065
Lithuania	Cigarettes	49,467	165,756	116,289
Luxembourg	Cigarettes	109,584	92,441	−17,143
Madagascar	Cigarettes	480	3	−477
Malawi	Cigarettes	4,864	0	−4,864
Malaysia	Cigarettes	62,962	171,027	108,065
Maldives	Cigarettes	13,235	0	−13,235
Mali	Cigarettes	13,355	29	−13,326
Malta	Cigarettes	18,977	35	−18,942
Mauritania	Cigarettes	16,264	0	−16,264
Mauritius	Cigarettes	38,010	5,463	−32,547
Mexico	Cigarettes	12,502	222,267	209,765
Mongolia	Cigarettes	33,977	50	−33,927
Montenegro	Cigarettes	28,148		−28,148
Morocco	Cigarettes	59,572	15,286	−44,286
Mozambique	Cigarettes	12,640	7	−12,633
Myanmar	Cigarettes	8,483	953	−7,530
Namibia	Cigarettes	4,865	29	−4,836
Nepal	Cigarettes	727	394	−333
Netherlands	Cigarettes	350,931	3,088,130	2,737,199
Netherlands Antilles	Cigarettes	3,100		−3,100
New Caledonia	Cigarettes	11,367	4	−11,363
New Zealand	Cigarettes	32,433	8,883	−23,550
Nicaragua	Cigarettes	20,520	4	−20,516
Niger	Cigarettes	39,568	7,754	−31,814
Nigeria	Cigarettes	19,172	23,472	4,300
Norfolk Island	Cigarettes	0		0
Norway	Cigarettes	88,252	626	−87,626

(continued)

Value of import, export, balance—cigarettes—2009—$1,000				
Countries	Item	2009 Imp	2009 Exp	Balance
Occupied Palestinian Territory	Cigarettes	12,942		−12,942
Oman	Cigarettes	82,509	45,050	−37,459
Pakistan	Cigarettes	439	311	−128
Panama	Cigarettes	7,531	0	−7,531
Papua New Guinea	Cigarettes	38	61	23
Paraguay	Cigarettes	26,312	21,015	−5,297
Peru	Cigarettes	27,643	3	−27,640
Philippines	Cigarettes	5,232	79,657	74,425
Poland	Cigarettes	43,803	1,352,660	1,308,857
Portugal	Cigarettes	40,618	421,154	380,536
Qatar	Cigarettes	26,107	0	−26,107
Republic of Korea	Cigarettes	11,027	466,990	455,963
Republic of Moldova	Cigarettes	76,539	4,790	−71,749
Romania	Cigarettes	77,891	503,988	426,097
Russian Federation	Cigarettes	114,745	326,078	211,333
Rwanda	Cigarettes	3,871	0	−3,871
Saint Kitts and Nevis	Cigarettes	346	0	−346
Saint Lucia	Cigarettes	3,929	457	−3,472
Saint Pierre and Miquelon	Cigarettes	787		−787
Saint Vincent and the Grenadines	Cigarettes	1,195		−1,195
Samoa	Cigarettes	9	15	6
Sao Tome and Principe	Cigarettes	151		−151
Saudi Arabia	Cigarettes	513,490	21,802	−491,688
Senegal	Cigarettes	2,198	39,318	37,120
Serbia	Cigarettes	48,655	29,769	−18,886
Seychelles	Cigarettes	625	618	−7
Sierra Leone	Cigarettes	7,855	0	−7,855
Singapore	Cigarettes	394,899	446,514	51,615
Slovakia	Cigarettes	66,184	0	−66,184
Slovenia	Cigarettes	96,468	209	−96,259
Solomon Islands	Cigarettes	32	0	−32
South Africa	Cigarettes	19,932	80,551	60,619
Spain	Cigarettes	1,512,900	125,477	−1,387,423
Sri Lanka	Cigarettes	889	427	−462
Sudan	Cigarettes	26,917	0	−26,917
Suriname	Cigarettes	491		−491
Swaziland	Cigarettes	2,846	6	−2,840
Sweden	Cigarettes	135,387	11,699	−123,688
Switzerland	Cigarettes	15,525	627,891	612,366
Syrian Arab Republic	Cigarettes	132,458	92	−132,366
Tajikistan	Cigarettes	1,600	1	−1,599
Thailand	Cigarettes	80,801	11,405	−69,396
The former Yugoslav Republic of Macedonia	Cigarettes	8,401	14,384	5,983
Timor–Leste	Cigarettes	91		−91

(continued)

Value of import, export, balance—cigarettes—2009—$1,000				
Countries	Item	2009 Imp	2009 Exp	Balance
Togo	Cigarettes	13,752	444	−13,308
Tonga	Cigarettes	1,654	23	−1,631
Trinidad and Tobago	Cigarettes	479	42,297	41,818
Tunisia	Cigarettes	73,485	31,720	−41,765
Turkey	Cigarettes	27	198,381	198,354
Turkmenistan	Cigarettes	9,874	0	−9,874
Tuvalu	Cigarettes	220		−220
Uganda	Cigarettes	11,784	5,800	−5,984
Ukraine	Cigarettes	90,844	159,845	69,001
United Arab Emirates	Cigarettes	198,170	386,070	187,900
United Kingdom	Cigarettes	245,652	407,410	161,758
United Republic of Tanzania	Cigarettes	903	3,647	2,744
United States of America	Cigarettes	187,425	453,209	265,784
Uruguay	Cigarettes	841	22,102	21,261
Uzbekistan	Cigarettes	7,367		−7,367
Vanuatu	Cigarettes	2,303	744	−1,559
Venezuela (Bolivarian Republic of)	Cigarettes	493	33	−460
Viet Nam	Cigarettes	351,155	19,491	−331,664
Yemen	Cigarettes	1,521	24,349	22,828
Zambia	Cigarettes	6,784	10	−6,774
Zimbabwe	Cigarettes	131	31,938	31,807

Value of import, export, balance—tobacco unmanufactured—2009—$1,000				
Countries	Item	2009 Imp	2009 Exp	Balance
Afghanistan	Tobacco, unmanufactured	0		0
Albania	Tobacco, unmanufactured	29	2,332	2,303
Algeria	Tobacco, unmanufactured	56,011	31	−55,980
American Samoa	Tobacco, unmanufactured	0		0
Angola	Tobacco, unmanufactured	4,224	381	−3,843
Antigua and Barbuda	Tobacco, unmanufactured	6		−6
Argentina	Tobacco, unmanufactured	14,285	359,250	344,965
Armenia	Tobacco, unmanufactured	11,865	797	−11,068
Aruba	Tobacco, unmanufactured	2	0	−2
Australia	Tobacco, unmanufactured	101,453	458	−100,995
Austria	Tobacco, unmanufactured	49,880	328	−49,552
Azerbaijan	Tobacco, unmanufactured	4,410	3,960	−450
Bahamas	Tobacco, unmanufactured	115	0	−115
Bahrain	Tobacco, unmanufactured	415	201	−214
Bangladesh	Tobacco, unmanufactured	9,200	41,257	32,057
Barbados	Tobacco, unmanufactured	37	1	−36
Belarus	Tobacco, unmanufactured	41,061	184	−40,877
Belgium	Tobacco, unmanufactured	596,730	401,065	−195,665

(continued)

Value of import, export, balance—tobacco unmanufactured—2009—$1,000				
Countries	Item	2009 Imp	2009 Exp	Balance
Belize	Tobacco, unmanufactured	87	0	–87
Benin	Tobacco, unmanufactured	327	0	–327
Bermuda	Tobacco, unmanufactured	0		0
Bhutan	Tobacco, unmanufactured	1		–1
Bolivia (Plurinational State of)	Tobacco, unmanufactured	2,008	0	–2,008
Bosnia and Herzegovina	Tobacco, unmanufactured	12,540	3,845	–8,695
Botswana	Tobacco, unmanufactured	2,613	110	–2,503
Brazil	Tobacco, unmanufactured	62,344	2,991,820	2,929,476
Brunei Darussalam	Tobacco, unmanufactured	531		–531
Bulgaria	Tobacco, unmanufactured	120,795	288,172	167,377
Burkina Faso	Tobacco, unmanufactured	45	0	–45
Burundi	Tobacco, unmanufactured	1,227	0	–1,227
Cambodia	Tobacco, unmanufactured	9,180	361	–8,819
Cameroon	Tobacco, unmanufactured	227	2,018	1,791
Canada	Tobacco, unmanufactured	47,441	56,123	8,682
Cape Verde	Tobacco, unmanufactured	777		–777
Central African Republic	Tobacco, unmanufactured	0	0	0
Chad	Tobacco, unmanufactured	96	27	–69
Chile	Tobacco, unmanufactured	11,333	1,775	–9,558
China	Tobacco, unmanufactured	806,504	533,301	–273,203
China, Hong Kong SAR	Tobacco, unmanufactured	74,944	22,578	–52,366
China, Macao SAR	Tobacco, unmanufactured	130	0	–130
Colombia	Tobacco, unmanufactured	3,128	18,076	14,948
Comoros	Tobacco, unmanufactured	7		–7
Congo	Tobacco, unmanufactured	0	0	0
Costa Rica	Tobacco, unmanufactured	5,166	608	–4,558
Côte d'Ivoire	Tobacco, unmanufactured	77,014	0	–77,014
Croatia	Tobacco, unmanufactured	20,671	16,427	–4,244
Cuba	Tobacco, unmanufactured	564	7,575	7,011
Cyprus	Tobacco, unmanufactured	0	0	0
Czech Republic	Tobacco, unmanufactured	69,083	4,663	–64,420
Democratic People's Republic of Korea	Tobacco, unmanufactured	29,725	0	–29,725
Democratic Republic of the Congo	Tobacco, unmanufactured	806	19,995	19,189
Denmark	Tobacco, unmanufactured	89,181	7,824	–81,357
Djibouti	Tobacco, unmanufactured	9,415		–9,415
Dominica	Tobacco, unmanufactured	123	0	–123
Dominican Republic	Tobacco, unmanufactured	129,631	783	–128,848
Ecuador	Tobacco, unmanufactured	2,196	38,329	36,133
Egypt	Tobacco, unmanufactured	23,000	366	–22,634
El Salvador	Tobacco, unmanufactured	123	0	–123

(continued)

Value of import, export, balance—tobacco unmanufactured—2009—$1,000				
Countries	Item	2009 Imp	2009 Exp	Balance
Equatorial Guinea	Tobacco, unmanufactured	0		0
Estonia	Tobacco, unmanufactured	2	0	−2
Ethiopia	Tobacco, unmanufactured	8,265	0	−8,265
EU(12)ex.int	Tobacco, unmanufactured	2,505,187	1,239,081	−1,266,106
EU(15)ex.int	Tobacco, unmanufactured	2,541,075	1,218,348	−1,322,727
EU(25)ex.int	Tobacco, unmanufactured	2,753,216	991,683	−1,761,533
EU(27)ex.int	Tobacco, unmanufactured	2,764,562	968,372	−1,796,190
Faroe Islands	Tobacco, unmanufactured	7		−7
Fiji	Tobacco, unmanufactured	156	0	−156
Finland	Tobacco, unmanufactured	0	0	0
France	Tobacco, unmanufactured	177,052	205,785	28,733
Gabon	Tobacco, unmanufactured	18,253	845	−17,408
Gambia	Tobacco, unmanufactured	103	0	−103
Georgia	Tobacco, unmanufactured	5,111	1	−5,110
Germany	Tobacco, unmanufactured	981,898	335,292	−646,606
Ghana	Tobacco, unmanufactured	0	3,120	3,120
Greece	Tobacco, unmanufactured	210,651	380,313	169,662
Grenada	Tobacco, unmanufactured	21		−21
Guatemala	Tobacco, unmanufactured	6,023	52,384	46,361
Guinea	Tobacco, unmanufactured	0	156	156
Guinea–Bissau	Tobacco, unmanufactured	394	133	−261
Guyana	Tobacco, unmanufactured	241	0	−241
Haiti	Tobacco, unmanufactured	1,973	0	−1,973
Honduras	Tobacco, unmanufactured	18,296	9,312	−8,984
Hungary	Tobacco, unmanufactured	29,242	11,023	−18,219
Iceland	Tobacco, unmanufactured	0	0	0
India	Tobacco, unmanufactured	7,804	748,553	740,749
Indonesia	Tobacco, unmanufactured	290,171	172,629	−117,542
Iran (Islamic Republic of)	Tobacco, unmanufactured	67,176	3,348	−63,828
Iraq	Tobacco, unmanufactured	34	299	265
Ireland	Tobacco, unmanufactured	15,163	0	−15,163
Israel	Tobacco, unmanufactured	6,301	0	−6,301
Italy	Tobacco, unmanufactured	57,447	284,800	227,353
Jamaica	Tobacco, unmanufactured	53	183	130
Japan	Tobacco, unmanufactured	400,572	8,370	−392,202
Jordan	Tobacco, unmanufactured	15,159	2,500	−12,659
Kazakhstan	Tobacco, unmanufactured	52,086	9,166	−42,920
Kenya	Tobacco, unmanufactured	37,147	50,121	12,974
Kuwait	Tobacco, unmanufactured	35	0	−35
Kyrgyzstan	Tobacco, unmanufactured	5,512	14,085	8,573
Lao People's Democratic Republic	Tobacco, unmanufactured	407		−407
Latvia	Tobacco, unmanufactured	1,760	2,752	992

(continued)

Value of import, export, balance—tobacco unmanufactured—2009—$1,000				
Countries	Item	2009 Imp	2009 Exp	Balance
Lebanon	Tobacco, unmanufactured	1,070	18,576	17,506
Liberia	Tobacco, unmanufactured	1,194	141	–1,053
Libya	Tobacco, unmanufactured	7,559	0	–7,559
Lithuania	Tobacco, unmanufactured	58,436	0	–58,436
Luxembourg	Tobacco, unmanufactured	32,675	4,125	–28,550
Madagascar	Tobacco, unmanufactured	3,943	47	–3,896
Malawi	Tobacco, unmanufactured	53,464	758,969	705,505
Malaysia	Tobacco, unmanufactured	206,143	16,710	–189,433
Maldives	Tobacco, unmanufactured	73		–73
Mali	Tobacco, unmanufactured	7	0	–7
Malta	Tobacco, unmanufactured	42	0	–42
Mauritania	Tobacco, unmanufactured	203		–203
Mauritius	Tobacco, unmanufactured	0	1,381	1,381
Mexico	Tobacco, unmanufactured	144,465	28,958	–115,507
Montenegro	Tobacco, unmanufactured	88	974	886
Morocco	Tobacco, unmanufactured	53,306	1,524	–51,782
Mozambique	Tobacco, unmanufactured	11,766	123,648	111,882
Myanmar	Tobacco, unmanufactured	1,659	560	–1,099
Namibia	Tobacco, unmanufactured	32	1,345	1,313
Nepal	Tobacco, unmanufactured	18,540	22	–18,518
Netherlands	Tobacco, unmanufactured	763,764	137,228	–626,536
Netherlands Antilles	Tobacco, unmanufactured	799		–799
New Zealand	Tobacco, unmanufactured	7,137	0	–7,137
Nicaragua	Tobacco, unmanufactured	10	5,141	5,131
Niger	Tobacco, unmanufactured	10	56	46
Nigeria	Tobacco, unmanufactured	45,485	0	–45,485
Norway	Tobacco, unmanufactured	0	0	0
Occupied Palestinian Territory	Tobacco, unmanufactured	6,500	0	–6,500
Oman	Tobacco, unmanufactured	11	551	540
Pakistan	Tobacco, unmanufactured	11,894	11,482	–412
Panama	Tobacco, unmanufactured	73	701	628
Papua New Guinea	Tobacco, unmanufactured	352	0	–352
Paraguay	Tobacco, unmanufactured	100,486	8,153	–92,333
Peru	Tobacco, unmanufactured	3	6,687	6,684
Philippines	Tobacco, unmanufactured	192,892	96,849	–96,043
Poland	Tobacco, unmanufactured	328,830	53,077	–275,753
Portugal	Tobacco, unmanufactured	30,381	94,833	64,452
Qatar	Tobacco, unmanufactured	17	0	–17
Republic of Korea	Tobacco, unmanufactured	242,882	7,194	–235,688
Republic of Moldova	Tobacco, unmanufactured	10,333	10,740	407
Romania	Tobacco, unmanufactured	154,063	4,380	–149,683
Russian Federation	Tobacco, unmanufactured	1,040,980	16,533	–1,024,447
Rwanda	Tobacco, unmanufactured	952		–952
Saint Kitts and Nevis	Tobacco, unmanufactured	11		–11

(continued)

Value of import, export, balance—tobacco unmanufactured—2009—$1,000				
Countries	Item	2009 Imp	2009 Exp	Balance
Saint Lucia	Tobacco, unmanufactured	97	1	–96
Saint Vincent and the Grenadines	Tobacco, unmanufactured	60	4	–56
Saudi Arabia	Tobacco, unmanufactured	6,307	4	–6,303
Senegal	Tobacco, unmanufactured	43,508	21,813	–21,695
Serbia	Tobacco, unmanufactured	3,704	20,753	17,049
Seychelles	Tobacco, unmanufactured	212	8	–204
Sierra Leone	Tobacco, unmanufactured	218	0	–218
Singapore	Tobacco, unmanufactured	53,169	15,354	–37,815
Slovakia	Tobacco, unmanufactured	2,761	466	–2,295
Slovenia	Tobacco, unmanufactured	35	279	244
Solomon Islands	Tobacco, unmanufactured	96		–96
Somalia	Tobacco, unmanufactured	24	0	–24
South Africa	Tobacco, unmanufactured	191,453	40,396	–151,057
Spain	Tobacco, unmanufactured	145,172	113,454	–31,718
Sri Lanka	Tobacco, unmanufactured	39,238	33,545	–5,693
Sudan	Tobacco, unmanufactured	12,930	15	–12,915
Suriname	Tobacco, unmanufactured	0		0
Swaziland	Tobacco, unmanufactured	3,051	1	–3,050
Sweden	Tobacco, unmanufactured	15,503	59	–15,444
Switzerland	Tobacco, unmanufactured	267,381	15,325	–252,056
Syrian Arab Republic	Tobacco, unmanufactured	0	1,662	1,662
Tajikistan	Tobacco, unmanufactured	200	370	170
Thailand	Tobacco, unmanufactured	23,625	81,366	57,741
The former Yugoslav Republic of Macedonia	Tobacco, unmanufactured	9,662	88,098	78,436
Togo	Tobacco, unmanufactured	0	0	0
Tonga	Tobacco, unmanufactured	101		–101
Trinidad and Tobago	Tobacco, unmanufactured	8,780	1	–8,779
Tunisia	Tobacco, unmanufactured	58,197	645	–57,552
Turkey	Tobacco, unmanufactured	289,876	491,087	201,211
Turkmenistan	Tobacco, unmanufactured	20	0	–20
Uganda	Tobacco, unmanufactured	11	56,572	56,561
Ukraine	Tobacco, unmanufactured	272,351	11,136	–261,215
United Arab Emirates	Tobacco, unmanufactured	1,101	3,438	2,337
United Kingdom	Tobacco, unmanufactured	300,948	14,469	–286,479
United Republic of Tanzania	Tobacco, unmanufactured	13,947	90,365	76,418
United States of America	Tobacco, unmanufactured	923,755	1,163,470	239,715
Uruguay	Tobacco, unmanufactured	29,689	10,415	–19,274
Uzbekistan	Tobacco, unmanufactured	19,270	17,058	–2,212
Venezuela (Bolivarian Republic of)	Tobacco, unmanufactured	14,801	53	–14,748

(continued)

Value of import, export, balance—tobacco unmanufactured—2009—$1,000				
Countries	Item	2009 Imp	2009 Exp	Balance
Viet Nam	Tobacco, unmanufactured	124,713	8,782	−115,931
Yemen	Tobacco, unmanufactured	35,573	244	−35,329
Zambia	Tobacco, unmanufactured	60	84,688	84,628
Zimbabwe	Tobacco, unmanufactured	32,902	241,775	208,873

Data are either official or unofficial or aggregated or estimated and are taken from FAOSTAT- FAO Statistics Division, March 2012. The Balance has been calculated by the authors

Index

G. La Torre, *Smoking Prevention and Cessation*, DOI 10.1007/978-1-4614-7046-5,

K

L

M

T

U

MIX
Papier aus verantwortungsvollen Quellen
Paper from responsible sources
FSC® C105338

If you have any concerns about our products,
you can contact us on
ProductSafety@springernature.com

In case Publisher is established outside the EU,
the EU authorized representative is:
Springer Nature Customer Service Center GmbH
Europaplatz 3, 69115 Heidelberg, Germany

Printed by Libri Plureos GmbH
in Hamburg, Germany